ual

DATE DUE

7-18-03			
MAR 2 8 2005			
5-4-5			
6-2-5			
6-16-5			
6/19/12			

D1532559

Notice

Medicine is an ever-changing science. As new research and clinical experience broaden our knowledge, changes in treatment and drug therapy are required. The editors and the publisher of this work have checked with sources believed to be reliable in their efforts to provide information that is complete and generally in accord with the standards accepted at the time of publication. However, in view of the possibility of human error or changes in medical sciences, neither the editors nor the publisher nor any other party who has been involved in the preparation or publication of this work warrants that the information contained herein is in every respect accurate or complete, and they disclaim all responsibility for any errors or omissions or for the results obtained from use of the information contained in this work. Readers are encouraged to confirm the information contained herein with other sources. For example and in particular, readers are advised to check the product information sheet included in the package of each drug they plan to administer to be certain that the information contained in this work is accurate and that changes have not been made in the recommended dose or in the contraindications for administration. This recommendation is of particular importance in connection with new or infrequently used drugs.

Trauma Manual

Ernest E. Moore, MD
Professor & Vice Chairman
Department of Surgery
University of Colorado Health Sciences Center
Chief of Surgery and Trauma Services
Denver Health Medical Center
Denver, CO

Kenneth L. Mattox, MD
Professor and Vice Chairman
Department of Surgery
Baylor College of Medicine
Ben Taub General Hospital
Houston, TX

David V. Feliciano, MD
Chief
Department of Surgery
Grady Memorial Hospital
Emory University School of Medicine
Atlanta, GA

McGRAW-HILL
Medical Publishing Division
New York   Chicago   San Francisco   Lisbon   London   Madrid   Mexico City
Milan   New Delhi   San Juan   Seoul   Singapore   Sydney   Toronto

Trauma Manual, 4/e

1234567890   DOCDOC   098765432

ISBN 0-07-136508-7

This book was set in Times Roman by Clarinda Company.
The editors were Susan R. Noujaim, Marc Strauss, and Regina Y. Brown.
The production supervisor was Richard Ruzycka.
The index was prepared by Jerry Ralya.
R.R. Donnelley & Sons Company was printer and binder.

This book is printed on acid-free paper.

Library of Congress Cataloging-in-Publication Data

Moore, Ernest Eugene—date
    Trauma manual/Ernest Moore, Kenneth Mattox, David Feliciano.
      p. ; cm.
    Includes bibliographical references and index.
    ISBN 0-07-136508-7
      1. Traumatology—Handbooks, manuals, etc. 2. Wounds and injuries—
Handbooks, manuals, etc. 3. First aid in illness and injury—Handbooks, manuals, etc. I. Mattox, Kenneth L. II. Feliciano, David V. III. Title.
    [DNLM: 1 Wounds and Injuries—diagnosis—Handbooks. 2. Wounds
and Injuries—therapy—Handbooks. WO 39 M444t 2003]
    RD93 .M386 2003
    617.1—dc21

                                                            2002021937

This book is dedicated to our families

Sarah, Hunter, and Peter – EEM

Wife, June and daughter, Kimberly – KLM

Grace S. Rozycki, MD, David J. Feliciano, and Douglas D. Feliciano – DVF

Contents

PART IV   SPECIAL PROBLEMS

PART V   MANAGEMENT OF COMPLICATIONS AFTER TRAUMA

CONTRIBUTORS

Maria E. M. Aaron, MD
Department of Ophthalmology
Emory University School of
Medicine
Chief of Service
Crawford Long Hospital
Atlanta, GA
(Chapter 14)

Edward Akelman, MD
Department of Orthopaedics
Brown University Surgery Program
in Medicine
Rhode Island Hospital
Providence, RI
(Chapter 37)

Juan A. Asensio, MD
Associate Professor of
Surgery
Department of Surgery
University of Southern California
Unit Chief
Trauma Surgery Unit
Los Angeles County Medical Center
Los Angeles, CA
(Chapter 25)

Arthur E. Baue, MD
Division of Cardiothoracic Surgery
St. Louis University School of
Medicine
St. Louis, MO
(Chapter 55)

Richard M. Bell, MD, FACS
University of South Carolina School
of Medicine
Department of Surgery
Richland Memorial Hospital
Columbia, SC
(Chapter 5)

Walter L. Biffl, MD
Chief
Pediatric Trauma
Denver Health Medical Center
Denver, CO
Thane Blinman
Department of Surgery
UCLA Medical Center
Los Angeles, CA
(Chapter 9)

L. D. Britt, MD, MPH
Brickhouse Professor and Chairman
Eastern Virginia Medical School
Department of Surgery
Norfolk, VA
(Chapter 16)

Geoffrey Broocker, MD
Professor of Ophthalmology
Chief of Service
Grady Memorial Hospital
Atlanta, GA
(Chapter 14)

Eileen M. Bulger, MD
Assistant Professor of Surgery
University of Washington, Seattle
Attending Surgeon
Harborview Medical Center and
University
University of Washington, Seattle
Seattle, WA
(Chapter 29)

Jon Burch, MD
Chief of General & Vascular
Surgery
Denver Health Medical Center
Professor of Surgery
University of Colorado Health
Science Center
Denver, CO
(Chapter 30)

Andrew R. Burgess, MD
Division of Orthopedic Surgery
University of Maryland Medical
System
Baltimore, MD
(Chapter 32)

William B. Cammarano, MD
Department of Anesthesiology
University of California,
San Francisco
San Francisco, CA
(Chapter 49)

André R. Campbell, MD
University of California, San
Francisco
San Francisco, CA

Charles Chandler
Department of Surgery
UCLA Medical Center
Los Angeles, CA
(Chapter 49)

Thomas H. Cogbill, MD
Department of Surgery
Gundersen Lutheran Medical
Center
LaCrosse, WI
(Chapter 19)

Martin A. Croce, MD
Professor of Surgery
University of Tennessee Health
Sciences Center
Memphis, TN
(Chapter 24)

H. Gill Cryer, MD
Department of Surgery
UCLA Medical Center
Los Angeles, CA
(Chapter 53)

Demetrios Demetriades, MD
Division of Trauma and Critical
Care
Department of Surgery
University of Southern California
Los Angeles, CA
(Chapter 25)

James C. Duke, MD
Associate Professor of Anesthesia
Department of Anesthesia
Denver Health Medical Center
Denver, CO
(Chapter 11)

Thomas J. Esposito, MD, MPH
Department of Surgery
Loyola University Medical Center
University Shock Trauma Institute
Maywood, IL
(Chapter 27)

Timothy C. Fabian, MD, MPH
Surgery
University of Tennessee
UT Medical Group, Inc.
Memphis, TN
(Chapter 24)

Eugen Faist, MD
Department of Surgery
LMU Munich
Klinikum Grosshadern
Munich, Germany
(Chapter 55)

David V. Feliciano, MD
Chief
Department of Surgery
Grady Memorial Hospital
Emory University School of
Medicine
Atlanta, GA
(Chapters 7,31,35,39, and 44)

Mitchell P. Fink, MD
Critical Care Medicine
UPMC
Pittsburgh, PA
(Chapter 51)

Scott B. Frame, MD
Director, Division of
Trauma/Critical Care
University of Cincinnati Medical
Center
Cincinnati, OH
(Chapter 3)

Donald E. Fry, MD
Professor and Chairman
Department of Surgery
University of New Mexico School
of Medicine
Albuquerque, NM
(Chapter 12)

Richard L. Gamelli, MD
Department of Surgery
Loyola University Medical Center
Maywood, IL
(Chapter 27)

Larry M. Gentilello, MD
Associate Professor
University of Washington School of
Medicine
Department of Surgery
Harborview Medical Center
Seattle, WA
(Chapter 46)

Kelly E. Green, MD
Department of Medicine
Denver Health Medical Center
Denver, CO
(Chapter 52)

Juliana E. Hansen, MD
Assistant Professor and Acting
Chief of Plastic and Reconstructive
Surgery
Oregon Health Sciences University
Medical Center
(Chapter 15)

Alden H. Harken, MD
Department of Surgery
Denver Health Medical Center
University of Colorado Health
Sciences Center
Denver, CO
(Chapter 9)

Geoffrey Hastings, MD
Associate Clinical Professor
University of California
San Francisco, CA
(Chapter 10)

Sharon M. Henry, MD
Associate Professor of Surgery
University of Maryland of Maryland
School of Medicine
Director
Wound Healing and Metabolism
R. Adams Cowley Shock Trauma
Center
Baltimore, MD
(Chapter 32)

Steven R. Hofstetter, MD
Department of Surgery
NYU Medical Center
New York, NY
(Chapter 26)

David B. Hoyt, MD
Division of Trauma, Burns, and
Intensive Care
Department of Surgery
University of California, San Diego
School of Medicine
San Diego, CA
(Chapter 2)

Rao R. Ivatury, MD, FACS
Professor of Surgery
Emergency Medicine and
Physiology
Virginia Commonwealth University
Director
Trauma and Critical Care

Medical College of Virginia
Hospitals
Richmond, VA
(Chapter 22)

Donald R. Kauder, MD, FACS
Associate Professor of Surgery
University Pennsylvania School of
Medicine
Vice Chief
Division of Rheumatology and
Surgical Critical Care Unit
Hospital of the University of
Pennsylvania
Philadelphia, PA
(Chapter 43)

Rachael Keilin, MD
Michael E. DeBakey
Department of Surgery
Baylor College of Medicine
Houston, TX
(Chapter 18)

Fernando J. Kim, MD
Division of Urology
University of Colorado
Assistant Professor of
Surgery/Urology
University of Colorado Health
Sciences Center
Denver, CO
(Chapter 33)

Ronald A. Kline, MD
Department of Surgery
Wayne State University
Detroit, MI
(Chapter 41)

M. Margaret Knudson, MD
Professor of Surgery
University of California San
Francisco
San Francisco General Hospital
San Francisco, CA
(Chapter 34)

Rosemary A. Kozar, MD, PhD
Assistant Professor
Department of Surgery
Attending Surgeon, Trauma
Memorial Hermann Hospital
Department of Surgery
University of Texas Houston
Medical School

Houston, TX
(Chapter 56)

Brent E. Krantz, MD, FACS
University of South Carolina School
of Medicine
Department of Surgery
Richland Memorial Hospital
Columbia, SC
(Chapter 5)

Kenneth A. Kudsk, MD
Professor of Surgery
Department of Surgery
University of Wisconsin Medical
School
Madison, WI
(Chapter 54)

Jeffrey Landercasper, MD
Department of Surgery
Gundersen Lutheran Medical Center
LaCrosse, WI
(Chapter 19)

Anna M. Ledgerwood, MD
Department of Surgery
Wayne State University
Detroit, MI
(Chapter 41)

Donald H. Lee, MD
Department of Orthopedics
University of Alabama
Birmingham, AL
(Chapter 36)

Scott A. LeMaire, MD
Assistant Professor of Surgery
Baylor College of Medicine
Houston, TX
(Chapter 23)

Howard G. Liang, MD
Department of Surgery
NYU Medical Center
New York, NY
(Chapter 26)

Alan Lisbon, MD
Chief
Division of Critical Care
Department of Anesthesia & Critical
Care
Harvard Medical School
Beth Israel Deaconess
Boston, MA
(Chapter 51)

Charles E. Lucas, MD
Department of Surgery
Wayne State University
Detroit, MI
(Chapter 41)

Robert C. Mackersie, MD
Professor of Surgery
University of California San
Francisco
Director of Trauma
San Francisco General Hospital
San Francisco, CA
(Chapter 49)

Donald W. Marion, MD
University of Pittsburgh School of
Medicine
Department of Neurological Surgery
Pittsburgh, PA
(Chapter 17)

Kenneth L. Mattox, MD
Professor and Vice Chairman
Department of Surgery
Baylor College of Medicine
Ben Taub General Hospital
Houston, TX
(Chapters 23 and 35)

Wren V. McCallister, MD
Resident in Orthopaedic Surgery
Department of Orthopaedics &
Sports Medicine
University of Washington Medical
Center
Seattle, WA
(Chapter 40)

Richard L. McGough, MD
Clinical Instructor
Brown University School of
Medicine
Attending Orthopedic Surgeon
Department of Orthopedics
Rhode Island Hospital
Providence, RI
(Chapter 38)

Norman E. McSwain, Jr., MD
Department of Surgery
Tulane Medical School
Charity Hospital
New Orleans, LA
(Chapter 4)

J. Wayne Meredith, MD, FACS
Director
Division of Surgical Sciences
Professor and Chairman
Department of General Surgery
Wake Forest School of Medicine
The Bowman Gray Campus
Winston-Salem, NC
(Chapter 20)

Andrew W. Mikulaschek, MD
University of California
San Diego Medical Center
San Diego, CA
(Chapter 2)

William J. Mileski, MD, FACS
Chief of Trauma Services
Department of Surgery
University of Texas Medical Branch
at Galveston
Galveston, TX
(Chapter 8)

Stuart E. Mirvis, MD
Professor of Radiology
MIEMSS/University of Maryland
Baltimore, MD
(Chapter 10)

Ernest E. Moore, MD
Professor & Vice Chairman
Department of Surgery
University of Colorado Health
Sciences Center
Chief of Surgery and Trauma
Services
Denver Health Medical Center
Denver, CO
(Chapters 9 and 56)

Frederick A. Moore, MD
James H. "Red" Duke, Jr.
Professor and Vice Chairman
Department of Surgery
Chief
General Surgery
Trauma & Critical Care
Medical Director
Trauma Services
Memorial Hermann Hospital
Department of Surgery
University of Texas-Houston
Medical School
Houston, TX
(Chapter 56)

John Morris, MD
Department of Surgery
Vanderbilt University Medical
School
Nashville, TN
(Chapter 1)

David S. Mulder, MD, FRCSC
Department of Surgery
Montreal General Hospital
Montreal, Quebec, Canada
(Chapter 6)

Richard J. Mullins, MD
Department of Surgery
Oregon Health Sciences University
Portland, OR
(Chapter 7)

Patrick J. Offner, MD, MPH
Department of Surgery
Denver Health Medical Center
Denver, CO
(Chapter 56)

H. Leon Pachter, MD
The Frank Spencer
Professor of Surgery
NYU School of Medicine
Director of Trauma and Shock Unit
NYU Bellevue Trauma/Critical Care
NYU Medical Center
New York, NY
(Chapter 26)

Norman E. Peterson, MD
Division of Urology
University of Colorado
Assistant Professor of
Surgery/Urology
University of Colorado Health
Sciences Center
Denver, CO
(Chapter 33)

Patrizio Petrone, MD
Division of Trauma and Critical Care
LAC+USC Medical Center
Los Angeles, CA
Chief of International Research
Fellows
Division of Trauma Surgery and
Critical Care
Department of Surgery
University of Southern California
Senior Attending Surgeon

University of Southern California
Medical Center
Los Angeles, CA
(Chapter 25)

Gregory J. Przybylski, MD
Associate Professor of Neurosurgery
Northwestern University School of
Medicine
Chicago, IL
(Chapter17)

Patrick M. Reilly, MD
East Carolina University
Brody School of Medicine
Greenville, NC
(Chapter 50)

J. David Richardson, MD
Department of Surgery
University of Louisville
Louisville, KY
(Chapter 21)

Ira E. Richterman, MD
Private Practice
Canton, OH
(Chapter 37)

Robert D. Riley, MD
Assistant Professor
Department of Cardiothoracic
Surgery
Wake Forest School of Medicine
The Bowman Gray Campus
Winston-Salem, NC
(Chapter 20)

Richard J. S. Robinson, MD
Department of Anesthesia
Montreal General Hospital
Montreal, Quebec, Canada
(Chapter 6)

Michael F. Rotondo, MD, FACS
Professor and Vice Chair
Department of Surgery
Chief
Trauma & Surgical Critical Care
East Carolina University
Brody School of Medicine
Greenville, NC
(Chapter 50)

Steven E. Ross, MD, FACS
Professor of Surgery
University of Medicine and
Dentistry

of New Jersey/Robert Wood
Johnson Medical School, Camden
Director of Trauma
Cooper Health Systems
Camden, NJ
(Chapter 47)

Grace S. Rozycki,MD, FACS
Associate Professor of Surgery
Emory University School of
Medicine
Director
Trauma/Surgical Critical Care
Grady Memorial Hospital
Atlanta, GA
(Chapter 34)

Thomas M. Scalea, MD
Professor of Surgery
Director
Program in Trauma
University of Maryland School of
Medicine
Physician-in-Chief
R Adams Cowley Shock Trauma
Center
(Chapter 10)

C. William Schwab, MD, FACS
Professor of Surgery
Chief
Division of Trauma and Surgical
Critical Care
University of Pennsylvania Medical
Center
Philadelphia, PA
(Chapter 43)

Alan E. Seyfer, MD, FACS
Professor of Surgery, Anatomy, and
Cell Biology
Department of Plastic Surgery
Oregon Health Sciences University
Portland, OR
(Chapter 15)

Michael B. Shapiro, MD, FACS
Assistant Professor
Department of Surgery
University of Pennsylvania School
of Medicine
Medical Director
Surgical Intensive Care Unit
Hospital of the University of
Pennsylvania
Philadelphia, PA
(Chapter 43)

David A. Spain, MD
Chief
Trauma & Surgical Critical Care
Stanford University School of
Medicine
Department of Surgery
Stanford, CA
(Chapter 21)

Christopher M. Stear, MD
Department of Emergency Medicine
Harbor-UCLA Medical Center
Torrance, CA
(Chapter 34)

Alison Steng, MD
Michael E. DeBakey
Department of Surgery
Baylor College of Medicine
Houston, TX
(Chapter 18)

Cameron M. Stone, MD
Western Carolina Retinal Associates
Asheville, NC
(Chapter 14)

Joseph J. Tepas, III, MD
Pediatric Surgery
University of Florida HSC
Jacksonville, FL
(Chapter 42)

Peter G. Trafton, MD
Professor of Orthopedics
Brown University School of
Medicine
Vice Chairman
Department of Orthopedics
Chief
Division of Orthopedic Trauma
Rhode Island Hospital
University Orthopedics
Providence, RI
(Chapter 38)

Thomas E. Trumble, MD
Professor and Chief
Hand and Microvascular Surgery
Department of Orthopaedics &
Sports Medicine
University of Washington Medical
Center
Seattle, WA
(Chapter 40)

Donald D. Trunkey, MD
Department of Surgery
Oregon Health Sciences University
Portland, OR
(Chapter 48)

Alex B. Valadka, MD, FACS
Associate Professor
Department of Neurosurgery
Baylor College of Medicine
Chief of Neurosurgery
Ben Taub General Hospital
Houston, TX
(Chapter 18)

Matthew J. Wall, Jr., MD
Michael E. DeBakey
Department of Surgery
Baylor College of Medicine
Houston, TX
(Chapter 18)

Arnold-Peter C. Weiss, MD
(Chapter 37)

Matthias W. Wichmann, MD
Munich, Germany
(Chapter 55)

Robert J. Winchell, MD
University of California
San Diego Medical Center
San Diego, CA
(Chapter 2)

David Wisner, MD
Professor of Surgery
University of California, Davis
Chief of Trauma
Davis Medical Center
Sacramento, CA
(Chapter 28)

Steven E. Wolf, MD
Assistant Professor
Department of Surgery
Director
Blocker Burn Unit
Assistant Chief of Staff
Shriners Burn Hospital
University of Texas Medical
Branch
Galveston, TX
(Chapter 45)

Preface

This Trauma Handbook is designed for and dedicated to all those who provide care for the injured patient. We have had numerous requests since the 1988 publication of the first edition of *Trauma* to extract the most critical information for patient management into a pocket manual. This critical information has been condensed into a volume that can be readily carried in a laboratory coat for immediate access in the ED, OR, SICU, floor or rehabilitation unit. The Trauma Handbook is organized in the same chronologic order as the parent textbook, the fourth edition of *Trauma*. Each of the chapter authors have selected the most relevant narrative, figures, tables, algorithms and references for acute decision making from their original chapters. This format allows the individual to read more extensively in the textbook, at a more convenient time, for further edification.

Acknowledgments

The editors would like to thank the authors for their extra effort in preparing this handbook. In addition to those individuals listed as authors, we are indebted to our administrative assistants: Victoria Martin (EEM), Mary K. Allen (KLM), and Vertis Walker (DVF) for their editorial expertise. Finally, we are tremendously grateful for the invaluable leadership, dedication and tenacity of Susan Noujaim, Senior Developmental Editor at McGraw-Hill.

EEM

KLM

DVF

Trauma Manual

I | TRAUMA OVERVIEW

1 | Injury Severity Scoring

Characterization of injury severity began in the 1950s as a method of quantifying diverse injuries of differing severity to predict patient outcomes. Emphasis was initially placed on blunt force injuries resulting from motor vehicle crashes. Numerous revisions have followed, incorporating various mechanisms of injury, subjective and objective responses to physiologic insult, and the heterogeneous nature of the critically ill and trauma populations.

The many applications of trauma scoring as a quantitative means of describing injury severity include:

- rational prehospital triage, including proper activation of air transport systems;
- appropriate referrals to regional trauma centers from rural hospitals;
- outcomes prediction;
- evaluation of injury prevention programs; and
- intrahospital quality improvement.

There are three major types of injury scoring systems: physiologic, anatomic, and combined or specialized systems. Each of these has its own advantages and drawbacks, and no clear consensus exists as to which is superior in any given clinical situation. Nevertheless, rational scoring systems are the only standardized tool available for epidemiologic studies and comparisons of treatment modalities and systems across the diverse trauma population.

PHYSIOLOGIC SCORES

Purely physiologic scores are widely employed in the prehospital arena for triage, as well as in the critically ill postinjury population, for evaluating injury treatment efficacy and outcome prediction. Certain scores can be rapidly calculated in the field using measures such as the *Glasgow Coma Score* (GCS, Table 1-1) and the *Trauma Score* (TS), and thus these are useful tools in the triage of the acutely injured patient. The TS, described by Champion in 1981, combines GCS values with measurements of systolic blood pressure, respiratory efforts, and capillary refill. The *Revised Trauma Score* (RTS, Table 1-2), derived from the trauma score, was designed for use both in field triage and for research purposes, and has proven to be a better predictor of in-hospital outcomes and mortality when compared to the TS.

The *Acute Physiology and Chronic Health Evaluation* (APACHE) classification system is a physiologic score employed extensively in assessment of both medical and surgical intensive care unit patients. The initial APACHE system and its subsequent revisions consider preadmission health status, age, and physiologic state during the first 24 hours of intensive care unit stay. The chronic health evaluation system incorporates major preexisting illnesses (diabetes mellitus, chronic renal failure, liver disease, malignancy, etc) that influence outcome. The physiologic section is composed of weighted variables derived from the body's principal systems (neurologic, cardiovascular, respiratory, renal, gastrointestinal, metabolic, and hematologic), and measurements of laboratory values indicative of physiologic derangements (e.g., pH, serum creatinine, hematocrit). While the APACHE system has been reported to perform poorly when characterizing trauma patients, it still has widespread use in general intensive care units and in the research arena for predictions of mortality and in the comparison of varied patient groups.

TABLE 1-1 Glasgow Coma Scale

Eye opening	Spontaneous	4
	To voice	3
	To pain	2
	None	1
Verbal response	Oriented	5
	Confused	4
	Inappropriate	3
	Incomprehensible	2
	None	1
Motor response	Obeys command	6
	Localizes pain	5
	Withdraws (pain)	4
	Flexion	3
	Extension (pain)	2
	None	1
	Glasgow Coma Scale total score	3–16

First described in 1992, the *Systemic Inflammatory Response Syndrome Score* (SIRS), calculated from patient temperature, heart rate, respiratory rate, and white blood cell count, has been shown to reliably predict mortality and hospital length of stay in trauma patients, with admission temperature (either >38°C or <36°C) as the most significant predictor of mortality. One of the greatest advantages of the SIRS system is its ease of calculation; future studies will help delineate its correlation with other, more complex scoring systems.

The measurement of base deficit in the critically injured, hypothermic, coagulopathic trauma patient is a useful adjunct to the Revised Trauma Score and Trauma Score and Injury Severity Score (TRISS; see below) for mortality prediction. Patients under age 55 with a postinjury base deficit exceeding 15 have been shown to have a mortality of over 25 percent. A base deficit of 15 or worse, core temperature less than 35°C, and development of coagulopathy identify the patient in extremis and mandate rapid termination of any surgical procedure, referred to as the "damage-control" concept. The damage-controlled patient is transported immediately to the intensive care unit, where physiologic reserve is restored and the patient is prepared for the completion of the operation once the physiologic parameters have normalized.

ANATOMIC SCORES

Numerous scores are based upon anatomic sites of injury. These include the Abbreviated Injury Score (AIS), Injury Severity Score (ISS), the New Injury

TABLE 1-2 Revised Trauma Score

A Glasgow Coma Scale	B Systolic blood pressure (mm Hg)	C Respiratory rate	Coded value (CV)
13–15	>89	10–29	4
9–12	76–89	>29	3
6–8	50–75	6–9	2
4–5	1–49	−1–5	1
3	0	0	0

Severity Score (NISS), the Anatomic Profile (AP), the Penetrating Abdominal Trauma Index (PATI), and the International Classification of Diseases, Injuries and Causes of Death (ICD)-based Injury Severity Score (ICISS). The *Injury Severity Score* (ISS), derived from the Abbreviated Injury Score first proposed in 1969, is the most widely used scoring system based purely on anatomy. The *Abbreviated Injury Score* (AIS) divides the body into six separate regions (head and neck, face, thorax, abdomen and visceral pelvic contents, bony pelvis and extremities, and external structures), and assigns each a severity value (from 1 [minor] to 6 [nearly always fatal]). The ISS is then calculated as the sum of the squares of the three highest AIS scores from different regions. Any trauma victim with a single body region AIS score of 6 is automatically assigned an ISS score of 75, and is considered to have a nonsurvivable injury. The ISS has been demonstrated to correlate reasonably well with probability of mortality, but it has limitations in that it cannot account for multiple severe injuries in a single region. Thus it is particularly problematic in evaluating penetrating torso trauma, as well as in the patient with multiple injuries to a single area. The *New Injury Severity Score* (NISS), introduced by Osler in 1997, attempts to overcome this limitation by inclusion of the three most severe AIS scores, regardless of body region, and has been shown to outperform the ISS in prediction of survival, as well as in the development of multiple organ failure in the postinjury period.

The *Anatomic Profile* (AP), like the NISS, allows inclusion of more than one serious injury per body region. The AP assigns relative weights to injuries in each of three body regions (brain and spinal cord, anterior neck and chest, and all other major injuries), as well as incorporating nonserious (AIS ≤2) injuries to calculate survival probability, but has not been reliably demonstrated to surpass the ISS in terms of mortality prediction.

Moore and coworkers described the *Penetrating Abdominal Trauma Index* (PATI) in 1981, designed to quantitate the risk of complications in patients with penetrating abdominal injuries requiring laparotomy. The trauma index score is calculated by assigning each intra-abdominal organ a risk factor (1 to 5), then multiplying this number by a severity grade (from 1 [minimal injury] to 5 [maximal injury]). The final penetrating abdominal trauma index is then obtained by adding together the individual organ scores. A PATI above 25 was associated with complication rates of roughly 50 percent for all patients studied, but significantly more gunshot victims than stab victims had a PATI in excess of 25.

In 1996, Rutledge and Osler introduced the *International Classification of Diseases Injury Severity Score* (ICISS), based on readily available ICD-9 discharge diagnoses within the injury categories. The system calculates Survival Risk Ratios (SRRs) for each ICD-9 diagnosis, and has also been used in predicting hospital length of stay and charges. ICISS is calculated from readily available computerizable data contained in hospital discharge summaries, without incurring the additional cost of calculating an AIS. Thus in theory it can be used to compare outcomes from both trauma centers and institutions lacking dedicated trauma registries, although in practice it remains incompletely validated. Newer ICISS systems based on ICD-10 codes are currently under investigation, and may outperform ICISS-9 in terms of survival prediction.

Finally, while not truly a scoring system for the patient as a whole, the American Association for the Surgery of Trauma Organ Injury Scaling provides a measure of consistency in the description of solid organ injuries.

COMBINED SCORING SYSTEMS

In 1984, the *Trauma Score and Injury Severity Score* (TRISS) was introduced by Champion and colleagues. The premise of the TRISS is that trauma outcome can be predicted by combining anatomic and physiologic derangements following injury. The scoring scheme is based on data obtained from the Major Trauma Outcome Study (MTOS) by the American College of Surgeons. The database consisted of 160,000 trauma patients from over 150 trauma centers. A multiple logistic regression model was used incorporating the RTS, patient age, ISS, and mechanism of injury to predict survival after trauma. The TRISS scoring system provides a rough predictor indicating whether mortality in a given patient is expected to be greater or less than 50 percent. The ASCOT (*A Severity Characterization of Trauma*) system was introduced in 1990 to overcome some of the criticisms with the TRISS methodology, namely its low predictive value in certain scenarios. However, despite its increased complexity, ASCOT has not consistently been shown to outperform the TRISS methodology.

SUMMARY

Injury scoring is far from an exact science. It is, however, the basis upon which we currently base triage algorithms, outcome analysis, system evaluation, and trauma research. Each scoring system, whether physiologic, anatomic, or a combined approach, has its strengths and weaknesses; the modern trauma surgeon must be familiar with these systems in order to critically read the literature and practice effectively.

ADDITIONAL READING

Hoyt DB: Is it time for a new injury score? *Lancet* 352:920, 1998.

Malone DL, Kuhls D, Napolitano LM, et al: Back to basics: validation of the admission systemic inflammatory response syndrome score in predicting outcome in trauma. *J Trauma* 51:458, 2001.

Osler T, Nelson L, Bedrick E: Injury severity scoring, in Trunkey DD, Lewis FR, (eds): *Current Therapy of Trauma,* 4th ed. St. Louis, Mosby, 1999, pp 10–17.

Rutledge R: Beyond TRISS: Improved methods of trauma severity scoring, in Trunkey DD, Lewis FR, (eds): *Current Therapy of Trauma,* 4th ed. St. Louis, Mosby, 1999, pp 352–359.

2 | Triage and Transfer

Triage is "the sorting out and classification of casualties and determining the priority of need and proper place of treatment." The aim of triage is to be selective because there are a finite amount of resources available for the care of patients within a given trauma system. War has been the general impetus for developing and refining the concept of medical triage. Civilian triage of trauma patients was not organized until the early 1970s.

The purpose of triage is to match the patient with the optimal resources necessary to adequately and efficiently manage the patient's injuries. Studies demonstrate that major trauma victims have better outcomes when treated at hospitals with the appropriate personnel and equipment. The difficulty is in correctly identifying which patient has injuries in need of a designated trauma center. Studies have shown that only 7 to 15 percent of all trauma victims have injuries that require the facilities of a dedicated trauma center. The goals of a triage system are shown in Table 2-1.

Once the decision has been made that the patient requires a trauma center for the care of injuries, the resources necessary to quickly and accurately diagnose and treat the patient must be determined. One way to do this is to bring these patients to a designated area of the emergency room where they are assessed by physicians and nurses, and a determination is then made as to where the patient must go next, (i.e., the operating suite, for diagnostic studies, or re-triaged to a lesser acute care setting). This type of triage is referred to as secondary in-hospital triage.

Undertriage is defined as a decision that incorrectly identifies a patient as not needing a trauma center, although retrospective analysis suggests that such care was needed. Undertriage results in potentially avoidable morbidity and mortality, the avoidance of which was one of the main reasons that trauma care systems were developed. *Overtriage* is a decision that incorrectly classifies a patient as needing a trauma center, although retrospective analysis suggests that such care was not needed. Overtriage has been said to result in overutilization of finite financial and human resources. An example would be the MVA victim taken to a level I trauma center who is found to have only minor abrasions and contusions.

Level of individual risk describes the amount of undertriage and overtriage within an individual trauma care system that the community is willing to accept. Depending on one's criteria, an acceptable level of undertriage may range between 1 and 5 percent. It is obvious that this figure should be reduced as much as possible, since the consequences include increased morbidity and potentially avoidable mortality. The safest way to triage trauma patients is to have a system with a high sensitivity for potential serious injury, and to accept the fact that there will be an inherently high overtriage rate, as much as 30 to 50 percent, which then can be addressed using in-hospital secondary triage.

SYSTEM RESOURCES

The definition of a trauma care system is a locally coordinated approach to swift identification of injured persons and their subsequent transportation to optimal care. Regionalized trauma care systems decrease the number of potentially avoidable deaths when compared to the number prior to regionalization. The resources of a trauma care system are shown in Table 2-2. These are described in the American College of Surgeons Committee on Trauma Systems Consultation Document.

TABLE 2-1 Goals of a Triage System

- Match patients to facilities
- Determine level of resource utilization
- Determine level of individual risk—overtriage vs. undertriage

The American College of Surgeons Committee on Trauma also publishes guidelines for hospitals called the "Resources for Optimal Care of the Injured Patient," which provides basic information needed for a hospital to become a designated trauma center

There are two types of patient transport in a trauma system: the prehospital transport of the acutely injured victim and the interhospital transport of injured patients. For regionalized trauma centers in the United States, prehospital assessment, initial therapy, and transport are carried out by the *emergency medical system* (EMS). EMS consists of personnel trained in the extrication, initial assessment and therapy, triage, and safe transport of the trauma victim. Ground ambulances remain the mainstay of patient transport; however, helicopters and fixed wing aircraft have been shown to safely and effectively extend the catchment area of a trauma center.

A *trauma center* is the physical plant, personnel, and resources necessary for the care of the trauma victim. The hospital must have 24-hour operation of the emergency department, operating room, postoperative recovery room, intensive care unit, radiologic facilities, and clinical laboratories, including all the equipment and personnel necessary to effectively run these areas, in order to care for the injury victim acutely.

The *trauma service,* headed by a *trauma director,* includes the trauma team and a trauma service coordinator. The trauma service should be a distinct and separate service which coordinates and is responsible for the primary management of all trauma patients, including coordination of care between the other subspecialties involved.

Multiple specialty and subspecialty services required around the clock include general surgery as well as the neurosurgery, orthopedics, plastic surgery, ENT, cardiovascular, ophthalmic, pediatric, ob/gyn, urologic, oral, and hand surgical specialties. There also must be physician specialists in the nonsurgical fields.

Nurses with special training and a commitment to the care of the trauma patient are required, as well as numerous ancillary support personnel.

CLINICAL TRIAGE

The initial care provider (first responder) assesses the patient according to the defined triage criteria for that particular regionalized trauma system. If the patient meets the criteria as a major trauma victim, then he or she should be transported to the nearest designated trauma center. With multiple patients the

TABLE 2-2 Resources of a Trauma Care Center

- Prehospital
- Transport capabilities
- Communications
- Facilities
- Personnel
- Cost
- Quality assurance

same essential precepts of trauma triage apply; however, major trauma victims are given priority over those who appear less injured.

With mass casualties, priorities are different. In the instance of a natural or man-made disaster, terrorist attack, or war, the resources of the designated trauma center, and perhaps the regional trauma system, may be overwhelmed. When resources are inadequate to meet the needs of all the victims, priority shifts from providing care to those with the most urgent need to providing care to those with the highest probability of survival.

COMPONENTS OF TRIAGE TOOLS AND DECISION MAKING

Triage decisions are facilitated by using a scoring system which identifies components associated with severe injuries. These components are combined into triage tools, which are used by the field personnel in making decisions as to whether a trauma victim should be transported to a designated trauma center (Table 2-3).

Physiologic criteria include measurements of basic vital signs such as heart rate, blood pressure, respiratory rate and effort, level of consciousness, and temperature. Patients who have sustained significant injury may not manifest physiologic changes immediately after the accident, and as a result are at risk of undertriage.

Anatomic criteria may include, but are not limited to: penetrating injury to the head, neck, torso, or proximal extremity; two or more proximal long bone fractures; pelvic fracture; flail chest; amputation proximal to the wrist or ankle; limb paralysis; or greater than 10 percent total body surface area burn or inhalation injury. The usefulness of anatomic criteria is limited because anatomic injury assessment may be difficult to reliably predict based on physical examination.

Mechanism of injury is an analysis of the type, amount, and direction of force or energy transfer. Mechanisms of injury felt to have a high potential for major trauma include falls of more than 15 feet; motor vehicle accidents with a fatality at the scene, passenger ejection, prolonged extrication, or major intrusion into the passenger compartment; pedestrians struck by a motor vehicle; motorcycle accidents of more than 20 mph; or any penetrating injuries to the head, neck, torso, or proximal extremities. Mechanism of injury improves the sensitivity and specificity of the triage process when combined with other triage components, such as physiologic/anatomic indices.

Age has been shown to impact on the outcome of trauma victims and should be taken into consideration when triaging a patient. Elderly trauma victims have been shown to have increased morbidity and mortality compared to younger trauma victims.

Chronic diseases have been shown to have a significant impact on morbidity and mortality independent of age and injury severity. Unfortunately, many times the associated medical condition of the patient cannot be ascertained in the prehospital setting.

TABLE 2-3 Components of Triage Tools and Decision Making

- Physiologic criteria
- Anatomic criteria
- Mechanism of injury
- Age and associated conditions
- Prehospital care provider judgment

Another important factor in assessing the trauma victim is the judgment of the on-site first responder, most often an emergency medical technician (EMT) or paramedic. Several studies have shown that judgment of prehospital field personnel can be as good or better than the available triage scoring methods commonly in use.

Current Field Methods

In order for a triage scoring method to be acceptable for use in the field, it must meet certain criteria. The first criterion is that the triage scoring scheme must correlate positively with outcome. Outcomes for major trauma victims are usually classified as death, need for urgent/emergent surgical intervention, length of hospital stay, or major single system or multi-system organ injuries. Second, the components of the scoring scheme must be credible, meaning that the system is logical for the injuries being described. Third, the scoring scheme must have intra- and interobserver reliability. That is, it should be consistently applied between observers and by the same observer at different points in time with the same results. Finally, the scoring scheme must be practical and easily applied.

Specific Scoring Systems

The Trauma Index

The Trauma Index was one of the earliest triage scoring methods, first published in 1971. It included measures of five variables: blood pressure, respiratory status, CNS status, anatomic region, and type of injury.

Glasgow Coma Scale

When the Glasgow Coma Scale (GCS) was first introduced, it was intended as a description of the functional status of the central nervous system, regardless of the type of insult to the brain. It was never intended to be used as a prehospital assessment tool, but it has become just that. The 3 components of the GCS score reflected different levels of brain function: eye opening corresponds to the brain stem, motor response corresponds to central nervous system function, and verbal response corresponds to CNS integration.

Triage Index/Trauma Score/Revised Trauma Score

The Trauma Score, first proposed in 1981, was actually a modification of the Triage Index, consisting of measurement of GCS, capillary refill, and respiratory effort. These were found to have the best predictive power for mortality. The Trauma Score was revised in 1989 due to concerns about accurate assessment of capillary refill and respiratory effort. The revised format consists of GCS, systolic blood pressure, and respiratory rate.

CRAMS Scale

CRAMS stands for Circulation, Respiration, Abdomen/chest, Motor, and Speech and was first proposed as a simplified method of field triage. These parameters are individually assessed and arbitrarily assigned a value corresponding to normal, mildly abnormal, or markedly abnormal. On a scale of 0 through 10, a score of 8 or less signifies major trauma.

Trauma Triage Rule

The most recent trauma field triage tool is the Trauma Triage Rule (TTR) proposed in 1990. The TTR consists of measurements of blood pressure, the GCS motor response, and the anatomic region and type of injury. Major trauma is a priori defined as a systolic blood pressure of less than 85 mm Hg, a GCS motor component score of 5 or less, or penetrating trauma to the head, neck, or trunk. The TTR was developed to potentially reduce overtriage while maintaining an acceptable undertriage rate.

ACS Field Triage System

The American College of Surgeons Field Triage System (Fig. 2-1), one that is widely used throughout the U.S., outlines indications for transport of the trauma victim to a trauma center based on specific physiologic and anatomic injury parameters. In addition, mechanism of injury and age, as well as comorbid factors and prehospital provider judgment are evaluated, and if the criteria are met, these become an indication for transport to a trauma center.

It is well accepted that a regionalized trauma system reduces the number of potentially avoidable deaths due to trauma. The regionalized trauma system is based on two principles: adequate resources at the in-hospital level and accurate assessment at the pre-hospital level. Trauma triage scoring schemes are used to improve accuracy in assessing whether a trauma victim should be taken to a designated trauma center for evaluation of the individual scoring systems, each has its advocates and its detractors; there is no gold standard. Studies have been published that question the ability of a specific element of triage or a triage scoring scheme to accurately identify a patient with major trauma.

It is clear that field triage of the trauma victim is not an exact science. The main problem is that there is no clear definition of what prospectively or retrospectively constitutes a major trauma victim. While most contemporary triage schemes have reasonable correlation with mortality, it could be argued that more sensitive indicators are necessary to avoid potential undertriage. At present, a combination of methods provides a more accurate field assessment of the seriously injured trauma victim and represents the current state of the art.

Assessment Physiological Criteria	→	+ Finding	→	Trauma Center
↓ (-)				
Assessment Anatomy Criteria	→	+ Finding	→	Trauma Center
↓ (-)				
Assessment Mechanism of Injury	→	+ Finding	→	Trauma Center
↓ (-)				
Assessment Age/Comorbid Disease	→	+ Finding	→	Trauma Center
↓ (-)				
Exercise Prehospital Provider Judgment	→	+ Finding	→	Trauma Center

FIG. 2-1. The American College of Surgeons Field Triage System

Interhospital Transfer

Many trauma victims who live in rural communities do not have immediate access to a designated trauma center or regional trauma system. While most are adequately cared for by local community facilities, there are a significant number of patients who will require the services found only at a hospital dedicated to the overall care of the trauma patient. Previous studies have shown that these patients are at an increased risk for death.

An interhospital transfer should occur when the patient requires resources beyond the capability of the initial receiving hospital. It is imperative that the initial contact physician be able to recognize that the trauma victim may have injuries requiring diagnostic or therapeutic modalities beyond the scope of the initial receiving hospital.

CRITERIA FOR TRANSFER

Criteria for transfer specify how to identify a situation in which a trauma victim may require transfer to a designated trauma center for the diagnosis and treatment of injuries. A number of factors must be considered when making this decision (Table 2-4).

The physiologic criteria used to determine transfer are the same as those used to identify major trauma in the prehospital arena. Ongoing deterioration of the patient's status despite resuscitative attempts requires urgent transfer. Specific types of injuries, when suspected or diagnosed, may be best treated at designated trauma centers. These include injuries that will require prompt attention by surgical subspecialty services.

The initial physician should also be aware of resources available at their receiving hospital and should also be able to recognize serious potential injuries based on mechanism of injury and significant comorbid factors that may need these resources.

Transfer agreements are protocols to ensure rapid and efficient passage of pertinent patient information prior to the actual transfer. These should include patient identification, history and physical examination findings, and diagnostic and therapeutic procedures performed and their results. The physicians involved should discuss the mode of transportation, as well as accompanying personnel and equipment that may be needed for optimal transfer. This discussion should also determine who will assume medical control of the patient during transport.

The mode of transportation is dependent on modes available as well as distance, geography, weather, patient status, the skills of the transport personnel, and equipment that will likely be needed during transport. The patient should have appropriate monitoring of physiologic indices and the patient should be accompanied by a transport team of at least 2 people in addition to the vehicle operator.

Careful attention must be given to the patient after the decision has been made to transfer to a center with a higher level of care. The resuscitation must

TABLE 2-4 Criteria for Transfer to a Trauma Center	Transport
• Physiologic	Essential Details
• Anatomic injury	• Transfer agreement
• Facility resources and personnel	• Transport modality
• Physician assessment	• Transport personnel

be ongoing, there may be unidentified potentially lethal injuries, and there are numerous mishaps that can potentially turn a routine transport into a tragic one.

ADDITIONAL READING

Champion HR, Sacco WJ, Copes WS, et al: A revision of the trauma score. *J Trauma* 20:188, 1989.

Emerman CL, Shade B, Kubincanek J: A comparison of EMT judgment and prehospital trauma triage instruments. *J Trauma* 31:1369, 1991.

Esposito TJ, Offner PF, Jurkovich GJ, et al: Do prehospital trauma center triage criteria identify major trauma victims? *Arch Surg* 130:171, 1995.

MacKenzie EJ, Steinwachs DM, Ramzy AI: Evaluating performance of statewide regionalized systems of trauma care. *J Trauma* 30:681, 1990.

Morris JA, MacKenzie EJ, Edelstein S: The effect of preexisting conditions on mortality in trauma patients. *JAMA* 263:1942, 1990.

Resources for Optimal Care of the Injured Patient:1999. Chicago, American College of Surgeons Committee on Trauma, 1999.

II

GENERALIZED APPROACHES TO THE TRAUMATIZED PATIENT

3 | Prehospital Care

Prehospital care of the trauma patient comes under the purview of the emergency medical services (EMS) system. EMS refers to an organized approach to the care of the acutely ill or injured patient during the period of time between the occurrence of the injury and the arrival of the patient at the hospital. The system concept encompasses the entire spectrum of trauma event recognition, system notification, system activation, response to scene, on-scene care, and transport to the hospital for definitive care.

INFECTIOUS DISEASE

In the prehospital setting, the emergency medical technician (EMT) will be commonly confronted with patients who either have, or have a high likelihood of having, a communicable disease. Often, there will be no overt indication that a communicable disease is present. The Occupational Safety and Health Administration (OSHA) and Centers for Disease Control and Prevention (CDC) have established guidelines for dealing with bloodborne and airborne pathogens.

Hepatitis

For over 40 years, the risk of acquiring hepatitis has remained one of the major occupational risks for infectious disease facing health care providers. There are currently six types of viruses that have been identified as pathogenic in humans: hepatitis A, B, C, D, E, and G.

Hepatitis A This type is best recognized for causing infection after the ingestion of contaminated food or water. It can be transmitted from an infected individual to an uninfected individual.

Hepatitis B This viral type poses the greatest risk for health care providers who are exposed to patient body fluids. Recombinant vaccines and plasma-derived vaccines are available and provide long-lasting immunity 95 to 98 percent of the time.

Hepatitis C Transmission is via exposure to infected blood. There is a 2.7 to 10% probability of infection in health care workers exposed to infected blood.

Hepatitis D This type is also known as the delta particle, because it is not a complete virus. It cannot cause infection by itself and requires the presence of hepatitis B. Transmission routes are the same as for hepatitis B, and vaccination for hepatitis B imparts immunity against hepatitis D.

Hepatitis E This viral type is transmitted via contaminated water and person-to-person fecal–oral contact. This virus is closely related to hepatitis A and behaves in a very similar fashion.

Hepatitis G This is a newly recognized viral type. It appears to be a chronic bloodborne pathogen in the blood donor population. Many patients are coinfected with hepatitis C. There is no immunization available.

Human Immunodeficiency Virus (HIV)

There are two currently recognized viral types: HIV-1 and HIV-2. Transmission of HIV-1 is through sexual contact, sharing of HIV-contaminated needles and syringes, and the infusion of contaminated blood and blood products. Contact with semen, blood, vaginal fluids, and associated tissues is accepted as high risk. The use of eye protection, masks, and impervious gowns is highly recommended in situations in which exposure to large volumes of body fluids is possible. There is no vaccine available at present.

Other Communicable Diseases

Tuberculosis Mycobacterium tuberculosis is transmitted via exposure to the bacteria in airborne droplets produced through coughing of individuals with pulmonary or laryngeal tuberculosis.

Meningococcal Meningitis Transmission of *Neisseria meningitidis* is via respiratory droplets from the nose and throat of an infected individual. Protective measures include body surface isolation for the EMS workers and surgical masks applied to patients demonstrating suggestive signs and symptoms. Immunizations are available which are effective in preventing outbreaks.

TRAUMA INCIDENT EVALUATION

The EMTs responding to the scene of a trauma incident have the responsibility to gather information that is important in the care of the trauma patient. The EMS personnel are literally the eyes and ears of the trauma surgeon in the field. The system of event evaluation is known as the three S's: safety, scene, and situation.

Safety

It is paramount that the EMTs do not enter into a situation that puts their health and well-being at risk. There is little to be gained by the reckless EMT who ventures into a dangerous circumstance and becomes a victim himself.

Scene

Once the incident site has been secured and deemed to be safe, the EMT must evaluate for the mechanism of injury.

Situation

The EMTs should attempt to gather any additional data on the patient, such as prior medical condition, current medications, allergies, and last meal.

MEDICAL CONTROL

A law commonly known as the Medical Practice Act governs the delivery of health care in the United States. This law spells out who may render care and under what circumstances. In order to implement the physician extender concept, prehospital care providers had to be given authority to deliver care through state laws or regulations. These laws and regulations placed the responsibility for EMT practice on a physician who agreed to supervise the prehospital providers. Many terms have been applied to this association, including *medical control, medical direction,* or *medical oversight.*

Components

Medical direction means that physicians determine what medical care will be provided in an EMS system and delineates how that care is to be provided.

How the physician is involved can occur in two distinct fashions: indirect (off-line/protocols) and direct (on-line).

Indirect (Off-Line/Protocols) This form of medical direction involves the development of written protocols and the review of EMT performance. Protocols are the overall steps in patient management that are to be followed by the prehospital provider at every patient contact. These plans for patient care are developed by the medical authority responsible for patient care within the particular community. Standing orders are those components of a protocol that the EMT initiates prior to establishing communications with medical control.

Protocols must address each step of prehospital care and include the most commonly encountered medical conditions. The protocols for the management of the trauma patient as developed by the American College of Surgeons Committee on Trauma are an example of a comprehensive protocol. The development of protocols for use in the prehospital arena should normally follow the condition or symptom approach. An accurate diagnosis will probably not be available in the field, so protocols are based on the patient's complaints, condition, or symptoms. Emergent management is necessary; establishing an accurate diagnosis is not. The primary goal of prehospital care is to evaluate and manage the patient's emergent condition while transporting to the appropriate facility for definitive care.

Direct (On-Line) This form of direction involves providing radio or telephone instructions to prehospital providers and direct observation of the system and individual performance; in some systems, the medical director may respond to the scene and provide prehospital patient care. Appropriate orders are provided for care in the field and en route to the hospital.

QUALITY ASSURANCE

In addition to looking at the system components, quality assurance includes evaluating each individual's training, performance, and patient care.

Care Rendered

The medical director and EMS staff must be able to objectively evaluate how well care is rendered by the EMTs. There are three basic methods used to evaluate quality: prospective, concurrent, and retrospective.

Prospective Evaluation This form of evaluation attempts to improve the level of care rendered prior to the actual delivery of the care skills.

Concurrent Evaluation Concurrent evaluation involves direct observation of the EMT during the delivery of care.

Retrospective Evaluation Chart audits, case reviews, and debriefings to review the events of any particular EMS call are all retrospective evaluation tools. Reviewing the quality of documentation and monitoring how closely established protocols are followed should also be performed.

System Efficiency

This type of evaluation process must look at the EMS activation system, notification time, response time, on-scene time, and transport time.

Notification Time The notification time for the EMS system involves two distinct components: the lay person–activated system and the EMS dispatch system. The lay person–activated system most commonly involves the 911 phone system. Once the initial call is made into the EMS system, there must be an efficient system to dispatch appropriate resources to the patient. Dispatchers must be properly trained to be able to provide prearrival instructions to the citizens activating the system and to determine the level of care required.

Response Time   Response time is defined as the period that starts when an emergency call is received into an EMS system and ends with the arrival of the ambulance at the scene. This time frame encompasses several actions: (1) The call must be physically received; (2) the dispatcher must analyze the call and decide on the appropriate response; (3) the ambulance must be contacted and dispatched; and (4) the ambulance must leave its current location and travel to the scene. The final factor, ambulance travel time, is a function of ambulance location and availability, weather, and traffic conditions.

Acceptable target response times by current standards should fall between 4 and 6 minutes in urban areas and no longer than 10 minutes in rural areas.

On-Scene Time   The time from the arrival of the EMTs at the scene of the incident to their departure from the scene en route to the receiving facility is called the on-scene time. This time will vary according to environmental conditions, geography of the scene and location accessibility of the patient, entrapment, injuries present, and patient packaging requirements.

Transport Time   The length of time required to transport the patient from the scene to an appropriate facility is the final phase of the total prehospital period. The factors that affect this time are distance from the facility, weather, and traffic conditions. For the critically injured patient, this time should be used to perform tasks that were inappropriate to take the time to perform on-scene.

PHASES OF PREHOSPITAL CARE

In 1965, the National Academy of Sciences/National Research Council described three phases of field medical care.

Prospective Phase

The initial phase of prehospital care includes the development, updating, and approval of treatment protocols; initial training and continuing education of personnel; purchasing, repairing, and equipping of vehicles; staffing of units; resupply of used resources in the units; and development of adequate and continuing sources of funding.

Immediate Phase

The immediate phase involves the period encompassing the actual EMS call and activities of the EMTs in the care of the patient. When an incident occurs, the EMS system is activated and an EMS unit is dispatched to the scene. During the on-scene and transport periods of the EMS response, medical control consists of supervision via monitoring of communications or on-the-scene observation by the system medical director. This phase also involves the orders carried out by the EMTs.

The situation sometimes occurs that a licensed physician who is not associated with the EMS system will be present at the scene and wish to assume medical control of the on-site care of the patient. This physician then becomes medically and *legally* responsible for the care of the patient until care is formally turned over to another physician, either by delivering the patient personally to another physician or by an on-line medical control physician's assuming care responsibility.

Retrospective Phase

This phase of prehospital care entails the review of run reports by the medical director to ensure that proper care has been given. This review may be physically performed by a designated representative of the medical director (eg, quality improvement nurse or paramedic), comparing the run report to accepted treatment protocols. Any report that deviates from the proposed guidelines is referred to the medical director's attention.

The retrospective phase also involves the development of a continuing education program to introduce new information or reinforce existing information that focused reviews have shown to be in need of attention. Continuing education in trauma care should include courses such as Pre-hospital Trauma Life Support or Basic Trauma Life Support.

SYSTEM DESIGN

It is generally recognized that there are two distinct levels of prehospital care that now exist: basic life support and advanced life support.

Basic Life Support

Basic life support (BLS) is a term used to describe a level of care that provides noninvasive emergency care. In other words, care rendered does not involve inserting any needles or tubes into the patient's body. BLS does involve cardiopulmonary resuscitation (CPR), basic control of external hemorrhage, splinting, spinal immobilization, normal childbirth, and other uncomplicated forms of emergency care.

Advanced Life Support

Advanced life support (ALS) usually involves the use of invasive procedures, such as intravenous lines and drug administration. The use of sophisticated equipment, including cardiac monitoring, pulse oximetry, and capnography, is also included. There are two nationally recognized levels of ALS training: Emergency Medical Technician–Intermediate (EMT-I) and Emergency Medical Technician–Paramedic (EMT-P).

Tiered Response System

An EMS system that is not purely BLS or ALS, but a combination of both, is called a *tiered response system.*

Single-Tiered Response The reasons for establishing a single-tiered response system, be it all-ALS or all-BLS, vary from community to community. Some rural communities do not possess the population or fiscal base to support an all-ALS system, or even a tiered system combining both ALS and BLS. These communities usually rely on all-volunteer personnel who possess neither the time nor financial assets to attain the training for ALS-level care, let alone maintain the training and skill level proficiency required.

Multitiered Response A hybrid system that involves both BLS and ALS responses is a multitiered response system. This system attempts to provide care in a cost-effective manner, providing ALS-level care only to those patients who require it.

Fire Department—Initial Responder In many communities, fire departments provide complete EMS services. The most common model at this time is for the fire agencies to function as the initial responders in a tiered response system.

Ambulance Service—ALS Response Once the initial responders assess the patient and determine the need for ALS services, a second unit is dispatched. The response times for these ALS units in a tiered system is usually allowed to be slightly longer, in the 6 to 8 minute time frame. The concept is that the BLS units can provide for initial, basic care to stabilize the patient until the ALS unit arrives. If transport time to the hospital is less than the response time of the ALS unit, then transport should be initiated without waiting for the ALS unit.

PERSONNEL

The National EMS Training Blueprint Project is an independent project that was financially supported by the National Registry of Emergency Medical Technicians (NREMT).

National Emergency Medical Services Education and Practice Blueprint

The goal of the blueprint project was to develop a national consensus on a framework for development of EMS training, education, and policies. The Blueprint recognizes four levels of prehospital EMS providers corresponding to various knowledge and skill levels in each of the defined core elements. The four levels of prehospital EMS providers are: First Responder, EMT-B, EMT-I, and EMT-P.

First Responder This prehospital caregiver uses a limited amount of equipment to perform initial assessment and rudimentary intervention. First Responders are also trained to aid other EMS providers.

Emergency Medical Technician–Basic The EMT-B has the knowledge and skills of the First Responder, but in addition, is qualified to function as minimum staff for an ambulance. The current course work required to achieve this level is successful completion of the 110-hour course developed by the U.S. Department of Transportation. After completion of the course, the prospective EMT-B takes a written and practical examination administered by either the NREMT or the state, or both.

Emergency Medical Technician–Intermediate The EMT-I possesses the knowledge and skills of the previous levels, but in addition, is trained to perform essential advanced techniques and administer a limited number of medications. The EMT-I must have completed the EMT-B course and have an additional 150 to 200 hours. The added training time is devoted to a more in-depth knowledge of shock management, advanced techniques of patient assessment, physiology and pathophysiology, and advanced airway management skills.

Emergency Medical Technician–Paramedic Once again, the EMT-P possesses the knowledge and skills of the three previous levels. Additionally, paramedics are trained in the use of a wider range of medications and the performance of a greater number of advanced skills. At the scene of the cardiac arrest, the paramedic would administer second-line advanced cardiac life support medications and use an external pacemaker. The new curriculum to train an EMT-P will require approximately 1000 hours of didactic course work and practical skills attainment.

Nurses

Nurses serve as prehospital providers (when dual trained), instructors, and quality improvement proctors. Nurses may also be employed by EMS services as field observers and on-site continuing education instructors.

Ground Nurses   When dual trained as a nurse and an EMT, the individual can function in the field as a prehospital provider under the auspices of EMT training. Nurses cannot, however, function in the field until they are trained in field skills such as extrication skills, splinting and bandaging skills, and endotracheal intubation.

Flight Nurses   Almost all aeromedical services in this country utilize nurses in the delivery of prehospital care and transport. Nurses who are dual trained as both an EMT and a nurse can provide care in the prehospital phase under the auspices of their EMT training.

Physicians

In the United States, it is unusual for physicians to directly participate in the provision of care to the injured patient in the field; however, in other countries, the use of physicians as primary field providers is commonplace.

Ground Units   Physicians are rarely associated with ground transport units in this country as primary members of the unit team. As previously described, physicians may happen upon a scene by chance and wish to assume on-site medical control of the patient. In this context, the physician must remain with the patient until care is formally turned over to another accepting physician, either by radio communication or by face-to-face turnover in the emergency department.

In other parts of the world physicians are commonly used as primary members of the EMS field care team. Physicians are members of the ambulance teams and/or are used in separate vehicles, carrying their own equipment, and responding emergently to the incident scene to work in conjunction with the ambulance crews.

Flight Physicians   The most common use of physicians in the emergent field care of patients in this country is as members of an aeromedical team. Often, the physicians assigned to the crews are senior emergency medicine residents who are rotated onto the aircraft as a formal part of their emergency medicine residency.

Medical Director

In 1986, Holroyd and coworkers recommended that the EMS medical director be a physician with the following qualifications: (1) knowledge and demonstrated ability in planning and operation of prehospital EMS systems, (2) experience in the prehospital provision of emergency care for acutely ill or injured patients, (3) experience in the training and ongoing evaluation of all levels of participants in the prehospital care system, (4) knowledge and experience in the application of medical control to an EMS system, and (5) a knowledge of the administrative and legislative processes affecting regional and/or state prehospital EMS systems.

EQUIPMENT

Currently, two national standard documents are available to aid in identifying the proper equipment. The American College of Surgeons Committee on Trauma (ACSCOT) publishes a document entitled Essential Equipment List for Ambulances. This publication identifies the standard equipment necessary to provide adequate care at the basic, intermediate, and advanced EMT levels. The American College of Emergency Physicians (ACEP) has developed a position paper defining the optimal advanced-level prehospital skills, medications, and equipment. Attempts are underway to ensure that the ACSCOT and ACEP documents are in agreement.

Airway Management

Advanced

Endotracheal Intubation All levels of EMTs have now been taught to safely insert endotracheal tubes. The use of this technique is almost universally accepted at the EMT-P level throughout the United States, while the EMT-1 level is experiencing growing knowledge of the technique. The success rate for endotracheal intubation in the field is greater than 90 percent. This rate is achieved without the benefit of muscle relaxants and in the adverse prehospital environment.

Basic

Esophageal Obturator Airway, Combitube, Pharyngotracheal Lumen Airway The esophageal obturator airway (EOA) was developed as an attempt to create a device that could be blindly inserted and provide adequate airway control and oxygen delivery. Several problems quickly arose with the EOA. First, the blind insertion technique led to incorrect placement, with ventilation of the stomach. If unrecognized, this has obvious disastrous consequences. Second, incomplete ventilation with pulmonary air trapping was common. Finally, mask seal around the face with air leakage was a major problem. The 1998 National Standard Curricula for both EMT-P and EMT-1 do not even address EOAs at all.

The pharyngotracheal lumen airway (PTLA) is basically an endotracheal tube encased in a large pharyngeal tube. There are two ventilation ports which provide a means to ventilate the patient regardless of the position of the distal endotracheal tube (either tracheal or esophageal). The Combitube® is a pharyngeal and endotracheal tube molded into a single unit. It is blindly inserted, and the dual ports allow ventilation regardless of position.

Breathing Adjuncts

Supplemental Oxygen If the patient does not require total airway control and is ventilating spontaneously, then equipment that delivers as much oxygen as possible should be supplied. This means that all trauma patients should have a nonrebreather mask with reservoir, that can supply up to 85 percent oxygen. There is no place in the care of the trauma patient for a nasal cannula.

Circulation

The choice between normal saline and lactated Ringer's as the preferred intravenous fluid remains an open question. Lactated Ringer's is a balanced electrolyte solution with components present in physiologic concentrations. The administration of large volumes of lactated Ringer's usually will not lead to electrolyte abnormalities. On the other hand, normal saline contains sodium chloride in concentrations much greater than are present in serum. The infusion of large volumes of normal saline can result in hypernatremia.

Adjuncts for Cardiopulmonary Resuscitation

Thoracic Compression Devices Pneumatically powered piston compression machines have been developed in an attempt to solve the problems of prolonged CPR. These devices are oxygen powered, so that they run off the internal oxygen supplies of the EMS unit. The piston is positioned over the midpoint of the sternum, and the device is activated. These devices have the added benefit of providing ventilation with 100 percent oxygen.

The device has gained moderate acceptance in both emergency departments and EMS services. The cost of the devices and storage space constraints in the back of units has limited the widespread use in the prehospital arena. Shorter response and transport times have also made the necessity for these devices less acute.

Defibrillators The prehospital application of defibrillation has become the standard of care for prehospital medical situations involving cardiac arrest. The automatic external defibrillator offers the advantage of eliminating the need for the EMT to read and interpret the patient's cardiac rhythm.

PATIENT PACKAGING

Preparation for transport is known as *patient packaging* and must be accomplished in a minimum amount of time and with maximum patient protection.

Cervical Immobilization

The trauma patient should be assumed to have a cervical spine injury, if the proper mechanism of injury is present, until proven otherwise. Stiff cervical collars are a useful device in the awake, cooperative patient as a reminder to not move their necks. As a sole source of cervical immobilization, they are completely inadequate. The degree of immobilization afforded by cervical collars alone is totally inadequate in the patient with known or potential cervical spine fracture. They must be used in conjunction with a long backboard.

Spine Immobilization

The spine in the human is considered a single, multiarticulated structure. The "joint above" is the atlanto-occipital junction, and the "joint below" is the hip joint. In order to achieve complete immobilization of the spine, the patient must be secured to a long backboard. As previously discussed, the neck should be placed in a hard cervical collar. The head must be securely fastened to the board and the legs likewise must be secured.

Fracture Immobilization

It must be kept in mind that the properly immobilized patient on a long back-board will by default have all of his or her extremities secured and stabilized.

TRANSPORT VEHICLES

Ground Vehicles

Basic Life Support Units These units should be equipped with medical devices and supplies recommended by the ACSCOT, and as defined by local medical direction and state requirements. BLS units should have radio communication providing for vehicle control, medical control, and consultation. Staffing should include at least two emergency medical technician–ambulance (EMT-A) personnel.

Advanced Life Support Units ALS units must contain all elements of a ground BLS unit. The staffing should consist of two EMTs trained beyond the EMT-A level to address specific clinical items in the medical service plan. Advanced communications to provide advanced biomedical telemetry is desirable. Additional equipment and supplies are provided as appropriate to support the defined scope of practice. In general, ALS units are staffed and equipped to provide advanced airway management, intravenous fluid administration, and defibrillation. Most commonly, ALS units now are staffed by at least one EMT-P.

Aeromedical Units

Rotor-Wing Aircraft Controversy exists as to the benefits of on-scene helicopter response in an urban setting when a well-trained ground EMS service is present. There seems to be little controversy that the transport of critically injured patients from a rural facility with limited resources to a major trauma center is beneficial for the patient. The two most common staffing patterns are two flight nurses, or a flight nurse and a paramedic. Helicopters are universally equipped as ALS units at a minimum, and more commonly as "flying intensive care units."

Fixed-Wing Aircraft When a transport radius of greater than 150 miles is required or helicopters are not available, fixed-wing aircraft are useful. Transfers of patients to regional specialized facilities, such as burn or transplant centers, are also commonly performed by fixed-wing aircraft.

PREHOSPITAL CARE

Basic Philosophy

The most basic philosophy in prehospital care, as it should be in all of medicine, is to first do no further harm. This may sound simple, but combined with the adverse conditions under which EMS personnel must work in the field, it can become a formidable task.

Definitive care for the cardiac patient is conversion from a malignant rhythm to an effective pumping action to perfuse the body. Unlike the cardiac patient, the goal of definitive care for the trauma patient is control of hemorrhage and reestablishment of normal circulating blood volume. Attempts to improve blood pressure without first achieving adequate control of hemorrhage have been demonstrated to increase blood loss.

The philosophy of prehospital care for the trauma patient, therefore, must include rapid movement of the patient to an appropriate facility where definitive care may be immediately provided. The standard has now been established to limit the prehospital field time to a maximum of 10 minutes in the severely, or potentially severely, injured patient.

Specific Injuries

Head   The two cornerstones of head injury management are providing maximal supplemental oxygen (including proper airway management) and maintaining cerebral perfusion. This includes avoiding unnecessary interventions that may raise intracranial pressure such as nasotracheal intubation. Blood pressure should be maintained with fluid resuscitation to preserve cerebral perfusion pressure.

Spine   The standard of care is to immobilize any patient involved in trauma with a mechanism of injury that may result in a spine injury. With proper immobilization, 15 percent of secondary spine injuries can be prevented.

Thorax   Controlling the airway and providing maximal oxygen supplementation is needed to treat thoracic injuries. Open pneumothorax should be treated with a three-sided occlusive dressing. Tension pneumothorax must be recognized and is treated in the field with needle decompression (large-gauge intravenous catheter, midclavicular line, second intercostal space). The needle is left in place and if transport will be prolonged, a one-way valve may be fashioned from the cut finger of a glove taped over the end of the catheter.

Abdomen   Definitive care for the patient with ongoing intra-abdominal hemorrhage is rapid surgical intervention at the hospital. Eviscerations should be covered with a moist dressing, and no attempt should be made to place the organs back into the abdomen. Impaled objects should be secured in place and removed only if absolutely necessary to extricate the patient for transport.

Pelvis   Patients with suspected pelvic injuries should be immobilized properly and rapidly transported to the closest appropriate hospital. The hemodynamically unstable patient may benefit from the application of a pneumatic antishock garment.

Extremities   The danger for the EMT encountering a trauma victim with extremity trauma is twofold. First, the EMT must not be distracted from the proper assessment of the patient by the horrible-appearing, but noncritical, extremity injuries. Second, life-threatening extremity injuries must not be overlooked. Properly securing a patient to a long backboard in the supine position can effectively support and splint every bone and joint.

TRIAGE CRITERIA

Triage is derived from the French term meaning "to sort." The definition now is to determine priority of need and proper place of treatment.

Transport to Trauma Center

The ACSCOT has developed triage criteria to determine those patients who should be taken to a trauma center. These criteria have been widely accepted and are integral components of most established trauma systems.

Transport of Dead or Apparently Dead Patients

Attempts have been made by the ACSCOT and the National Association of EMS Physicians (NAEMSP) to define conditions that, when present, should indicate that resuscitation should not be attempted:

- Dependent lividity
- Rigor mortis
- Decapitation
- Decomposition
- Hemicorporectomy
- Trauma Score of 1 for 10 minutes
- Complete incineration
- Multiple extremity amputations without signs of life
- Penetrating cranial injuries with extrusion of brain matter and no signs of life
- Underwater submersion for more than 2 hours
- Evisceration of the heart
- Severe crush injury

PREHOSPITAL CONTROVERSIES

The provision of care in the prehospital setting is not always well defined, and complete agreement does not exist on all aspects of trauma care.

Airway Management

Circumstances may occasionally arise when endotracheal intubation is indicated, but accomplishing the task is difficult. When these rare circumstances arise, alternative techniques for airway management have been proposed.

Surgical Cricothyroidotomy

Surgical cricothyroidotomy in the prehospital setting has been utilized by aeromedical crews for several years. Aeromedical crews who have been allowed to perform this procedure have demonstrated a limited need and desire to utilize it.

Rapid Sequence Intubation   When paramedics are well trained in and experienced with endotracheal intubation, the adjuvant use of rapid sequence intubation allows safe intubation in the small subset of patients who may not otherwise have had a definitive airway established. Included are patients with uncooperative behavior due to hypoxia, head injury, hypotension, or drugs/alcohol.

Percutaneous Transtracheal Catheter Ventilation   Percutaneous transtracheal catheter ventilation (PTCV) possesses the following advantages: it does not require paralysis, as with rapid sequence intubation; it is less invasive than surgical cricothyroidotomy; it affords easy access and insertion; it requires minimal education; and it requires very basic equipment.

Fluids

Controversies exist along a number of fronts with regard to fluids in the prehospital care of the trauma patient.

Normotensive Versus Hypotensive Resuscitation Versus No Fluids The basis of the controversy is whether the improvement in tissue perfusion with oxygenated red blood cells (RBCs) is worth the cost of increased bleeding secondary to uncontrolled hemorrhage brought about by the increased blood pressure. Currently, there is no evidence in the literature that demonstrates with statistical significance that either of these treatment strategies affects outcome.

Pneumatic Antishock Garment

The use of a PASG has been severely curtailed in recent years in the prehospital care of the trauma patient.

Urban The use of PASGs in an urban setting with an efficient EMS service (short response and transport times) applied to penetrating torso trauma patients does not affect outcome.

Rural Many feel that if the PASG can be of benefit in the catastrophic intra-abdominal hemorrhage seen with ruptured abdominal aortic aneurysms, it must be of benefit in traumatic intra-abdominal bleeding, given the prolonged transport time involved; however, there are no specific studies that support this supposition.

Specific Injuries The PASG has been shown to have detrimental effects on patients with thoracic injuries, particularly those due to penetrating causes. They are also contraindicated in patients with diaphragmatic rupture. Current recommendations are for use in hypotension due to suspected pelvic fracture, otherwise uncontrollable lower extremity hemorrhage, and severe traumatic hypotension.

"Load and Go" Versus "Stay and Play"

All of the preceding discussions highlight the need for definitive control of hemorrhage as the primary therapy for hemorrhagic shock. This may only be provided by the rapid transport of the critically injured patient to the nearest appropriate hospital. This means limiting on-scene care to a bare minimum, with only necessary interventions provided in the field. The goal of prehospital trauma care is to limit on-scene time to 10 minutes.

Composition of Emergency Medical Services Systems: Firefighters Versus Paramedics

Fire services have strategically-placed bases available 24 hours a day from which to dispatch to all areas of a community. They have personnel who are often already trained in basic EMS skills, and the transition to more advanced levels is relatively easy and inexpensive. They also have budgets that may be easily converted to an EMS mission. As communities wrestle with who will provide EMS in the future, the fight between hospital-based, privately run, and fire-based systems will heat up.

PREHOSPITAL TRAUMA EDUCATION

Two courses currently exist that are nationally and internationally available for continuing education in prehospital trauma care: The PHTLS course and the BTLS course.

Prehospital Trauma Life Support Course

This course is a combined effort of two national organizations with interest in the care of the trauma patient. PHTLS is provided by the National Association of Emergency Medical Technicians (NAEMT) with the cooperation of the ACSCOT. The tenets of the ATLS course are reflected in the PHTLS curriculum, with changes to meet the needs of the patient in the prehospital setting. A new edition of the course is produced every 4 years, 1 year after the introduction of the new ATLS edition.

Basic Trauma Life Support Course

This course was developed by the Alabama Chapter of the ACEP. It is now administered by an independent, private corporation, the BTLS Foundation. BTLS also incorporates the philosophies of the ATLS, with the unique needs of the prehospital environment taken into account. As with the PHTLS course, the basic philosophies of prehospital trauma care are taught: rapid assessment, appropriate airway management, field control of hemorrhage, stabilization of fractures, and initiation of volume replacement en route to the hospital. The course is suitable for both basic- and advanced-level EMTs.

ADDITIONAL READING

American College of Surgeons Committee on Trauma: *Advanced Trauma Life Support,* 6th ed. Chicago, American College of Surgeons, 1997.

McSwain NE Jr: The physician in EMS: The medical director, in McSwain NE Jr, White RD, Paturas JL, et al (eds): *The Basic EMT: Comprehensive Prehospital Patient Care.* St. Louis, Mosby Year Book, 1997, pp 299–310.

National Highway Traffic Safety Administration: *Implementation Guide: Emergency Medical Services: Agenda for the Future.* Washington, DC, U.S. Department of Transportation, 1998.

Patient assessment and management, in McSwain NE Jr, Frame SB, Paturas JL (eds): *Pre-Hospital Trauma Life Support,* 4th ed. St. Louis, Mosby Year Book, 1998, pp 36–55.

U.S. Department of Transportation: *National Standard EMT—Basic Curriculum.* Washington, DC, U.S. Government Printing Office, 1994.

U.S. Department of Transportation: *National Standard EMT—Intermediate Curriculum.* Washington, DC, U.S. Government Printing Office, 1998.

U.S. Department of Transportation: *National Standard EMT—Paramedic Curriculum.* Washington, DC, U.S. Government Printing Office, 1998.

4 | Kinematics of Trauma

Trauma is a wound or injury characterized by structural alteration or physiologic imbalance resulting from acute exposure to mechanical, thermal, electrical, or chemical injury, or from the absence of such essentials such as heat or oxygen. A briefer definition is: *energy exchange with the human body that produces injury.* Precrash (prevention), crash (initial impact), and postcrash (medical care) are the three components, regardless of mechanism. This chapter is concerned with and discusses events that occur in the crash phase. There are many factors which affect the final outcome for the patient, such as distance from the hospital, quality of hospital care, age of the patient, preexisting conditions, and ambient or environmental conditions, and these are addressed in other parts of the book.

PHYSICS OF ENERGY EXCHANGE

Laws of Motion and Energy

This energy exchange is dependent on several laws of physics. The exact calculations are not important, but the concepts that are described by these energy laws are critical.

- *Newton's First Law of Motion:* An object at rest or an object in motion will tend to remain in that state until acted upon by some outside force.
- *Newton's Conservation of Energy Law:* Energy can be neither created nor destroyed, but its form can be changed.
- *Newton's Second Law of Motion (Force):* Force equals mass times acceleration ($F = MA$).

Force is required to put an object in motion. Once in motion, according to Newton's First Law, the object will continue in the same motion in the same direction and with the same force until a force that is equal to the starting force acts on the object to stop it.

$$\text{Mass} \times \text{acceleration} = \text{FORCE} = \text{Mass} \times \text{deceleration}$$

The force that puts an object in motion must be absorbed before the object will stop. The absorption of energy into the tissues of the body produces injury. To stop that object's forward motion requires a force equal to that which created it. Striking the percussion cap of a round in the chamber of a weapon creates an explosion inside the shell, which drives the bullet out. Once this acceleration has driven the missile to its peak speed, an explosion of equal intensity will occur as the object comes to rest. If this explosion occurs inside the human body, an injury is produced in the patient.

Kinetic energy: $KE = \text{mass}/2 \times \text{velocity}^2$

Therefore, the kinetic energy is dependent on the weight (mass) of the moving object and its speed. The weight is a linear relationship but the speed is logarithmic. Doubling the mass of the projectile results in doubling the resultant kinetic energy; however, doubling the velocity results in a quadrupling of the kinetic energy.

Cavitation

In the game of pool, the cue ball is driven down the table into the rack of balls, scattering them away from the point of impact. Bowling produces a similar cavitation at the end of a wooden lane.

When an object strikes the human body, tissue particles are knocked from their positions and crash into other tissue particles. This creates an explosion in which the energy of the moving object is passed onto tissue particles that in turn pass on this energy to the other tissues until all of the energy has been absorbed.

Two cavities are created: a permanent one, seen when the patient is examined, and a temporary one, which exists for only a fraction of a second, at the time of impact (crash). The temporary cavity expands rapidly at the time of the impact. When the period of the initial impact ends, the tissue particles will return to (as nearly as possible) their original positions. The amount of movement back to the original position depends to a great extent on the elasticity of the tissue involved. Muscle contains elastic-type fibers and tends to easily spread without tearing. Thus it may return to near its normal position. On the other hand, the liver and spleen are very inelastic and tend to fracture as the energy exchange occurs.

The outcome that is seen at the time of exploration is tissue crushed by the initial impact. As an object goes through (or impacts) the human body, a certain number of tissue particles are struck directly and will be crushed by the object. This creates a permanent cavity. The permanent cavity is visible to the examiner, whereas a temporary cavity is not.

An analogy is to take a baseball bat and swing it with equal force into either a roll of foam rubber or an aluminum barrel. After removing the bat from the aluminum barrel, a large cavity can be seen on the side of the barrel, but none is seen in the foam rubber when the bat is removed. The foam rubber is very elastic while the barrel is inelastic.

The other variable that affects the amount of energy exchange imparted to the tissue is the number of particles that are impacted by the moving object. The higher the number of particles impacted, the more instant energy exchange will occur. There will be more tissue particles in contact at the collision point of a very dense part of the human body as compared with a less dense part of the body. Although the differences in tissue density are on a continuum without absolute limit, they can be divided into air density such as is found in the lungs, parts of the small intestine, and sinuses; liquid density tissue such as muscle, vessels, and the solid organs; and the very dense bone. The energy exchange that occurs at the collision interface between these three types of tissues will vary, based on the density (number of tissue cells per volume of tissue). The frontal area of the moving object will also affect the number of tissue particles impacted. An ice pick, a baseball bat, and an automobile will exchange energy over increasingly wider areas, with increasing cavitation occurring at the interface.

BLUNT TRAUMA

Physics

Three separate types of forces in blunt trauma produce injury to the body and the organ. These three types are compression, shear, and overpressure.

Compression

Crushing disruption and cavitation cause injuries to tissues and organs. Compression forces are similar to laying an organ on a solid steel table and hitting it with a hammer. At every point that the head of the hammer touches the organ, those cells will be compressed and crushed. Some cavitation may occur in the surrounding tissue.

Shear

Shear forces occur as an organ and the organ's attachment do not accelerate or decelerate at the same time and at the same rate of speed, or two parts of the organ accelerate or decelerate at different rates, e.g., the thoracic aorta may be involved in this differential motion of uneven acceleration or deceleration in motor vehicle crashes. The descending aorta is firmly fixed to the vertebral bodies of the spine, but the arch of the aorta is not fixed. When the human body is struck from the side in a pedestrian/automobile collision, or in a frontal or side impact collision, the occupant is accelerated away from the point of impact. The descending aorta is attached to the spine and is accelerated at the same rate of velocity as the spine. The arch of the aorta, however, because its attachments are not directly to the bone, is accelerated slower when pulled along by the attachments of the descending aorta. The shear forces that occur at the interface between the attached and unattached parts can exceed the tensile strength of the aorta. The result can be full-thickness disruption with immediate exsanguination, or disruption of the intima and media alone producing a pseudoaneurysm.

Similar exchanges occur between the spleen and its attachments to the splenic artery and splenic vein, or to the kidney along its pedicle. Other organs may be similarly involved.

Overpressure

When a body cavity is compressed at a faster rate than the surrounding tissue, the muscular and fascial walls of the body cavity stretch much like the walls of a toy balloon when squeezed. An example is hitting a closed inflated paper bag with the open hand and noting that the bag pops. During a frontal impact of a vehicle, overpressure of the abdominal cavity is produced by impact with the steering column. Rupture of the diaphragm into the thoracic cavity is the outcome. Such overpressure events can and do take place in other cavities as well (e.g., bladder, bowel, and lungs).

VEHICULAR COLLISIONS

The five different types of collisions that produce different patterns of injury are: (1) head-on collisions, (2) lateral collisions, (3) off-center collisions, (4) rear impact collisions, and (5) rollovers.

After the initial impact, known as vehicular collision, is a secondary collision in which the vehicle occupant impacts some part of the inside of the vehicle. The third collision involves either compression or shear of the abdominal organs.

Frontal Impact Collisions

The vehicle and its occupants are moving at the same rate of speed. The vehicle (bullet vehicle) strikes an object (target vehicle or inanimate object) that is moving at a slower rate of speed or is not moving at all. There is a speed differential between the bullet vehicle and the target object struck. The bullet vehicle rapidly decelerates as the metal, plastic, and other parts of the car absorb the energy of the impact to bring the bullet vehicle to a stop or significantly reduce its speed. The unrestrained occupants in the target vehicle continue to move forward at the same rate of speed as the vehicle just prior to the moment of impact. Newton's First Law of Motion indicates that unless the occupants are somehow tied to the vehicle, their motion is not slowed until they impact the front of the passenger compartment, the steering wheel, or the back of the front seat, depending on their position just prior to the crash. As the occupants move forward, they do so in two different patterns, although these patterns frequently overlap.

Down-and-Under Pathway

The occupant continues to move forward in a down-and-under motion so that the legs first impact the dash. Most occupants sit in the car with their knees bent such that it is not the foot and lower leg that absorbs the energy, but the knee. As the knee impacts the dash, the energy can be absorbed by the tibia, which allows the femur to override, dislocating the knee and producing an unstable joint and damage to the popliteal vessels.

If the femur is the major point of impact, the continued force of the torso from behind fractures the femur somewhere along the shaft, or the pelvis overrides the head of the femur, producing an anterior dislocation with potential fracture of the acetabulum. The lower part of the body then comes to rest.

The upper part of the body continues in motion, colliding with the steering column or dash at the center of the chest, or perhaps the upper part of the abdomen. The front of the abdominal compartment, or the sternum, will stop, but the posterior abdominothoracic wall continues forward. In the abdomen, the organs are trapped and compressed between the stopped anterior abdominal wall and the continued motion of the posterior abdominal wall.

If the posterior abdominal wall stops before reaching the anterior abdominal wall, then the organs attached posteriorly can continue in motion and stretch or tear their attachments. These attachments are usually vascular, such as with the spleen, kidney, or intestine, but can be structural, such as the ligamentum teres.

In the thoracic cavity, the continued forward motion of the posterior thoracic wall is initially absorbed by the ribs. As the tensile strength of the ribs is exceeded, fractures result, producing a flail chest or compression of the lung or heart. A "paper bag effect" rupture of the lung is a frequent cause of pneumothorax.

As the posterior thoracic wall (vertebral column) with the attached descending aorta stops its forward motion, the unrestrained arch and heart continue in motion, producing shear forces at the junction between the unrestrained arch and the restrained descending aorta. The resulting injury ranges from an intimal tear to complete transection of the aorta as previously described.

Up-and-Over Pathway

The head becomes the lead point of the human missile as the occupant moves forward in the stopped vehicle. It strikes the windshield or the steel supporting structures for the windshield. The head stops its forward motion, but the brain and torso do not. The impact may damage the skull like the front of the car was damaged on impact. Part of the brain impacts the inside of the skull, resulting in contusion and lacerations, while the opposite end of the brain is separated from the skull. The spinal cord may remain in the spinal canal, with the brain separated from the brain stem.

Once the head has stopped its forward motion, the continued pressure of the torso on the unsupported cervical spine produces compression, hyperextension, or hyperflexion injuries. This may occur in the thoracic and lumbar spine as well. Approximately 10 percent of fractures of the cervical spine have an associated fracture in another part of the spine.

The chest and abdomen go forward into the steering column, producing similar injuries as those seen in the down-and-under pathway. The difference is that the impact is usually lower on the chest or completely in the abdomen.

Lateral Impact Collisions

These collisions usually occur at an intersection when one or both of the vehicles are trying to "beat" the traffic light. The collision will be a frontal collision to the bullet vehicle with injuries as described above. The target vehicle is hit in the side and accelerated rapidly at 90° to its previous direction of travel.

The impact on the target vehicle changes its direction from a purely forward motion to a combined forward-lateral motion, with the amount of the lateral motion determined by the speed and weight of the bullet vehicle in relation to that of the target vehicle. The first component of this collision is the intrusion into the passenger compartment. The second component is the lateral motion of the vehicle itself. If the occupant is restrained, he or she will begin lateral motion at the same time the vehicle moves away from the impacted door.

If the occupant is unrestrained, his or her lateral motion begins when the occupant is impacted from the side by his or her own vehicle. It is this impact that starts the cascade of injuries that are both compression and shear (acceleration or deceleration). The first element of this energy exchange moves the target vehicle laterally and out from under the occupants. As the motion of their own vehicle crashes into the occupant, they are first hit in the side and then begin to move away from the impact point at the same speed as the passenger compartment is moving.

The change in direction of the motion of the occupants is done by friction contact between the occupant's upper legs, buttock area, and back; by the lap and shoulder belt restraints; and by the door if there is intrusion into the passenger compartment or if the restraint devices are not properly worn. As intrusion into the passenger compartment occurs, the occupant on the side of the impact receives the major force, and thus the most severe injuries. The impact points by the door or "B" pillar are usually to the arm and shoulder, the lateral chest wall, and the proximal portion of the femur at the greater trochanter.

The shoulder impact can produce a fractured clavicle. This usually occurs as the concavity collapses into the center. The bone protrudes anteriorly into the overlying skin and not posteriorly into the vessels.

The intrusion into the organ compartments of the patient is similar to the intrusion of the vehicle wall into the passenger compartment. The occupant may receive inward compression of the ribs and intrusion into both the thoracic and abdominal cavities. The thoracic injuries can include multiple rib fractures, pulmonary contusion, and flail chest. Lateral collisions account for approximately 25 percent of aortic injuries; frontal impact collisions account for the rest. As the torso is accelerated, shear injuries to the aorta, spleen, and kidneys can become apparent later. The greatest shear force is at the junction between the fixed descending aorta and the mobile arch. The abdominal injuries can include compression of the spleen to the occupant on the driver's side and compression of the liver in the passenger. Acceleration injuries are caused in solid abdominal organs that are tethered on the side opposite the impact. In addition, the lateral impact on the femur drives the femoral head through the acetabulum. Further intrusion into the ilium produces compression fractures of the pelvis itself. The cervical spine is the fourth area that is affected in lateral impact collisions. The change in direction of the vehicle accelerates the torso rapidly to the side. Injuries to the cervical spine in lateral collisions are different than the compressive injuries seen in a frontal collision. As the torso (and thoracic spine) is accelerated laterally, the head, whose center of gravity is anterior to and cephalad to the pivot point, remains in position until the torso has already begun its motion. The head is flexed laterally and rotated toward the impact. This tends to open, then rotate and dislocate the vertebra, and finally lock the facets on the side opposite the impact.

Rear Impact Collisions

Vehicles are moving at different speeds in a frontal impact. Therefore the forces are additive because the vehicles are in direct opposition to each other. In rear impact collisions, the two vehicles are generally heading in the same direction; therefore the forces are decreased. Vehicles in a frontal impact, going at 20 and 30 miles per hour (mph) respectively, can produce an energy exchange equal to a barrier impact speed of 50 mph. In a rear impact, a target vehicle moving at 20 mph and a bullet vehicle moving at 30 mph will produce an energy exchange equal to a barrier impact speed of 10 mph.

Rear impact collisions move the frame of the target vehicle forward. All the contents that are attached to the frame move forward at the same rate of acceleration. Those that are unattached, such as the occupant, move at a rate associated with their relationship to the fixed parts of the vehicle. A seated occupant will move forward initially at a slower acceleration as the springs in the seat and the seat back absorb part of the energy of acceleration. As the seat back transfers energy to the posterior surface of the occupant, the torso will start to accelerate.

The head will move forward only when pulled by the neck musculoskeletal attachments or by the head restraint. If the forward motion of the head has not reached the same point of forward motion as the torso when the head restraint impacts the head, then the head restraint will provide support to prevent severe hyperextension of the neck. The acceleration of the torso, neck, and head will eventually equalize with that of the vehicle.

Off-Center or Rotational Collisions

When an off-center part of the vehicle strikes an object of significantly slower speed, the striking part of the bullet vehicle rapidly decelerates. The opposite side of this vehicle continues its forward motion according to Newton's First Law of Motion, but its attachment to the impacted side acts as a lever to pull it around in a circle. The differential motion will cause the vehicle to rotate around the point of impact, i.e., clockwise rotation with right frontal off-center impacts and counterclockwise rotation when the impact is on the left frontal area. The occupants inside the vehicle continue in their original direction until acted upon by the changed motion in the vehicle itself, when they impact the inside of the passenger compartment.

Off-center lateral and rear collisions will produce similar rotation. A little time taken when the patient presents in the emergency department to discuss the circumstances at the time of the crash will aid in effective patient care.

Rollover

The abrupt changes in motion of the occupant inside a rolling vehicle produces shear interactions between the body organs and their attachments, as well as compression of the body parts that collide with the inside of the passenger compartment.

OCCUPANT PROTECTION

The two components that provide protection to the occupants in a motor vehicle crash are (1) vehicular construction that prevents intrusion into the passenger compartment, and (2) devices that prevent ejection of the occupant and prevent or reduce the forces of contact with the interior of the vehicle. Although the design changes that have occurred in vehicles in the last 30 years have significantly reduced the chances of an occupant being injured, no device is perfect. When the energy exchange of the vehicle is large enough, the safety afforded by these protective designs can be exceeded and injuries can result. This is not a condemnation of the safety design, but an acceptance of the reality of injury exchange. Given enough energy, any protective device can be defeated. Therefore the individual taking care of the patient must understand these limitations and address the most likely causes of injury.

CRASHES INVOLVING OPEN VEHICLES: MOTORCYCLES, BICYCLES, AND MOPEDS

The laws of physics are the same as in other kinds of collisions, but the motions that the riders undergo will deviate some from those of closed vehicle collisions. These motions are described as frontal, angular, or ejection.

Type of Collision

Frontal

The motorcycle's center of gravity is above and behind the front axle, which is the pivot point in frontal collisions. Open vehicles will tip forward, and the rider will crash into the handlebars or continue the forward motion over the bars. The rider may receive injuries to the head, chest, abdomen, or pelvis, depending on which part of the body is involved. If the rider's feet remain on the pegs of the motorcycle and his or her thighs hit the handlebars, the forward motion will be absorbed by the midshaft of the femur.

Angular

If the open vehicle hits an object at an angle, the cycle folds on the object like a pair of scissors and crushes the rider between the cycle and the object struck. This results in injuries to the lower extremities. Injuries to the chest wall and abdomen are similar to the injuries sustained in a lateral closed vehicle collision as previously described.

Ejection

The rider continues over the open vehicle with the same speed that the vehicle was traveling just prior to impact. He or she travels like a missile until the head, arms, chest, abdomen, or leg strikes another object, such as a motor vehicle, a telephone pole, or the road. Injury will occur at the point of impact and will radiate to the rest of the body as the energy is absorbed. As with the occupant ejected from an automobile, the potential for serious injury is very high for this essentially unprotected rider.

PEDESTRIAN COLLISIONS

Pedestrian collisions are divided into three stages: initial impact, roll onto the vehicle, and impact with the ground. The initial impact on an adult involves either the lower extremities or the hips; the second component can cause chest and abdominal injuries; and the third component can result in injuries to the head and neck.

FALLS (FAILURE TO FLY SYNDROME)

In general, falls from greater than three times the height of the victim are severe. The surface on which the victim lands, and its degree of compressibility (ability to be deformed by the transfer of energy) have an effect on stopping distance and the severity of injury.

Determining which part of the body hit first is important because it will help to predict the injury pattern. The pattern that often occurs when victims fall or jump from a height and land on their feet is called the "Don Juan" syndrome. Fractures, dislocations, and shear injuries are part of the syndrome. The feet and especially the calcanei impact the ground, asphalt, or concrete and stop. The compressive forces of the continued motion of the torso produce fractures of the calcaneus and/or ankle.

The legs are the next body part to absorb energy. Knee injuries, long-bone fractures, and hip fractures/dislocations result. The spine is forced into flexion on the convex side by the weight of the still-moving head and torso. This can cause compression fractures of the spinal column in the thoracic and lumbar areas on the concave side, and opening on the convex side at each bend of the S-shaped spine. If the victim falls forward onto his outstretched hands, the forearms can absorb significant energy, producing fractures.

When the head is the lead point of the human missile, such as commonly occurs in shallow-water diving injuries, then the entire weight and force of the moving torso, pelvis, and legs are compressed on the head and cervical spine.

BLASTS

A blast can be broken down into primary, secondary, and tertiary effects.

Primary

The heat or light from the blast first affects any unprotected part of the skin. Clothing that can burn or melt causes secondary injury from the heat source. Structures that are between the blast and the individual can provide protection from the heat and light.

The pressure wave follows the blast, producing overpressure to all gas-filled or hollow organs, such as the sinuses, lungs, or gastrointestinal tract.

Secondary

Projectiles thrown through the air by the blast become missiles that can produce injury to the victim.

Tertiary

The pressure force of the blast knocks the individual down and perhaps into another structure, causing injuries similar to those of ejection from a vehicle or fall from a height.

PENETRATING INJURIES

Energy Exchange

As a bullet leaves the muzzle of a weapon, a significant amount of kinetic energy (KE = mass/2 $\times$ velocity^2) is produced. Based on Newton's First Law of Motion, this bullet will continue its travel until something acts on it to decrease its energy. Since energy can neither be created nor destroyed, the interaction between the bullet and the tissue will decrease the energy of the bullet by transfer of the energy to the tissues of the body.

The amount of energy exchanged to the surrounding environment depends on the amount of interaction between the bullet and the tissue. This in turn depends on the density of the medium through which the bullet is traveling, and to the frontal area of its path, as long as few particles are present to slow the bullet. When the bullet begins to interact with the human body, the density or the number of tissue particles present slow its forward motion. This energy from the missile is subsequently transferred to the victim.

If the bullet hits a thick sheet of steel that it cannot penetrate, the bullet itself will be deformed significantly to absorb its energy. On the other hand, if it hits something softer, such as skin, subcutaneous tissue, muscle, or even bone, the bullet does penetrate and create a hole or cavity. In order to create this cavity, tissue particles must be knocked out of their position. The motion of energy of the bullet is passed on to the tissue particles, setting them into motion (energy exchange). The tissue immediately in front of and in contact with the bullet is then crushed. The exchange of energy creates a cavity that stretches tissues on either side of the bullet's pathway. The amount of energy exchanged, and therefore the size of the explosion produced, are dependent on the number of tissue particles that come in contact with the bullet. This is dependent on the density of the tissue, the frontal area of the bullet, and the energy of the bullet. The frontal area is determined by the profile or shape of the bullet, any tumbling or unstable motion, and finally whether it breaks up into smaller pieces (fragmentation).

Cavitation

The process of stretching the tissue produces two types of cavities, as described earlier in the chapter. One that is temporary enlarges to produce damage as great as 20 to 25 times the diameter of the frontal area of the bullet. These tissue particles rapidly return to their previous position, leaving a more permanent cavity that is visible to the examiner.

The size of the cavity and the destruction caused by this cavitation are dependent to a great extent on the amount of elastic fibers present in the tissue through which the bullet is passing. For example, muscle contains a significant amount of elastic tissue and is able to stretch and reform with only a moderate amount of damage. On the other hand, the solid intra-abdominal organs, such as the kidney, spleen, and liver, contain few elastic fibers; therefore, when stretched, they tend to fracture and remain in a visibly damaged condition.

Size and Profile

The profile or frontal area of an ice pick is much smaller than that of a baseball bat, which in turn is much smaller than that of a truck. As a bullet travels through the air, its frontal area is kept small and streamlined by its conical shape. Therefore, it will strike fewer air particles and maintain most of its energy. If that missile strikes the skin and becomes deformed, covering a larger area, there will be a much greater energy exchange than if its frontal surface area does not expand.

The soft-pointed missile or dum-dum type bullet, if crushed and deformed as a result of striking the body, will have a much larger frontal area than it did before its shape was changed. A hollow-point bullet flattens and spreads on impact. This enlarges the frontal area, hitting more tissue particles and producing greater energy exchange. This in turn leads to a larger cavity being formed and more injury produced.

Tumble

A wedge-shaped bullet's center of gravity is located nearer to the base than to the nose of the bullet. When the nose of the bullet strikes something, it slows rapidly. Momentum continues to carry the base of the bullet forward. The center of gravity seeks to become the leading point of the bullet. This movement causes an end-over-end motion or tumble. As the bullet tumbles, the normally horizontal sides of the bullet will become its leading edges, thus striking far more particles than when the nose was the leading edge. This in turn produces more energy exchange, and therefore greater tissue damage.

Fragmentation

Bullets such as those with soft noses or vertical cuts in the nose, and Glazer safety slugs, increase body damage by breaking apart on impact. The mass of fragments produced comprises a larger frontal area than the single solid bullet, and energy is dispersed rapidly into the tissue. If the missile shatters, it will spread out over a wider area, with two results: (1) more tissue particles will be struck by the larger frontal projection; and (2) the injuries will be distributed over a larger portion of the body because more organs will be struck and more damage done. Fackler pointed out that the tissue disruption was significantly greater ($p < 0.001$) when the bullet fragmented than when it did not. The shotgun also uses this principle.

Exploding Bullets

Bullets that explode after entering the body can produce more injury than if the missile simply passes through intact.

DAMAGE AND ENERGY LEVELS

Damage caused by a penetrating injury is based on the energy of the wounding agent. Low-energy weapons include hand-driven weapons such as a knife or an ice pick. These objects produce damage only with their sharp point or cutting edge. Because these are low-velocity injuries, less secondary trauma is usually associated with them. Injury in these victims can be predicted by tracing the path of the weapon into the body. If the weapon has been removed, the examiner should identify the type of weapon used and the gender of the attacker whenever possible. Men tend to stab with the blade on the thumb side of the hand and with an upward thrust, whereas women tend to stab downward and hold the blade on the little-finger side.

When evaluating a patient with a stab wound, it is important to look for more than one wound. Multiple stab wounds are possible and should not be ruled out until the patient is completely exposed and closely examined. This close inspection may take place at the scene or en route to or at the hospital, depending on the circumstances surrounding the incident and the condition of the patient.

The attacker may stab his victim and then move the knife around inside the body. A simple entrance wound may therefore give a false sense of security. The entrance wound may be small, but the damage inside may be extensive. This cannot be determined in the field, but the possibility must always be suspected, even in seemingly minor injuries. The potential scope of the movement of the inserted blade is an area of possible damage. Evaluation of the patient for associated injury is important. For example, the diaphragm can reach as high as the nipple line on deep expiration. A stab wound to the lower chest can injure intrathoracic and intra-abdominal structures as well.

Firearms can be divided into two groups: Medium-energy and high-energy. Medium-energy weapons include handguns and some rifles. As the amount of gunpowder in the cartridge increases, the speed of the bullet, and therefore its kinetic energy, increases.

The difference in the damage done by medium-energy and high-energy firearms is in the size of the temporary cavity and of the residual permanent cavity. Generally, these weapons damage not only the tissue directly in the path of the missile but also the tissue on each side of the missile's path. The variables of tumble, fragmentation, and profile will influence the extent and direction of the injury. The pressure on tissue particles, which are moved out of the direct path of the missile, compresses and stretches the surrounding tissue. A temporary cavity is always associated with weapons in the medium-energy classification. This cavity is usually 3 to 6 times the size of the missile's frontal surface area.

High-energy weapons include assault weapons, hunting rifles, and other weapons that discharge high-velocity missiles. These missiles not only create a permanent track, but produce a much larger temporary cavity than lower-velocity missiles. This temporary cavity expands well beyond the limits of the actual bullet track and damages and injures a wider area than is apparent during the initial assessment. Tissue damage is far more extensive with a high-energy penetrating object than with one of medium energy. The vacuum created by this cavity pulls clothing, bacteria, and other debris from the surrounding area into the wound as well.

ANATOMY

The anatomy of penetrating trauma can be approximately identified by defining the wound of entrance and the wound of exit and drawing a line between the two. It is obvious that this line is not straight, as the bullet's pathway is deflected by its contact with organs and bones and that the cavitation produced inside the body will also vary. On the other hand, one can get a general idea of the organs that will potentially be injured and more specifically identify the regions that are involved. As an example, if the entrance wound is in the right chest and the exit wound is in the left chest, one has to be concerned about damage to midline structures. Alternatively, when the wound of entrance and wound of exit are both on the same side of the chest and fairly lateral, one can assume that, unless there is excessive bleeding from the chest tube, the injuries are not going to require surgical intervention. When the wound of entrance and the wound of exit are on opposite sides of the buttocks, one has to be concerned about rectal injuries.

As less and less mandatory exploration is done and more selectivity is added, identifying the difference between wound of entrance and wound of exit becomes extremely important. In most instances, it is easy to distinguish between a wound of entrance and a wound of exit simply by paying attention to the details of the physical appearance of the wound.

Entrance and Exit Wounds

Evaluating wound sites can provide one with valuable information to direct management of the patient. Do two holes in the victim's abdomen indicate that a single missile entered and exited, or that two missiles are both still inside the patient? Did the missile cross the midline (usually causing more severe injury) or remain on the same side? In what direction did the missile travel? What organs are likely to have been in its path?

An entrance wound lies against the underlying tissue, but an exit wound has no support. The former is a round or oval wound, whereas the latter is a stellate (star-shaped) wound.

Because the missile is spinning as it enters the skin, it leaves a small area of abrasion (1 to 2 mm in size) that is black or pink. There is none on the exit side. If the muzzle is directly against the skin at the time of discharge, the expanding gases will enter the tissue and produce crepitus on examination. When the muzzle is within 5 to 7 cm of the skin, the burning gases will burn the skin; at 5 to 15 cm, the smoke will adhere to the skin; and closer than 25 cm, the burning cordite particles will tattoo the skin with small (1- to 2-mm) burned areas.

ADDITIONAL READING

Barnes FC: Cartridge nomenclature, in Bussard M (ed): *Cartridges of the World,* 7th ed. Northbrook, IL, DBI Books, 1993, pp 8–12.

Bellamy RF, Zajtchuk R: The physics and biophysics of wound ballistics, in Bellamy RF Zajtchuk R (eds): *Conventional Warfare: Ballistic, Blast and Burn Injuries.* Washington, Office of the Surgeon General, Department of the Army, 1990, pp 107–162.

McSwain NE Jr: Mechanisms of injury in blunt trauma, in McSwain NE Jr, Kerstein MD (eds): *Evaluation and Management of Trauma.* Norwalk, CT, Appleton-Century-Crofts, 1985.

Nahum AM, Melvin J (eds): *The Biomechanics of Trauma.* Norwalk, CT, Appleton-Century-Crofts, 1985.

National Safety Council: Injury Facts, 1999. Chicago, National Safety Council, 1999.

5 | Initial Assessment

Care of the injured patient begins with *preparation:*

- Prehospital plans, training of personnel.
- Identify closest *appropriate* medical facility.
- Enhanced communications between trauma team and hospital.
- Disaster plans that are practiced and refined.
- On-site in-hospital teams of health care professionals committed to the care of the injured patient.
- Periodic check of equipment.
- Practice management skills to insure proficiency.
- Prearranged agreements to transfer patients for specialty care not available locally.
- Periodic outcome review to improve the structure of patient care.
- Verification of performance.

THE PRIMARY SURVEY

The algorithm in Fig. 5-1 pertains to the evaluation and resuscitation of patients with potentially serious or multiple injuries. The primary survey is designed to identify injuries that may be immediately life-threatening and to treat them as they are identified. This systematic approach is designed to identify injuries that are likely to result in poor outcome, in the order of their propensity to do so. Prior to the patient's arrival, all health care providers should ensure that they are protected against the transmission of infectious diseases and bodily fluids.

Airway and Protection of Spinal Cord

Diagnostic Pearls

- Loss of airway can kill within 3 minutes.
- Head, facial, neck, and inhalation injuries have potential to cause airway loss.
- Patients who can speak generally do not have an immediate need for airway management.
- Noisy respiration frequently indicates obstructed respiration.
- Patients with a Glasgow Coma Scale score <9 usually need airway protection.
- Laryngeal injury can be subtle; a hoarse or weak voice can indicate serious injury.

Treatment Pearls

- Practice skills to maintain proficiency.
- Use of chin lift, jaw thrust, and nasopharyngeal airway sometimes helpful.
- Have suction immediately available.
- If chemical paralysis is needed for intubation, ensure that someone is available who can perform a surgical airway.
- Chemically paralyzed patients cannot respond; neurologic examination is not possible.
- Confirm proper tube positioning.
- Secure tubes appropriately.

Cautions

- Anticipate problems, including equipment failure.
- Do not fail to recognize the potential for airway compromise.

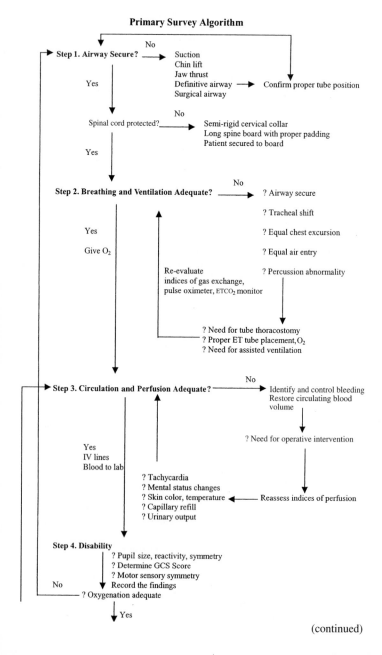

Primary Survey Algorithm

Step 1. Airway Secure? → No → Suction / Chin lift / Jaw thrust / Definitive airway / Surgical airway → Confirm proper tube position

Yes

Spinal cord protected? → No → Semi-rigid cervical collar / Long spine board with proper padding / Patient secured to board

Yes

Step 2. Breathing and Ventilation Adequate? → No → ? Airway secure / ? Tracheal shift / ? Equal chest excursion / ? Equal air entry / ? Percussion abnormality

Yes

Give O₂

Re-evaluate indices of gas exchange, pulse oximeter, ETCO₂ monitor

? Need for tube thoracostomy / ? Proper ET tube placement, O₂ / ? Need for assisted ventilation

Step 3. Circulation and Perfusion Adequate? → No → Identify and control bleeding / Restore circulating blood volume

? Need for operative intervention

Yes / IV lines / Blood to lab

? Tachycardia / ? Mental status changes / ? Skin color, temperature / ? Capillary refill / ? Urinary output ← Reassess indices of perfusion

Step 4. Disability

? Pupil size, reactivity, symmetry / ? Determine GCS Score / ? Motor sensory symmetry / Record the findings

No — ? Oxygenation adequate

Yes

(continued)

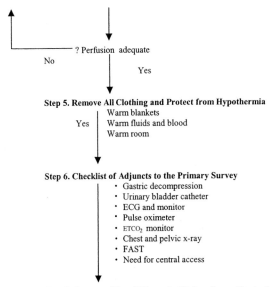

? Perfusion adequate

No

Yes

Step 5. Remove All Clothing and Protect from Hypothermia

Yes

Warm blankets
Warm fluids and blood
Warm room

Step 6. Checklist of Adjuncts to the Primary Survey
- Gastric decompression
- Urinary bladder catheter
- ECG and monitor
- Pulse oximeter
- ETCO₂ monitor
- Chest and pelvic x-ray
- FAST
- Need for central access

Step 7. Re-assess Steps 1 Through 6 Before Proceeding to the Secondary Survey

> **Periodic monitoring of vital functions during the Secondary Survey is *critical*!**

FIG. 5-1. Algorithm for the primary survey for trauma assessment and treatment. ECG, electrocardiogram; ET, endotracheal; $ETCO_2$, end-tidal carbon dioxide concentration; FAST, focused abdominal sonography for trauma; GCS, Glasgow Coma Score.

- Do not mistake ventilation difficulty for airway problems.
- In children, use of tubes that are too small can obstruct clearance of secretions.
- Patient movement can dislodge tubes or result in malposition.
- Prepare for contingency of inadvertent extubation during patient transport.
- A combative patient may be hypoxic.

Protect the entire spinal cord until injury has been excluded by radiography or clinical examination in patients with the potential for spinal injury. Complete spinal protection requires that the entire spine be immobilized, from head to toe.

Diagnostic Pearls

- Potential spinal fractures are treated before they are diagnosed; immobilize first, diagnose later.
- Diagnosis of spinal fracture should not precede resuscitation of the patient's vital functions.
- Motor vehicle crashes and falls are most commonly associated with spinal injury.
- Evidence of paralysis equates to instability of the spine.

- Evaluation of motor and sensory function is not possible after the use of chemical paralytics.
- Observe extremity movement before administration and document.

Treatment Pearls

- Spinal protection requires that the entire spine be immobilized.
- Spine boards that are not appropriately padded can destabilize lower thoracic and lumbar spine fractures.
- Patients must be strapped to the board to be protected.
- Manual immobilization of the patient's neck during patient movement is prudent.
- Immobilization in a neutral position is the goal, not in-line traction.
- The use of beanbags or other devices that conform to the patient's body contours have found utility in some parts of the world.

Cautions

- Soft cervical collars offer no protection.
- Reliance on a semirigid cervical collar alone is insufficient for protection of the spine.
- When used alone, strapping the patient to a long spine board does not protect the spinal cord.
- The utility of the spine board is the ability to move the patient without excessive spinal column motion.
- Health care providers should be especially attentive to the patient who is restless and combative.
- Coma and an altered level of consciousness are frequently associated with spinal injury.
- Children and the elderly are at risk for spinal cord injury without radiographic abnormalities.

Breathing and Ventilation

Inadequate gas exchange is as serious as an inadequate airway.

Diagnostic Pearls

Conditions	Frequently associated clinical findings
Tension pneumothorax	Absent breath sounds, air hunger, percussion hyperresonance, ± distended neck veins, ± tracheal shift (contralateral)
Tension hemothorax	Absent breath sounds, ± tracheal shift, percussion dullness, hemodynamic instability
Large flail segment	Paradoxical chest wall motion (seen without positive pressure ventilation)
Open pneumothorax	Sucking chest wound
Cardiac tamponade	Hemodynamic instability, fear of impending death, distended neck veins (unless volume depleted), often seen in transient or nonresponders to volume infusion

Treatment Pearls

- The above conditions are diagnosed by physical examination and are managed without the need for radiographic confirmation.

- Oxygen is essential for life, is a powerful inotrope, and should be given liberally.
- Endotracheal and thoracostomy tubes are definitive management tools for 85 to 90 percent of all immediately life-threatening chest injuries.
- Chest tube placement in the fifth intercostal space and directed posteriorly is generally adequate for immediate management.
- Massive hemothorax usually requires blood transfusion.
- Consider blood salvage with a suitable collection system for reinfusion into the patient.
- Pulse oximetry is invaluable.
- Capnography is very helpful to ensure adequate ventilation.
- Absence of breath sounds in a hemodynamically abnormal patient requires immediate chest decompression with a needle followed by tube thoracostomy.
- After any intervention, reassess the adequacy of ventilation.
- Arterial blood gas analysis is very helpful in monitoring the adequacy of oxygenation and ventilation.
- Confirm appropriate positioning of all tubes, radiographically if necessary.
- Cardiac tamponade may be temporized by volume infusion or pericardiocentesis, but generally requires an emergent sternotomy or thoracotomy.

Cautions

- Do not await radiographic confirmation of the suspected diagnosis before initiating treatment.
- Pulse oximetry is less effective in patients with poor perfusion, an inflated blood pressure cuff proximal to the monitoring device, in hypothermic patients, or when placed on a pulseless extremity.
- Chest tubes can be removed inadvertently during patient movement or transport; plan for contingencies and secure tubes appropriately.
- Inform transport personnel what to do if tubes become dislodged, obstructed, or nonfunctional during transport.

Circulation

Shock is a clinical diagnosis. Consider all injured patients who manifest signs of shock to have hemorrhagic shock.

Diagnostic Pearls

- Evaluate the patient for signs of inadequate organ perfusion (pale skin color, cool, clammy skin, delayed capillary refill, altered level of consciousness, inadequate urine output [<0.5 mL/kg/h for adults, <1 mL/h for children], weak or thready pulse).
- *Tachycardia is the most common sign of hemorrhagic shock.*
- *Find the source of bleeding!*
- Examine every part of the patient: front, back, and sides, from head to toe.
- Palpate for pelvic pain.
- Inspect extremities for fracture.
- Chest and pelvic radiographs are helpful.
- Consider diagnostic peritoneal lavage or focused abdominal sonography for trauma.

- If distended neck veins are identified, look for a source in the chest: massive hemothorax, tension pneumothorax, or tamponade.
- Celiotomy or thoracotomy may be necessary for diagnosis and control of hemorrhage; involve the surgeon early.
- Consider preinjury events such as myocardial infarction or cerebrovascular accident as etiology of shock.
- Transient response, as seen in patients who improve then deteriorate or who do not respond as anticipated may indicate ongoing blood loss or an incorrect diagnosis.
- For patients who do not respond to interventions, consider surgical intervention.
- Patients with pure neurogenic shock usually have warm extremities and a normal heart rate.
- Patients with septic shock usually have warm extremities.

Treatment Pearls

Stop the Bleeding

- Apply direct pressure.
- Arterial bleeders in open wounds can be ligated if visualized and isolated.
- Scalp lacerations can be temporarily closed with skin staples.

Close the Pelvic Volume in Patients with Open-Book or Vertical Shear Pelvic Fractures

- A bed sheet wrapped tightly around the pelvis is effective.
- An external fixation device applied by an orthopedist is helpful.

Restore Circulating Blood Volume to Normal

- Initiate two large-bore intravenous lines; peripheral access is preferable.
- All infused fluids should be warmed.
- Adults: crystalloid fluid bolus (Ringer's lactate or normal saline, 2 L infused rapidly).
- Children: crystalloid fluid bolus 20 mL/kg infused rapidly.
- *Administer blood products as needed;* consider transfusion of type-specific or uncrossmatched, emergency release blood: O^+ for men, O^- for women.

Other Important Points

- Immobilize fractures.
- Re-expand the lungs with a chest tube.
- In transient responders (patients who respond initially but deteriorate, or those who do not respond to interventions to the degree anticipated) search for ongoing blood loss.
- In nonresponders (those who do not respond to interventions) consider an alternative diagnosis (i.e., tamponade, spinal cord injury, etc) or the need for operative intervention.
- *Frequent reassessment of indices of perfusion is essential!*

Cautions

- Do not rely on blood pressure as the only indicator of shock.
- Children demonstrate a fall in blood pressure as the *last* clinical indicator of the shock state.
- Children who demonstrate hypotension have lost a significant portion of their blood volume and may require early transfusion.

- Elderly patients may be in profound shock with relatively normal blood pressure.
- Athletes may have significant hemodynamic reserve and may not demonstrate the classic signs of shock.
- A fetus may be in serious jeopardy with relatively normal maternal vital signs.
- Chronic medication use may mask the classic findings of shock (i.e., beta-blockers, digitalis, calcium channel blockers, etc).
- Plan for contingencies during patient transport or movement (in case the patient's hemodynamic status deteriorates during transport, or intravenous lines become nonfunctional or become disconnected).
- Elderly patients need to be treated aggressively but cautiously; invasive monitors such as central venous pressure lines or flow-directed pulmonary artery catheters may be useful.
- Vasopressors have a limited role in the initial normalization of a patient's perfusion indices.
- Sodium bicarbonate has no role in the resuscitation of patients from hemorrhagic shock.
- Restoration of normal perfusion corrects the metabolic acidosis.
- Pericardiocentesis is not always effective in temporizing the pathophysiology of tamponade; surgical intervention is usually necessary.

Disability

The baseline neurologic examination is essential in order to determine deterioration in neurologic function and to determine "asymmetry" in the examination that may indicate the need for emergent neurosurgical intervention!

Diagnostic Pearls

Determine the Glasgow Coma Scale (GCS) score:

Eyes Open	Spontaneously	4
	To verbal command	3
	To pain	2
	No response	1
Best Motor Response	Obeys verbal command	6
	Localizes pain	5
	Withdraws from pain	4
	Flexion to pain	3
	Extension	2
	No response	1
Verbal Response	Oriented/conversant	5
	Disoriented/confused	4
	Inappropriate words	3
	Incomprehensible	2
	No response	1

- Determine pupil size, reactivity, and briskness of response to light.
- Determine gross motor movement and symmetry of movement.
- If asymmetry is detected upon examination, the presence of extra-axial intracranial hemorrhage is likely and neurosurgical intervention may be required.
- A precise diagnosis is not necessary at this point in the evaluation.

- *Document the findings.*

Hypoxia and hypotension are the leading causes of secondary brain injury and it is essential to prevent them and correct them rapidly when identified!

Treatment Pearls

- *Ensure cerebral oxygenation and perfusion!*
- Repeat the ABCs as outlined above if necessary.
- Stop the bleeding from scalp wounds.
- A deterioration in the GCS score requires efforts to reduce intracranial pressure and maintain cerebral oxygenation and perfusion.
- *Involve the neurosurgeon early!*
- See secondary survey for steps to lower intracranial pressure.

Cautions

- *Hypotension is rarely caused by isolated traumatic brain injury!* Look for another source, usually hemorrhagic shock.
- Do not ascribe mental status changes to alcohol or drugs until all other causes have been excluded.
- A detailed neurologic examination is not necessary during the primary survey.
- Patients chemically paralyzed cannot have an adequate neurologic evaluation by physical examination.
- Coma and altered level of consciousness are associated with cervical spine injury.
- Patients with a GCS score of <9 usually need airway protection.
- *Frequent neurologic re-evaluation is essential!*

Exposure and Control of the Environment (Prevention of Hypothermia)

Hypothermia is potentially lethal to injured patients!

Diagnostic Pearls

- Remove *all* clothing. If injuries cannot be seen they cannot be diagnosed.
- Determine the patient's temperature. A urinary bladder catheter with a temperature probe is very helpful.

Treatment Pearls

- *Hypothermia is easier to prevent than it is to treat!*
- Control of hemorrhage is the most effective measure to prevent hypothermia.
- Keep everything warm; the patient with warm blankets and a warm room, and use fluid and blood warmers for infusion of fluids and blood.

Table 5-1 describes several procedures and two radiographic studies that are useful during the primary survey to monitor the patient's response to resuscitation and identify the source of bleeding from body cavities that are somewhat obscure (i.e., chest, abdomen, and pelvis). Diagnostic procedures to identify specific injuries are performed during the secondary survey and must not impede efforts to restore vital functions to normal.

General Rules

- Do not proceed to the secondary survey until the patient's vital functions are normal or showing improvement.

TABLE 5-1 Diagnostic Procedures and Studies

Procedure	Rationale	Cautions
Gastric decompression	Reduces, *but does not eliminate,* the risk of aspiration. Gastric distention and delayed gastric emptying commonly accompanies major injury. Gastric distention can result in hemodynamic deterioration, especially in children and the elderly. The course of the gastric tube through the esophagus and stomach as seen on chest x-ray can suggest aortic or diaphragmatic injury (i.e., deviation of the tube to the right or seen in the hemithorax on the left).	Facial fractures, especially of the mid-face. Basal skull fracture and fracture of the cribriform plate—use oral-gastric route. Placement may prompt vomiting. Have suction available. Gastric decompression is essential for patients who are intubated and mechanically ventilated.
Urinary bladder catheter	Diagnostic—hematuria or use for cystogram. Determination of urinary output is a helpful monitor of index of perfusion status. Relieves bladder distention that may modify the abdominal examination. Relieves bladder distention that may induce hemo-dynamic aberrations in some patients—reflex autonomic dystrophy.	Urethral injury—blood at urinary meatus, perineal or scrotal hematoma, open-book or vertical shear pelvic fracture, mobile or high-riding prostate. Perform rectal exam-ination prior to insertion of the catheter. Urethral strictures or benign prostatic hyperplasia may make catheter placement difficult or impossible—do not force the catheter. Obtain retrograde cystourethrogram if there is concern.
Electrocardio-graphic monitor and electro-cardiogram	Monitors cardiac rhythm and rate. Assists in the detection of baseline cardiac abnormalities (i.e., infarction, left ventricular hypertrophy, conduction disturbance, etc)	None known other than equipment failure.
Pulse oximetry	Continuous reading of hemo-globin oxygen saturation and heart rate. Allows early detection of oxygen desaturation. May be useful in determining peripheral perfusion—may be helpful in evaluation of patients with suspected vascular injury.	Do not place sensor on extremity distal to the blood pressure cuff—inflation of the cuff will result in temporary occlusion of blood flow and cause the alarm to sound. Less reliable in hypo-thermic patients. Bright ambient light may interfere with the sensor.

TABLE 5-1 continued

Chest radiograph	Identification of pneumo- or hemothorax. Assessment of contour of diaphragm. Screening evaluation of aortic integrity. Identification of skeletal injury. Identification of tracheal deviation. Determine size and contour of cardiac shadow. Identification of subcutaneous or mediastinal emphysema. Assist in determination of proper endotracheal, chest, or gastric tube placement.	Do not delay the placement of a chest tube for radiographic confirmation of a life-threatening tension or hemothorax. Manually protect the spinal cord if repositioning of the patient is necessary to obtain the x-ray.
Pelvic radiograph	Identification of pelvic fracture as a potential source of blood loss and possible associated urethral injury.	Attempts at manual manipulation of the pelvis to determine stability are ill-advised, as this may promote additional hemorrhage— palpation of the pelvis may demonstrate pain. Manually protect the spinal cord if repositioning of the patient is necessary to obtain the x-ray.
Baseline laboratory studies	Type and crossmatch of blood. Baseline hemoglobin determination. Coagulation parameters useful in those with massive blood loss or brain injury or to identify those patients taking anticoagulants when a history is not available. Drug and alcohol screening *may* provide clues as to the etiology of hemodynamic changes or altered level of consciousness. Serum chemistries *may* guide fluid and electrolyte replacement in patients with chronic medical conditions or those using chronic medications, ie diuretics. Arterial blood gases determine the adequacy of oxygenation, ventilation and perfusion status (base excess and pH).	Confusing blood samples when multiple patients are being evaluated.
End-tidal CO_2 monitor	Continuous assessment of the adequacy of ventilation.	Equipment failure. Obstruction of the sensor by secretions.

TABLE 5-1 continued

Central venous access—flow-directed pulmonary artery catheter	Assessment of filling pressures and ability of the heart to accept additional fluid. Assessment of cardiac function—may be especially useful in the elderly. Occasionally helpful in determination of the etiology of the shock state when there is uncertainty in the diagnosis. Supplemental ports for volume infusion.	Risk of iatrogenic pneumothorax or hemothorax. Risk of infection in a relatively uncontrolled environment. Cardiac rhythm disturbances. Placement requires special equipment, training of personnel, and time.
Focused abdominal sonogram for trauma (FAST)	Rapid determination of intraperitoneal, pericardial, or intrathoracic fluid, presumed to be blood. Noninvasive examination. Portable and repeatable.	Extremely dependent on the skill of the individual performing the examination—requires training and practice. Equipment failure.

- Repeat the primary survey for patients who deteriorate during subsequent evaluation.
- Resuscitation should never be delayed to obtain a specialized diagnostic test.
- Prompt control of hemorrhage is the key to management of hemorrhagic shock; therefore, consider the possible need for operative intervention.
- Early involvement of the surgeon is essential.
- The decision to transfer a patient is often made during the primary survey, when the needs of the patient exceed the capabilities of the health care team or the institution. Once the decision to transfer has been made, all further efforts should be directed toward: improving the patient's vital functions with all available local resources; avoiding further diagnostic tests that would not add to the resuscitation and only delay the transfer process; and planning for contingencies that may occur during transfer and providing adequate instruction and equipment for transfer personnel to deal with the problems encountered.

THE SECONDARY SURVEY

This survey is performed after the primary survey is completed and resuscitation is well on the way to success. On occasion, the secondary survey cannot be completed until the patient has undergone an operation to control hemorrhage. The secondary survey includes a history and head-to-toe physical examination done rapidly to avoid delay of definitive care. Adjuncts to the secondary survey are used as appropriate. If hemodynamic instability recurs, the primary survey should be redone.

History

The AMPLE history is obtained from the patient by first responders before they leave the facility, and history is also obtained from the family.

Allergies—Tetanus toxoid, contrast media, and antibiotics may be used early in trauma patients and may cause adverse reactions in an allergic patient.

*M*edications—Sedatives, illegal drugs, anticonvulsants, and insulin can all change the level of consciousness. Anticoagulant thrombopathy can aggravate head injury and otherwise increase bleeding. Miotic and mydriatic eye drops may affect the pupillary examination.

*P*revious illnesses—Chronic diseases such as diabetes mellitus, arteriosclerotic heart disease, renal failure, morbid obesity, and immunosuppression may be comorbid conditions. Children younger than 2 years and adults older than 55 have special issues when injured.

*L*ast meal—Alcohol and injury can cause delayed gastric emptying and all patients should be treated as if the stomach is full.

*E*vents associated with the injury—Hypo- and hyperthermia may affect treatment. Mechanisms of injury are important in determining the type of injury (see Chapter 4).

Physical Examination

Head

A rapid, careful neurological examination including GCS, pupillary evaluation, and symmetry of function should be performed. Careful inspection and palpation of the scalp for bleeding lacerations and evidence of open skull fracture is also useful (see Chapter 13).

Diagnostic Pearls

- Brain injury may become manifest after the primary survey is completed and GCS and pupillary examinations should be repeated.
- Anisocoria associated with a low GCS should be considered a brain injury until proven otherwise.
- Brain and spine injuries can coexist and cause a confusing examination.
- Computed tomography (CT) of the brain is important in patients who have lost consciousness, whether the GCS is low or not.
- Palpation may detect skull fracture.

Cautions

- Pressure ulcers may start to form in the emergency department, so the backboard should be removed as soon as possible.
- Eye prostheses can cause confusion on examination.
- Do not insert a finger into the brain.
- A patient who belongs in the operating room should not be in the CT scanner.
- Persistent scalp bleeding should be controlled (stapled) before completion of the exam.

Eyes

The eyes should be protected, particularly in an unconscious patient. "Can you see normally?" is a useful question to ask an alert patient (see Chapter 14).

Diagnostic Pearls

- Restriction of upward gaze, infraorbital hypesthesia, and diplopia suggest a blowout fracture.
- Anisocoria in the absence of brain injury may represent eye injury or be normal.

Cautions

- Contact lenses should be considered foreign bodies and should be removed.
- Failure to protect the eyes during resuscitation may cause serious abrasions.
- Consult an ophthalmologist early.

Ears

The external ears, external auditory canals, and tympanic membranes should be inspected and gross auditory acuity evaluated.

Diagnostic Pearls

- Identify exposed cartilage of the external ear.
- Disruption of external auditory canal, cerebrospinal fluid otorrhea, Battle's sign (bruise over the mastoid), and hemotympanum are associated with basilar skull fracture.
- Hearing the sound made by rubbing together the thumb and index finger of the examiner indicates reasonable hearing.

Cautions

- Cover exposed cartilage to avoid chondritis.
- Document deafness associated with basilar skull fracture as soon as possible.

Maxillofacial Area

The airway should be reevaluated as resuscitation progresses to identify swelling or bleeding that may cause delayed airway obstruction. Careful palpation and inspection of the maxillofacial region should be done to identify fractures. CT provides excellent identification of fractures and other deformities (see Chapter 15).

Diagnostic Pearls

- Noisy breathing is obstructed breathing.
- Edema and hemorrhage prevent accurate diagnosis without a CT scan.
- Serosanguineous drainage from the nose may be cerebrospinal fluid from a cribriform plate fracture.
- Gentle upward pressure on the hard palate may detect midface mobility.
- Teeth that do not appear to meet normally (malocclusion) may indicate midface or mandibular fracture.

Cautions

- Consider cervical spine injury.
- The airway may be suddenly lost due to edema.
- The nasogastric tube may be passed into the brain with cribriform plate injury; an orogastric tube should be used instead.

Neck

The neck was examined in the primary survey to determine if any injury is present that might affect the airway. A spinal immobilization collar is usually in place and needs to be carefully removed for further examination. An assistant must hold the head in neutral position to avoid injury. The anterior neck is examined for swelling and palpated for crepitus and laryngeal tenderness. The posterior neck is palpated for deformity and/or tenderness. Imaging studies are mandatory for evaluation of the cervical spine in patients with neurological deficits and pain or tenderness in the neck. Penetrating injuries are examined for penetration of the platysma muscle (see Chapter 16).

Diagnostic Pearls

- Hoarseness may develop late and may indicate a laryngeal injury.
- Penetration of the platysma in unstable patients must be explored in the operating room.
- Penetration of the platysma in a stable patient may require endoscopy, arteriography, and contrast studies to search for vascular and visceral injury.
- Tenderness of the cervical spine or neurological deficit mandates spinal imaging.
- High-quality lateral, anteroposterior, and odontoid x-rays that visualize the craniocervical junction and the top of vertebra T1 are required.
- Inadequate or indeterminate x-rays should be followed by CT of the cervical spine.
- Magnetic resonance imaging (MRI) is indicated in the presence of spinal cord injury.

Cautions

- Do not overlook a significant laryngeal injury.
- Consult a surgeon if the platysma is penetrated.
- Do not delay exploration of the neck with penetrating injury of the platysma in an unstable patient.
- Do not accept inadequate x-rays to "clear the cervical spine."

Chest

Inspection, palpation, percussion, and auscultation are performed on the injured patient. A chest x-ray is critical to adequately diagnose intrathoracic injury (see Chapters 18 through 23 and Chapter 25).

Diagnostic Pearls

- Inspection: sternal contusion may indicate cardiac or great vessel injury.
- Palpation: subcutaneous air or tenderness may indicate lung or chest wall injury.
- Percussion: dullness suggests hemothorax or diaphragmatic hernia; hyperresonance suggests pneumothorax.
- Auscultation: asymmetric breath sounds may indicate hemothorax or pneumothorax; pleural or pericardial rubs may indicate hemothorax or cardiac tamponade; bowel sounds in the chest suggest diaphragmatic rupture.
- Review of the chest x-ray may reveal a small pneumothorax, a widened mediastinum (great vessel injury), abnormal cardiac silhouette (cardiac tamponade), a ruptured diaphragm, or mediastinal air (esophageal or airway injury).
- Stable patients with traversing mediastinal injury need a focused abdominal sonography for trauma (FAST) exam, contrast studies, angiography, and endoscopic evaluation.
- An abnormal electrocardiogram (ECG) may indicate blunt cardiac injury.

Cautions

- Maintain a high index of suspicion in patients with a rapid deceleration

injury to avoid missing life-threatening great vessel injury or blunt myocardial injury.
- An abnormal ECG in a young patient needs to be investigated by echocardiography.
- Beware of small diaphragmatic injuries because positive-pressure ventilation may obscure the x-ray findings.

Abdomen and Pelvis

Shock from intra-abdominal and bony pelvic injury is addressed in the primary survey. The abdomen extends from the nipples to the groin creases, and is usually divided into the thoracic abdomen, abdomen, pelvic abdomen, and retroperitoneum. Physical examination of the abdomen has a significant rate of false positive and negative findings. Though it is a good study, diagnostic peritoneal lavage (DPL) is invasive and has largely been replaced by the FAST exam. CT of the abdomen and pelvis gives the most specific information (see Chapters 26 through 34).

Diagnostic Pearls

- Penetrating injury to the abdomen requires the attention of a surgeon.
- Serial physical examinations are not as helpful as diagnostic imaging for identifying bleeding and detecting peritoneal signs of hollow viscus injury.
- Thoracic abdominal (splenic and hepatic) injury may be detected by CT scan.
- Abdominal (small bowel and colon) injury with leak of fluid or stool may be identified by CT, ultrasound (US), or DPL.
- Pelvic abdominal (rectal) injury may be associated with pneumoperitoneum and fluid in the abdomen; bladder injury may be associated with gross hematuria; female reproductive organs are well protected.
- Gentle palpation of the pelvis that elicits tenderness may suggest a fracture. Avoid compression of the pelvis. X-ray and CT are useful in decision making.
- Retroperitoneal abdominal (renal) injury is often associated with gross hematuria, and pancreatic injury is occasionally associated with elevated lipase. Both are best diagnosed with CT, but pancreatic injury may be subtle.

Cautions

- Consult a surgeon early to facilitate management.
- Penetrating injury of the thorax at the nipples or below and from the scapular tips to the infragluteal creases should be considered abdominal injuries until proven otherwise.
- Seat belt marks suggest hollow viscus injury.
- Observation of patients with solid organ injury must be done under the supervision of a surgeon.
- Advantages of the FAST exam are its portability, repeatability, and the ability to identify new fluid collections.

Genitalia, Perineum, and Anorectum

The external genitalia, perineum, and anorectum must be inspected and palpated in injured patients to avoid missing potentially serious injury. Imaging studies with contrast are used to identify disruption of all but the vagina (see Chapter 33).

Diagnostic Pearls

- Blood on the urethral meatus, scrotal hematoma, and a high-riding prostate on rectal exam indicate urethral injury. A urethrogram is indicated.
- Vaginal and perineal lacerations associated with a pelvic fracture may indicate an open fracture of the pelvis; significant bleeding may be associated.
- Testicular and scrotal hematomas may need operative evaluation, but ultrasound can aid in the diagnosis.
- Rectal examination may demonstrate blood and bony fragments when pelvic fracture is present.
- Absence of sphincter tone in the absence of chemical paralysis may indicate spinal cord injury.
- Sensation testing in the perianal area may demonstrate sacral sparing in a patient with spinal cord injury.

Cautions

- Gross blood on the examiner's finger indicates rectal injury.
- A positive hemoccult examination is irrelevant with respect to the recognition of acute injury.
- Deferred exams can lead to missed injuries.
- Avoid urinary catheterization in a patient suspected of urethral injury.

Musculoskeletal

Each extremity must be evaluated carefully with neurovascular assessment before and after manipulation of an injured extremity (see Chapters 38 and 39).

Diagnostic Pearls

- Search for swelling and deformity.
- Check neurovascular status.
- Crush injury and extensive soft-tissue injury can be elucidated by a good history.
- X-ray painful areas.
- Consider compartment syndrome with extensive injuries to the soft tissues and bone in an unconscious patient.
- Promptly identify open fractures.
- Immobilize fractures as they are identified to control hemorrhage, provide comfort, and reduce possibility of further injury.

Cautions

- Consult an orthopedic surgeon early to facilitate care.
- Do not rely on the absence of distal pulses to diagnose compartment syndrome. The only beneficiaries of neglected compartment syndrome are attorneys.
- Reevaluate extremities at risk for compartment syndrome after *any* surgical procedure.
- Always reassess neurovascular status after manipulation of fracture.

Back and Spine

The back is inspected and palpated when the patient is log-rolled. The backboard is removed while the patient is rolled to the side, allowing the patient to rest on a firm but padded examining bed to avoid pressure sores. The cervical collar remains in place until spinal injury is excluded (see Chapter 17).

Diagnostic Pearls

- Palpation of deformity and/or tenderness suggests injury.
- X-ray of the thoracolumbar spine is indicated for tenderness, deformity, paralysis, decreased level of consciousness, and if a cervical fracture is present.
- Evaluate for any open injury.

Cautions

- Do not defer examination of the back because injuries may be missed.
- Pressure sores may develop after as few as 30 minutes on the backboard, particularly in the paralyzed and unconscious patient.

Nervous System

The neurological examination is done throughout the secondary survey. Treatment factors, chemical paralysis, and sedatives sometimes make the exam difficult. This examination to evaluate spinal cord function should be done as soon as the patient can cooperate. Symmetry of strength and sensation are assessed (see Chapter 17).

Diagnostic Pearls

- The patient must be able to cooperate for an accurate examination to be made.
- If the patient has a good hand grasp and can spread his fingers with good strength, he is not quadriplegic.
- An anomalous examination that shows patchy sensation and upper extremity paralysis and lower extremity weakness may be a central cord syndrome.
- Brown-Séquard's syndrome is a partial cord injury that is manifested by paralysis with sensation on one side and abnormal sensation and motor function on the other.
- Lax anal sphincter tone may be a clue to cord injury.
- Priapism is a bad prognostic sign.

Cautions

- Do not try to perform this examination in a chemically-paralyzed patient.
- Consult a neurosurgeon early.
- Cord syndromes are confusing and rarely "pure."

THE TERTIARY SURVEY

This survey involves repeated examinations of the injured patient, usually after the initial evaluation and resuscitation seems to be complete, and often after definitive care has been given. All newly discovered pain, tenderness, and areas exhibiting edema should be investigated for injury.

Diagnostic Pearls—Delayed Diagnoses

- Any injury in the unconscious patient that requires the patient to respond for the injury to be detected.
- Hollow viscus injury.
- Compartment syndrome.

- Diaphragmatic rupture.
- Missed spinal fracture.
- Ligamentous injuries.
- Distal extremity fractures.
- Peripheral nerve injuries.
- Scalp lacerations.

ADDITIONAL READING

American College of Surgeons Committee on Trauma: *Advanced Trauma Life Support.* Chicago, American College of Surgeons, 1997.

Bell RM, Krantz BE: Initial assessment, in Mattox KL, Feliciano DV, Moore EE, (eds): *Trauma,* 4th ed. New York, McGraw-Hill, 2000, pp 153–170.

Krantz BE: Secondary assessment, in Trunkey DD, Lewis FR, (eds): *Current Therapy of Trauma,* 4th ed. St. Louis, Mosby, 1999, pp 136–139.

Lewis FR: Primary assessment, in Trunkey DD, Lewis FR, (eds): *Current Therapy of Trauma,* 4th ed. St. Louis, Mosby, 1999, pp 131–135.

6 | Airway Control

Advanced trauma life support (ATLS) guidelines stress immediate airway management with cervical spine immobilization as the first treatment of trauma patients. ATLS-trained physicians and paramedics follow an algorithm for airway management of victims of blunt trauma (Fig. 6-1) which was first adopted in 1989 by the American College of Surgeons Committee on Trauma (ACSCOT) and is reviewed every 4 years.

SPECIAL PROBLEMS OF AIRWAY MANAGEMENT FOR THE TRAUMA VICTIM

Suspected Cervical Spine Injury

Approximately 1.5 to 3 percent of survivors of blunt trauma have a cervical spinal injury, 25 to 75 percent of which are unstable. Patients with clinically significant head injury have a greater risk of cervical spine injury (4.9 percent vs. 1.1 percent without head injury), and the incidence increases to 7.8 percent in trauma victims with a Glasgow Coma Score under 8. Neurologic deficits are present in 30 to 70 percent of patients with significant cervical spine fracture, and cord compression is commonly associated with fracture dislocations of C5 to C7, where the vertebral canal is at its narrowest. All trauma patients in a high-risk category should be managed as if they had a cervical spine injury; emergency intubation should never wait for a cervical x-ray, and cervical immobilization should be maintained until the spine is clinically cleared.

At the trauma scene, the cervical spine is immobilized by application of a Philadelphia collar, and the patient is secured on his or her back to a trauma board. Sandbags are placed on either side of the head, and the forehead is then taped to the board with 3-inch tape. Once a patient is immobilized per ATLS protocol, cervical movement is restricted to about 5 percent of normal. A Philadelphia collar used alone does not adequately immobilize the c-spine; it restricts lateral movement of the neck to 50 percent, and extension to 30 percent of normal.

AIRWAY MANAGEMENT WITHOUT INTUBATION

Administration of oxygen and relief of airway obstruction by manual removal or suction of mucus, blood, and debris from mouth and pharynx; the use of a well lubricated nasal or oropharyngeal airway; or the insertion of a laryngeal mask airway may allow time for transport of the spontaneously breathing patient to the trauma center, but will not guarantee the airway or protect against aspiration.

The Laryngeal Mask Airway (Fig. 6-2)

When used by paramedics, the LMA can be inserted with the head strapped in the neutral position, and it provides a clearer airway with improved oxygenation and a lower incidence of obstructive incidents than a face mask. An LMA can ventilate a patient with a difficult airway and can be used when endotracheal intubation proves difficult or impossible. Airway obstruction of an immobilized patient in a moving ambulance can be difficult to manage, and guidelines by the American College of Critical Care Medicine suggest that appropriately sized LMAs should be available for use during patient transport.

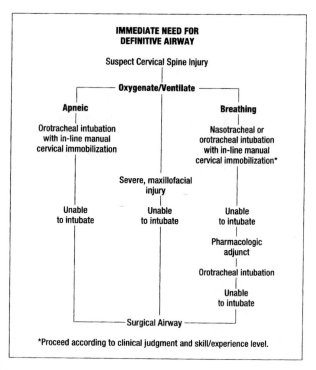

FIG. 6-1.   Airway management algorithm.

The Esophageal-Tracheal Combitube (Fig. 6-3)

The Combitube® is especially useful when vomitus or blood obscures the larynx during direct laryngoscopy. It can be placed correctly by paramedics in 69 percent of patients, and preliminary studies show it provides adequate ventilation and oxygenation with few complications. The Combitube can be inserted without causing movement of the neck, can be used when intubation fails, and is an alternative airway rescue device recommended by the American Society of Anesthesiologists, the American Heart Association, and the European Resuscitation Council for managing patients impossible to intubate or ventilate. One case of esophageal perforation has been reported. The pressure exerted by the pharyngeal balloon can also cause swelling of the tongue if left in place for more than 30 minutes. The Combitube should be left in place, and only the proximal cuff needs to be deflated when proceeding to subsequent direct oral intubation; the distal lumen will then direct any vomitus away from the intubating field.

AIRWAY MANAGEMENT USING INTUBATION

Direct Orotracheal Intubation

Direct orotracheal intubation with rapid sequence induction (RSI) and manual in-line stabilization (MILS) of the cervical spine is the most reliable and

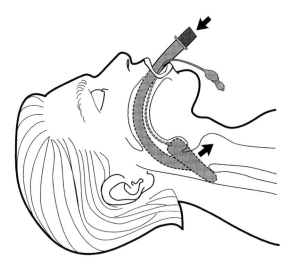

FIG. 6-2. Anterior and lateral drawing of the Bain laryngeal mask airway (LMA). The LMA in position. The LMA is inserted blindly with the cuff deflated or partly inflated over the tongue and pushed as far as it will go. The cuff is inflated with 20 to 30 mL of air. When correctly placed, the cuff lies in the pharynx, its tip obstructing the upper esophageal lumen, and the mask interposed between the base of the tongue and the posterior pharyngeal wall to open the airway. Patients can breathe spontaneously through it (when it is used to reduce upper airway obstruction) or can be ventilated via the LMA if apneic.

quickest way of securing the airway of an apneic or unstable patient. The patient is carefully placed in the supine position, with the head in the neutral position (not on a pillow). A pulse oximeter is placed on the finger. The anterior portion of the Philadelphia collar (or the whole collar) is removed because it reduces mouth opening to a mean value of 2 cm, and will interfere with subsequent cricothyroidotomy. An assistant applies manual in-line stabilization of the neck with his or her hands placed flat along the sides of the head, fingers grasping the mastoid process, to resist extension of the cervical spine with laryngoscopy. Usually the assistant kneels at the left side of the laryngoscopist. The patient is preoxygenated if still breathing, and with loss of consciousness, cricoid pressure is applied by a second assistant standing to the right. Cricoid pressure should be maintained until intubation has been successfully confirmed. The assistant applying cricoid pressure should use the other hand to support the neck posteriorly, as concern has been expressed that cricoid pressure may dislocate cervical vertebrae when applied without the posterior cervical support of the Philadelphia collar. Hypnosis is provided by intravenous midazolam, propofol, or ketamine, and the patient is paralyzed with succinylcholine. Fasciculations of the patient's muscles indicate the onset of paralysis. The patient is intubated with the most commonly used curved (Macintosh) laryngoscope blade designed to be placed into the right side of the mouth, displacing the tongue to the left. The tip of the blade is placed into the vallecula at the base of the tongue, and upward traction is applied. Direct laryngoscopy in the neutral position (i.e., the head not placed on a pillow) makes laryngoscopy more difficult and produces a grade 3

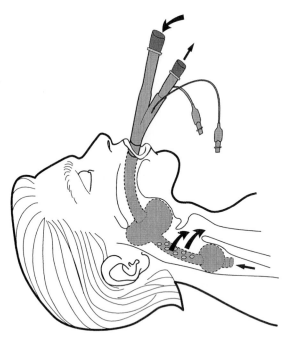

FIG. 6-3. Lateral view of the Combitube double lumen tube. The Combitube in place for emergency airway control. The tube is inserted blindly by lifting the jaw and tongue upward until the two printed rings are at the teeth. The tip of the tube usually enters the esophagus. The pharyngeal cuff is inflated with 100 mL of air, and when correctly placed, seals off the nasopharynx and oral cavity. The distal cuff is inflated with 15 mL of air. Ventilation through the longer (blue) connecting tube will inflate the lungs via the 8 side holes in the pharyngeal portion of the Combitube (as illustrated). If no breath sounds are heard, ventilation is attempted through the other lumen (the shorter tube) as the distal tube and cuff has probably entered the larynx.

laryngoscopy (only the epiglottis seen) in 22 percent of patients compared to 1.3 percent of patients placed in the optimal position.

In an adult, a smaller-than-usual internal diameter (ID) 7-mm endotracheal tube is often used with a stylet placed in the tube bent to curve the tip of the tube anteriorly (like a hockey stick). Backward, upward, and right sided pressure (BURP maneuver) applied to the thyroid cartilage may bring a difficult-to-visualize larynx into view. If unsuccessful, the curved tip of a lubricated gum elastic bougie is then placed under the epiglottis through the cords. The laryngoscopist will feel the bougie rubbing up against the tracheal rings and a #7 ID endotracheal tube can then be inserted over it. Resistance is felt as the endotracheal tube abuts against the epiglottis and the tube may have to be rotated 90° to pass into the larynx. If there is no resistance to intubation, the bougie and tube may well lie in the esophagus. Repeated unsuccessful attempts at intubation may cause laryngeal edema, bleeding, airway obstruction, and severe hypoxia. Following oropharyngeal suction, the physician may use a laryngeal mask airway or bag and mask ventilation to provide oxygenation during the time taken to create a surgical airway with or without ketamine for analgesia/anesthesia. When orotracheal intubation failed in one study, 12 patients with maxillofacial fractures and 7 with cervical spine injury were successfully managed at the trauma site at the first attempt by retrograde intubation (Fig. 6-4).

Alternative devices used to assist intubation include a light wand, Bullard laryngoscope, CLM laryngoscopy blade, and fiberoptic bronchoscope. The laryngoscopist needs to be experienced and familiar with this equipment before using it in the trauma patient.

Muscle paralysis should not be used by the inexperienced physician. An unconscious patient can often be intubated without sedation or paralysis. The airway can be inspected with MILS to assess difficulty of intubation prior to using paralysis; awake direct orotracheal intubation with MILS can be used when the laryngoscopist is concerned that paralysis could cause loss of the airway. In a pediatric patient, awake intubation is impractical, and blind nasotracheal intubation is rarely successful because of the acute nasopharyngeal angle. Young children may have spinal cord injury with a normal cervical radiograph, and direct orotracheal intubation, MILS, and hypnosis with and without paralysis is the best method to secure the airway. A younger child has

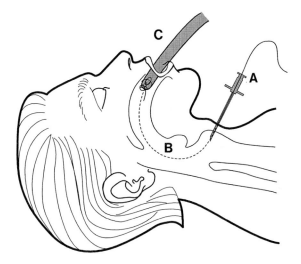

FIG. 6-4. Retrograde intubation. An epidural size 17 Tuohy needle is inserted through the cricothyroid membrane as close to the upper border of the cricoid cartilage as possible and angled cephalad (*A*). An epidural catheter (*B*) is advanced through the vocal cords into the oropharynx and pulled out of the mouth. The epidural needle is withdrawn, and the catheter is tied to the Murphy's eye of a size ID 7- to 8-mm endotracheal tube (*C*), which is then pulled through the vocal cords. Once through or at the vocal cords, the endotracheal tube is pushed into the trachea, and once in position, the epidural catheter can be cut at the skin. Modifications include threading the endotracheal tube or a tube changer over the catheter or a J wire, and inserting the endotracheal tube into the trachea over it; or feeding the distal end of a J wire through the suction port of a bronchoscope over which an endotracheal tube has been loaded.

a large occiput, which produces cervical flexion in the neutral position, and a rolled up towel is therefore placed under the shoulder blades before intubation. The size (ID) of tube needed in a child can be calculated with this formula: ID = 4 + age ÷ 4.

The technique of direct oral endotracheal intubation, with RSI, cricoid pressure, and MILS is the recommended method of intubation of all trauma patients at the R Adams Cowley Shock Trauma Center, in Baltimore, Maryland. At the trauma scene, 307 of 310 patients in one study were successfully managed with this technique by the London Helicopter Emergency Medical Service. A study by Stewart and coworkers reported a 58 percent success rate of oral intubation by trained paramedics at the trauma scene at the first attempt and a 79 percent overall success rate with subsequent attempts.

Blind Nasotracheal Intubation

Blind nasotracheal intubation is included in the ATLS algorithm as an alternative to direct oral intubation in the breathing patient. However, Dronen and colleagues, in a study of patients with drug overdose, showed only a 65 percent success rate versus 100 percent with oral intubation. Blind nasal intubation took a mean 276 seconds compared to 64 seconds for direct oral intubation. Multiple intubation attempts were not unusual, and they produced an 86 percent complication rate (epistaxis, vomiting, and aspiration), and there are two reports of death resulting from airway obstruction with repeated attempts at blind nasal intubation in trauma patients.

Following topical anesthesia to the nasopharynx, a well lubricated, softened, small (ID 6 to 7 mm) endotracheal tube is gently advanced into the nasopharynx; overly aggressive advancement may cause epistaxis or push the tube submucosally into the retropharyngeal space. The tube is advanced, guided by breath sounds heard by the physician at the proximal end of the tube. Maximal breath sounds are heard when the tube is close to the glottic opening. Usually at this point, the head is flexed or the larynx is manipulated and the tube is pushed through the glottis. When flexion is not allowed (e.g., with cervical spine injury), the endotracheal tube may hang up anterior to the glottis. Inflation of the endotracheal cuff in the oropharynx may help direct the tube towards the larynx, or use of a light wand to illuminate the larynx can help with blind nasotracheal placement. If available, a capnograph can be attached to the endotracheal tube, or fiberoptic bronchoscopy can be performed when breath sounds are loudest.

MAXILLOFACIAL TRAUMA

Airway problems are particularly common with fractures of the mandible. Bilateral fractures or shotgun wounds may result in a floating mandible or blow the jaw apart. Such victims characteristically must sit upright leaning forward so that the no longer suspended tongue and suprahyoid muscles fall out of the airway. Attempts to lay the patient down for laryngoscopy or creation of a surgical airway will cause airway obstruction. In the seated, cooperative patient, suction of the airway, blind nasal intubation, or fiberoptic nasal intubation may secure the airway. A blow to the inferior surface of the mandible can cause a bimandibular fracture at the level of the first and second molars. This causes a foreshortened appearance of the mandible (the Andy Gump Fracture), as the distracted segment is pulled inferiorly and posteriorly by the muscles of the floor of the mouth to compromise the airway. Airway obstruction can often be relieved by applying steady forceful anterior traction to the mandible, or direct laryngoscopy can lift the segment, allowing endotracheal intubation.

Subcondylar fractures and bone fragments from posteriorly displaced zygomatic fractures can involve the temporomandibular joints or impact on the coronoid process and cause physical limitation of jaw opening. If time allows, such patients are best managed by nasotracheal fiberoptic intubation. Radiographs or a CT scan can differentiate impaction from the more common limitation of mouth opening caused by pain and masseter muscle spasm (trismus), which will relax with anesthesia and paralysis. Unfortunately, intubation is often required for an unstable patient before radiographs are available. When managing severe mandibular fractures, respirations should be maintained and muscle paralysis and sedation should be avoided unless direct prior laryngoscopy shows intubation to be simple. If endotracheal intubation is too difficult or too dangerous to attempt, the patient should be managed with a surgical airway.

Maxillary fractures may compromise the airway by causing severe bleeding from the fracture sites or from laceration of ethmoidal arteries. Nasal packing, insertion of Foley catheters to tamponade the nasopharynx, good suction, and head down position will help clear the airway. Le Fort III fractures are usually associated with basilar skull fractures. Attempts at nasal intubation may force the endotracheal tube through the cribriform plate. Airway management involving Le Fort III fractures is often managed by awake tracheostomy.

LARYNGEAL INJURY AND TRACHEOBRONCHIAL DISRUPTION

Injury is usually caused by a direct anterior blow to the neck by a hockey puck or against dashboards or steering wheels in motor vehicle crashes, or impaction of the larynx against handlebars or cables in motorbike or snowmobile accidents. Such hyperextension injury may be associated with cervical fractures and esophageal injury. Patients may have minimal complaints of hoarseness or dyspnea, which may rapidly progress to severe upper airway obstruction because of increasing edema or an expanding hematoma. Because of the close proximity of the trachea to carotid and jugular vessels, high-velocity missile injuries and knife wounds to the anterior neck may cause aspiration of blood into disrupted airways and drown the patient, or may cause a rapidly expanding hematoma which tracks under the fascial planes of the neck to compress the airway.

Diagnosis of injuries to the larynx depends on inquiring about the mechanism of injury and examining the anterior neck for subcutaneous emphysema, swelling, contusion, and localized tenderness. If suspected, the airway should be examined in the awake, spontaneously breathing patient with a bronchoscope, and a small endotracheal tube (ID 6 or 7 mm) can be advanced over a 4-mm bronchoscope to secure the airway. Or a tracheostomy (which may be difficult because of subcutaneous emphysema or hematoma) should be created below the laryngeal injury. Cricothyrotomy may aggravate laryngeal injury. Blind nasal or direct orotracheal intubation is contraindicated in laryngeal trauma as the endotracheal tube can create a false passage and cause fatal airway obstruction. Cricoid pressure applied before intubation may disrupt the airway.

Approximately 1 to 3 percent of patients with acceleration/deceleration or crush injuries to the chest suffer tracheobronchial disruption, 80 percent of which occur within 2.5 cm of the carina. In a study by Bertelsen and Howitz, 6 of 33 patients with intrathoracic tracheobronchial disruption were admitted to the hospital alive. Five died within 45 to 120 minutes. The probable cause of death in these patients is either associated injury or positive pressure ventilation by the rescuers using an endotracheal tube, which preferentially ventilates through the tracheobronchial tear to cause a tension pneumothorax. This diagnosis should be suspected in a patient whose pneumothorax does not resolve with pleural suction. The airway should be examined by awake bronchoscopy. Methods used to secure the airway depend on lung isolation and subsequent one-lung ventilation using an endobronchial or Univent tube.

HYPNOTICS, ANALGESICS, AND NEUROMUSCULAR BLOCKING AGENTS

Intravenous, usually short-acting hypnotics, analgesics, and muscle relaxants are used in the multiply injured patient to facilitate rapid endotracheal intubation. Hypnosis and paralysis is especially indicated in the head injured patient showing signs of raised intracranial pressure (ICP). Following preoxygenation, head-injured patients are intubated by RSI and MILS after intravenous propofol (1.5 to 3 mg/kg IV) or sodium thiopentone (3 to 5 mg/kg IV) which reduce ICP, followed by succinylcholine (1.5 mg/kg), with or without lidocaine 1.5 mg/kg to obtund the hypertensive response to intubation. Although there is debate as to whether or not succinylcholine raises ICP, it provides the quickest onset and most reliable and briefest duration of muscle paralysis of any agent and is widely used for intubation of head-injured patients. If a contraindication to the use of succinylcholine exists, or the physician is worried that ocular muscle fasciculations could expel the contents of an open eye injury, then rocuronium 1.2 mg/kg IV will provide total paralysis within a mean 75 seconds. Intubation is timed when total paralysis occurs as monitored by a nerve stimulator (a train of four applied stimuli to the ulnar nerve shows no twitch response). However, rocuronium (1.2 mg/kg) causes paralysis for 38 to 150 minutes and does not have the advantage of the rapid recovery time of succinylcholine (6 to 17 minutes).

Hypotension and apnea will occur in patients intubated with thiopentone or propofol. Alternatives include intravenous midazolam (5 to 10 mg), which may cause airway obstruction with loss of consciousness, or a short-acting IV narcotic such as remifentanil 2 to 3 μg/kg IV bolus, which can offer an alternative when given just prior to succinylcholine. It causes apnea, analgesia, and sedation but does not guarantee loss of consciousness. Hypotension negatively affects outcome of patients with severe head injury. Before intubation, preparation of an infusion of phenylephrine (20 mg in 500 mL NS), or infusion by pump of norepinephrine (8 mg in 500 mL NS) can be used to support blood pressure and brain and organ perfusion until the effects of the drugs wear off, or until hemorrhage is arrested in the operating room. Vasoconstrictors lose their effectiveness in patients with a low hematocrit, and large doses may be needed.

In the hypotensive patient intravenous ketamine (1 to 2 mg/kg), a potent analgesic and dissociative general anesthetic, can be used prior to succinylcholine. Furthermore, it can be used to anesthetize patients without airway obstruction who are agitated or combative, while maintaining respirations and usually the airway (its use may not prevent the risk of aspiration). The patient can then be preoxygenated and paralyzed for rapid sequence intubation or positioned for cricothyroidotomy. When ventilation is controlled, ICP is not elevated when ketamine is used.

Succinylcholine causes an increase in serum potassium, and should be avoided for 24 to 48 hours after an acute burn or denervation injury. Severe hyperkalemia >8 mEq/mL was noted in patients crushed in the Kyoto earthquake, and succinylcholine should be avoided in such patients, or if it is used, serum K should be measured before or after its use, and hyperkalemia treated initially with sodium bicarbonate. Its use is contraindicated in patients with malignant hyperthermia, in patients untested with a family history of malignant hyperthermia, and in patients with muscular dystrophy. Succinylcholine may cause bradycardia in children, and asystole if used repeatedly (treat with atropine).

SURGICAL CONTROL OF THE AIRWAY

Cricothyroidotomy

Cricothyroidotomy is the first procedure to consider for any patient who has a strong indication for intubation and in whom the trachea cannot be intubated for any reason. It is felt to be contraindicated in the pediatric trauma patient because of concern about a greater risk of subglottic stenosis. This contraindication is relative, depending particularly on the patient's age and the availability of other acceptable options for airway management.

The subcutaneous cricothyroid membrane is identified by palpation, the larynx is stabilized, and a short incision (either transverse or vertical) is made at the level of the membrane. After the position of the membrane is reconfirmed with the tip of a gloved finger, a small incision is made in the cricothyroid membrane and is then bluntly enlarged. Although a scalpel handle is sometimes used for this purpose, it is far preferable to spread the tissue with a hemostat, surgical scissors, or ideally, a Trousseau's dilator. When the opening has been adequately expanded, a standard tracheostomy tube of approximately 7 to 8 mm outer diameter (OD) is inserted into the tracheal lumen.

Any tube selected for placement through the cricothyroid space should not exceed 7 to 8 mm in OD in the average sized adult. Smaller tubes should be chosen for smaller patients, especially women.

The procedure for cricothyroidotomy is generally described as a simple one, but has probably been overrated for technical ease in airway emergencies. In patients whose cervical landmarks may be obscured by hemorrhage or edema, or who may be hypoxic and struggling, the procedure is far from trivial. McGill and colleagues' excellent report cites an overall complication rate of 39 percent. This included a 13 percent incidence of incorrect placement of the tube (most commonly through the supraglottic thyrohyoid membrane) and an 11 percent incidence of having the procedure take more than 3 minutes. The most serious complication was fracture of the thyroid cartilage during the forced insertion of a no. 9 Shiley tracheostomy tube that had an outer diameter of 12 mm.

Cricothyroidotomy in the Prehospital Environment

Gerich and colleagues have reported on a prospective analysis of 383 patients requiring prehospital airway control. Only 8 patients required cricothyroidotomy on site, due to the nature of injury in 6 patients, and a failure of intubation in 2 patients. The most difficult aspect of the procedure is inserting the tracheostomy tube into the airway in a patient who is awake and may be struggling. Ketamine can be used to anesthetize the patient. Paramedics attached to large trauma centers are now performing oral intubation and cricothyroidotomy with increasing frequency at the trauma site.

Tracheostomy

With few exceptions, tracheostomy is a poor choice of procedure for acute airway control in the trauma victim. The trachea lies deeper in the neck than is commonly appreciated, it is surrounded by a number of veins that are capable of alarming hemorrhage, and the location for the recommended tracheal incision is frequently obscured by the isthmus of the thyroid gland. Also, the necessary light, instruments, and assistance are rarely available in the emergency setting.

Tracheostomy may be indicated in patients with acute laryngeal trauma in whom placement of a tube through the cricothyroid space can contribute to the patient's existing laryngeal injury, and in those under age 12 in whom cricothyroidotomy is not recommended. The patient who has an open wound of the neck with a large tracheal laceration will frequently be best served by an endotracheal tube or tracheostomy tube inserted directly through the tracheal wound if an emergency airway is required.

When tracheostomy is contemplated in the trauma patient, it should be preceded by endotracheal intubation whenever possible, having first established airway control. We prefer a midline incision for these rare occasions, and enter the trachea by excising a segment of the second or third tracheal rings to insert a tracheostomy tube.

Experience in performing 100 percutaneous tracheostomies has been reported. One death in an obese patient was attributed to use of the technique. The device was placed paratracheally in 6 patients.

CONCLUSION

This chapter has presented an approach to airway control in the trauma victim that reinforces the ATLS algorithm (Fig. 6-1). Airway control is pivotal to successful resuscitation after major injury.

ADDITIONAL READING

Anonymous. Guidelines for the transfer of critically ill patients. *Crit Care Med* 21:931, 1993.

Blostein PA, Koestner AJ, Hoak S: Failed rapid sequence intubation in trauma patients: esophageal tracheal Combitube is a useful adjunct. *J Trauma Injury Infection Crit Care* 44:534, 1998.

Criswell JC, Parr MJA: Emergency airway management in patients with cervical spine injuries. *Anaesthesia* 49:900, 1994.

Crosby E, Lui A: The adult cervical spine: Implications for airway management. *Can J Anaesth* 37:77, 1990.

Desjardins G, Varon AJ: Airway management for penetrating neck injuries: the Miami experience. *Resuscitation* 48:71, 2001.

Gofrit ON et al: Ketamine in the field: the use of ketamine for induction of anaesthesia before intubation in injured patients in the field. *Injury* 28:41, 1997.

Hatley T et al: Flight paromedic scope of practice: current level and breath. *J Emerg Med* 16:731, 1998.

Isaacs JH, Pedersen AD: Emergency cricothyroidotomy. *Am Surgeon* 63:346, 1997.

Pennant JH, Walker MB: Comparison of the endotracheal tube and the LMA management by paramedical personnel. *Anesth Analg* 74:531, 1992.

7 | Management of Shock

Shock is ultimately dysfunction of cellular biochemistry. Resuscitation from shock is restoration of adequate oxygen delivery to mitochondria. After shock, organs fail in proportion to the hypoxic damage to constitutive cellular function. To effect a full recovery from shock often requires a patient's progress through a series of stages. Thus, during the period when their patients are recovering from shock, surgeons focus therapy on enhancing cellular recovery. As the patient recovers, anticipated complications related to cellular dysfunction can be at least minimized, if not avoided. Finally, the surgeon must recognize that treatments that reverse shock may produce a new set of abnormal circumstances.

PATHOPHYSIOLOGY OF SHOCK

Pathophysiology of Acidosis

The fundamental risk to a patient in shock is failure of cellular bioenergetics. For energy, cells depend on hydrolysis of the high-energy phosphoanhydride bonds in adenosine triphosphate (ATP) by the reaction

$$ATP + H_2O \Rightarrow ADP + P_i + H^+ + Energy$$

where
$$ADP = \text{adenosine diphosphate,}$$
$$P_i = \text{inorganic phosphate, and}$$
$$H^+ = \text{hydrogen ion (proton).}$$

Acidosis—the accumulation of unbuffered protons in cytosol—ensues in shock because oxidative phosphorylation (aerobic metabolism), which reclaims the proton in resynthesis of ATP from ADP, is slowed. Patients in shock have a critical reduction in nutritive blood flow in the microcirculation, and the partial pressure of oxygen available to mitochondria declines. In these hypoxic circumstances, ATP can be synthesized by anaerobic glycolysis; however, without oxygen, the rate of high-energy bond production is 5 to 10 percent of normal. Thus, H^+ concentration in extracellular fluid is a quantitative indicator of the magnitude of the shock insult to cellular bioenergetics.

During shock, hydrogen ions are shifted to the extracellular fluid compartment. While the decline in blood pH is buffered, principally by bicarbonate, a metabolic acidosis ensues. Acidemia can stimulate sensitive central chemoreceptors, and the reflex response is hyperventilation, which drops the $Paco_2$ and reduces acidemia. The plasma pH measured with an arterial blood gas analysis is the sum effect of respiratory and metabolic physiology. A method of interpretation of blood gas results, which attempts to separate the metabolic and respiratory effects, has been developed. Standard base excess reported in a whole blood gas analysis is the predicted quantity (mM) of strong acid or base that would be required to titrate the sample to a pH of 7.40, if the sample had a $Paco_2$ of 40 mm Hg and the blood had a hemoglobin of 5 g/dL. The change in standard base excess is a quantitative index of the metabolic consequences of shock and may predict the magnitude of resuscitation needed (Table 7-1).

The response to the metabolic acidosis of shock involves several organs. Buffers other than bicarbonate bind excess protons when acidosis develops. A principal buffer in blood is hemoglobin. Renal function is important in the reversal of acidosis. In glomerular filtrate, the anions sulfate and phosphate bind protons, and these anions are important buffers in urine excretion of excess H^+. In addition, intracellular macromolecules with anionic sites are

71

TABLE 7-1 Volume Requirements (Ringer's Lactate and Blood) in Base Deficit Groups*

BD Group	N	Hours after admission			
		1	2	4	24
Mild (2 to −5)	70	2966 ± 335	4030 ± 520	5881 ± 817	7475 ± 766
Moderate (−6 to −14)	110	3893 ± 322	7522 ± 642	8120 ± 718	13007 ± 1078
Severe (<−15)	29	6110 ± 589	9800 ± 982	10909 ± 1435	16396 ± 3252
		$p < 0.001$	$p < 0.001$	$p < 0.008$	$p < 0.001$

*Values expressed as mL ± SEM.
Source: Reproduced, with permission, from Davis JW et al: Base deficit as a guide to volume resuscitation. J Trauma 28:1464, 1988.

buffers of excess protons. One biochemical consequence of anaerobic glycolysis is that pyruvate accumulates. As pyruvate concentration increases, it is dehydrogenated in the cytosol and converted to lactate. In the acidosis of shock, as protons leak from the cell, extracellular lactate buffers the hydrogen and is converted to lactic acid. The ratio of lactate to pyruvate is a sensitive indicator of cellular hypoxia, with a normal value of 10:1 driven to a larger ratio during cellular hypoxia. Normally, the liver clears lactate from plasma.

Clinical Measures of Acidosis

Either arterial or venous blood samples can be used to determine the patient's base deficit. Experimental studies in animals with adequate tissue perfusion report a good correlation between arterial and venous base excess, with the base excess of venous blood 4 mEq/L less than the base excess in arterial blood. An important exception is patients with very low flow states. A venous sample might be more reliable than an arterial sample in indicating the acid-base status of a patient who has a low cardiac output.

Several studies of injured patients have demonstrated that the magnitude of metabolic acidosis has prognostic value. For the clinician monitoring a patient, a rising base deficit may be the first indication that a patient whose blood pressure is "normal" has a "low-flow" state and is in shock.

In contrast to a global index of hypoxia such as measurement of base deficit, recent clinical reports of gastric mucosal pH have been advocated as providing a precise and tissue-specific indication of a localized hypoxic insult. Gastric mucosal pH (pHi) is a calculated value. The measured values are the bicarbonate concentration (HCO_3^-) in an arterial blood gas and the P_{CO_2} in fluid instilled into a Silastic bag that is in contact with gastric mucosa. The pathophysiologic concept that is advanced as explaining the predictive value of low pHi is that ischemia of the bowel is an early manifestation of shock.

Treatment of Patients With Acidosis

If adequate tissue perfusion can be achieved in patients with shock, lactic acidosis can be resolved rapidly through normal metabolic pathways that depend on hepatic metabolism and alveolar ventilation. It should be noted, however, that injured patients with improved perfusion immediately following resuscitation may have a transient further increase in base deficit as there is reperfusion of ischemic areas.

Infusion of sodium bicarbonate in repeated scheduled doses into the venous side of the circulation during arrest situations may transiently buffer protons in blood, but generate more CO_2. Because CO_2 is more diffusible than bicarbonate, intracellular acidosis may be exacerbated while the blood pH increases. This paradoxical exacerbation of intracellular acidosis is a rationale for avoidance of universal bicarbonate therapy in cardiac arrest situations. For an acidotic patient to benefit from intravenous sodium bicarbonate, there must be adequate pulmonary blood flow and alveolar ventilation. Bicarbonate for patients with an arterial pH less than 7.20 has been advocated. This recommendation is based on experimental studies, which indicate that cardiac performance is reduced when blood pH drops below 7.20. If excessive amounts of bicarbonate are given during the phase of anaerobic metabolism, however, patients develop post resuscitation alkalemia. Alkalemia is associated with more severe adverse effects than acidemia on cardiac function and oxygen-hemoglobin interactions. In these circumstances, the bicarbonate load is cleared by the slow process of renal excretion, unless a neutralizing acid is administered.

Alternative buffers including Tris-(hydroxymethyl) aminomethane (TRAM), sodium carbonate, acetate, and combinations of these have been studied. They have the advantage of buffering protons without stoichiometrically producing carbon dioxide and respiratory acidosis. A novel alternative to buffers for treating patients with acidosis that is being investigated is administration of dichloroacetate (DCA), which accelerates intermediate carbohydrate metabolism. Specifically, pyruvate entry into the tricarboxylic acid cycle is increased by the influence of DCA on pyruvate dehydrogenase. As pyruvate concentration declines within the cell, there is less lactate released into the extracellular fluid.

Trauma patients rarely have alternative causes for acidosis other than cellular hypoxia from underperfusion. Patients with diabetic ketoacidosis will have elevated serum ketones and should be given intravenous insulin and glucose. Trauma patients can be poisoned with methanol, acetaminophen, ethylene glycol, cyanide, or carbon monoxide because of inadvertent consumption or suicide attempts. These forms of acidosis require specific treatment. Lactic acidosis does occur in alcoholic patients and is managed with repletion of thiamine, vitamins, glucose, and supportive care, including intravascular volume expansion.

SPECIFIC CAUSES OF SHOCK: DIAGNOSIS AND TREATMENT

Hemorrhagic Shock

Physiology

Patients who hemorrhage into shock have critically reduced cardiac filling pressures. As their cardiac output declines, organ perfusion becomes inadequate. The severity of hypovolemic shock is proportional to blood volume deficits. Loss of up to 10% of the blood volume is tolerated because compensatory physiologic mechanisms sustain perfusion and restore intravascular volume. Cardiac output declines significantly when 20 to 40 percent of the blood volume is lost, and this amount of hemorrhage produces a measurable decline in blood pressure. Hemorrhage of 40 percent or more of blood volume causes shock that is imminently life threatening.

Vasoconstriction in response to hypovolemia occurs in venous capacitance vessels and systemic arterioles. Circulating endogenous vasoconstrictors include epinephrine, angiotensin II, and vasopressin. The plasma concentrations of these quickly increase after hemorrhage in humans. Autonomic reflexes increase norepinephrine release from the terminal sympathetic nerves, which contributes to arteriolar vasoconstriction. The vasoconstrictive response is variable, with skin, bowel, and muscle blood flow reduced in deference to flow to the brain and heart.

The decline in blood volume can be partially replaced by a shift of fluid and proteins from the extravascular compartments back to the intravascular compartment. Interstitial fluid may move directly from the abluminal to the luminal side of the microvascular membrane, or through lymph flowing into veins.

Clinical Diagnosis of Shock

Clinical findings of compensated hemorrhagic shock include postural hypotension, diaphoresis, restlessness, and pallor from cutaneous vasoconstriction. Tachycardia is commonly reported in patients in hemorrhagic shock. Nevertheless, clinical studies of the admitting pulse rate of patients with substantial blood loss have consistently revealed that pulse rates vary widely.

Patients with significant blood loss compensate through neuroendocrine reflexes, which cause vasoconstriction of the cutaneous circulation. Plasma vasopressin—a powerful cutaneous vasoconstrictor—levels increase in the hypovolemic patient. One clinical manifestation of shock is cool, pale skin and slow reperfusion of capillaries beneath nail beds after they are compressed.

Severely hypotensive patients often have a depressed level of consciousness and a sense of dread, and may be agitated. Patients in profound shock are unconscious and should have endotracheal intubation and mechanical ventilation; however, intubation has risks. Hypovolemic patients may have a further decline in blood pressure with positive pressure ventilation or, rarely, experience cardiac arrest. For patients in shock, lower tidal volumes of 5 mL/kg, delivered at respiratory rates of 20 to 30 breaths per minute in adults, are appropriate.

Resuscitation From Hemorrhagic Shock

Injured hypovolemic patients need two interventions: reversal of hypovolemia and control of hemorrhage. Adult hypotensive patients will often have an increase in systolic blood pressure after rapid intravenous infusion of 2 L of balanced electrolyte solution. Children should receive a bolus of 20 mL/kg. The blood pressure response to the initial attempts at resuscitation must be determined. Patients who remain hypotensive should have a rapid evaluation to determine whether there is continuing hemorrhage. Simultaneously, a second bolus infusion of balanced electrolyte fluid is appropriate. Patients who do not respond to a second bolus will usually need an operation to control hemorrhage, as well as a blood transfusion of type O or type-specific blood.

Lucas described three phases of treatment of injured patients resuscitated from shock. After the first phase of active bleeding and equivalent blood volume replacement, there is a second phase of fluid uptake when extravascular fluid sequestration occurs. The patients commonly gain weight equivalent to 10 percent of their total body weight. After a mean of 40 hours for phase 2, a spontaneous diuresis occurs in most patients. Several reasons are proposed to explain the gain in weight during phase 2, including dilution of plasma colloid oncotic pressure, increased microvascular membrane permeability, alteration of the interstitial matrix, or expansion of the intracellular space. Failure to sustain a hyperdynamic circulation by inadequate isotonic fluid administration during phase 2 impairs recovery from shock and increases the risk of organ failure (Table 7-2).

Increased Oxygen Requirement After Resuscitation

Clinical evidence indicates that patients need to consume supranormal amounts of oxygen after resuscitation. The oxygen debt hypothesis proposes that patients resuscitated from shock have a residual bioenergetic deficit because during the period of shock, cellular oxidative metabolism was altered. As oxygen becomes plentiful during recovery from shock, there is a period of greater-than-normal oxygen consumption that is mandatory for cellular recovery. Successful resuscitation and optimal patient recovery depends on supranormal oxygen delivery.

The hypothetical relationship of oxygen delivery and oxygen consumption can be usefully presented in graphic form (Fig. 7-1). Considerable experimental evidence indicates that as oxygen delivery decreases during shock, there is a linearly correlated decrease in oxygen consumption. Deterioration below a critical level of deficiency causes death. In a normal patient receiving adequate oxygen delivery, the physiologic response to a further increase in oxygen delivery is represented on the graph as a plateau, where the oxygen extraction ratio (oxygen consumption/oxygen delivery, normally approximately 20 percent) declines, and consumption remains unchanged. The hypothesis that increased oxygen needs occur after patients are resuscitated from shock is graphically represented as the shift upward and to the right of the threshold point, corresponding to the point with which consumption becomes independent of delivery.

Table 7-2 Sequential Fluid and Protein Changes (MEAN $\pm$ SD) (During Lucas' Second and Third Phases of the Treatment of Shock)

	Phase 2		Phase 3	
	1st Half	2nd Half	1st 48 h	2nd 48 h
Plasma volume, L	2.8 ± 0.6	3.2 ± 0.5	$3.5 \pm 0.6^*$	$3.2 \pm 0.7^*$
Extracellular volume, L	18 ± 1.5	21 ± 1.4	21 ± 1.3	$15 \pm 1.1^*$
PV-ECF†	0.15 ± 0.01	0.15 ± 0.01	$0.165 \pm 0.02^*$	$0.21 \pm 0.05^*$
Serum albumin, g/dL	2.9 ± 0.1	2.8 ± 0.3	2.85 ± 0.15	3.2 ± 0.5
Total intravascular albumin, g	81 ± 3.3	91 ± 4.6	$100 \pm 2.9^*$	$103 \pm 3.3^*$
Albumin leak, %/h	6.0 ± 0.7	6.4 ± 1.2	$6.9 \pm 0.5^*$	$8.0 \pm 0.6^*$
Serum colloid oncotic pressure, mOsm/L	11.9 ± 0.4	10.6 ± 0.3	$13 \pm 0.5^*$	$14.1 \pm 0.5^*$

$^*p < .05$ when compared with early phase 2 data by student's t test for independent variables.
†Plasma volume:extracellular fluid ratio.
Source: Reproduced, with permission, from Lucas CE, Benishek DJ, Ledgerwood AM: Reduced oncotic pressure after shock. *Arch Surg* 117:675, 1982.

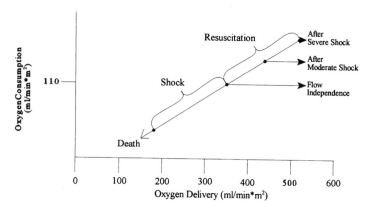

FIG. 7-1. A hypothetical model demonstrating the variability of the relationship between oxygen delivery and oxygen consumption. There is a linear decline in the two variables during shock. Flow independence occurs when further increases in delivery are not associated with greater oxygen consumption. The threshold for achieving flow-independent delivery shifts upward during resuscitation from shock, and in proportion to the severity of the shock insult.

Identification of the Site of Bleeding

Significant hemorrhage in injured patients will occur from five locations, and each site has unique considerations for diagnosis and hemostasis. The five sites are external hemorrhage, intracavitary bleeding into the pleural space or peritoneal cavity, bleeding into the muscle and subcutaneous tissue from contusion and fracture, and bleeding into the retroperitoneum, usually from pelvic fracture.

External Hemorrhage External hemorrhage from wounds may be obvious, and direct pressure will usually control bleeding. If the bleeding is in a distal extremity, a blood pressure cuff inflated proximally can stop the bleeding while the patient is promptly transported to the optimal resources of the operating room for wound exploration and repair or ligature of bleeding vessels. Actively bleeding lacerations of the scalp may be best managed with a rapidly accomplished running suture, which is revised later.

Pleural Space Bleeding into the pleural space from a large artery or the aorta is usually immediately lethal. Chest bleeding from the lung, or smaller chest wall vessels, such as intercostal branches or the internal mammary artery, produce a hemothorax. A chest x-ray or pleural ultrasound provides a prompt diagnosis. A commonly accepted guideline for requiring thoracotomy is an initial blood loss of greater than 20 mL/kg, or a continuing blood loss at a rate exceeding 2 to 3 mL/kg/h.

Peritoneal Cavity Substantial intra-abdominal blood loss can occur without obvious external signs. Hemoperitoneum can be promptly identified with diagnostic peritoneal lavage, ultrasound, or, in hospitals in which they are immediately available, CT scans. A laparotomy is the procedure of choice in patients in shock with significant hemoperitoneum.

Extremity Fracture   The volume of blood lost into the extremities or the muscle layers of the torso can be deceptively large. Large subfascial hematomas in extremities and the torso are usually associated with fractures; however, liters of blood can be lost into contusions.

Retroperitoneal Space   Liters of blood can fill the compliant tissues of the retroperitoneum in patients with pelvic fracture, renal injuries, or lumbar vessel disruption. Patients in shock with suspected active hemorrhage from arterial disruption associated with pelvic fracture are best managed by diagnostic angiography and transvascular embolization.

Neurogenic Shock

Spinal Cord Injury

Injury to the spinal cord at the level of the cervical or thoracic vertebrae can cause sympathetic denervation. Neurogenic shock is the consequence of the sudden loss of vasomotor tone. Without alpha-adrenergic tone in the arteriolar vessels, vasodilation occurs, leading to a drop in systemic vascular resistance. The hemodynamic response is a fall in systolic and diastolic pressure and an increase in cardiac output. Vasodilation of the venous capacitance vessels enlarges what is already a substantial reservoir, and the treatment is intravascular volume expansion. The hypotensive patient with neurogenic shock will characteristically not be tachycardic, will have weakly palpable peripheral pulses, and will exhibit pink nail beds with good capillary fill. These patients have a wide pulse pressure, and hypotensive patients may be alert. Heart rates below 100 beats per minute, even in the sinus bradycardia range, occur in patients with neurogenic shock and are attributed to uncompensated vagal tone to chronotropic areas of the heart in a patient who has loss of sympathetic innervation.

Most adult patients with neurogenic shock will respond to intravenous infusion of 2 L of balanced electrolyte solution. Volume expansion may replete losses from hemorrhage, and also "fill" the dilated venous reservoirs. Paraplegic or quadriplegic adults may achieve a systolic blood pressure of only 90 mm Hg after infusion of isotonic fluid.

Brain Injury

Brain injury should not be considered the primary cause of hypotension in multiply-injured patients, even though a brain stem injury may cause cardiovascular instability. Furthermore, large blood loss from scalp lacerations or open facial fractures can occur.

A unique problem in trauma patients with lethal head injury is preservation of adequate perfusion pressure until organs can be harvested for transplantation. Loss of the normal brain stem–mediated reflexes leads to irreversible hypotension and cardiac arrhythmias. Donors must have adequate perfusion if harvested organs are to function after transplantation. Organ donors in shock should receive intravenous fluid and blood to treat shock. Judicious use of vasopressors may be indicated; however, these vasoconstrictive drugs may compromise the suitability of organs for transplantation.

Compressive Shock

Compressive shock occurs when cardiac output is low due to extrinsic pressure from fluid, air, or hemorrhaged blood on the heart or lungs, impairing vena cava blood flow during diastolic filling of the right chambers of the heart.

Tension Pneumothorax

Tension pneumothorax occurs when air trapped in the pleural space between the lung and chest wall achieves sufficient pressure to compress the lungs and shift the mediastinum. Many patients with a tension pneumothorax have a hemothorax as well. The diagnosis of tension pneumothorax is suspected on the clinical examination of a hypotensive patient who has chest tympany on percussion of the anterior chest, ipsilateral absent breath sounds, deviation of the trachea away from the injured lung, distended neck veins, and penetrating chest trauma or a blow to the chest sufficient to have fractured ribs. Although most patients with tension pneumothorax have easily identified findings on chest x-ray, rarely patients with pleural adhesions holding the lung to the chest wall develop loculated air pockets not evident on a routine chest x-ray. These can be identified with CT scans. In situations in which a chest tube cannot be immediately inserted, patients with a tension pneumothorax can be emergently decompressed with a large needle inserted into the third or fourth intercostal space at the midclavicular line. Hypotension may dramatically reverse as air is heard to decompress through the needle. The definitive management of a tension pneumothorax is insertion of a chest tube into the pleural space.

Cardiac Tamponade

Cardiac tamponade is a cause of shock because compression of the cardiac chambers limits ventricular filling. Three factors influence the magnitude of shock that develops in a patient with tamponade: (1) the volume of blood in the pericardial sac, (2) compliance of the pericardium, and (3) central venous pressure (CVP).

Physical findings are hypotension, distended neck veins, and distant or muffled heart sounds in a patient with extreme anxiety. In stable patients, a surgeon-performed ultrasound will confirm the diagnosis of fluid in the pericardial sac. More formal echocardiographic features of cardiac tamponade include right atrial compression and right ventricular diastolic collapse. Transesophageal echocardiography can be performed during laparotomy or thoracotomy and improves visualization of the posterior heart.

Treatment of most adults suspected of cardiac tamponade should begin with intravenous infusion of 500 to 1000 mL of balanced electrolyte solution and evaluation of the hemodynamic response. In the moribund patient with a penetrating chest injury, who has lost his or her vital signs within minutes of arrival in the emergency department, and whose cardiac rhythm is agonal contractions, endotracheal intubation and an immediate left anterolateral thoracotomy are indicated.

An alternate diagnostic and therapeutic approach when ultrasound is not available is to perform a subxiphoid pericardial window. This procedure has low morbidity and can safely enable the surgeon to establish whether the suspected diagnosis of hemopericardium is correct. The pericardial window should be performed with the patient anesthetized and equipment and personnel ready to proceed with exploration of the heart. Induction of a general anesthetic in a patient with cardiac tamponade who is marginally compensated can precipitate profound hypotension or a cardiac arrest. Thus, before administration of drugs and beginning positive pressure ventilation in a patient suspected of having cardiac tamponade, it is prudent to have the patient fully prepped and draped and the surgical team prepared to proceed immediately. During a laparotomy, either a subxiphoid or transdiaphragmatic pericardiotomy can be used. When the subxiphoid window drains pericardial blood, the patient's tamponade is decompressed and there is usually time to proceed with a median sternotomy, providing excellent exposure of the heart.

Cardiogenic Shock

In physiologic terms, cardiogenic shock is the circumstance of low cardiac output despite ventricular end-diastolic volumes which should be adequate to prime the ventricle for vigorous contraction and ejection of an ample stroke volume. In clinical circumstances, cardiogenic shock may reflect several concurrent adverse influences, including deficient myocardial power, valvular dysfunction, and arrhythmias. Perfusion to multiple organs is inadequate in cardiogenic shock, including delivery of oxygen to the myocardium itself, which exacerbates a critical failure in myocardial performance. The combination of myocardial pump failure and declining coronary perfusion are synchronous insults that can deteriorate quickly to cause death.

Blunt Cardiac Injury

While a contusion to the heart may occur commonly in patients with substantial blunt torso trauma, cardiac contusion is an example of blunt cardiac injury that is infrequently a cause of serious myocardial dysfunction and shock in hospitalized injured patients. The diagnosis of a cardiac contusion is confirmed by new-onset abnormalities on the admission ECG or hypotension that is not explained by the injuries sustained. Autopsy findings in patients who have expired with blunt cardiac injury include lacerations of the heart, disruption of valves, transmural myocardial hematoma, or, rarely, evidence of a traumatically induced main coronary artery occlusion. Severely disabled patients with cardiac contusion have been salvaged by an intra-aortic balloon pump during periods of hypoxia, associated surgery, and refractory cardiogenic pump failure.

Preexisting Heart Failure

Cardiovascular deterioration in a patient with preexisting heart failure is a common problem among geriatric trauma patients. Causes of preexisting heart failure are previous myocardial infarctions, cardiomyopathy from lifelong hypertension, valvular disease, and viral cardiomyopathy. These patients have limited reserves available to enable them to respond to the stress of injury. When a low cardiac output is confirmed with use of a Swan-Ganz catheter, intravascular volume loading, inotropic drugs, and afterload reduction are indicated. Inotropic drugs that have been successfully used to increase contractility include dopamine, dobutamine, and amrinone.

Myocardial Infarction

Shock in a trauma patient can be secondary to a myocardial infarction (MI) caused by acute coronary artery occlusion. In some cases, the MI is precipitated by the stress, pain, and surge in endogenous production of catecholamines that follow an injury. Alternatively, an acute MI was the event responsible for the patient losing control of a vehicle or falling. In either case, the trauma surgeon must promptly recognize that a MI is the cause of shock and proceed to not only resuscitate the patient, but also consider practicable options for reperfusion therapy (thrombolysis, bypass surgery, angioplasty). It often is impossible to differentiate angina pectoris from chest pain caused by injuries to the chest wall. The diagnosis of an MI can be established by a characteristic ECG finding of a new Q-wave or changes in the ST segment. Laboratory tests can confirm significant myocardial damage. A rise within 6 hours of creatine kinase-MB isoenzyme or cardiac troponin I is an indication of myocardial damage. Cardiac troponin I may be an optimal diagnostic test in patients with musculoskeletal trauma because the enzyme is found only in heart muscle. Treatment of patients with an acute myocardial infarction is based principally on anticoagulation, which is a therapy that may be contraindicated in a patient with multiple bleeding wounds. Thrombolytic agents reduce frequency of cardiac death and improve recovery of functional myocardium. Aspirin does have benefit in patients with an acute myocardial infarction and can usually be administered. Emergent coronary angioplasty can restore blood flow and salvage myocardium, particularly in patients who have unstable angina and an impending MI. Randomized controlled trials have confirmed the value of adjunctive pharmacologic therapy with use of beta-adrenergic antagonists and angiotensin-converting enzyme inhibitors in patients during an acute MI.

Directed Resuscitation of the Failing Heart

Therapies for cardiogenic shock can be divided into four categories: intravascular volume expansion, inotropic support for the failing ventricle, drugs to alter the systemic vascular resistance, and devices that assist pumping. In complex situations, a thermodilution pulmonary artery catheter can supply critical additional information to the measurement of filling pressures for the right heart. The optimal filling pressure depends on the patient. Patients with mitral stenosis may require central venous pressure or pulmonary arterial wedge pressure (PAWP) levels that in normal individuals would be associated with pulmonary edema. Several studies using pulmonary artery catheters with volumetric oximetry have calculated a right ventricular end-diastolic volume index (RVEDVI). This measure is used to guide cardiac preload expansion until maximum stroke volume index is achieved. Supranormal levels of RVEDVI have been associated with better outcome. The superiority of RVEDVI to PAWP has been demonstrated in mechanically ventilated patients, in whom positive airway pressures may produce effects that reduce reliability of PAWP.

Inotropic drugs can increase cardiac contractility and, for a given preload, achieve greater cardiac output. These drugs are infused continuously, and dosage is adjusted to achieve the desired effect. Inotropic drugs differ from each other in hemodynamic effects and can vary in mechanism of action, depending on the dosage. Furthermore, patients may differ in their response. Thus, use of inotropic drugs must always be empirical, and the following are intended only as guidelines. Dopamine or epinephrine is given to patients with adequate intravascular volume but a low systolic blood pressure. At lower doses, they increase contractility and may vasodilate some vascular beds. At higher doses, both drugs cause arterial vasoconstriction. For patients with an adequate systolic blood pressure but low cardiac output, dopamine or dobutamine can increase cardiac contractility, vasodilate, and increase cardiac index. In most cases with epinephrine and dobutamine, heart rate will increase at the doses that increase contractility, and tachycardia may be part of the benefit. However, tachycardia can exacerbate myocardial ischemia, and drugs with a chronotropic effect may be detrimental in patients with coronary artery disease. Amrinone is an inotropic agent that also vasodilates. The principal indicator of benefit from inotropic agents is an increase in cardiac index.

Two categories of drugs can be used to change systemic vascular resistance (SVR): vasodilators and vasoconstrictors. Directed use of these medications requires measurements of SVR. The adverse effects of a high SVR include increased workload for the myocardium and the risk of MI. Intravenously infused nitroprusside lowers SVR. Aggressive narcotic administration for pain control and adequate sedation are indirect methods of reducing catecholamine levels and reducing SVR.

Shock Related to Adrenal Insufficiency

Primary adrenal insufficiency is caused by a pathologic condition of both adrenal glands. The most common cause of primary decline in adrenal function is autoimmune adrenalitis.

Among trauma patients, rapid onset of adrenal insufficiency can be the consequence of hemorrhage or infarction of both adrenal glands, a condition called adrenal apoplexy. Administration of heparin or endogenous coagulopathies are associated with a predisposition to adrenal hemorrhage, which patients can experience as sudden epigastric pain that radiates into the flanks. While loss of adrenal function in both glands is lethal, unilateral adrenal hemorrhage is common and adrenal insufficiency rarely a complication.

Secondary adrenal insufficiency is caused by a defect in ACTH secretion. A common cause of secondary adrenal insufficiency, chronic administration of glucocorticoids for a medical condition, suppresses normal feedback loops of hypothalamic stimulation.

Addison's disease is chronic adrenal insufficiency in which the low cortisol production is adequate to sustain life. Patients with chronic adrenal dysfunction develop signs and symptoms of adrenal insufficiency in proportion to the deficiency in cortisol and the magnitude of stress.

For an adult, the usual adrenal replacement dose is 100 mg of hydrocortisone sodium succinate given intravenously every 6 to 8 hours. Pharmacologic doses of steroids do not benefit patients in shock. Hypoadrenal patients may not respond immediately, and intravenous fluid infusions with inotropic agents to augment cardiac contractility are sometimes required. After resuscitation from a suspected adrenal insufficiency, the patient should continue to receive glucocorticoid therapy until the diagnosis is confirmed. Cosyntropin is a synthetic ACTH used to diagnostically stimulate glucocorticoid synthesis and release from the adrenal cortex. A normal glucocorticoid response should be a more than twofold increase in serum cortisol concentration.

Septic Shock

Injured patients can present to the hospital in shock caused by infection. This rare circumstance is often accounted for by a delay between injury and onset of treatment. Death from septic shock in injured patients usually occurs days to weeks after hospital admission, and is commonly associated with multiple organ failure. Severe infection, particularly when associated with bacteremia, can be a cause of rapidly lethal shock with characteristic cardiovascular findings if administration of fluid resuscitation has been prompt and vigorous: hypotension, high cardiac output, and low systemic vascular resistance.

Septic shock is categorized as distributive, a term which emphasizes that despite increased delivery of oxygen to cells by a hyperdynamic circulation, the availability of that oxygen to sites of aerobic metabolism is impaired.

The resuscitation of patients in septic shock involves three steps. First, intravenous fluid is infused to restore intravascular volume and optimize the end-diastolic filling pressures in the right and left ventricles. Fluid resuscitation is accomplished with isotonic solutions. Second, because myocardial contractility is impaired in patients with septic shock, inotropic support is usually required. The third treatment for septic shock that may be required for patients with an unremitting low SVR is vasoconstrictors, which increase mean systemic arterial pressure.

Unusual Conditions Influencing Shock in Trauma Patients

Thiamine Deficiency

Beriberi heart disease—characterized by biventricular myocardial failure, peripheral vasodilation, and high cardiac outputs—develops in patients with inadequate thiamine intake (alcoholics) or malabsorption. Injured patients at risk for thiamine deficiency (e.g., alcoholics, food faddists, elderly persons with diet deficiencies, long-term furosemide use) should receive 100 mg of thiamine intravenously followed by an oral daily dose of 200 mg.

Alcohol-Related Conditions

Alcoholic cardiomyopathy is a chronic deterioration of ventricular function, often connected to atrial and ventricular dysrhythmias associated with a frequency of sudden cardiac death. Acute ethanol intoxication may exacerbate hemorrhagic shock because ethanol depresses cardiac contractility.

Preexisting Medications

Beta blockers are used to treat several cardiovascular conditions, and many geriatric patients take these medications. Slowed pulse rate and decrease in myocardial contractility may prevent compensatory changes to hypovolemia. After adequate intravascular volume expansion, infusion of epinephrine to maintain perfusion pressure can be effective in some patients. Patients who take calcium channel blockers, alpha-adrenergic blocking or depleting agents, and angiotensin inhibitors are vasodilated and may not have a compensatory increase in systemic vascular resistance in response to blood loss. Patients on diuretics have a contracted intravascular volume and develop hypotension after a smaller blood loss from hemorrhage. Most hypotensive patients on antihypertensive medications respond to intravascular volume expansion. Negative inotropic effects of drugs can be compensated for by dopamine or dobutamine.

Anaphylactic Shock

Anaphylactic shock is a systemic reaction precipitated by exposure of a sensitized patient to an antigen. In anaphylactic shock, there is a life-threatening histamine release, which is manifest as urticaria, angioedema, laryngeal edema, nausea, vomiting, diarrhea, and bronchospasm. The hypotension in anaphylaxis is the result of vasodilation, and substantial losses of intravascular fluid and plasma proteins are caused by an increase in permeability of the microcirculation. Epinephrine has remained the principal treatment of anaphylactic shock, along with restoration of intravascular volume deficits. In severe reactions, epinephrine is immediately administered intravenously and can rapidly reverse hypotension. Antihistamines and steroids have been advocated as beneficial; however, evidence of efficacy is limited.

ADDITIONAL READING

Cairns CB, Moore FA, Haenel JB, et al: Evidence for early supply independent mitochondrial dysfunction in patients developing multiple organ failure after trauma. *J Trauma* 42:532, 1997.

Crile GW: *An Experimental Research Into Surgical Shock.* Philadelphia, JB Lippincott, 1899.

Crile GW: *A Physical Interpretation of Shock, Exhaustion, and Restoration.* London, Henry Frowde, Oxford University Press, 1921.

English PC: *Shock, Physiological Surgery and George Washington Crile: Medical Innovation in the Progressive Era.* Westport, CT, Greenwood Press, 1980.

Ivatury RR, Simon RJ, Islam S, et al: A prospective randomized study of end points of resuscitation after major trauma: Global oxygen transport indices versus organ-specific gastric mucosal pH. *J Am Coll Surg* 183:145, 1996.

Natanson C, Hoffman WD, Suffredini AF, et al: Selected treatment strategies for septic shock based on proposed mechanisms of pathogenesis. *Ann Intern Med* 120:771, 1994.

Peitzman AB, Billiar TR, Harbrecht BG, et al: Hemorrhagic shock. *Curr Probl Surg* 32:925, 1995.

Velanovich V: Crystalloid versus colloid fluid resuscitation: A meta-analysis of mortality. *Surgery* 105:65, 1989.

8 | Transfusion, Autotransfusion, and Blood Substitutes

Blood products remain a vital and limited resource. Increased awareness of the potential risks of transfusion-transmitted diseases (TTDs) has not reduced the number of transfused units of blood, which has remained steady at over 14 million units of blood components per year since 1986. Responsible utilization of this limited commodity is an additional factor mandating judicious transfusion therapy.

In this chapter, we will discuss the types of blood products available, and the characteristics of these products. Then we will outline a strategy to match appropriate products with the specific indications.

BLOOD PRODUCTS AVAILABLE

The majority of blood is collected with anticoagulant and is rapidly separated into the following components: packed red blood cells (PRBCs), platelets, plasma, cryoprecipitate, leukocytes, and more concentrated clotting factors (Table 8-1). The separation of blood into components and improvements in anticoagulant/preservation solutions has significantly increased storage life and the efficiency of utilization of this important resource. The anticoagulants currently in use depend on calcium chelation by citrate.

PRBCs are the most frequently administered blood component, representing approximately 50 percent of the 14.8 million units of blood products administered each year. This consists primarily of RBCs (hematocrit 60 to 80 percent), with 10 percent of the plasma, 30 percent of the platelets, and 10 percent of the leukocytes present in the initial volume of whole blood. As a result of the isolation process, PRBCs contain insignificant amounts of clotting factors and platelets, and those that remain are nonfunctional.

Fresh frozen plasma (FFP), as the name indicates, is stored in a frozen state. FFP typically has a volume of 200 to 250 mL and contains levels of the coagulation factors found in fresh whole blood except for factors V and VIII. It is important to avoid delays in administration of FFP once thawed; delays beyond 2 hours postthawing result in progressive decreases in the levels of other coagulation factors. To correct coagulation abnormalities following injury, 10 to 15 mL/kg of FFP should be administered initially. This will restore clotting factors to within 25 percent of normal in most situations, and repeat coagulation parameters should be obtained prior to additional administration.

Platelet concentrates are stored at room temperature in gas-permeable plastic bags with gentle agitation for up to 5 days. The administration of platelet concentrate will raise the circulating platelet count for 6 to 7 days in the absence of consumptive coagulopathy or platelet-specific antibodies in the recipient. An "adult dose" of platelets is considered to be 3×10^{11}, because this number will provide a rise in platelet count of 30,000 to 60,000/μL. For this reason, random platelet concentrates obtained by centrifugations are frequently "pooled" in quantities of 6 to 8 units.

In addition to the more commonly used blood components, others such as recombinant factors, cryoprecipitate, and granulocyte concentrates, as well as derivatives obtained by further manufacture, are available. Recombinant factor VIII is available and is the preferred method of treatment for patients with hemophilia A, because the content of the factor is known, the volume of

84

Table 8-1 Summary Chart of Blood Components

Component	Major indications	Action	Special precautions	Rate of infusion
Whole blood	Symptomatic anemia with large volume deficit	Restoration of oxygen carrying capacity, restoration of blood volume	Must be ABO identical; Labile coagulation factors deteriorate within 24 hours after collection	For massive loss, as fast as patient can tolerate
Red blood cells (RBCs)	Symptomatic anemia	Restoration of oxygen-carrying capacity	Must be ABO compatible	As patient can tolerate but less than 4 hours
Red blood cells (RBCs), leukocytes removed	Symptomatic anemia, febrile reactions from leukocyte antibodies	Restoration of oxygen-carrying capacity	Must be ABO compatible	As patient can tolerate but less than 4 hours
Fresh frozen plasma (FFP)	Deficit of labile and stable plasma coagulation factors and thrombocytopenia	Source of labile and stable plasma factors	Should be ABO compatible	Less than 4 hours
Cryoprecipitated antihemophilic factor (AHF)	Hemophilia A, von Willebrand's disease, hypofibrinogenemia, factor XIII deficiency	Provides factor VIII, fibrinogen, von Willebrand factor, factor XIII	Frequent repeat doses may be necessary	Less than 4 hours
Platelets (pheresis)	Bleeding from thrombocytopenia or platelet-function abnormality	Improves hemostasis	Should not use some microaggregate filters (check manufacturer's instructions)	Less than 4 hours
Granulocytes (pheresis)	Neutropenia with infection	Provides granulocytes	Must be ABO compatible, do not use depth-type microaggregate filters	One unit over 2–4 hour period; observe closely for reactions

administration is less, and the risk of TTD is eliminated. Factor VIII activity disappears rapidly, with a half-life of 12 hours, and measurement of factor VIII levels is important following major injury in patients with hemophilia to maintain factor VIII levels at 30 to 50 percent of normal values.

Prothrombin complex concentrate contains prothrombin and factors VII, IX, and X. It is used in the care of patients with known deficiencies of these factors. Specific factor IX is now available and provides an alternative to the administration of prothrombin complex for those with this deficiency.

BLOOD TYPES AND CROSSMATCHING

Of the many blood group systems currently recognized, the ABO and the Rh systems are of primary importance when discussing blood types for emergent transfusions.

The safest type of blood to administer has gone through the usual routine of full compatibility testing. Full compatibility testing includes selection of ABO and Rh type, as well as screening for the presence of other antibodies (including Lewis, Kell, Kidd, MNS, and Duffy), and finally crossmatching of recipient and donor specimens. Blood that has been through full compatibility testing has the lowest risk of causing a major hemolytic reaction. It takes over 30 minutes to obtain full compatibility-tested blood in most situations, and it may not be possible to delay transfusion while waiting for this degree of testing in cases of major hemorrhage.

Type O PRBCs are used when it is necessary to emergently transfuse recipients of unknown blood type. It is recommended that the number of type O units transfused be limited to a maximum of 4, or if this is not possible, that transfusion with type O blood be continued until the patient is stable.

Type-specific blood is ABO and Rh compatible and can be made available for administration in less than 15 minutes in circumstances in which the transfusion services are involved and supportive. Experience with type-specific blood has shown it to be as safe as type O blood for emergency resuscitation in both military and civilian practice.

LOGISTIC CONSIDERATIONS

The establishment of protocols for blood request and administration, including specimen identification, processing of blood requests, and transportation, can reduce confusion and limit delays in blood administration. Physicians attending to the injured patient should be familiar with the protocols for emergency transfusion, particularly the mechanisms for obtaining type O and/or type-specific blood.

MATCHING BLOOD PRODUCTS AND SPECIFIC INDICATIONS

Restoration of Intravascular Volume

When considering the administration of blood to restore intravascular volume, an initial assessment of the injured patient's hemodynamic stability is made to determine the need for transfusion, as outlined in the algorithm presented in Fig. 8-1. For patients who have sustained injury and blood loss, but have a stable and normal blood pressure and heart rate, the administration of modest amounts of balanced salt solution (1 to 2 L) and monitoring may be all that is required. Patients with blood loss between 15 and 30 percent of their blood volume (class II shock) may initially respond to administration of

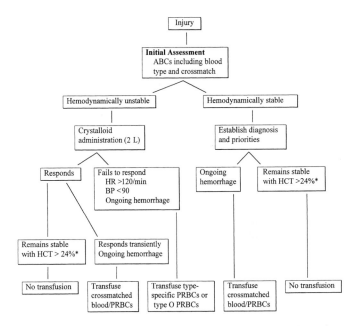

FIG. 8-1. Algorithm for transfusion to restore intravascular volume following injury. (*24 percent reflects usual practice. In less stable patients and those with preexisting cardiovascular or pulmonary disease, a higher hematocrit may be desirable.)

balanced salt solution and require no blood transfusion if the source of hemorrhage is controlled.

Trauma patients frequently present in a hypotensive and tachycardic state, with clear evidence of hypoperfusion (classes III and IV shock). When cardiogenic and thoracic causes of severe shock (tension pneumothorax and pericardial tamponade) are eliminated, transfusion is generally indicated for restoration of intravascular volume and oxygen-carrying capacity during the initial resuscitation. Under such circumstances, the administration of up to 4 units of PRBCs, either type O or type-specific, may be life-sustaining while definitive control of hemorrhage is pursued.

Oxygen-Carrying Capacity

Traditional teaching has been to maintain a hemoglobin of >10 g/dL or a hematocrit of >30 percent as optimal, but these guidelines are under considerable scrutiny. In a previously healthy individual, if intravascular volume is maintained with balanced salt solutions, hemoglobin levels of 7 g/dL and hematocrits as low as 20 to 21 percent may be well tolerated in the acute postoperative phase of care. In such situations, transfusion to maintain oxygen delivery should be guided by the patient's signs and symptoms, including heart rate, respiratory rate, and activity tolerance. The transfusion trigger is much less clear when the situation is complicated by extremes of age, preexisting medical illness (e.g., atherosclerotic heart disease), multiple injuries, or the subsequent development of complications such as sepsis or the systemic inflammatory response syndrome (SIRS). Under such conditions, the administration of blood products should be guided by indicators such as oxygen delivery.

Correction of Documented Coagulation Abnormalities

Thrombocytopenia is the most common disorder resulting from massive transfusion. The platelet count should be monitored in trauma patients requiring large volumes of blood transfusion, but the function of the platelets under such circumstances is unpredictable. Thus while circulating platelet counts of $20,000/mm^3$ and less may be adequate in nonbleeding patients, platelet transfusion is indicated in the early postoperative period following trauma when the platelet count is below $100,000/mm^3$ and there is evidence of ongoing microvascular bleeding.

When massive blood loss occurs and is ongoing, it is possible to perform coagulation studies and platelet counts concurrently with requests for the preparation of FFP and/or platelets. The preparation time for these components (30 to 45 minutes) is roughly equivalent to the time it takes for the laboratory results to be obtained. If abnormalities are detected, they may be rapidly treated without additional preparation time. If the laboratory results are not available by the time the components are and the microvascular bleeding is continuing, it may be best to give the first dose empirically. This allows a specific approach to therapy with a minimal delay and a minimal exposure of the patient to the risks of blood transfusion.

When a history of a specific deficit is known, monitoring of the factor levels involved (e.g., factor VIII, von Willebrand factor, or components of the prothrombin complex) and evidence of bleeding should be used to guide treatment. Replacement should be administered with the goal of maintaining circulating factor levels at 50 to 100 percent of normal when there is evidence of ongoing blood loss, and at roughly 50 percent of normal when bleeding is controlled.

COMPLICATIONS

Transfusion-Transmitted Diseases

TTDs are the most common cause of late death from transfusion (Table 8-2). Increased awareness of TTDs, particularly HIV infection, has contributed substantially to the reconsideration of indications for blood transfusion. The most common infectious complication at present is hepatitis B. Prior to testing for hepatitis C, non-A non-B hepatitis was the most frequent infectious complication.

Transfusion Reactions

Transfusion reactions can be thought of in two broad categories: hemolytic (involving the hemolysis of RBCs) and nonhemolytic. Major hemolytic transfusion reactions result from the interaction of antibodies in the plasma of the recipient with antigens in the red cells of the donor. The majority of hemolytic reactions are the result of clerical error in which mistakes are made in the identification of blood samples or in the administration of appropriately cross-matched blood to the wrong patient. The urgent nature of trauma may contribute to human error, as suggested by the fact that more than half of the

Table 8-2 Relative Incidence of Transfusion-Transmitted Disease (TTD)

Hepatitis C	1:103,000	HCV transmission risk per screened unit
		50% of posttransfusion HCV becomes chronic
HTLV	1:641,000	HTLV-I/II transmission risk per screened unit
		HTLV-I infection: 4% lifetime risk of associated disease (adult T-cell leukemia; tropical spastic paraparesis)
Hepatitis B	1:200,000	HBV transmission risk per screened unit
		50% of posttransfusion HBV is symptomatic
		4% of posttransfusion HBV requires hospitalization
HIV	1:450,000	HIV transmission risk per screened unit
Other	<1:1,000,000	Transmission rate for *Yersinia*, malaria, *Babesia*, Chagas
Overall	3:10,000	Risk that blood recipient will contract a serious or fatal TTD

Source: Reed RL et al: Prophylactic platelet administration during massive transfusion. *Ann Surg* 203:40, 1986.

major reactions in trauma patients occur in the operating room and the emergency department. Meticulous attention must be directed to the proper labeling of blood specimens sent to the blood bank and to checking the identification of the blood and the recipient prior to its administration to the trauma patient.

Nonhemolytic reactions are more common than hemolytic reactions, with an incidence of 2 to 10 percent. They are related to reactions to leukocytes or plasma proteins and can be significantly reduced by the use of leukocyte-filtered blood products and premedication with antipyretics and antihistamines. The vast majority of nonhemolytic reactions are relatively mild, consisting of fever, hives, or mild bronchoconstriction; however, rare severe reactions, including glottic edema and severe bronchoconstriction or anaphylaxis with circulatory collapse, can be life-threatening.

Recognizing and addressing significant transfusion reactions is fundamental to the safe administration of blood and blood products.

Metabolic Complications

The rapid administration (1 unit every 5 minutes) of large quantities (>12 units) of blood has been a source of theoretical concern for some time. During prolonged storage of anticoagulated blood, levels of potassium, lactate, ammonia, and free hemoglobin increase and pH decreases.

In patients with significant hypothermia, uncontrolled acidosis, and shock, as well as in those with major crush and/or soft tissue injuries and those with renal insufficiency, significant hyperkalemia can occur. In these situations, electrocardiographic monitoring and frequent measurement of potassium levels should be performed. If there is evidence of significant hyperkalemia (K >5.5 mEq/L) and there are indications for transfusion of red cells to maintain volume of oxygen-carrying capacity, the use of blood within its first week of storage or washed red cells that have little if any potassium should be considered.

In the "shocky" hypothermic patient and patients with hepatic injury or insufficiency, accumulation of citrate in the plasma can lead to reduced calcium availability, which can result in cardiac effects, including ventricular fibrillation and depression in cardiac contractility. Citrate toxicity can be monitored by measuring ionized calcium levels during administration of large quantities of blood, with supplemental calcium given to maintain ionized calcium levels above 3.8 mg/dL.

Macroaggregates and Hypothermia

The administration of blood products should be accomplished with large-bore intravenous tubing containing a 140- to 170-μm inline filter to remove macroaggregate particles and prevent pulmonary microembolization. The rapid administration of cold crystalloid solutions and PRBCs can cause hypothermia and the additional complication of cardiac arrhythmias, as well as coagulopathy. When large volumes of blood and crystalloid solutions are required in a resuscitation, the use of countercurrent fluid-warming devices and careful monitoring of the patient's environment and temperature can be helpful in limiting the development of hypothermia.

SUMMARY

Heightened concern for the risks of transfusion, including TTDs, along with sensitivity to the decreased availability of blood products, have focused acute attention on the clinical decisions involving transfusion of blood products. In general, but particularly in the care of the injured, for whom loss of blood is a principal component of the pathophysiology, it is important not to allow the momentum of fear of TTDs to obfuscate the goals of restoring and maintaining perfusion. The consideration of specific indications for transfusion and the judicious use of appropriate components allow a reasonable balance of risk and benefit in the application of blood transfusion in the injured patient. Coordination with hospital transfusion services makes it possible to have effective mechanisms in place to provide for rapid availability and safety of blood for transfusion.

ADDITIONAL READING

Simon TL, Alverson DC, AuBuchon J, et al. Practice parameters for the use of red blood cell transfusions. *Arch Pathol Lab Med* 122:130, 1998.
Wudel JH, Morris JA Jr, Yates K, et al: Massive transfusion: Outcome in blunt trauma patients. *J Trauma* 31:1, 1991.

9 | Emergency Department Thoracotomy

Advances in prehospital care of the critically injured have increased the number of patients arriving at the hospital in extremis. Salvage of these individuals often demands immediate control of hemorrhage as an integral component of their initial resuscitation. The optimal use of emergency department (ED) thoracotomy as a component of this initial resuscitation requires a thorough understanding of the physiologic objectives, technical maneuvers, systemic consequences, and selective indications for this procedure.

HISTORIC PERSPECTIVE

Based on reports of successful open cardiac massage and management of penetrating cardiac wounds in the late 1800s, emergent thoracotomy came into routine use for the treatment of heart wounds and anesthesia-induced cardiac arrest in the early 1900s. Over the ensuing 50 years, indications for emergent thoracotomy changed as resuscitative techniques (e.g., closed chest compression, external defibrillation) improved and patient outcomes were critically analyzed. By the late 1960s, refinements in cardiothoracic surgical techniques had reestablished the role of immediate thoracotomy for salvaging patients with life-threatening chest wounds. The indications for this procedure were further expanded to temporary thoracic aortic occlusion in patients with exsanguinating abdominal trauma. However, critical analysis of patient outcomes following postinjury thoracotomy in the ED has tempered the unbridled enthusiasm for this technique, and a more selective approach has evolved.

DEFINITION OF EMERGENCY DEPARTMENT THORACOTOMY

ED thoracotomy refers to that performed in the ED for patients in extremis. The value of ED thoracotomy for acute resuscitation is unclear from the literature, because of the variety of indices used to characterize the patient's physiologic status. We define "no signs of life" as no detectable blood pressure, pupillary activity, respiratory effort, or cardiac electrical activity (i.e., clinical death). "No vital signs" refers to the absence of palpable blood pressure, but with pupillary reactivity or respiratory effort.

PHYSIOLOGIC RATIONALE FOR EMERGENCY DEPARTMENT THORACOTOMY

The primary objectives of ED thoracotomy are to (1) release pericardial tamponade, (2) control intrathoracic bleeding, (3) control air embolism or bronchopleural fistula, (4) permit open cardiac massage, and (5) allow for temporary occlusion of the descending thoracic aorta.

Pericardial Tamponade

Prompt pericardial decompression and cardiac repair are essential to improving survival following cardiac wounds. Rising intrapericardial pressure produces abnormalities in hemodynamic and cardiac perfusion that can be divided into three phases. Initially, increased pericardial pressure restricts ventricular diastolic filling and reduces subendocardial blood flow. Cardiac

91

output is maintained by compensatory tachycardia and increased systemic vascular resistance. In the intermediate phase, rising pericardial pressure further compromises diastolic filling, stroke volume, and coronary perfusion, resulting in diminished cardiac output. Although blood pressure may be maintained, clinical signs of systemic shock (e.g., anxiety, diaphoresis, pallor) soon become evident. During the final phase of tamponade, compensatory mechanisms fall precipitously as intrapericardial pressure approaches ventricular filling pressure. Cardiac arrest ensues as profound coronary hypoperfusion occurs. Aggressive airway management, volume loading, and pericardiocentesis are key components in the management of the first two phases of cardiac tamponade. The patient presenting with profound hypotension in the third phase, however, should undergo ED thoracotomy as part of his or her initial management.

Intrathoracic Hemorrhage

Bleeding from thoracic great vessel lacerations is often fatal because of the lack of containment by adjacent tissue tamponade or vessel spasm. Either hemithorax can rapidly accommodate more than half of a patient's total blood volume before the physical signs of hemorrhage become obvious. Patients arriving with such exsanguinating wounds generally require ED thoracotomy if they are to be salvaged.

Bronchovenous Air Embolism

Major air embolism can be a subtle clinical entity following thoracic trauma, and is no doubt more common than recognized. The typical scenario for its occurrence involves a patient sustaining a penetrating chest wound who develops precipitous shock after endotracheal intubation and positive-pressure ventilation. The shock results from global myocardial ischemia produced by coronary arterial air emboli arising from traumatic alveolovenous communications. The process is enhanced by a relatively low intrinsic pulmonary venous pressure and by a positive bronchoalveolar pressure resulting from assisted ventilation; this combination increases the gradient for air transfer across bronchovenous channels. A similar process may also occur in patients with blunt lacerations of the lung parenchyma. Immediate thoracotomy with pulmonary hilar cross-clamping is essential to prevent further pulmonary venous air embolism. The left ventricle is vented of air with the patient in Trendelenburg position. In addition, vigorous cardiac massage may assist movement of air out of the coronary arteries, and venting of air from the root of the aorta prevents further egress into the coronary arteries.

Open Cardiac Massage

External chest compression provides approximately 25 percent of baseline cardiac output and 10 to 20 percent of cerebral and coronary perfusion. This vital organ perfusion results in reasonable salvage after 15 minutes, but only limited survival after 30 minutes in euthermic patients. Furthermore, in models of inadequate intravascular volume (hypovolemia) or restricted ventricular filling (pericardial tamponade), external chest compression failed to augment arterial pressure or provide adequate systemic perfusion. In addition, associated low diastolic pressure resulted in inadequate coronary perfusion. Open cardiac massage is superior to closed compression in maintaining cardiac output and providing cerebral as well as coronary perfusion. In normovolemic models of cardiac arrest, open massage generates aortic pressures of approximately 60 percent of control values, and coronary and cerebral perfusion may be maintained at an adequate level for up to 30 minutes. This encourages the timely and aggressive use of thoracotomy in the resuscitative protocol for patients sustaining traumatic cardiopulmonary arrest.

Thoracic Aortic Cross-Clamping

In theory, the rationale for temporary thoracic aortic occlusion in the patient with massive hemorrhage is to redistribute a limited blood volume to the myocardium and brain, as well as to reduce subdiaphragmatic blood loss. Indeed, aortic occlusion enhances both coronary and cerebral perfusion by maintaining aortic diastolic pressure and augmenting the carotid systolic blood pressure. In hypovolemic shock, increased diastolic pressure resulting from aortic occlusion increases the left ventricular stroke-work index and myocardial contractility. These experimental observations imply that temporary aortic occlusion may be valuable in the patient with continued shock following the repair of cardiac or other exsanguinating wounds. On the other hand, thoracic aortic cross-clamping may be deleterious in the normovolemic patient because of increased myocardial oxygen demands resulting from the increased systemic vascular resistance. Furthermore, blood flow to the abdominal viscera, spinal cord, and kidneys is reduced to 10 percent of normal, and femoral systolic blood pressure reduced to 10 mm Hg. Consequently, profound anaerobic metabolism and secondary lactic academia are induced. The resultant hypoxia of distal organs, white blood cells, and endothelium induces the elaboration, expression, and activation of inflammatory cell adhesion mechanisms and mediators that have been linked to organ dysfunction and multiple organ failure. Moreover, although thoracic aortic occlusion has been tolerated for as long as 75 minutes without spinal sequelae, clinical experience with elective thoracic aortic procedures indicates that 30 minutes is generally the threshold for reversible normothermic ischemia. In sum, although the routine use of thoracic aortic occlusion in patients with massive intra-abdominal hemorrhage makes intuitive physiologic sense, its association with a significant improvement in the overall survival of these patients has yet to be clearly established.

RISKS OF EMERGENCY DEPARTMENT THORACOTOMY TO THE TRAUMA TEAM

The use of ED thoracotomy in the resuscitation of acutely injured patients by necessity involves the rapid use of sharp surgical instruments and exposure to patients' blood. Even during elective procedures in the OR, the contact rate of patients' blood with the surgeon's skin is as high as 50 percent. The overall seroprevalence rate of human immunodeficiency virus (HIV) among patients admitted to the ED for trauma has been shown to range from 2 to 9 percent, and may be as high as 20 percent among the subgroup of patients most likely to require ED thoracotomy (i.e., urban patients with penetrating chest trauma). Thus the likelihood of a health care worker sustaining a significant HIV-seropositive blood exposure is a matter of concern. Fortunately, occupation-related HIV seroconversions have so far remained infrequent. Nevertheless, the risk of contagion from exposure to HIV and other bloodborne pathogens can be minimized by the use of appropriate precautions and the selective use of ED thoracotomy.

TECHNICAL DETAILS OF EMERGENCY DEPARTMENT THORACOTOMY

The technical skills needed for optimal outcome following ED thoracotomy include the ability to perform rapid thoracotomy, pericardiotomy, cardiorrhaphy, and thoracic aortic cross-clamping, as well as familiarity with vascular repair techniques and exposure of the pulmonary hilum for cross-clamping. The equipment needed for accomplishing these objectives is limited (Table 9-1).

Thoracic Incision

A left anterolateral thoracotomy incision is preferred for resuscitation of the acutely injured patient in extremis. Advantages of this incision in the trauma patient include (1) rapid access with simple instruments, (2) applicability to the patient in the supine position, and (3) ready extension into the contralateral hemithorax for the exposure of both pleural spaces as well as mediastinal structures. Moreover, the key resuscitative maneuvers of pericardiotomy, open cardiac massage, and thoracic aortic occlusion are best achieved through this approach. The initial use of a right thoracotomy is reserved for hypotensive patients with penetrating injuries to the right chest, for direct access to massive blood loss or air embolism resulting from a pulmonary wound. If an associated cardiac wound is encountered in such a case, trans-stemal extension into the left chest should be done promptly.

An incision is made at the level of the fourth or fifth intercostal space. In women, the breast should be retracted superiorly to gain access to this interspace, corresponding to the inferior border of the pectoralis major muscle. The skin, subcutaneous fat, and chest wall musculature are incised with a knife to expose the proper intercostal space. Intercostal muscles and the parietal pleura are then divided in one layer with heavier scissors, coursing along the superior margin of the rib to avoid the intercostal neurovascular bundle. Chest wall bleeding is minimal in these patients and should not be a concern at this point. Once the incision is completed, a standard rib retractor is inserted, with the handle directed inferiorly toward the axilla. Resistance encountered in opening the retractor can usually be alleviated by division of intercostal muscles, but may require transection of the costal cartilages above and below the opened interspace. Wide exposure of both pleural

Table 9-1 Emergency Department Thoracotomy Tray

Scalpel with no. 10 blade	DeBakey's aortic clamp
Mayo's scissors (curved)	Long needle holder (Hegar's) (2)
Finochietto's chest retractor	Tonsil clamps (4)
Lebsche's knife and mallet	Teflon pledgets—different sizes (5)
Laparotomy pads (8)	2-0 silk strands (multiple)
Metzenbaum scissors	3-0 cardiovascular ethibond suture (multiple)
Satinsky's vascular clamps (large and small) (2 each)	Internal defibrillator paddles
DeBakey's vascular forceps (long) (2)	Tooth forceps (2)

cavities may be achieved by transecting the sternum and performing a concomitant right anterolateral thoracotomy—a "clamshell" or "butterfly" incision. This extension can be accomplished quickly with a Lebsche knife. In this instance, the internal mammary vessels must be ligated. When exposure of penetrating wounds in the aortic arch is needed, the superior sternum is split in the midline.

Pericardiotomy and Hemorrhage Control

A knife or scissors is often required to initiate the pericardiotomy incision in the presence of tense cardiac tamponade. Blood clots should be completely evacuated and cardiac bleeding sites should be controlled with digital pressure (ventricle) or partially occluding vascular clamps (atrium or great vessels). In the beating heart, efforts at cardiorrhaphy should be delayed until initial resuscitative measures have been completed. In the nonbeating heart, suturing is done prior to defibrillation. Although temporary control of bleeding can often be achieved with a skin stapling device, cardiac wounds are best repaired with 3-0 nonabsorbable horizontal mattress sutures. Buttressing with Teflon pledgets is done routinely in the right ventricle, but is required only selectively in the left. Low-pressure venous and atrial lacerations can be repaired with simple running sutures. Posterior cardiac wounds may be particularly treacherous when they necessitate elevation of the heart for exposure. Closure of these wounds is best accomplished in the operating room with optimal lighting and equipment. For a massive wound of the ventricle, or for inaccessible posterior wounds, temporary inflow occlusion of the superior and inferior vena cavae may be employed to facilitate repair. If coronary or systemic air embolism is present, further embolism is prevented by placing a vascular clamp across the pulmonary hilum. Vigorous cardiac massage helps move air through the coronary arteries. Additionally, air is evacuated by needle aspiration of the elevated left ventricular apex and the aortic root.

Cardiac Massage and Thoracic Aortic Occlusion

In the event of cardiac arrest, bimanual internal massage of the heart should be instituted promptly. We prefer to do this with a hinged clapping motion of the hands, with the wrists apposed and ventricular compression proceeding from the apex to the base of the heart. The one-handed massage technique poses the risk of myocardial perforation with the thumb. If internal defibrillation does not restore vigorous cardiac activity, the descending thoracic aorta should be occluded to maximize coronary perfusion. We prefer to cross-clamp the thoracic aorta inferior to the left pulmonary hilum. Exposure of this area is best provided by elevating the left lung anteriorly and superiorly. Dissection of the thoracic aorta is optimally performed under direct vision by incising the mediastinal pleura and bluntly separating the aorta from the esophagus anteriorly and from the prevertebral fascia posteriorly. The aorta should not be completely encircled, but rather occluded with a large Satinsky's or DeBakey's vascular clamp.

Technical Complications

Technical complications of ED thoracotomy involve virtually every intrathoracic structure. Previous thoracotomy virtually assures technical problems from the presence of dense pleural adhesions, and is therefore a relative contraindication to ED thoracotomy. Additional postoperative morbidity among ultimate survivors of ED thoracotomy includes recurrent chest bleeding, infection of the pericardium, pleural spaces, and chest wall, and postpericardiotomy syndrome.

CLINICAL RESULTS OF EMERGENCY DEPARTMENT THORACOTOMY

The results of ED thoracotomy vary considerably, owing to the heterogeneity of patient populations reported. As discussed above, critical determinants of survival include the mechanism of injury and the patient's condition at the time of thoracotomy. We have attempted to elucidate the impact of these factors in ascertaining the yield of ED thoracotomy by collating data from a number of recent clinical series based on patient status at the time of presentation to the ED (Table 9-2). The data demonstrate that ED thoracotomy permits the salvage of 30 to 57 percent of adult patients presenting with signs of life following isolated cardiac injury. In contrast, only 1 to 2 percent of patients requiring ED thoracotomy following blunt injuries are salvaged, regardless of their clinical status on presentation. Following penetrating noncardiac injuries, 18 percent of patients requiring ED thoracotomy are salvaged if they present in a hypotensive state with detectable vital signs, whereas 6 percent of those who show only signs of life on presentation and 5 percent of those without signs of life are salvaged.

A growing body of data exists on the use of ED thoracotomy in children. The expectation that children have a more favorable outcome than adults after resuscitative thoracotomy in the ED has not been borne out in these studies. In our 11-year experience at the Denver Health Medical Center, 83 patients less than 18 years old underwent ED thoracotomy. Survival by injury mechanism was 9 percent (1 of 11) following stab wound, 4 percent (1 of 25) following gunshot wound, and 2 percent (1 of 47) following blunt trauma. Among 69 patients presenting to the ED without vital signs, only 1 patient (1 percent) survived (with a stab wound). This contrasted to a salvage of 2 (14 percent) among 14 patients with vital signs. Thus as in adults, outcome was largely determined by injury mechanism and physiologic status on presentation to the ED (Table 9-2).

SELECTIVE APPLICATION OF EMERGENCY DEPARTMENT THORACOTOMY

The value of ED thoracotomy in resuscitation of the viable patient in profound shock but not yet dead is unquestionable. Its indiscriminate use, how-

Table 9-2 Survival Following Emergency Department Thoracotomy

Injury Pattern	Shock	No vital signs	No signs of life	Total
Adult				
Cardiac	28/49 (57%)	36/120 (30%)	18/135 (13%)	95/412 (23%)
Penetrating	158/870 (18%)	81/1292 (6%)	38/775 (5%)	290/3237 (9%)
Blunt	8/373 (2%)	6/718 (0.8%)	3/428 (0.7%)	17/1558 (1%)
Pediatric				
Penetrating	2/8 (25%)	4/20 (20%)	0/28 (0%)	6/56 (11%)
Blunt	1/17 (6%)	0/35 (0%)	0/30 (0%)	1/82 (1%)

ever, renders it a low-yield high-cost procedure. Although originally described for penetrating thoracic wounds, ED thoracotomy has become a nearly obligatory procedure before declaring any trauma patient unsalvageable in some centers. This practice has been effectively challenged by a critical analysis of patient outcome in multiple trauma centers. Based on our collective experience and that reflected in the current literature, we have formulated a decision algorithm for resuscitation of the moribund trauma patient (Fig. 9-1). At the scene, patients in extremis and without electrical cardiac activity are declared dead, unless they have sustained a penetrating thoracic wound. Patients in extremis but with electrical cardiac activity are intubated, supported with CPR, and rapidly transported to the ED. In the ED, patients arriving in extremis following blunt injury undergo thoracotomy only if they show electrical cardiac activity. Patients who exhibit electrical cardiac activity or who have sustained thoracic wounds undergo resuscitative thoracotomy.

Upon opening of the chest, patients without cardiac activity who do not have blood in the pericardium are declared dead. All other patients are treated according to the injury mechanism. Pericardial tamponade is decompressed and bleeding from cardiac wounds is controlled. Suspected air embolism is treated by the application of a pulmonary hilar cross-clamp, vigorous cardiac massage, and aortic root and left ventricular aspiration of air. Intrathoracic hemorrhage is controlled. Cardiopulmonary collapse from suspected intra-abdominal hemorrhage is temporized by occlusion of the descending thoracic aorta. Those patients with intra-abdominal hemorrhage who respond to occlusion of the thoracic aorta with a blood pressure above 70 mm Hg, as well as all other surviving patients, are rapidly transported to the OR for definitive treatment of their injuries.

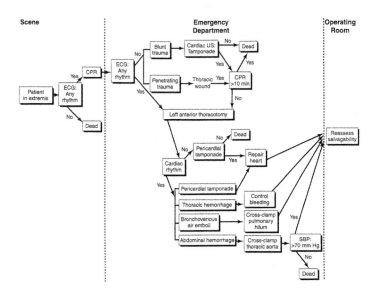

FIG. 9-1.   Decision algorithm for the selective use of resuscitative thoracotomy in the emergency department.

FUTURE CONSIDERATIONS

Defining Nonsalvageability

As we face increasing scrutiny over appropriation of resources, it is critical to identify the patient who faces mortality or permanent neurologic morbidity. However, we do not want to abandon resuscitative efforts prematurely in the potentially salvageable patient. Our algorithm moves us closer to that endpoint, but we must continue to evaluate outcomes, searching for more definitive predictors of neurologic outcome.

ADDITIONAL READING

Boczar ME et al: A technique revisited: Hemodynamic comparison of closed- and open-chest cardiac massage during human cardiopulmonary resuscitation. *Crit Care Med* 23:498, 1995.

Branney SW et al: Critical analysis of two decades of experience with postinjury emergency department thoracotomy in a regional trauma center. *J Trauma* 45:87, 1998.

Campbell NC et al: Review of 1198 cases of penetrating cardiac trauma. *Br J Surg* 84:1737, 1997.

Dunn EL, Moore EE, Moore JB: Hemodynamic effects of aortic occlusion during hemorrhagic shock. *Ann Emerg Med* 11:238, 1982.

Wall MJ Jr et al: Acute management of complex cardiac injuries. *J Trauma* 42:905, 1997.

10 | Diagnostic Imaging in the Trauma Patient

Diagnostic imaging plays a major role in the initial work-up of trauma patients and in establishing management and treatment priorities. Radiography serves as a major diagnostic study performed in the acute trauma setting, but other modalities including sonography, spiral (fast) computed tomography (CT), diagnostic and interventional angiography, and magnetic resonance imaging (MRI) have become vital for the definitive diagnosis or exclusion of many traumatic injuries. Advances in diagnostic imaging technology have increased the accuracy and speed of identification of traumatic injuries, while improvements in interventional angiographic techniques have offered a definitive nonsurgical alternative for treatment of some vascular injuries.

Selection of diagnostic imaging studies depends on several factors that may be unique to a given clinical setting including:

- Proximity and availability of the imaging technology to the patient resuscitation area
- Quality and speed of the imaging equipment available
- Experience and availability of radiology technologists to perform emergent imaging
- Availability of expert interpretation of imaging studies
- Ability to communicate that interpretation in a timely fashion
- Capacity to accurately monitor vital signs, maintain appropriate physiologic support, and respond therapeutically to sudden clinical deterioration both during transport to an imaging facility and during the diagnostic study.

Physiologic stability of the patient is the single most important factor in determining if the opportunity exists to perform diagnostic studies and to what extent. A patient admitted in profound shock who fails to respond to initial resuscitation may not be safely imaged at all or may only undergo a quick abdominal bedside sonogram for detection of gross hemoperitoneum. A patient who is admitted in hemodynamic shock, but responds well to aggressive and ongoing resuscitation, may safely undergo rapid portable radiographic screening, but would be at high risk for transport to a distant site for CT or MRI scanning. A trauma patient who is initially hemodynamically stable and maintains stability in the resuscitation area may be an appropriate candidate for off-site imaging studies as CT or MRI, depending on the clinical concern. *Close cooperation and open communication between the trauma team physicians, nurses, imaging technologists, and radiologists is always necessary to optimize any imaging assessment.* The radiologist can and should be a valuable ally in selecting the type and order of diagnostic procedures to most efficiently answer particular clinical questions.

IMAGING THORACIC TRAUMA

The AP (anteroposterior) chest radiograph is accurate for the diagnosis of pneumothorax, pneumomediastinum, pulmonary contusion, moderate to large pleural effusion, simple and tension pneumothorax, pneumopericardium, thoracic skeletal injury, and aspiration. Technical limitations include lack of patient cooperation, portable equipment with limited exposure, motion, and lack of study contrast. Significant diagnostic limitations include missing diagnoses such as cardiac injury, mediastinal injury, lung laceration, small pneumothorax, subtle thoracic spine injury, about 50 percent of left diaphragm injuries, and most right diaphragm injuries.

Diagnostic Caveats

Pleural Effusion (Hemothorax)

Layers posteriorly and produces a uniform increase in density over the hemithorax. Accumulations of pleural fluid displace the lung away from the chest wall at the lung apex and laterally, producing a radiodense fluid band.

Pneumothorax

Supine patient: Accumulates in the *anterior inferior* aspect of the chest producing basal hyperlucency, a deepened lateral costophrenic sulcus, or a "double-diaphragm" appearance. May see visceral pleura at base of lung if subpulmonic in location. Erect patient: Pneumothorax will collect in the superior aspect of the hemithorax and outline the visceral pleura of the upper lobe. The shape and location of a pneumothorax can be altered due to pleural adhesions, atelectasis, and patient positioning.

Lung Contusion

Usually a nonlobar "geographic" homogeneous density typically in peripheral lung without air-bronchograms. Rib fractures often not present in young patients.

Lung Laceration

Elliptical lucent area typically within contusion, with 2- to 3-mm pseudo-capsule. Becomes more apparent as contusion fades over 3 to 5 days. Complications: Bronchopleural fistula, infection, bleeding, enlargement with compression of adjacent lung.

Extrapleural Hematoma

Indents the parietal pleura and lung with a convex margin toward the lung, has obtuse margins with chest wall, typically associated with multiple and displaced rib fractures. Consider intercostal, internal mammary, subclavian, or branch arterial injury as potential source.

Hemidiaphragm Rupture (Left)

Suspicious signs: Apparent elevation of diaphragm, ill-defined contour, contralateral mediastinal and cardiac shift, left pleural effusion. Diagnostic signs: Tapering of stomach gas shadow at point of tear ("collar sign"), nasogastric tube within stomach in left lower thorax. Mimics: Diaphragm eventration, left lower lobe atelectasis, phrenic nerve paresis or palsy, diaphragm contusion, subpulmonic fluid, chronic Bochdalek hernia, lung contusions, and lacerations in lower lobe.

Hemidiaphragm Rupture (Right)

Rarely diagnostic radiographically due to hepatic protection of diaphragm. Signs on plain film include elevation of the apparent hemidiaphragm, pleural effusion and mass effect, rarely gas-containing structures seen over the right lower lung.

Hemopericardium

In the acute setting, hemopericardium is rarely evident radiographically; chronic accumulation of fluid increases size of the cardiac shadow globally with loss of usual contours ("water-bottle heart"). May observe distension of superior vena cava. Pneumopericardium produces lucent arc around entire heart ending superiorly at reflection of pericardium at aortic root. With tension, a small heart shadow may be apparent compared with prior studies. Pneumopericardium may be concurrent with and difficult to distinguish from pneumomediastinum. Sources of pericardial air include dissection from pulmonary veins, trachea, esophagus, and penetrating injury. Typically occurs in setting of severe lung injury and high ventilatory support pressure.

Pneumomediastinum

Usually results from lung injury with interstitial dissection of air into hilum, mediastinum, and pleural space. Typically seen as lucent lines extending vertically close to mediastinum and into the neck. White parietal pleural line seen paralleling mediastinal border mainly on left side and descending below diaphragm. Straight lucent line under heart (continuous diaphragm sign) also may occur. Leads to very sharply defined aortic outline, cardiac apex, and pericardial fat pads. Consider tracheobronchial injury (see below) if severe, progressive pneumomediastinum.

Mediastinal Hemorrhage (MH) and Major Arterial Injury

The assessment of MH is based upon understanding and recognition of the normal mediastinal contours. An absolute measurement of the mediastinal width or the mediastinal-width to chest-width ratio *is not reliable* in determining the presence or absence of mediastinal blood (an indirect sign of major vascular injury). Only about 20 percent of patients with MH have a major thoracic arterial injury. Main radiologic signs suggesting MH include:

- Poor delineation of the aortic arch and descending aorta
- Rightward deviation of the nasogastric or endotracheal tube
- Wide left paraspinal stripe that ascends above the aortic arch
- A right paratracheal soft tissue density not due to normal anatomy

While there are other radiologic signs that have been described, these four in the authors' experience provide the best accuracy to predict MH. If the mediastinum has a normal contour, the chance of aortic injury is extremely low. In many cases an abnormal mediastinum on a supine radiograph will appear normal on the "true erect" view with the patient leaning forward 15 percent from vertical and this maneuver should be tried when possible. Given an abnormal or equivocal chest x-ray, further work-up is needed. Spiral CT has become the standard secondary screening test and is usually definitively negative or positive for direct vascular injury. The algorithm in Fig. 10-1 delineates our current approach.

Positive CT findings for traumatic aortic injury include:

- Pseudoaneurysm—most common (usually at aortic isthmus)
- Intimal flaps
- Intraluminal thrombus
- Variation in aortic diameter over a short distance

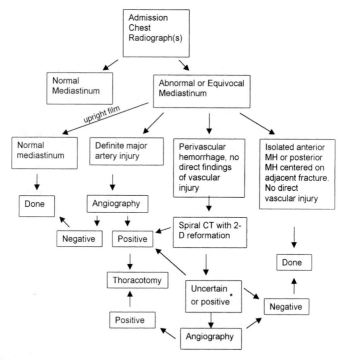

FIG. 10-1. Imaging approach to the patient with potential aortic injury. (*Decision to proceed directly to thoracotomy after a positive CT depends on the experience of the institution with CT, the level of diagnostic confidence in the CT findings, and the experience of the surgical team.)

- Abnormal aortic contour
- Extravasation of contrast from the aorta (rare)
- Periaortic hemorrhage (almost all cases)

Diagnostic difficulties for CT diagnosis of aortic injury include:

- Ductus diverticulum
- Aberrant aortic branching
- Atherosclerotic disease
- Aortic ulceration
- Chronic aortic pseudoaneurysm
- Atypical location of injury
- Subtle (small) injuries

When the CT is unequivocally positive for a typical-appearing aortic injury, some surgeons will operate on the basis of the CT. Others prefer confirmation by thoracic angiography. CT angiography with newer systems provides information in a format similar to angiography. It is vital with either modality to exclude a second vascular lesion that might alter the surgical approach. If the CT study shows perivascular hemorrhage around the aorta or its major branches, angiography is performed. In the vast majority of cases in the authors' experience the angiogram will be normal if there is no direct CT evidence of aortic injury. Transesophageal echocardiography (TEE) can serve as an alternative screening test for aortic injury, but is operator-dependent and can be compromised by air in the trachea blocking portions of the arch and false positive interpretations due to atherosclerosis. Optimal application may be in the intraoperative setting when the aorta cannot be definitely assessed prior to emergent surgical intervention.

Tracheal Injury

Consider in setting of persistent major air leak. Diagnostic radiologic signs include:

- Ectopic endotracheal tube (ETT) position
- Overdistended ETT balloon
- "Fallen lung" (collapsed in gravity-dependent location)
- Abrupt cut-off or tapering of mainstem bronchus air column.

CT may show mediastinal air immediately around tracheal walls (suggestive) or direct communication between airway and mediastinal air (diagnostic).

Esophageal Injury

Extremely rare in blunt trauma. Nonspecific findings are left pleural effusion, pneumomediastinum (limited), and abnormal mediastinal contour. Requires either endoscopy and/or esophagram to exclude.

Penetrating Thoracic Trauma

In a stable patient, obtain chest radiography to detect pneumothorax, pleural effusion, pneumomediastinum, foreign body localization, and potentially pneumoperitoneum. CT may be useful to determine path of injury *specifically regarding mediastinal involvement or transdiaphragmatic penetration.* If there is potential mediastinal involvement, work-up requires endoscopic assessment of airway and esophagus or esophagram and aortography to include the great vessels. Injury to the diaphragm may be suggested by CT findings, but typically requires thoracoscopy or open inspection for confirmation.

Potential Rupture of the Diaphragm—Blunt Trauma

Both helical CT and MRI have been successfully utilized to diagnose or exclude rupture of the hemidiaphragm if suspected radiographically. The algorithm in Fig. 10-2 is in current use in the author's institution (see also textbook Fig. 14-6).

IMAGING BLUNT ABDOMINAL/PELVIC TRAUMA

The ideal use of diagnostic imaging to evaluate the abdomen and pelvis of blunt trauma victims is controversial. Both diagnostic peritoneal lavage (DPL) and bedside sonography, particularly focused abdominal sonography for trauma (FAST), have been shown in many studies to be highly accurate for detection of intraperitoneal fluid. Both methodologies have well-known limitations. Limitations of DPL include:

- Insensitive to retroperitoneal injury
- Overly sensitive to minimal hemorrhage related to minor intraperitoneal injuries

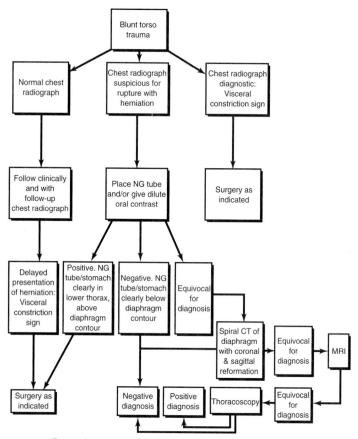

*Repeat after discontinuation of positive pressure ventilatory support.

FIG. 10-2. Assessment of potential diaphragm rupture following blunt torso trauma.

- Falsely positive from retroperitoneal hemorrhage that leaks into peritoneal cavity
- Limited ability to detect injuries that are contained within solid organs
- Propensity to be falsely negative for injuries to the hemidiaphragm
- Debate over what lavage RBC count constitutes a "positive" result
- Contraindicated in advanced pregnancy and patients with numerous prior abdominal surgeries
- Can be falsely negative or positive due to improper technique
- Introduction of air and fluid into the abdomen compromises post-DPL CT

Indications for CT after blunt abdominal trauma are listed in Table 10-1 (see textbook Table 14-1). Based on these considerations, the algorithm shown in Fig. 10-3 describes the recommended imaging assessment of blunt abdominopelvic trauma based on clinical presentation (see textbook Fig. 14-12).

TABLE 10-1 Indications for CT After Blunt Abdominal Trauma

Baseline Conditions
  1. Hemodynamically stable patients or those responsive to resuscitation
  2. Physiologic monitoring available and full physiologic support and resuscitation available in CT suite
  3. CT in close proximity to admissions area and recent technology available (spiral CT preferred)
  4. Radiologic expertise available
Previous abdominal surgery
Pelvic fractures
Gross hematuria or likely retroperitoneal injury (i.e., substantial fall from height, direct impact)
Mid- or late-term pregnancy
Coagulopathy (DPL)
Positive DPL
Positive or technically inadequate FAST (obesity, bowel gas, open wounds, etc)
Negative FAST unless 6+ h of observation and repeat FAST performed
Unreliable clinical examination
Multiple CT studies required of other body regions (head, spine, face, pelvis, etc)
Technically failed or equivocal DPL result
Abdominal pain/guarding and negative FAST or DPL
Lumbar and lower thoracic vertebral injuries

DPL, diagnostic peritoneal lavage; FAST, focused abdominal sonography for trauma.

Caveats of CT assessment in blunt abdominal trauma:

- Free intraperitoneal fluid without an obvious source must be regarded with suspicion and followed clinically or with a repeat CT (6 to 8 hours later).
- Liquid blood has a CT density of 35 to 45 H and blood clot is 70 to 90 H. The clot with the highest density is nearest the site of bleeding.
- Active bleeding typically measures within 10 H of an adjacent vessel and is surrounded by lower-density clot (sentinel clot sign).
- The presence of a parenchymal contrast blush or pseudoaneurysm is an indication for intervention by angiography or surgery due to increased risk of delayed bleeding.
- Diagnostic indications of full-thickness bowel injury include pneumoperitoneum without another known source (chest), direct visualization of bowel discontinuity, or oral extravasation of contrast. Other CT signs of bowel/mesenteric injury include bowel wall thickening, increased bowel wall enhancement, and mesenteric stranding or hematoma adjacent to the bowel. Triangular-shaped fluid collections in the mesenteric folds are also a clue to potential bowel and mesenteric injury, but are not specific.
- "Shock-bowel" secondary to hypoperfusion results in a small IVC and aorta diameter, thick-walled dilated bowel (usually small bowel), mesenteric edema, and abnormal patchy enhancement of the bowel wall.
- Elevated IVC pressure can be caused by overresuscitation, cardiac tamponade, tension pneumothorax, or hepatic hematoma obstructing the IVC. CT findings include distension of the IVC and renal veins with a small aorta, periportal lymphatic distension, mesenteric and bowel wall edema, pericholecystic fluid, and retroperitoneal edema.
- Mesenteric injuries requiring surgery include active bleeding in the mesentery, mesenteric hematoma enveloping the bowel, and mesenteric contusion or hematoma adjacent to abnormal-appearing bowel.

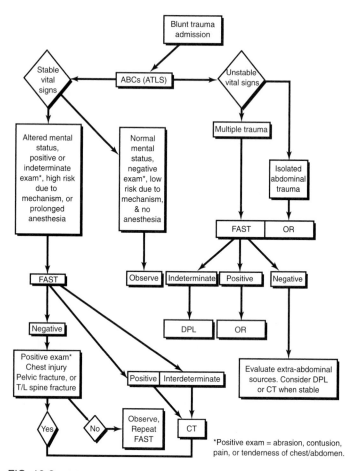

FIG. 10-3.   Initial evaluation of blunt abdominal trauma.

- Extraperitoneal bladder rupture causes streaks of contrast in the soft tissues around the bladder and the site of injury is often seen on CT. Intraperitoneal bladder rupture may cause contrast to spill into the peritoneal recesses.
- Typical helical CT is not adequate to exclude bladder injury, and this requires either formal CT-cystography or a radiographic cystogram.
- CT has a well-established role in the assessment of penetrating trauma to the flank and back in stable patients. A potential role for possible tangential wounds and penetrating gunshot wounds to the right upper quadrant is being explored.

ANGIOGRAPHY AND INTERVENTIONAL RADIOLOGY IN TRAUMA

In recent years the use of angiographic intervention for trauma has increased dramatically in many centers. Diagnostic angiography guides the selection of appropriate management in many clinical situations, and therapeutic techniques, especially selective distal embolization, have been useful in supporting nonoperative management of selected injuries. *Major* applications of angiography include:

- Diagnosis or confirmation of major thoracic vascular injury
- Diagnosis and treatment of pelvic hemorrhage following blunt trauma
- Diagnosis and potential selective embolization of actively bleeding hepatic, splenic, and renal vessels, or treatment of vascular injuries such as pseudo-aneurysm, "cut-off," or arteriovenous fistula
- Diagnosis and embolization of bleeding thoracic branch vessels such as the internal mammary or intercostal artery
- Diagnosis and embolization of selected abdominopelvic branch vessels such as the lumbar, epigastric, phrenic, or adrenal arteries
- Diagnosis and possible treatment of injuries to craniocervical arteries
- Diagnosis of injuries to the peripheral (extremity) arteries and assessment of postsurgical repair

In addition to techniques of vascular occlusion, recent developments in stent and stent-graft technology permit either temporary or permanent intravascular repair of selected injuries to vessels such as the renal or carotid arteries.

In the authors' institution there has been increasing use of angiographic embolization of hepatic and splenic injuries sustained from blunt trauma. Typically, angiography is performed urgently in stable patients for injury grade 3 or higher or for evidence of active bleeding by CT (contrast blush). Angiographic signs of vascular injury such as vessel occlusion, active bleeding (blush or pseudoaneurysm), or arteriovenous fistula mandate intervention. In splenic trauma, diffuse splenic injuries are typically treated with proximal coil embolization of the splenic artery to decrease splenic perfusion pressure, while distal lesions are treated by selective distal embolization. Both methods appear to be effective in controlling further hemorrhage with minimal rebleeding and infection rates. Distal embolization appears to infarct a larger amount of splenic tissue due to lack of collateral flow. Use of CT combined with angiography has lead to a reduction in the need for surgical repair for hepatic and splenic trauma.

It is imperative that close communication and cooperation exist between the trauma team and angiography team since the course of patient management may evolve rapidly. In many cases both surgical and angiographic intervention may be required to control severe injuries.

ADDITIONAL READING

Hagiwara A, Yukioka T, Ohta S, et al: Nonsurgical management of patients with blunt hepatic injury: Efficacy of transcatheter arterial embolization. *Am J Roentgenol* 169:1151, 1997.

Sclafani SJ, Shaftan GW, Scalea TM, et al: Nonoperative salvage of computed tomography-diagnosed splenic injuries: Utilization of angiography for triage and embolization for hemostasis. *J Trauma* 39:818, 1995.

Shanmuganathan K, Mirvis SE: Imaging diagnosis of nonaortic thoracic injury. *Radiol Clin North Am* 37:533, 1999.

Shanmuganathan K, Mirvis SE, Boyd-Kranis R, et al: Nonsurgical management of blunt splenic injury: use of CT criteria to select patients for splenic arteriography and potential endovascular therapy. *Radiology* 217:75, 2000.

Shanmuganathan K, Mirvis SE, Sover ER: Value of contrast-enhanced CT in detecting active hemorrhage in patients with blunt abdominal trauma. *Am J Roentgenol* 161:65, 1993.

11 | Anesthesia

ANESTHETIC ASSESSMENT AND MANAGEMENT

The limited time available requires the anesthesiologist to be aggressive and methodical in assessment. All severely injured patients should be considered at risk for aspiration, cervical spine and closed head injury, hypovolemia, and being potentially difficult to intubate. Pertinent information includes prior medical history with cardiovascular and pulmonary disease being particularly important. Hepatic and renal dysfunction will alter the choice and dosage of anesthetic agents and muscle relaxants. Current medications, allergies, previous surgeries, and history of diabetes is also notable. Gastroparesis is assumed after any traumatic event.

The American Society of Anesthesiologists (ASA) has developed a five-category classification system based on preoperative assessment of physical status (Table 11-1). The higher the ASA class the greater the risk for perioperative cardiopulmonary complications and death, especially if surgery is performed emergently.

Establishing a patent airway is critical and is discussed in Chapter 6. Resuscitating intravascular volume is important and multiple large-gauge intravenous lines should be inserted (14 and 16 gauge or 8 and 9 French catheters). Lower extremity access should be considered if there is severe upper extremity or thoracic injury. Intravenous infusions should be warmed, isotonic, and compatible with blood products.

Prior to the administration of anesthetic and paralytic medications, one should estimate the likelihood of difficulty ventilating or intubating the patient. The "Cannot Ventilate, Cannot Intubate" scenario must be avoided at all costs. About 1 percent of patients with seemingly normal airways may prove difficult to intubate, even by experienced personnel.

MONITORING

Pulse Oximetry

Contemporary pulse oximeters measure light absorbance at visual red (660 nm) and infrared (940 nm) wavelengths; oximetry calibration curves convert the absorbance ratio into an estimate of hemoglobin saturation. Four hemoglobin species may be found in normal adult blood: oxyhemoglobin (HbO_2), reduced hemoglobin (RHb), methemoglobin (MetHb), and carboxyhemoglobin (COHb). Methemoglobin results in spurious pulse oximetry values while carboxyhemoglobin does not, but in both instances true hemoglobin saturation is compromised. To accurately measure these four hemoglobin species, it is necessary to measure absorbance at four different wavelengths. Co-oximeters have this capacity.

Capnography

Carbon dioxide monitoring is considered the best method of verifying correct placement of the endotracheal tube. Carbon dioxide measurement throughout the respiratory phase may assist in the diagnosis of such conditions as pulmonary embolism, obstructive lung disease, increased dead space, hyperventilation, and malignant hyperthermia.

CHOICE OF ANESTHETIC

An anesthetic should be appropriate for the planned procedure and the condition of the patient. Choices include local anesthetic infiltration of the sur-

TABLE 11-1 American Society of Anesthesiologists (ASA) Physical Status Classification

Status	Disease state
ASA class I	No organic, physiologic, biochemical, or psychiatric disturbance
ASA class II	Mild to moderate systemic disturbance that may or may not be related to the reason for surgery
ASA class III	Severe systemic disturbance that may or may not be related to the reason for surgery
ASA class IV	Severe systemic disturbance that is life threatening with or without surgery
ASA class V	Moribund patient who has little chance of survival but is submitted to surgery as a last resort
Emergency	Any patient in whom an emergency operation is required

gical site with sedation, spinal or epidural anesthesia, and general anesthesia. General anesthesia will be the technique of choice for most injured patients. Recommended local anesthetic doses for infiltration can be found in Table 11-2.

Advantages of spinal/epidural anesthesia include avoidance of manipulation of the airway, reduction in the risk of pulmonary aspiration, the ability to follow mental status, and reduction in the physiologic stress response. There may be decreased blood loss, more rapid return of bowel function, improved blood flow to the extremities, and a decreased incidence of deep venous thrombosis. A major disadvantage is hypotension due to sympathetic blockade, particularly if the patient is hypovolemic. One should always administer a fluid challenge before performing regional anesthesia. If local anesthetics are injected into the circulation, there is a risk of seizures or cardiovascular collapse. Side effects of epidural infusions include motor blockade, nausea, vomiting, pruritus, and urinary retention. There is also a risk of epidural abscess or hematoma, and regional anesthesia is contraindicated when low molecular weight heparin is given. Coagulation status should always be assessed prior to considering these procedures.

General anesthesia with endotracheal intubation will be the anesthetic choice for most injured patients as noted above. It is appropriate and indicated for any patient undergoing significant fluid resuscitation; those requiring oxygen therapy or in need of hyperventilation or mechanical ventilation for any reason; in the obtunded patient; and in anyone at risk for aspiration or experiencing significant metabolic abnormalities. As opposed to regional anesthesia, general anesthesia can be titrated to the severity of the surgical stimulus.

TABLE 11-2 Maximal Recommended and Typical Doses for Local Anesthetics for Infiltration

Drug	Plain solution		Epinephrine-containing solution*		
	Concentration (%)	Max dose (mg)	Duration (min)	Max dose (mg)	Duration (min)
Chloroprocaine	1–2	800	15–30	1000	30–90
Lidocaine	0.5–1.0	300	30–60	500	120–360
Mepivacaine	0.5–1.0	300	45–90	500	120–360
Bupivacaine	0.25–0.5	175	120–240	225	180–420

* Suggested epinephrine concentration is 1:200,000 (5 μg/mL).

As the patient is intubated and ventilated, muscle relaxants may be administered to improve operating conditions.

ANESTHETIC AGENTS

Injudicious use of anesthetic agents in trauma may result in disastrous respiratory or cardiovascular complications. All anesthetic agents have significant hemodynamic impact, and their therapeutic indices are much lower in the trauma patient (Table 11-3).

Etomidate is a cardiostable anesthetic induction agent, having little effect on cardiac contractility or sympathetic function. It has high hepatic extraction and is rapidly eliminated. Side effects include pain on injection, myoclonus, and transient, though clinically unimportant, adrenal depression.

Sodium thiopental has a rapid hypnotic effect but is a potent cardiovascular depressant secondary to negative inotropism, impairment of sympathetic activity, and increases in venous capacitance. Few would consider it first-line treatment in the injured patient. For similar reasons, the utility of propofol is limited.

Ketamine is an intravenous anesthetic agent producing analgesia, and in larger doses, unconsciousness. Ketamine is a bronchodilator and has sympathomimetic effects that support blood pressure and heart rate, making it desirable in trauma. It also has direct myocardial depressant effects, usually seen only in catecholamine-depleted patients.

Benzodiazepines produce anxiolysis and amnesia and induce anesthesia in high doses. They are cardiostable, though they may act synergistically with opioids and volatile anesthetics, resulting in hypotension and apnea. If necessary, the benzodiazepine effect may be reversed by the competitive antagonist flumazenil. Flumazenil should be titrated to effect, because injudicious use may result in seizures, particularly in chronic users. Profoundly hypovolemic trauma patients are sometimes administered scopolamine to minimize recall, though this is less reliable than benzodiazepines.

Commonly used opioids include morphine, hydromorphone, and fentanyl and its congeners sufentanil, alfentanil, and remifentanil. The opioid's principal analgesic action occurs within the spinal cord. The substantia gelatinosa is dense with opioid receptors. Opioids are cardiostable agents, though factors such as volume status, associated medications, and ventricular function may modify cardiostability. They reduce surgically-induced stress response. They are respiratory depressants, decrease gastrointestinal motility and cause nausea and vomiting. The rapid onset of action of alfentanil and remifentanil may be used to blunt brief but highly stimulating noxious stimuli. Remifentanil is the first ultra-short acting opioid and is administered by infusion. As its effect

TABLE 11-3 Cardiovascular Effects of Induction Agents

Agent	MAP	HR	SVR	CO	Contractility	Venodilation
Thiopental	−	+	0 to +	−	−	+
Ketamine	+ +	+ +	+	+	+ or −	0
Midazolam	0 to −	0 to +	0 to −	0 to −	−	+
Propofol	−	+	−	0	−	+
Etomidate	0	0	0	0	0	0

MAP, Mean arterial pressure; HR, heart rate; SVR, systemic vascular resistance; CO, cardiac output; (+) increases; (0) no effect; (−) decreases. Ketamine's effect depends on patient's catecholamine levels.

terminates precipitously, the clinician must provide other means of analgesia whenever postprocedural pain is anticipated.

Opioids have pharmacologic antagonists (e.g., naloxone). Respiratory depression may be reversed but analgesia dissipates as well. Injudicious use may result in sympathetic storm, pulmonary edema, and an out-of-control patient. Under some circumstances it may be prudent to secure the airway and support ventilation rather than reverse the opioid effect.

Common inhaled halogenated anesthetics include isoflurane, desflurane, and sevoflurane. These agents are titratable and produce unconsciousness, amnesia, analgesia, and a degree of muscle relaxation. They are all vasodilators and have cardiac depressant effects in larger doses. They increase cerebral blood flow while decreasing oxygen consumption. Desflurane and sevoflurane are the most insoluble; their effects diminish rapidly upon discontinuance. Nitrous oxide is contraindicated in the trauma patient because it will diffuse into and enlarge an untreated pneumothorax, intracranial air, or an air embolus.

NEUROMUSCULAR BLOCKING AGENTS

Neuromuscular blockers (NMBs) relax skeletal muscle, facilitating endotracheal intubation, mechanical ventilation, and surgical exposure. NMBs either depolarize or block the neuromuscular junction. The only depolarizing agent currently available is succinylcholine (SCH), an agonist at the neuromuscular junction. Due to its short onset (approximately 45 seconds) and duration of action (5 to 8 minutes), SCH is primarily used to facilitate emergent endotracheal intubation and lessen the chance of aspiration. In conjunction with induction agents, the process of rapidly securing the airway is known as "rapid sequence induction."

Risks of SCH administration include anoxic injury and death if the patient cannot be ventilated. Arrhythmias may occur, particularly bradyarrhythmias. Succinylcholine may cause rhabdomyolysis and masseter muscle spasm, is a trigger for malignant hyperthermia, and increases intracranial and intraocular pressure. SCH normally causes a small, transient rise in serum potassium levels (0.5 to 1.0 mEq/L). Patients having sustained major trauma, burns, spinal cord injuries, or major crush injuries, however, are susceptible to profound potassium efflux from skeletal muscle, and are at risk for hyperkalemic cardiac arrest after SCH administration.

Nondepolarizing relaxants are competitive antagonists and are divided into two groups based on chemical structure: the aminosteroid compounds (vecuronium, rocuronium, rapacuronium, and pancuronium), and the benzylisoquinoline group (atracurium, cisatracurium, and mivacurium). Rapid-onset, short-acting, nondepolarizing NMBs may be used in lieu of SCH as long as the airway is believed to be manageable, and their duration is longer than that of SCH. Mivacurium and rocuronium are examples. Vecuronium and the atracurium compounds are of intermediate duration, are workhorses in the operating room, and are administered as infusions in the intensive care unit. Pancuronium is a long-acting muscle relaxant that induces tachycardia. Many agents in the benzylisoquinoline group may produce histamine release with bronchospasm and hypotension, especially if administered rapidly or in large doses. With the exception of atracurium, which breaks down spontaneously, the effect of nondepolarizing relaxants may be prolonged with hepatic and renal dysfunction. Table 11-4 suggests doses of relaxants to facilitate endotracheal intubation.

Table 11-4 Suggested Doses of Muscle Relaxants for Rapid Intubation

Drug	Intubating dose (mg/kg)	Intubation time (sec)	Full recovery* (min)
Succinylcholine	0.7–1.5	60	12–15
Mivacurium	0.16–0.3	90	40–60
Atracurium	0.6–0.8	90	60–90
Vecuronium	0.7–0.15	90	75–120
Rocuronium	0.9–1.2	60	60–160
Pancuronium	0.15–0.2	90	210–270

*Full recovery is considered return of twitch height of 95% of control.

ANESTHETIC IMPLICATIONS IN INJURY TO SPECIFIC BODY REGIONS

Traumatic Brain Injury

Cerebral blood flow is lowest in the hours following the injury, and maintaining cerebral oxygenation and perfusion are fundamental priorities. Isotonic crystalloids are the fluids of choice because of their superior osmotic effects. Hypertonic solutions decrease brain water and are useful for lowering intracranial pressure. Glucose-containing solutions are avoided in the absence of hypoglycemia, as hyperglycemia is associated with poor neurologic outcome. Table 11-5 reviews the cerebrovascular effects of some anesthetic agents.

Etomidate is a superior agent for induction/intubation when intracranial pressure is elevated, especially if volume status is uncertain. Lidocaine (1.5 mg/kg IV) decreases the sympathetic response to intubation. Current guidelines recommend avoiding prophylactic hyperventilation during the first 24 hours after severe traumatic brain injury. Brief hyperventilation may be necessary during intubation, when there is acute neurologic deterioration, and when elevated intracranial pressure fails to respond to other measures.

SPINAL CORD INJURY

All forms of airway control, including chin lift, jaw thrust, and oral and nasopharyngeal airway insertion, result in some motion of the cervical spine. In-line stabilization is the current recommendation for limiting cervical motion while performing direct laryngoscopy. Straight and curved laryngoscope blades do not differ substantially in the motion they produce, though the Bullard laryngoscope causes less extension of the cervical spine than conventional laryngoscopy. Flexible fiberoptic intubation is an excellent technique

Table 11-5 Cerebrovascular Effects of Induction Agents

Agent	CBF	ICP	CPP	CMRO$_2$
Thiopental	− −	− −	− −	− −
Ketamine	+ +	+	+	+
Midazolam	−	−	−	−
Propofol	− −	− −	− −	− −
Etomidate	− −	− −	0	− −

CBF, cerebral blood flow; ICP, intracranial pressure; CPP, cerebral perfusion pressure; CMRO$_2$, cerebral metabolic oxygen rate; (+) increases; (0) no effect; (−) decreases.

for avoiding cervical motion, but its utility in an acutely compromised patient is questionable.

Spinal cord injuries can produce hypotension due to loss of sympathetic tone, but only after hemorrhagic shock is ruled out can neurogenic shock be considered. If fluid resuscitation does not result in hemodynamic improvement, a pulmonary artery catheter should be placed to guide therapy. Fluid administration should be limited to pulmonary artery diastolic pressures of approximately 18 mm Hg. Spinal cord injuries cephalad to midthoracic levels interrupt sympathetic cardioaccelerator fibers, resulting in bradycardia. If accompanied by hypotension, atropine should be administered. Infusions of phenylephrine or another vasopressor may be required. Anesthetic agents should be titrated carefully, anticipating that doses of 30 to 50 percent of normal are likely to be sufficient. Succinylcholine may be administered in patients sustaining cord injuries in the first 24 hours after injury, but should be avoided thereafter to avoid the potential for life-threatening hyperkalemia.

THORACIC INJURY

Lung Isolation and Single Lung Ventilation

Double-lumen endotracheal tubes (DLET) possess both a tracheal and a bronchial ventilating channel. Isolation is achieved by inflating tracheal and bronchial low-pressure cuffs. A major disadvantage of a DLET is that it must be exchanged for a single lumen endotracheal tube at the conclusion of an operation unless differential lung ventilation is planned. A patient undergoing major fluid resuscitation may be too edematous to perform this exchange safely.

An alternative to avoid the risk of such airway loss is use of a bronchial blocker. The Univent® tube (Fuji Systems Corp., Tokyo, Japan) has a balloon-tipped hollow stylet contained within the wall of a single-lumen endotracheal tube that is inserted under endoscopic guidance. Failure of lung inflation is sometimes a problem, especially with contused and non-compliant lungs.

The Arndt endobronchial blocker (Cook Critical Care, Bloomington, IN) is inserted through a conventional single lumen endotracheal tube. A multiport airway adapter is attached to the proximal endotracheal tube connector and the ventilating circuit remains connected and continues to deliver ventilation. The blocker is inserted and has an endoscopic snare that is passed around the advancing bronchoscope. This may be the optimal method of obtaining lung separation when postoperative ventilation is planned.

The patient in the lateral decubitus position with an open chest is likely to have considerable ventilation-perfusion (V/Q) imbalance due to injury and single-lung ventilation. To facilitate optimal V/Q matching, the following practices are suggested: maintain two-lung ventilation as long as possible; begin one-lung ventilation with tidal volumes of 10 mL/kg; adjust respiratory rate to maintain normocarbia (FIO_2 of 1.0); and utilize frequent blood gas analysis. Positive end-expiratory pressure to the dependent lung may be added, but should not exceed 10 cm H_2O. Continuous positive airway pressure to the nondependent lung may be applied. Low levels (5 to 10 cm H_2O) will inflate nondependent alveoli slightly, allowing for some gas exchange while not impairing the surgical procedure.

Cardiac Tamponade

An acutely distending pericardium is noncompliant, and as pericardial pressure reaches right atrial pressure, cardiac filling diminishes. Only through augmentation of preload can cardiac output be maintained. As pericardial pressure approaches left ventricular diastolic pressure, however, acute cardiac decompensation ensues (see Chap. 22).

Anesthetic agents should be administered with great caution in untreated acute tamponade. Insertion of invasive monitors is useful, but only if the patient is hemodynamically stable. It is rarely necessary to perform pericardiocentesis or subxiphoid pericardial drainage under local anesthesia before anesthetic induction. Intravenous fluid augmentation is usually necessary. Once pericardial drainage has occurred, general anesthesia can be cautiously induced, and ketamine is recommended. Once intubated, high airway pressures and positive end-expiratory pressure should be avoided as both impair venous return to the heart. Tachycardia is a compensatory mechanism and should not be overtreated. Bradycardia should be treated aggressively with atropine. Contractility is ordinarily intact and inotropes are rarely beneficial. Vasodilator therapy may be catastrophic in the hypovolemic patient.

ABDOMINAL INJURY

These patients often undergo significant volume resuscitation and may develop the abdominal compartment syndrome as the incision is closed. Early recognition is important because the treatment is surgical decompression. Increases in intra-abdominal pressure are transmitted to intrathoracic compartments, spuriously elevating the measured occlusion pressure. When confronted with a patient with pathologically increased intra-abdominal pressure, a trial of volume expansion is indicated despite seemingly normal intravascular status (see Chap. 35).

ADDITIONAL READINGS

American Society of Anesthesiologists: Practice guidelines for management of the difficult airway. *Anesthesiology* 78:597, 1993.
Go AS, Browner WS: Cardiac outcomes after regional or general anesthesia: Do we have the answer? *Anesthesiology* 84:1, 1996.
Hastings RH: Airway management of patients with cervical spine injury, in Prough DS, Zornow MH (eds): *Problems in Anesthesia,* Vol. 9, Philadelphia, Lippincott-Raven, 1997, pp 25–37.
Zornow MH, Prough DS: Fluid management in patients with traumatic brain injury. *New Horiz* 3:488, 1995.

12 | Prevention, Diagnosis, and Management of Infection

Infection continues to be a major source of morbidity and death in the trauma patient. This chapter will describe commonly identified infections in the trauma patient and emphasize prevention, diagnosis, and best treatment modalities.

WOUND INFECTION

Infection in any wound in the trauma patient is the consequence of the interplay and biological summation of the following four determinants of infection: (1) the quantity of bacteria that contaminate the wound; (2) the virulence of the wound contaminant; (3) amplification factors in the wound which increase bacterial virulence (e.g., hematoma, necrotic tissue, foreign bodies, etc); and (4) the integrity of host defenses. The dynamic interaction among these four separate determinants underscores the complex clinical conundrum in which infection may or may not occur in trauma patients.

Traumatic Wound Infection

The prevention of infections in traumatic wounds is principally one of mechanical debridement and cleansing of the injury site. Devitalized tissue is debrided, while hematoma and foreign bodies are removed. Topical antiseptics (e.g., povidone iodine) in the open wound are not of value and may injure the tissue. The use of a single dose of a systemic antibiotic with activity against *Staphylococcus aureus* (e.g., cefazolin) is logical at the time of wound debridement and irrigation, but should not be continued thereafter. A critical decision in prevention is whether the wound should be primarily closed. Well-vascularized tissues that have been adequately debrided can be primarily closed. Severely contaminated wounds and those from traumatic avulsions or high-energy disruptions should have delayed or secondary closure.

The diagnosis of a wound infection after trauma is a clinical one. Wound erythema, induration, and disproportionate pain are evidence of infection. The discharge of pus is definitive evidence. Severe cellulitis and/or necrosis of the wound edge is evidence of severe infection. Cultures are commonly helpful in treatment and will show gram-positive organisms (e.g., *S. aureus* or group A streptococcus) in soft tissue injuries, or polymicrobial infection when enteric contamination has been present.

Necrotizing fasciitis may be a consequence of an initial traumatic injury. The diagnosis of necrotizing fasciitis should be suspected when there is rapidly developing skin necrosis, blistering, and bullae formation about the wound. Group A streptococcal infection should be suspected with rapidly advancing cellulitis with pain and tenderness that extends in a wide perimeter around the wound. Actual pus from the wound itself may be minimal or not in evidence at all. The patient will commonly have a systemic toxemia that is far greater than one would expect from a simple wound infection. The microbiology of necrotizing fascial infections can be group A streptococci, or a polymicrobial microflora of aerobic and anaerobic species. The polymicrobial infections are usually less aggressive.

Deep penetration of *Clostridium perfringens* from puncture wounds or other traumatic injuries can result in the rapid emergence of gas gangrene.

115

Infection due to clostridial myonecrosis is commonly associated with fairly mild signs of inflammation at the site of the puncture wound, but the patients have severe toxemia. With clostridial myonecrosis after an injury to an extremity, rapid loss of function of the extremity occurs as the tense deep compartment syndrome develops. Wound drainage may be quite minimal and have a "dishwater" appearance. Gram stains of any exudate or drainage from the wound will confirm the gram-positive rod.

The management of traumatic wound infections is to open the wound, drain pus, and mechanically remove fibrin and other infected debris. Systemic antibiotics may not be necessary in simple wound abscess, but when cellulitis or advancing necrosis is present, they are warranted. Invasive group A streptococcal infection requires systemic antibiotic therapy with penicillin and clindamycin. These necrotizing infections with group A streptococci will dissect along the anterior planes of fascia without fascial necrosis, particularly if the initial injury did not penetrate the fascia. Extensive debridement until only bleeding viable tissue remains behind is essential for survival. Polymicrobial necrotizing infections similarly need to be treated with extensive local debridement and antibiotic therapy appropriate for aerobic and anaerobic pathogens. Both group A streptococcal and polymicrobial necrotizing infections may require daily debridement until complete arrest of the infection has been achieved.

Rapidly advancing clostridial infections require immediate and extensive debridement. High-dose penicillin therapy is used for these patients, but is of limited value in the absence of complete eradication of dead tissue. Hyperbaric oxygen is used, but remains of unproven value.

Open Fracture Wounds

The prevention of infection in open fractures is achieved by immediate and thorough irrigation and debridement of the wound. A large volume (8 to 16 L) of warm pulsed lavage of the fracture site removes hematoma, debris, and fibrin. Systemic antibiotics appropriate for staphylococcal coverage are warranted at debridement, but infection rates are not reduced by continuation of the antibiotics after the procedure. The general practice has been to not primarily close the open fracture wound. The diagnosis of infection in the open fracture is the recognition of purulence within the wound (Table 12-1). On occasion, infection is diagnosed by nonunion of the fracture. The management of open fracture infections requires continued local debridement and irrigation as well as prolonged systemic antibiotics. Infected internal fixation hardware will usually need to be removed. Systemic antibiotics are obviously an important feature in the management of these patients and need to be focused on the culture and sensitivity data.

Surgical Wounds

Surgical wound infections follow the same general clinical guidelines as traumatic wounds. The prevention of wound infection in surgical incisions requires preoperative antiseptic preparation of the skin at the surgical site. A decision for wound closure at the conclusion of the procedure should be predicated upon the degree of intraoperative contamination. Preoperative systemic antibiotics will reduce wound infection rates, but should not be continued beyond 24 hours postoperatively. The diagnosis of surgical wound infection is similar to that detailed for the traumatic wound, with signs of inflammation

Table 12-1 Microflora from Infected Open Fractures in 32 Infections, with the Identification of 48 Separate Pathogens

Culture bacterial species	No. of isolates
Enterococcus spp.	14
Pseudomonas spp.	11
Staphylococcus spp.	9
Klebsiella/Enterobacter spp.	9
E. coli	2
Serratia spp.	2
Proteus spp.	1

Source: Roth AE, Fry DE, Polk HC Jr: Infectious morbidity in extremity fractures. *J Trauma* 26:757, 1986.

seen to suggest that infection is present, and the discharge of pus for confirmation. The management of the infected closed wound is to open, drain, and debride the infection. Antibiotics are only required if there is severe cellulitis or evidence of wound necrosis.

INTRA-ABDOMINAL INFECTION

Intra-abdominal infection in the trauma patient begins with injury to the intestinal tract, especially the colon, or the biliary tree. The prevention of acute peritonitis in the trauma patient begins with prompt laparotomy, management of the source of contamination (e.g., resection, oversewing, exteriorization), and removal of intraperitoneal contamination. Systemic antibiotics should be initiated preoperatively and should have a spectrum to cover enteric aerobic and anaerobic species. With massive contamination, antibiotics are continued for a therapeutic course and are discontinued based upon clinical criteria. Intraperitoneal antibiotics at the time of celiotomy have not been shown to add any value to appropriately employed systemic antibiotics. The diagnosis of acute peritonitis following traumatic disruption of the intestinal tract is a clinical one, based upon the patient having fever and leukocytosis after the laparotomy. It is a diagnosis of presumption since the physical examination of the traumatized abdomen after a laparotomy is of limited value. The microbiology of acute peritonitis following traumatic injury of the intestinal tract will be those microbes consistent with the level of the intestinal injury. The management of the acute peritonitis phase following its presumptive recognition consists of systemic antibiotics against the likely aerobic and anaerobic contaminants from the initial injury (Table 12-2).

Abdominal Abscess

An abdominal abscess may occur despite all the attempts at prevention noted above, including the use of drains of any kind. The diagnosis of abdominal abscess is suspected with fever, leukocytosis, prolonged ileus, hyperglycemia, or any evidence of early organ failure (e.g., arterial desaturation, chemical hyperbilirubinemia). The diagnosis of an abdominal abscess is confirmed by an abdominal CT scan. Abscesses generally will be found in the dependent areas of the abdominal cavity (e.g., subphrenic, pericolic, and pelvic spaces). Cultures of abscess are necessary since prior antibiotics may affect the isolates that are identified. The management of abdominal abscess and its sequelae is summarized in the algorithm (Fig. 12-1).

Table 12-2   Advantages and Disadvantages of Antibiotic Options for the Treatment of Patients with Acute Peritonitis After Penetrating Trauma of the Abdomen

Antibiotic choice	Advantages	Disadvantages
Cefoxitin	Combined aerobic-anaerobic coverage; good activity against non-fragilis *Bacteroides* spp. Non-toxic.	Short half-life; some reported resistance among gram-negatives and *B. fragilis.*
Cefotetan	Combined aerobic-anaerobic coverage; long half-life (3.5–4 h), allows twice-a-day dosing. Non-toxic.	Less activity against *B. fragilis* and non-fragilis *Bacteroides* spp.
Ceftizoxime	Clinically effective against aerobic/anaerobic infections; longer half-life (1.7–2 h) allows every 8–12 h dosing. Non-toxic.	Limited clinical data; highly variable in vitro activity against anaerobes.
Ampicillin/ sulbactam	Activity against *E. coli* and *B. fragilis;* enterococcal coverage favored by some.	Short half-life; gram-negative resistance.
Ticarcillin/ clavulanate	Combined aerobic/anaerobic coverage; enterococcal activity.	Short half-life.
Piperacillin/ tazobactam	Very good combined aerobic/anaerobic coverage, including *Pseudomonas* spp; enterococcal activity.	Short half-life.
Imipenem	Superb coverage of all potential pathogens.	Short half-life makes every 8 h therapy suspect; neurologic toxicity.
Meropenem	Superb coverage of all potential pathogens; no neurologic toxicity.	Short half-life makes every 8 h therapy suspect.
Gentamicin or tobramycin	Considered gold standard for gram-negative coverage; inexpensive.	Renal and ototoxicity; high costs for monitoring; unpredictable pharmacology in the critically-ill; require a second drug for anaerobic coverage.
Aztreonam	Good gram-negative coverage; avoids toxicity of aminoglycosides.	Limited clinical data; requires a second drug for anaerobic coverage.
Ciprofloxacin	Good gram-negative coverage; avoids toxicity of aminoglycosides.	Limited clinical data; requires a second drug for anaerobic coverage.
Clindamycin	Sustained *B. fragilis* activity over two decades; also covers aerobic gram-positive pathogens.	Expensive compared to alternative choices; requires a second drug for gram-negative coverage.
Metronidazole	Excellent anaerobic coverage; inexpensive.	Requires a second drug for gram-negative coverage.

Pleural Space Infections

Infections in the pleural space may occur due to external contamination from injury, but most are consequences of chest tubes inserted to remove blood and air. Clotted blood and undrained fluids are an ideal environment for infection. The prevention of infection in the pleural space requires adherence to the

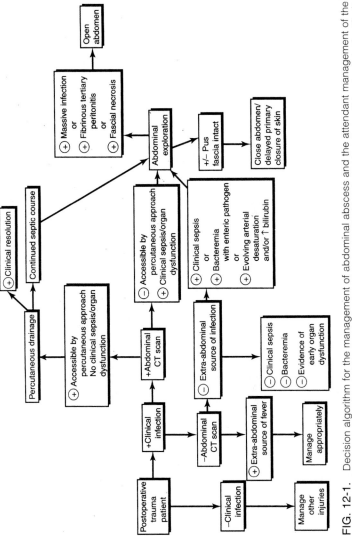

FIG. 12-1. Decision algorithm for the management of abdominal abscess and the attendant management of the reoperated abdominal wound. −, clinical entity is absent or suggested treatment is not possible; +, clinical entity is absent or suggested treatment is not possible.

principles of infection control, with sterile insertion of chest tubes, complete evacuation of blood and clot from the pleural space, and removal of the tube once its purpose has been served. Systemic antibiotics at the time of tube placement may reduce the risk of empyema. The diagnosis of empyema is a concern, with fever, leukocytosis, and purulent drainage from the chest tube. It is often established with a chest roentgenogram and is usually confirmed with a chest CT scan. *Staphylococcus aureus* remains the most common pathogen, but any bacterial colonist of the trauma patient may be present. Gram stains and cultures are necessary. The management of empyema requires drainage of the pus by placement of a drainage tube directly into the cavity. CT-directed drainage may be necessary. Tubes remain in place until the cavity has completely collapsed and drainage ceases. Some empyemas require weeks of drainage to resolve and are managed by tube drainage without suction. Complex empyemas may require rib resection to afford complete drainage, and still others require decortication, especially if restricted pulmonary ventilation is documented. Antibiotics are employed and must be active against the documented pathogen.

NOSOCOMIAL INFECTIONS

Nosocomial infections in this discussion will refer to those that occur remote from the sites of injury or operation. Pneumonia, urinary tract infection, and infections of indwelling intravascular catheters are the most common. Always examine the febrile trauma patient for common sites of nosocomial infection, and always carefully examine areas that have been touched.

Pneumonia

Pneumonia may be (1) non-ventilator-associated, (2) ventilator-associated, or (3) aspiration-associated.

Non-Ventilator-Associated Pneumonia (N-VAP)

Chest injury, closed head injury, use of narcotics, and general anesthesia result in reduced tidal volumes and atelectasis. If atelectasis is untreated, pneumonia is the result. To prevent N-VAP, increase tidal volume and keep alveoli and small airways expanded. Coughing, deep breathing, early ambulation, and postural changes are important, while preventive antibiotics are not indicated. The diagnosis of N-VAP is suspected with fever, leukocytosis, productive cough, and new or expanding chest infiltrates on a chest roentgenogram. The infectious agent in N-VAP early after injury and operation will often be *Streptococcus pneumoniae* or *Haemophilus influenzae*. Patients who have been hospitalized for more than a week and those following a course of antibiotics will tend to have hospital-acquired pathogens. Thus, *Pseudomonas* spp., *Enterobacter* spp., and other resistant hospital-acquired pathogens will predominate as pathogens. The treatment of N-VAP requires culture and sensitivity data to direct antibiotic therapy. Infection secondary to *Streptococcus pneumoniae* can still be treated with penicillin, but emerging resistance may make wide-spectrum beta-lactams or quinolones preferable. *Haemophilus influenzae* may still be treated with second-generation cephalosporins (e.g., cefuroxime) or ampicillin/sulbactam. Supportive care of the N-VAP patient requires pulmonary toilet and maintenance of oxygenation.

Ventilator-Associated Pneumonia (VAP)

VAP occurs because a need for ventilator support clearly indicates an impaired lung from injury or postresuscitative edema, and the endotracheal tube affords both a direct route into the lung and creates a foreign body effect in the airway. The prevention of VAP is extraordinarily difficult. The endotracheal tube must be handled within accepted standards of infection control. Suctioning of airway secretions, humidification of lung and airway, and early weaning are important preventive strategies.

The diagnosis of VAP is also very difficult. Injured patients often have noninfectious infiltrates, which are dynamic processes even without infection. Conventionally-obtained lung aspirates may represent colonization and not infection; hence, the use of protected brush samplings or bronchoalveolar lavage is required for isolation of a probable pathogen. The diagnosis of VAP requires the clinical synthesis of all available information to arrive at an accurate conclusion. The microbiology of VAP in the trauma patient reflects nosocomial pulmonary pathogens, and requires good culture and sensitivity data to guide therapy (Table 12-3). The treatment of VAP is principally with systemic antibiotic therapy, but suctioning with appropriate infection control practices and humidification of the airway remain important. Because of resistant organisms, combinations of antibiotics with different modes of action (e.g., an aminoglycoside and a wide-spectrum penicillin) are frequently employed. The duration of antibiotic administration remains a difficult decision and should be based upon clinical improvement of the patient and not bacteriological clearance or complete resolution of pulmonary infiltrates on a chest x-ray.

Aspiration-Associated Pneumonia (AAP)

Pneumonia due to aspiration may be secondary to either gross or microscopic aspiration. The altered sensorium of trauma patients always makes

Table 12-3 Pathogens Identified in Trauma Patients Who Developed Postoperative Pneumonia

Cultured pathogen	Rodriguez	Fink
Gram-positive		
Staphylococcus aureus	37 (27%)	48 (13%)
Others	0	26 (7%)
Gram-negative		
Pseudomonas spp.	38 (22%)	70 (19.5%)
Haemophilus spp.	16 (9%)	53 (15%)
Enterobacter spp.	26 (15%)	32 (9%)
Klebsiella spp.	13 (7.5%)	38 (10.5%)
E. coli	7 (4%)	24 (7%)
Acinetobacter spp.	12 (7%)	11 (3%)
Proteus spp.	10 (6%)	11 (3%)
Serratia spp.	14 (8%)	0
Others	0	46 (13%)
Total	173	359

Source: From Rodriguez JR, Gibbons KJ, Bitzer LG, et al: Pneumonia: incidence, risk factors, and outcome in injured patients. *J Trauma* 31:907, 1991 and from Fink MP, Snydman DR, Niederman MS, et al: Treatment of severe pneumonia in hospitalized patients: results of a multicenter, randomized, double-blind trial comparing intravenous ciprofloxacin with imipenem-cilastatin. *Antimicrob Agents Chemother* 38:547, 1994.

gross vomiting and aspiration an issue. Microscopic aspiration of oropharyngeal secretions is yet another mechanism. The prevention of gross aspiration pneumonia is by elevation of the head of the bed and early evacuation of the stomach. Gross aspiration is initially a chemical event, and when suspected should not be treated with preventive antibiotics. Prevention of AAP in the patient with suspected microaspiration remains elusive. Antacids via the nasogastric tube probably increase aspiration events and should not be used. Restricting histamine or proton pump inhibitors because they promote alkalinization of the aerodigestive tract has diminished as a preventive strategy. The diagnosis of acute gross aspiration usually requires bronchoscopy, and the transition from a chemical to an infectious event requires bronchoalveolar lavage for identification of a pathogen. The causative pathogens are similar to those of VAP. The diagnosis of microaspiration AAP may be indistinguishable from N-VAP and should follow the same guidelines. The microbiology is the same as for other hospital-acquired nosocomial pneumonias. The management of gross AAP is antibiotic administration similar to the strategy employed in the VAP patient. The supportive care of the trauma patient with pneumonia is similar regardless of the cause.

Urinary Tract Infection

Urinary tract infection (UTI) in the trauma patient is ordinarily a consequence of bladder catheterization. Prevention of UTI requires sterile placement and maintenance of the catheter and removal as soon as clinically appropriate. Preventive systemic antibiotics only change the pathogen but not the frequency of UTI. The diagnosis is established with quantitative cultures that document $>10^5$ bacteria/mL of urine in patients with pyuria. The bacteriology of UTI in the surgical patient is very different than that seen in community-acquired infections (Table 12-4). The treatment of UTI is with antibiotics against the cultured pathogen. Sterilization of the urine will not be possible until the catheter is discontinued. Short courses of antibiotics (3 to 5 days) will prove successful in most trauma patients.

Intravascular Device Infection

The numerous intravascular devices inserted in the trauma patient are all portals for microbial colonization and are potential sites for device-associated bacteremia or suppurative thrombophlebitis. Prevention requires placement of the device with standard infection control practices, occlusive dressings at the site, and early removal of the device. Peripheral devices should be rotated every 48 to 72 hours. Topical antibiotics at the site are of no value. The diagnosis of intravascular device infection is associated with acute spiking fevers and should be suspected in every trauma patient with a positive blood culture. *Staphylococcus aureus, Staphylococcus epidermidis,* and *Candida albicans* identified in blood cultures suggest intravascular device infection. When suspected, the devices are removed and distal tip of the catheter is cultured by the semiquantitative technique (>15 colony-forming units define the diagnosis). Positive catheter cultures without positive blood cultures should not be the basis for diagnosis and treatment. Suppurative thrombophlebitis (STP) is defined as active suppuration within the vessel even after the device has been removed. The diagnosis is confirmed by local exploration of the catheter site and documentation of suppuration within the vein. The microbiology of intravascular device infection is described in Table 12-5. A positive blood

Table 12-4 Microbiology of Postoperative UTI Among 212 Infections in 153 Surgical Patients

Cultured pathogens	No. of isolates
E. coli	56
Klebsiella spp.	38
Pseudomonas spp.	37
Proteus spp.	30
Enterobacter spp.	22
Enterococcus spp.	22
Serratia spp.	16
Citrobacter spp.	10
Other bacteria	22
Candida spp.	3
Total	256

Source: From Asher EF, Oliver BG, Fry DE: Urinary tract infections in the surgical patient. *Am Surg* 54:466, 1988.

culture for *Staphylococcus* spp. in the trauma patient should be considered an intravascular device infection until proven otherwise. The treatment of device infections is removal of the device and systemic antibiotics. It is not appropriate to give antibiotics and keep an infected device in place. Antibiotics for gram-negative organisms are continued until the bacteremia has cleared (2 to 5 days). With *Staphylococcus aureus,* the antibiotics need to be continued for 2 weeks because of the risk of endocarditis. When a diagnosis of suppurative thrombophlebitis is confirmed, the entire infected segment of the vein requires surgical removal. Persistence of bacteremia after vein excision means inadequate removal of infected venous tissue, or endocarditis may have already developed.

Candida Sepsis

Sepsis due to *Candida* spp. is the result of colonization of the trauma patient following use of broad-spectrum systemic antibiotics, combined with acquired immunosuppression of the host due to injury, illness, or multiple operations. Infection may arise from central catheters, primarily from the gastrointestinal tract, or uncommonly from an anatomic site (e.g., peritoneal

Table 12-5 Pathogens Cultured from Documented Intravascular Device Infections

Cultured pathogens	No. of isolates
Staphylococcus aureus	78
Staphylococcus epidermidis	33
Serratia spp.	18
Candida spp.	11
Klebsiella spp.	11
Enterococcus spp.	8
Proteus spp.	6
Enterobacter spp.	5
Other	6
Total	176

Source: From Fry DE, Fry RV, Borzotta AP: Nosocomial blood-borne infection secondary to intravascular devices. *Am J Surg* 167:268, 1994.

cavity). Prevention of candidemia is best achieved by restricting use of antibiotics and by use of enteral feeding, since the gut is the reservoir for this organism. Systemic anticandidal prophylaxis in the patient at risk is used by some, but is not widely recommended. The diagnosis of *Candida* sepsis is by positive blood cultures or by culturing the fungus from two or more anatomic sites. Treatment is with either fluconazole or amphotericin B. Fungemia may arise from central catheters and require removal of the catheter and documentation of the suspected infection by semiquantitative cultures of the catheter tip.

Clostridium difficile Enterocolitis

Antibiotic-associated enterocolitis due to *Clostridium difficile* is a diagnostic consideration in every trauma patient who has received a course of antibiotics and has diarrhea. Prevention is best achieved with shorter courses of antibiotic administration, particularly with preventive strategies. Diagnosis is by detection of the toxin in the diarrheal discharge of the patient. Treatment is equally effective with either oral metronidazole or vancomycin, with metronidazole generally preferred because of its lower cost. If intravenous therapy is necessary, metronidazole is preferred to vancomycin because of better intraluminal concentrations. Particularly severe cases associated with toxic megacolon may require surgical decompression or resection of the affected segment of colon.

ADDITIONAL READING

Brown DL, Hungness ES, Campbell RS, et al: Ventilator-associated pneumonia in the surgical intensive care unit. *J Trauma* 51:1207, 2001.
Centers for Disease Control and Prevention: *HIV/AIDS Surveillance Report* 9:15, 1997.
Fallon WF Jr, Wears RL: Prophylactic antibiotics for the prevention of infectious complications including empyema following tube thoracostomy for trauma: Results of meta-analysis. *J Trauma* 33:110, 1992.
Feliciano DV, Gentry LO, Bitondo CG, et al: Single agent cephalosporin prophylaxis for penetrating abdominal trauma. Results and comments on the emergence of the enterococcus. *Am J Surg* 152:674, 1986.
Maki DG, Botticelli JT, LeRoy ML, et al: Prospective study of replacing administration sets for intravenous therapy at 48- versus 72-hour intervals. 72 hours is safe and cost-effective. *JAMA* 258:1777, 1987.
Nichols RL, Smith JW, Robertson GD, et al: Prospective alterations in therapy for penetrating abdominal trauma. *Arch Surg* 128:55, 1993.
Roth AI, Fry DE, Polk HC Jr: Infectious morbidity in extremity fractures. *J Trauma* 26:757, 1986.

III | MANAGEMENT OF SPECIFIC INJURIES

13 | Injury to the Cranium

SIGNIFICANCE AND EPIDEMIOLOGY OF TRAUMATIC BRAIN INJURY (TBI)

- TBI contributes significantly to the outcome in one-half of all deaths from trauma.
- Almost 75 percent of victims of fatal traffic accidents demonstrate postmortem evidence of brain injury.
- The annual financial burden of TBI in terms of both lost productivity and cost of medical care exceeds $75 billion in the United States alone.
- Motor vehicle accidents are the most common cause of TBI, especially in teenagers and young adults. Falls are responsible for the next biggest group of injuries and are more common in the pediatric and geriatric populations. In some areas, gunshot wounds account for more traumatic brain injuries than do automobile accidents.

PATHOLOGY

Although traumatic intracranial lesions are easily demonstrated by computed tomography (CT), less obvious diffuse processes (e.g., ischemia, diffuse axonal injury, excitotoxicity, apoptosis) are often more important in influencing outcome after trauma (Table 13-1).

PREHOSPITAL AND EMERGENCY CENTER MANAGEMENT OF SEVERE TBI

Figure 13-1 summarizes the initial management of patients with severe TBI.

Neurologic Assessment

A detailed neurologic assessment should be done as soon as possible, but valuable information can be gained in just a few seconds by determining the Glasgow Coma Scale (GCS) score (Table 13-2) and by assessing pupillary reactivity.

Glasgow Coma Scale

- Three components: best motor, verbal, and eye-opening responses.
- List scores for each component separately (as well as sum).
- Maximum score is 15. Most severe injury: one point in each category (total of 3).
- Document inability to assess component(s) (e.g., verbal score in intubated patients), but proceed with scoring other components.
- Beware of confounding systemic factors (e.g., hypotension, hypoxia, hypothermia, hypoglycemia, sedating drugs) which may depress neurologic function.
- GCS score of 13 to 15 is mild TBI; 9 to 12 is moderate TBI; and 8 or below is severe TBI. Do not assume that "mild TBI" automatically indicates a trivial injury, especially if abnormalities are present on CT scan.

Pupillary Response

A dilated pupil that does not constrict in response to bright light may indicate transtentorial herniation (the ipsilateral uncus of the medial temporal lobe compresses and inactivates the pupilloconstrictor fibers on the periphery of

TABLE 13-1 Pathology of Traumatic Brain Injury*

Mass lesions	Diffuse processes	Other entities
Subdural hematoma	Diffuse axonal injury	Subarachnoid hemorrhage
Epidural hematoma	Ischemia (global)	Intraventricular hemorrhage
Intracerebral hematoma	Excitotoxicity	Shear injury
Cerebral contusion	Apoptosis	Depressed skull fracture
Ischemia (causing		Penetrating brain injury
focal infarction)		

*Many patients may demonstrate more than one type of pathology.

the third nerve). Immediate CT scanning is needed to identify any surgically treatable mass lesions, but remember that a fixed and dilated pupil may also result from direct injury to the orbit and its contents.

NEUROSURGICAL INTENSIVE CARE

Goals: (1) Prevent secondary cerebral insults (i.e., any deviation from normal homeostasis), which are especially harmful after severe TBI; (2) provide

PREHOSPITAL AND EMERGENCY CENTER MANAGEMENT OF SEVERE TBI

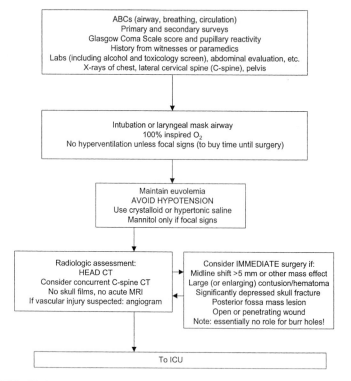

FIG. 13-1.   Basic steps in the initial assessment and resuscitation of head-injured patients.

TABLE 13-2 Glasgow Coma Scale

Score	Motor	Verbal	Eye opening
6	Obeys commands	—	—
5	Localizes stimulus	Oriented	—
4	Withdraws from stimulus	Confused	Spontaneously
3	Flexes arm	Words/phrases	To voice
2	Extends arm	Make sounds	To pain
1	No response	No response	Remain closed

optimal physiologic environment for the brain's own reparative processes. Cardiovascular, pulmonary, renal, and other organ systems must be monitored vigilantly, with aggressive support and intervention as necessary.

Neurologic Management

The single most important indicator of a patient's neurologic status is the neurologic examination, but in comatose patients, in whom the exam is limited, valuable information can be gained by using different techniques to monitor cerebral metabolism (Table 13-3).

Principles of Intensive Care Unit Management

- Treat intracranial hypertension aggressively (Table 13-4).
- Prevent or immediately correct hypotension and hypoxia (keep systolic blood pressure at least 80 mm Hg and arterial oxygen saturation at least 90 percent).

TABLE 13-3 Techniques of Monitoring Cerebral Metabolism

Physiologic parameter	Monitor	Global or regional monitor	Critical value
Intracranial pressure (ICP)	Ventriculostomy Intraparenchymal catheter	Global	ICP >20 mm Hg
Cerebral blood flow (CBF)	Xenon-enhanced CT scan	Both	Ischemic threshold: 18 mL/100 g/min
	Nitrous oxide clearance	Global	
	PET (positron emission tomography) scan	Both	
	SPECT (Single photon emission computed tomography) scan	Both	
	Thermal diffusion probe	Regional	
	Laser Doppler probe	Regional	
	Transcranial Doppler sonogram	Regional	Normal values vary for different arteries
Brain parenchymal oxygen tension ($PbtO_2$)	Intraparenchymal PO_2 catheter	Regional	$PbtO_2$ <15 mm Hg?
Jugular venous oxygen saturation ($SjvO_2$)	Jugular bulb oximetric catheter	Global	Saturation <50%
Cerebral perfusion pressure (CPP)*	Arterial blood pressure and ICP monitors	Global	CPP <60 mm Hg?
Arterial oxygen saturation	Pulse oximeter	Global	<90%?

*CPP = mean arterial pressure (MAP) minus ICP

TABLE 13-4 Control of Elevated Intracranial Pressure
_____

Eliminate factors that can elevate ICP
- Straighten head to prevent kinking of jugular vein, raise head of bed slightly (no more than 30°), eliminate hypercarbia, etc.
- Repeat CT (if not done recently) to look for mass lesion requiring surgical intervention.

Treat pain with narcotics, e.g., morphine 2–10 mg IV for adults. Sedating effects may also help lower ICP. If response inadequate, consider benzodiazepines or propofol infusion (watch blood pressure).

If ICP still elevated: neuromuscular blockade. Monitor depth of paralysis with nerve stimulator.

Note: Try to hold sedation and paralysis at least once a day (such as before morning rounds) so that a valid neurological examination can be perfomed.

If ICP still elevated: drainage of cerebrospinal fluid (CSF) via ventriculostomy.

If CSF drainage fails or is not possible: mannitol 0.25–1.0 gm/kg bolus. May repeat as needed as long as fluid balance is followed closely and serum osmolality stays below 320 mOsm/L.

If ICP elevation persists: may try mild hyperventilation (keeping $Paco_2$ >30 mm Hg), especially if cerebral oxygenation is monitored by $SjvO_2$ cathether and/or by $PbtO_2$ monitor.

Next step: pentobarbital-induced coma. Meticulous attention must be paid to avoiding arterial hypotention. Consider having pressors hanging and ready to be infused as pentobarbital is given.

Other treatments.
- Hypothermia was not beneficial when tested in a multicenter trial, but it is possible that select subgroups of patients may benefit.
- Decompressive craniectomy may be an option in some cases (especially with unilateral pathology), but this treatment still awaits validation in a rigorous trial.
_____

- Give prophylactic phenytoin or other anticonvulsant only for the first 7 to 8 days in patients who have no seizures. If seizures occur, continue anticonvulsants and reevaluate after a prolonged interval (e.g., 6 to 12 months).
- Consider broad-spectrum antibiotics for at least several days in patients with contaminated injuries or gunshot wounds, with special emphasis on coverage against gram-negative bacilli and anaerobes.
- Keep blood glucose levels as close to normal as possible.
- Investigate temperature spikes and treat aggressively.
- Initiate enteral feedings as soon as possible. Parenteral nutrition should be considered in patients who still cannot tolerate enteral feedings after several days.
- Do not administer steroids for brain injury; they do not help and may have undesirable side effects. They should be used if indicated for other problems.
- Do not deliberately dehydrate patients in hopes of preventing cerebral edema, but treat hyponatremia aggressively with hypertonic saline to prevent diffusion of water into the brain.

Prevention and Management of Complications

Coagulopathy

Coagulopathy occurs frequently after severe TBI. Treat aggressively with fresh frozen plasma (and other blood products as needed) to prevent delayed hemorrhages or enlargement of existing intracranial bleeds.

Thromboembolic Events

During prolonged stays in the intensive care unit (ICU), TBI patients are at increased risk of deep venous thrombosis and pulmonary embolism because lack of spontaneous movement promotes venous stasis and thrombosis.

- Use intermittent pneumatic compression devices on the lower extremities.
- Low molecular weight heparin combined with pneumatic compression has been reported to be more effective than pneumatic compression alone in general neurosurgery patients, and has been reported to be safe and effective in trauma patients (including those with head injury).
- Treatment of thromboembolic events in TBI patients: full anticoagulation is probably best deferred for 1 to 2 weeks after craniotomy or after injury producing intracranial hemorrhage or contusion. Consider inferior vena cava filter (IVCF) instead. We have not found it necessary to use prophylactic IVCFs routinely.

Gastrointestinal Ulceration

Optimal method of prophylaxis remains controversial. Our standard practice: initiate therapy with parenteral H_2 blockers as soon as patient arrives in ICU. If patients exhibit thrombocytopenia or other possible side effects of these agents, we switch to sucralfate.

OUTCOME

Outcome after TBI is commonly described with the Glasgow Outcome Scale (GOS) (Table 13-5).

- Approximate distribution of outcomes in patients with severe TBI: death 30 to 36 percent, persistent vegetative state 5 percent, severe disability 15 percent, moderate disability 15 to 20 percent, good recovery 25 percent or more.
- Approximate distribution of outcomes in patients with moderate TBI: death or persistent vegetative state 7 percent, severe disability 7 percent, moderate disability 25 percent, good recovery 60 percent.
- Gunshot wounds: up to 90 percent mortality. If patient arrives at hospital alive, mortality is 60 percent, vegetative or severe disability is <10 percent, moderate disability or good recovery is 30 to 40 percent.

TABLE 13-5 Glasgow Outcome Scale

Score	Category	Description
5	Good recovery (GR)	Able to live and work independently despite minor disabilities.
4	Moderate disability (MD)	Able to live independently despite disabilities. Can use public transportation, work with assistance/supervision, etc.
3	Severe disability (SD)	Conscious but dependent upon others for self-care. Often institutionalized.
2	Persistent vegetative state (PVS)	Not conscious, but may appear "awake."
1	Death (D)	Self-explanatory.

- Even among apparently good recoveries, the psychological and social sequelae of head injury are often overwhelming for both patients and families.

GUIDELINES FOR THE MANAGEMENT OF SEVERE HEAD INJURY

The Guidelines for the Management of Severe Head Injury, published jointly by the Brain Trauma Foundation and the American Association of Neurological Surgeons, have attracted a great deal of attention.

The Guidelines are simply a review of the literature relevant to specific aspects of head injury, (i.e., evidence-based medicine). They classify various therapeutic practices according to the strength of the available evidence. Unfortunately, the Guidelines have on occasion been misinterpreted as rigid requirements. They were never intended to replace the judgment of the individual practitioner.

MILD TBI

The main diagnostic concern is to determine if a patient with mild TBI is one of the small minority who proceed to neurologic deterioration from a delayed intracerebral hematoma. Neurological examination often not reliable. The safest approach is liberal use of CT scanning, but the criteria for ordering a CT scan are not well defined. Patients with mild TBI generally do well, although some prolonged problems with memory, attention deficits, headaches, dizziness, and other neuropsychological deficits are not uncommon.

ADDITIONAL READINGS

Clifton GL, Miller ER, Choi SC, et al: Lack of effect of induction of hypothermia after acute brain injury. *N Engl J Med* 344:556, 2001.

Marshall LF et al: The outcome of severe closed head injury. *J Neurosurg* 75:S28, 1991.

Robertson CS et al: Prevention of secondary ischemic insults after severe head injury. *Crit Care Med* 27:2086, 1999.

Teasdale G, Jennett B: Assessment of coma and impaired consciousness. A practical scale. *Lancet* 2:81, 1974.

The Brain Trauma Foundation, The American Association of Neurological Surgeons, The AANS/CNS section on neurotrauma and critical care: guidelines for the management of severe traumatic brain injury. *J Neurotrauma* 17:453, 2000.

14 | Injury to the Eye

Ocular trauma is a major cause of monocular blindness and visual impairment in the United States. An estimated 2.4 million eye injuries occur annually, with 90,000 of these injuries resulting in some degree of disabling visual impairment.

DIAGNOSIS

Figure 14-1 presents a schematic overview of ocular injury diagnosis and initial management.

HISTORY

- Detailed description of the traumatic event
- Visual symptoms (level of vision, flashes, floaters, laterality, diplopia, pain, discharge)
- Previous ocular disease or surgery
- Blunt injury (nature of the offending object, the force, and the direction of impact)
- Penetrating injury (composition of a potentially retained foreign body)

EXAMINATION

Visual Acuity

- Test each eye independently
- Test with glasses correction if available
- Use standard eye chart or near-vision card if possible (if not available, use a newspaper, magazine, package label, or even an identification badge)
- If the patient cannot read print, record distance the patient can count fingers, see gross movements of the examiner's hands (hand motion), or perceive light

External Examination: Orbit and Eyelids

- Exophthalmos/enophthalmos
- Orbital rim step-off or subcutaneous emphysema (orbital floor fracture)
- Hypesthesia involving the cheek or upper lip (injury to the infraorbital nerve)
- Lid laceration involving either the margin of the lid or the lacrimal drainage system (canaliculi) located near the nasal aspect of the lid
- Eversion of the upper lids (foreign bodies embedded in the conjunctivae of the inner surface of the upper lids)

Pupils

- Size, shape, and reactivity
- Relative afferent pupillary defect (Marcus-Gunn pupil). The "swinging flashlight" test is performed by shifting a bright light back and forth from pupil to pupil while observing the initial pupillary response. A normal pupil will immediately constrict in response to the light, but an eye with a relative afferent pupillary defect (RAPD) will cause an initial dilation of the pupil when the light is swung from the fellow eye to the eye in question.

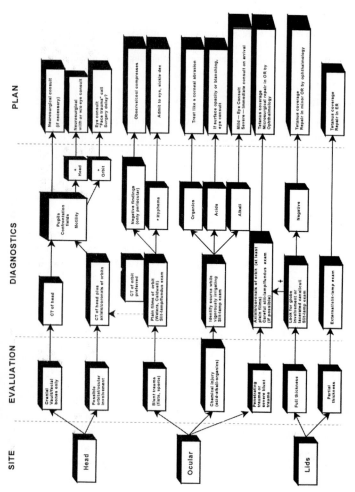

FIG. 14-1. Algorithm for diagnosis and treatment of ocular injuries. (+ head = positive CT of head; + orbit = positive CT of orbit; + hyphema = presence of hyphema; sickle dex = sickle cell preparation.)

Globe

- Position
- Rupture: stop examination and shield the eye. Clues to rupture include the following: Uveal prolapse (iris or ciliary body on the surface of the eye or protruding through a laceration); irregular or peaked pupil; excessively shallow or deep anterior chamber; hyphema (blood in the anterior chamber) or vitreous hemorrhage; suffused subconjunctival hemorrhage

Anterior Segment

- Sclera and conjunctiva: lacerations, subconjunctival hemorrhage
- Cornea: corneal abrasion or laceration; evaluate with fluorescein staining
- Depth and contents of the anterior chamber: hyphema, traumatic subluxation of the lens

Ophthalmoscopy

- Red reflex: decreased or absent with a media opacity (hyphema or vitreous hemorrhage), cataract, or large retinal detachment
- Optic nerve, blood vessels, and macula: swelling of optic nerve, retinal hemorrhages

Other Components of the Examination

- Intraocular pressure: do not check if suspicious for open globe
- Extraocular muscle function
- Confrontation visual fields

Diagnostic Testing

Radiography and Echography

- Orbital x-rays: orbital fractures and radiopaque intraorbital or intraocular foreign bodies.
- Computed tomography (CT): orbital fractures, globe rupture, presence and location of intraocular or intraorbital foreign bodies. Request axial and coronal views (may be reconstructed) of the orbits. If suspicious for intraocular foreign body (IOFB) request 1 to 1.5 mm cuts.
- Magnetic resonance imaging (MRI): contraindicated in the setting of trauma especially if a foreign body is suspected.
- Echography: detection and localization of foreign bodies and gross anatomy of intraocular tissues. Best performed by ophthalmic personnel to avoid globe pressure and manipulation.

Injuries to the Eye

Corneal Abrasion

Based on an appropriate history and diagnostic findings (corneal fluorescein uptake), a corneal abrasion can be treated in the emergency department. Non-contact lens-related traumatic corneal abrasions may be treated adequately with instillation of a topical cycloplegic agent (e.g., 5 percent homatropine) and topical antibiotic ointment (erythromycin or polysporin ophthalmic ointment) three times per day until the lesion is healed. Follow-up should include daily reexamination of the eye. In general, a clean, noninfected corneal abrasion will heal completely in 2 to 3 days, and long-term visual loss is rare.

Corneal Foreign Bodies

In the majority of cases, corneal foreign bodies are very superficially embedded and easily visible on slit-lamp examination. A moistened, sterile cotton swab may be rolled across the cornea in an attempt to loosen and remove the foreign body. If this is unsuccessful, ophthalmic consultation should be obtained. Following removal of the foreign body, the eye should be treated for the residual corneal abrasion (as noted previously).

Chemical Injuries

While both acids and alkalis are capable of causing significant damage to the eye, alkalis tend to cause the most severe injury. The primary treatment of any ocular chemical exposure is copious irrigation to minimize the concentration and contact time of the offending agent. Lavage should begin immediately in the field with tap water, saline, lactated Ringer's, or any commercially available irrigant with a neutral pH, and then continued in the emergency department. During irrigation, the lids should be held open and the stream of irrigating fluid directed into the superior and inferior conjunctival fornices in an attempt to wash away any particulate matter. Topical anesthesia will better facilitate irrigation. The fornices should be swept with moistened swabs in order to loosen and dislodge any retained particulate matter. An ophthalmologist should be called immediately unless the injury is clearly the result of a nonalkali, innocuous compound and the damage sustained is no more than a mild corneal abrasion. Irrigation should continue until the pH of the tear lake remains neutral (7.4) at least 5 minutes after cessation of active infusion of irrigant.

Severe chemical burns, most often the result of alkali exposure, require prolonged management that is directed at reducing ocular inflammation and ischemia, and toward detection and treatment of complications. It is important to remember that the outcome in such cases is often determined by the expediency with which the initial treatment is given.

Blunt Ocular Trauma

Severe concussive injury to the globe and orbit can produce damage to almost every ocular tissue. A concussive force striking the eye causes a shortening of the anteroposterior dimension and a compensatory increase in the circumference at the equator. This in turn can produce damage to the soft lining tissues of the globe (choroid, iris, ciliary body, retinal pigment epithelium, and retina), which are subjected to stretching vectors, in addition to causing fractures of the thin medial orbital wall and floor (blowout fractures).

Scleral rupture following severe blunt trauma may be difficult to clinically detect because intraocular or subconjunctival hemorrhage may obscure visualization of a wound. Some predictors of scleral rupture include an abnormally deep or shallow anterior chamber, peaked pupil, lowered intraocular pressure, severe ocular hemorrhage (intraocular or periocular), and media opacity preventing a view of the fundus. When a ruptured globe is suspected, a fox shield or other rigid device (such as a Styrofoam cup) should be placed over the eye, ophthalmology contacted, and further ocular manipulation avoided.

Orbital Fracture

Orbital fractures are a relatively common injury, usually involving either the thin inferior or medial (lamina papyracea) orbital walls, often sparing the orbital rim. Herniation of orbital tissue into the maxillary sinus or, less commonly, the ethmoid sinus may complicate a blowout fracture and cause muscle entrapment and/or contusion, or cranial nerve dysfunction, both of which result in clinical diplopia. Signs suggestive of orbital blowout fracture include crepitus, orbital emphysema, enophthalmos, restrictive or paretic extraocular muscle function, and hypesthesia in the distribution of the infraorbital nerve.

High-resolution CT is the modality of choice when investigating a potential orbital fracture. Both axial and coronal slices less than or equal to 1.5 mm in thickness through the entire orbit, optic canal, and cavernous sinus are recommended for optimal evaluation. Bone windows are especially useful to detect the more subtle fractures.

Orbital fractures are not considered an ophthalmic emergency unless visual impairment or globe injury has occurred. Indications for surgical repair of an isolated orbital wall fracture include persistent diplopia in primary gaze, enophthalmos greater than 2 mm, symptomatic restrictive entrapment of extraocular muscles, and greater than 50 percent disruption of the orbital floor as noted by CT imaging. Because most patients have significant soft tissue swelling concurrent with orbital wall fractures, most ophthalmic surgeons advocate observation for a minimum of 7 days, during which time most swelling will resolve.

Subconjunctival Hemorrhage

Although they are dramatic in appearance and often prompt patients to seek urgent medical attention, subconjunctival hemorrhages are most often benign. Typically, they are associated with Valsalva maneuvers or trauma, but may arise in the setting of severe hypertension and bleeding diatheses. Clinically, a subconjunctival hemorrhage appears as a flat, bright red area noted on the bulbar conjunctiva. Visual acuity is not affected, and the hemorrhage will resolve spontaneously in 2 to 4 weeks. If subconjunctival hemorrhage is associated with significant antecedent trauma and chemosis (edema of the conjunctiva) is present, the suspicion of more serious globe injury should be high and subsequently investigated.

Hyphema

Hyphema is the presence of blood in the anterior chamber of the eye. The overall treatment strategy for management of hyphemas is directed at reducing the chance for secondary hemorrhage (rebleed) and lowering intraocular pressure. Rebleeding into the anterior chamber usually occurs within 3 to 5 days. Metal-shield protection and bedrest with ambulation are essential mainstays of management. Even with such measures, rebleeds occur in 10 to 30 percent of cases and significantly complicate the management and worsen the overall prognosis of patients with hyphema.

Prolonged, elevated intraocular pressure is primarily responsible for the morbidity associated with hyphema. Patients with hyphema and concurrent sickle hemoglobinopathies (including trait) are at a particular risk for developing elevated intraocular pressure because sickled red blood cells do not easily clear from the anterior chamber. All susceptible patients should have a sickle cell preparation (sickle dex), followed by hemoglobin electrophoresis. Elevated intraocular pressure associated with hyphema is usually managed with topical beta blockers, carbonic anhydrase inhibitors, and osmotic agents. Carbonic anhydrase inhibitors, however, should not be used in those patients with sickle hemoglobinopathies as they aggravate red blood cell sickling in the anterior chamber, thus slowing the egress of blood from the eye by actually clogging the trabecular meshwork. Other frequently used medications for the management of acute, nonclotted hyphema include cycloplegics to reduce the possibility of synechiae formation and topical steroids for their anti-inflammatory effects. In the event of a persistently elevated intraocular pressure or early corneal blood staining, blood in the anterior chamber should be surgically removed.

Traumatic Iridocyclitis

Blunt trauma may result in irritation to the iris and ciliary body, which subsequently causes inflammation in the anterior chamber. Symptoms are often delayed and typically begin 24 to 48 hours following injury. Patients present with pain, photophobia, and blurred vision. Examination reveals a red eye (perilimbal injection); a small, poorly reactive pupil; and an inflammatory reaction in the anterior chamber. Treatment should include cycloplegic drops (homatropine 5 percent three times a day) and, in severe cases, steroid drops with close ophthalmology follow-up.

Injuries to the Lens

The lens is suspended behind the iris by zonular fibers that attach to the ciliary body. With blunt trauma, the zonules may break, resulting in a partially subluxed or completely dislocated lens. The edge of a dislocated lens may be visible following dilation of the pupil, while a totally dislocated lens may be seen in the anterior chamber or posteriorly on the retina. Typically, treatment is not emergent unless an anteriorly dislocated lens is causing corneal endothelial damage or obstructing aqueous outflow through the pupil, causing acute angle-closure glaucoma.

Trauma is the most common cause of unilateral cataract in young individuals. Traumatic cataracts may form acutely or develop over a period of weeks to months.

Retinal Tears and Detachment

Direct contusive injury to the globe may cause retinal breaks. Symptoms include a sudden "shower" of vitreous floaters, flashing lights, and visual field deficits. A fully dilated fundus exam is necessary to rule out peripheral retinal tears. If a retinal detachment is suspected, the patient should be positioned in order to prevent progression. Emergent consultation is indicated.

Retrobulbar Hemorrhage

Blunt trauma to the globe may also produce a retrobulbar hemorrhage. An orbital hematoma may cause proptosis, periorbital edema and ecchymoses, subconjunctival hemorrhage and chemosis, corneal edema (from raised intraocular pressure), disk edema, and rarely central retinal artery occlusion (from raised intraorbital pressure causing nerve and vascular compression). An orbital CT scan should be obtained to confirm the diagnosis; however, if there is visual loss, raised intraocular pressure, or a relative afferent pupillary defect in the presence of a tense orbit, the scan should be delayed until immediate therapy is instituted. Treatment with lateral canthotomy and cantholysis permits anterior displacement of the globe with acute orbital decompression. Following the cantholysis, the vision, intraocular pressure, and pupils are reassessed and followed closely. Lid and canthal repair may be required at a later time.

Traumatic Optic Neuropathy

Optic nerve injury may be divided into direct and indirect injuries. Direct injuries result from compression or laceration from bony fragments, foreign bodies, and hematoma; indirect injury results from contusion and disruption of vascular supply. Signs and symptoms of traumatic optic neuropathy include severely decreased vision with an afferent pupillary defect and poor color vision (test with a red bottle cap). Evaluation should include CT of the brain and orbits to study each segment of the optic nerve. Treatment may entail admission and high-dose intravenous steroids for indirect injury, and rarely surgical decompression for direct optic neuropathies.

Penetrating Trauma

Corneoscleral Lacerations

While less common than contusion, penetrating injuries may also result in severe visual impairment. Penetrating injury refers to a wound through the eye wall into the globe; perforation implies the presence of both an entrance and exit wound.

Signs and symptoms of penetrating injury include an appropriate history (e.g., high-velocity foreign body), shallow anterior chamber, leakage of clear fluid from the wound, lower intraocular pressure and exposed uveal tissue (iris or ciliary body) with or without a teardrop-shaped or eccentric pupil. A CT scan with axial and direct coronal views may aid in the diagnosis. Once the diagnosis of a penetrating ocular injury is made, further manipulation should be deferred until the time of surgical repair. A fox shield should be placed over the eye while ophthalmology is contacted.

The prognosis is related to a number of factors, including initial presenting visual acuity, type and extent of injury, presence or absence of retinal detachment, and presence or absence of intraocular foreign body. In general, the more posterior the penetration and the larger the laceration or rupture, the worse will be the prognosis.

Intraocular Foreign Body

When penetrating ocular injuries are associated with intraocular foreign bodies (IOFBs), the composition of the foreign body should be identified because it may influence treatment decisions. In the absence of infection, inert, sterile foreign bodies (e.g., stone, glass, stainless steel, porcelain, plastic, and sand) may be left in place if not obstructing vision. On the other hand, iron, copper, lead, aluminum, and zinc may cause an inflammatory response and require removal. If any instrument such as a knife or wire is still impaled in the eye or orbit, it should not be removed until surgery. Injury with organic or vegetable foreign matter (e.g., branches, wood) carries a higher risk of infection and mandates removal.

If the possibility of an IOFB exists, plain films, CT scans, and ultrasonography may facilitate localization. If an IOFB is suspected, broad-spectrum intravenous antibiotics should be initiated prophylactically. Traumatic endophthalmitis associated with *Bacillus cereus* infection (soil-contaminated injuries) has a rapid and severe course which often requires the addition of intravitreal antibiotics. With prompt recognition and improved intraocular surgical techniques, the prognosis for penetrating ocular injuries has greatly improved.

Lid Lacerations and Ocular Adnexa

Lid lacerations may be divided into three groups: (1) nonmarginal, (2) marginal, and (3) canalicular.

Nonmarginal lid lacerations that involve only the superficial skin and do not violate the orbital septum may be closed primarily in the emergency department. Those that involve deeper tissues with or without fat prolapse (a clinical indication of penetration of the orbital septum), the canalicular system, or other major ocular adnexa such as the medial or lateral canthal tendon should be referred to ophthalmology.

Those lesions involving the lid margin should be closed by the ophthalmology service in order to obtain proper lid margin alignment and prevent notching. Any laceration involving the medial third of the lid, near the medial canthus, is likely to cause damage to the lacrimal outflow system. These should be referred to ophthalmology because they often require careful reapproximation of the canaliculi and prolonged intubation with silicone tubes to prevent epiphora.

Surgical delay with cool saline compresses may reduce swelling, facilitating proper anatomic repair. When a full-thickness lid laceration is present, the integrity of the globe must be carefully assessed. Regardless, shield the globe and use aggressive lubrication in the presence of marginal lacerations or avulsions.

ADDITIONAL READING

Hutton WL, Fuller DG: Factors influencing final visual results in severely injured eye. *Am J Ophthalmol* 97:715, 1984.

Trauma, section XV, in Albert DM and Jakobiec FA (eds): *Principles and Practice of Ophthalmology.* Philadelphia, WB Saunders, 1994, pp 3359–3502.

Blunt trauma, vol. (3)31, in Tasman W (ed): *Duane's Clinical Ophthalmology,* Philadelphia, Lippincott, Williams and Wilkins, 2000, pp 1–14.

Penetrating trauma—anterior segment, vol. (6)39, in Tasman W (ed): *Duane's Clinical Ophthalmology,* Philadelphia, Lippincott, Williams and Wilkins, 2000, pp 1–13.

Posterior segment, vol. (6)66, in Tasman W (ed): *Duane's Clinical Ophthalmology,* Philadelphia, Lippincott, Williams and Wilkins, 2000, pp 1–21.

Trauma, in Jakobiec FA, Navon SE, Rubin PAD (eds): *Int Ophthalmol Clin,* Boston, Little, Brown and Company, 35(1), Winter 1995.

Linden J, Renner G: Trauma to the globe. *Emerg Med Clin North Am* 13:581, 1995.

Thomas MA, Parrish RK, Fener WJ: Rebleeding after traumatic hyphema. *Arch Ophthalmol* 104:206, 1986.

Zagelbaum BM, Tostenoski JR: Urban eye trauma: A one year prospective study. *Ophthalmology* 100:851, 1993.

15 | Facial Trauma

INITIAL ASSESSMENT

Although often dramatic in appearance, maxillofacial injuries of themselves are seldom life threatening, Most patients with facial injuries, however, also have significant associated injuries or medical problems that require immediate attention. Foremost among these are airway obstruction, head and/or cervical spine injury, and hemorrhage.

Early death can result from airway obstruction and is most likely to occur with multiple mandibular fractures or combined maxillary, mandibular, and nasal fractures. Soft-tissue swelling around injured oronasal structures, especially when combined with unconsciousness, can result in a catastrophic loss of airway patency and the rapid demise of the patient. Nasal intubation, whether nasotracheal or nasogastric, may be contraindicated because of midfacial instability and the possibility of the tube being inadvertently forced through the fractured base of the cranium and into the brain. Likewise, swelling and hemorrhage within the hypopharynx may make endotracheal intubation impossible. Under these circumstances, a surgical airway may have to be created to prevent death by asphyxiation.

All trauma patients should be considered to have cervical spine instability until the cervical spine is cleared by physical or radiographic examination. If one cannot demonstrate normality of the entire cervical spine, the patient must be treated as if a cervical fracture exists.

Profuse bleeding through the nares may occur with nasal fractures, maxillary fractures, and cranial base fractures. Emergent placement of nasal packing both anteriorly and posteriorly be required. Full-thickness lacerations of the scalp can cause life-threatening bleeding if not controlled. These can often be controlled quickly and easily by surgical stapling of the skin. Serious tongue lacerations may also cause profuse bleeding and compromise the airway in an obtunded patient. Access and exposure are the most difficult obstacles for these injuries. These can be overcome by placing a bite block between the teeth at the corner of the mouth and using a towel clip or large stitch to secure the tongue and provide traction. Once exposed, the lingual artery can be ligated easily.

Other injuries that, though not life threatening are surgical emergencies, include globe injuries, severe avulsion injuries, and septal hematoma. Ophthalmologic consultation should be obtained immediately for any concerns of globe rupture. Severe scalp, ear, or nasal avulsion-type injuries for which there is a possibility of replant or replacement grafting should be referred immediately to a plastic surgeon. Any completely amputated parts should be kept cold in an iced saline bath. Direct contact with ice should be avoided to prevent burn. Exposed areas of cartilage or bone should not be allowed to become desiccated.

All nasal injuries should have complete nasal speculum examinations to rule out a septal hematoma, which is an emergency and should be treated immediately. Hematomas in this location can expand to produce airway occlusion and can cause pressure necrosis of the septal cartilage. Late consequences of severe septal necrosis may include saddle-nose deformity or nasal obstruction. Treatment is by immediate drainage with a single incision through the nasal mucosa in a dependent position.

DIAGNOSIS

During the initial trauma survey, the diagnosis of facial fractures can be achieved by a rapid and focused examination. If the patient is able to cooperate, ask him or her to follow a penlight that is moved through the cardinal fields of gaze and observe globe movement from the extraocular muscles. Entrapment of the inferior ocular muscles can occur with orbital floor (blowout) fractures, which will limit motion. Visual acuity should routinely be checked.

Palpation of the orbital rims, nose, and upper and lower jaws should be performed, checking for bony step-offs and instability. The midface as well should be assessed for instability, by placing a finger in the mouth and grasping the upper jaw. Ask the patient if the teeth fit together normally when he or she bites down. If there is subjective malocclusion, the presence of a jaw fracture is likely.

A neurologic exam of cranial nerves V and VII should be performed. Zygomatic fractures are associated with infraorbital nerve damage. Decreased sensation of the cheek, side of the nose, upper lip, and upper teeth is frequently seen with these injuries. The frontal branch of the facial nerve courses in a superficial plane and is vulnerable with lacerations in the temporal area and over the zygomatic arch. Inability to raise the brow on the affected side and the lack of forehead wrinkles are seen on examination of the conscious patient. Fractures through the temporal bone can cause injury to the facial nerve as it runs through the bony facial canal, and is associated with hemifacial paralysis.

Deep lacerations of the cheek may transect the parotid duct. When this is suspected, the diagnosis is made by placing a probe or Silastic tubing through Stinson's duct intraorally. If the duct is lacerated, the probe may pass out through the cheek wound. Irrigation through the cannula may demonstrate the injury in occult cases.

RADIOGRAPHIC STUDIES

In the patient with an exam consistent with facial fractures, both axial and coronal CT scans should be routinely performed. A panographic x-ray of the mandible is extremely helpful for visualizing the body, ramus, angle, and condylar areas.

TREATMENT

Early soft-tissue management of facial injuries consists of sharp debridement of ragged edges or devitalized tissue and meticulous, layered closure. Care must be taken to precisely align borders of anatomic structures such as the eyebrow, the vermilion border of the lip, and the nostril. Parotid duct and lacrimal canalicular injuries must be suspected with lacerations in the vicinity and repaired immediately. Skin should be closed with fine (6-0) monofilament sutures. Antibiotics are usually administered because of the contaminated nature of these injuries. A first-generation cephalosporin is adequate for skin and scalp injuries. Gentamicin should be added for severely contaminated wounds, and penicillin should be used when there is intraoral involvement.

Figure 15-1 shows an algorithm for management of facial injuries.

MANAGEMENT OF SPECIFIC INJURIES

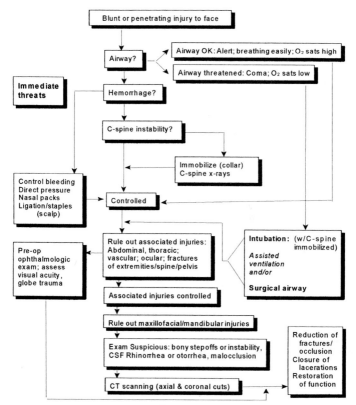

FIG. 15-1   Algorithm for management of facial injuries.

GENERAL PRINCIPLES IN THE MANAGEMENT OF FACIAL FRACTURES

Fracture reduction should be carried out as soon as possible after injury. Often in multiply injured patients, other medical issues such as brain injury or cervical spine fracture precludes a long anesthetic or manipulation of the head. Open reduction and external fixation should be scheduled when it can be safely performed (Table 15-1).

Maxilo-Mandibular Fixation (MMF)

One of the prime requirements in the successful management of facial fractures is the reestablishment of effective occlusion of the teeth in any fracture involving the occlusal plane.

Arch bars are wired to the stable teeth using the molars to provide strength. Once firmly attached to the upper and lower jaws, the bars can be wired together to achieve alignment and stabilization. Alternatively, two MMF

TABLE 15-1 Surgical Approaches to Facial Fractures

Fracture	Incision
Frontal	Coronal; through existing forehead lacerations
Nasal	Closed reduction
Nasal (complex)/ nasoethmoid	Coronal; existing glabellar lacerations; lateral nasal
Orbit	Transconjunctival; subciliary
Lateral orbit	Lateral brow; coronal
Maxilla	Upper buccal sulcus
Zygomatic arch—simple	Temporal (Gillies)
Zygomatic arch—complex	Coronal
Mandible—body, parasymphyseal	Lower buccal sulcus
Mandible—angle	Intraoral
Mandible—condylar	Preauricular

screws can be placed in each jaw and wires or rubber bands attached to the screw heads for stabilization. This is a much quicker method of obtaining MMF and is useful in patients with simple (noncomminuted) ascending ramus fractures or isolated, simple parasymphyseal fractures. Following this preliminary and indispensable step, the underlying fractures are exposed and realignment accomplished.

Zygoma

Most zygoma fractures are associated with a direct impact on the cheek. The force drives the bone posteriorly and medially. The zygomaticomaxillary buttress and inferior orbital rim are fractured, and the energy is transmitted to the floor of the orbit. This type of fracture can be managed by approaching the zygoma through a ciliary or transconjunctival incision, a lateral brow incision, and a gingivobuccal sulcus incision. Subperiosteal dissection is used to visualize the fractures of the inferior orbital rim, lateral orbit, maxilla, and zygomaticomaxillary buttresses. The orbital floor is in most instances routinely explored. Significant orbital floor defects require repair to restore the normal orbital volume and prevent enophthalmos.

It is of utmost importance to reestablish the normal cheekbone projection of the zygoma in relation to the base of the cranium and the opposite zygoma. The normal articulations of the zygoma with the frontal bone and maxilla are established at the lateral and inferior orbital rims, respectively. At the same time, the lateral structural pillar (the zygomaticomaxillary buttress) is precisely aligned, and all three articulations are secured with microplates for the orbital rims and a miniplate for the lateral maxillary buttress.

If a fracture of the zygomatic arch cannot be reduced, a coronal incision may be needed to expose the arch, reduce the fracture, and stabilize the arch with a microplate. Alternatively, the endoscope may be utilized to gain access to a difficult arch fracture without the need for a coronal incision.

Nasoethmoidal/Orbital Region

The nasoethmoidal/orbital fracture usually involves the lower portions of the medial orbital rim and may also result in displacement of the medial canthal ligaments. It is of utmost importance to accurately diagnose involvement of the medial canthal ligaments because this area is exceedingly difficult to reconstruct at a later time. The medial canthal ligaments maintain the almond shape of the palpebral fissure of the eye and have important roles with regard to facial symmetry, eyelid appearance, and lacrimal function.

If the medial canthal tendon is detached or attached to an unstable, free-floating piece of bone, exposure of the nasal root and medial orbital area will be required, usually by a coronal incision. Alternatively, existing lacerations over the glabella or lateral nasal incisions can be used.

Treatment of such fractures requires the use of wire sutures passed directly into the canthal tendon and reinsertion of the canthal tendon through a transnasal wiring technique. Occasionally, the tendon insertion remains attached to a large enough segment of bone that adequate bony reduction and fixation will pull the canthal tendon into the correct position without the need for a transnasal wire suture. Restoration of the margin of the medial orbital rim and canthal support system with autogenous bone grafts may also be necessary in high-energy fractures.

Such midfacial fractures may also be telescoped posteriorly and impacted on the cranial base. Fractures of this type require the use of vigorous disimpaction techniques with specially constructed forceps (Rowe/Killey forceps) in order to reestablish midfacial projection. Following this maneuver, dental occlusion is reestablished through intermaxillary fixation with arch bars and rubber bands. The fractures are then exposed, reduced, and stabilized as noted above.

Nasal Fractures

Nasal fractures can sometimes be managed by closed reduction and the application of a nasal splint. More extensive injuries that demonstrate telescoping or a saddle-nose deformity usually involve both nasal bones. In these cases, the nasal bones require disimpaction and reduction of fracture. Once aligned, internal packing and external splinting is done. If there is extensive telescoping of the nasal bones or comminution that results in extensive fragmentation, bone grafting may be required.

Orbit

Direct force over the globe can cause fracture of the orbital floor as the orbital contents "blow-out" this thin bone into the air-filled maxillary sinus below. This blow-out fracture becomes problematic when large defects increase the orbital volume. This allows the globe to drop down and back, resulting in enophthalmos and dystopia. Diplopia may develop. Smaller defects or trap-door type fractures can cause entrapment of orbital fat and of the inferior or medial rectus muscles. Limitation of ocular motion is seen clinically. Entrapment mandates surgical release.

Orbital floor defects are approached by ciliary or transconjunctival incisions. Floor reconstruction is accomplished with autogenous bone graft, titanium mesh, or other alloplastic implants.

Alveolar Ridge/Palate

Segmental tooth-bearing fragments of the maxilla should be reduced and stabilized with interdental wiring and placement of an arch bar and/or acrylic splint. Depending on the size of the fragment, it may be appropriate to employ plates and screws. Such fractures may also involve the hard palate.

Such fractures should be precisely reduced and plated through an intraoral approach, which may be supplemented with the application of a transverse plate across the lower pyriform aperture. Avulsed teeth should be replanted into the empty sockets and stabilized with arch bars.

Mandibular Fractures

Fractures of the mandible are most often low- or intermediate-energy fractures. Low-energy fractures usually require MMF with arch bars, local exposure using intraoral incisions, and small plate fixation. MMF may not be required postfixation. High-energy mandibular fractures may be segmental and often involve the symphysis or parasymphyseal areas. They usually require multiple intraoral approaches and open reduction of fractures using large reconstruction plates. Preauricular incisions may be used for reduction of fractures involving the ramus, condyle, and/or subcondylar regions. MMF is generally maintained for stabilization of complex mandibular fractures.

Older methods of close reduction and 6 weeks of intermaxillary fixation have largely been replaced by open reduction and internal fixation, using either rigid fixation with compression plates or semirigid fixation with miniplates. Intraoral incisions are used whenever possible; skin incisions may be needed in severely comminuted or infected cases, especially in the region of the angle.

Frontal Sinus

Fractures that cause obstruction of the nasofrontal drainage system of the frontal sinus and extensive comminution of the anterior table may require exenteration of the frontal sinus in order to prevent recurrent suppurative and obstructive sinusitis. This is accomplished by removing the lining of the frontal sinus through an anterior approach, sealing off the nasofrontal duct with bone, fat, or dermal graft, and returning the anterior table to its precise position. The anterior table can be secured with microplates for stability.

Le Fort Fractures

Although René Le Fort identified certain patterns of fracture in a series of cadaver experiments, such classic patterns rarely occur clinically as isolated findings. The classification, however, remains useful as a descriptive tool (Table 15-2).

The Le Fort I separates the maxilla from the face and skull by a fracture line passing horizontally across the upper jaw and into the pyriform aperture. The Le Fort II (nasomaxillary fracture) crosses the maxilla and extends through the inferior and medial orbital walls and across the nasal root, separating the nasomaxillary complex from the upper face and skull. The Le Fort III (true craniofacial separation) fractures across the zygomatic arches and the lateral and medial orbits, connecting along the inferior orbits below the optic nerves, joining in the midline at the nasal root. All of the Le Fort fractures extend posteriorly through the pterygoid plates. These fractures may be present unilaterally or bilaterally or in combination in panfacial fractures.

GENERAL COMMENTS ON POSTOPERATIVE CARE

Antibacterial ointment is usually the only dressing applied to facial wounds. Antibacterial mouthwash is used with any intraoral incision. Facial sutures should be removed within 5 days.

TABLE 15-2 Le Fort Fractures

I Maxillary fracture	
II Nasomaxillary fracture	
III Craniofacial separation	

Hardware used for fixation of fractures can be left in place permanently, and no special postoperative care is needed. Titanium plates do not require removal unless they cause local problems, such as exposure or infection.

ADDITIONAL READING

Evans GR, Clark N, Manson PN, et al: Role of mini- and microplate fixation in fractures of the midface and mandible. *Ann Plast Surg* 34:453, 1995.

Gruss JS, Bubak PJ, Egbert MA: Craniofacial fractures and algorithm to optimize results. *Clin Plast Surg* 19:195, 1992.

Manson PN, Clifford CM, Su CT, et al: Mechanisms of global support and post-traumatic enophthalmos: 1. The anatomy of the ligament sling and its relation to intramuscular cone orbital fat. *Plast Reconstr Surg* 77:193, 1985.

Manson PN, Hoopes JE, Su CT: Structural pillars of the facial skeleton: An approach to the management of LeFort fractures. *Plast Reconst Surg* 66:54, 1980.

Markowitz BL, Manson PN, Sargent L, et al: Management of the medial canthal tendon in nasoethmoid orbital fractures: The importance of the central fragment in classification and management. *Plast Reconstr Surg* 87:843, 1991.

McDonald WS, Thaller SR: Priorities in the treatment of facial fractures for the millennium. *J Craniofacial Surg* 11:97, 2000.

16 | Neck Trauma

PENETRATING NECK TRAUMA

Significant debate continues to surround several aspects of the management of penetrating neck injuries, including the following:

- Should the mechanism of injury dictate the specific management approach?
- The diminishing role of selective management and the emerging expectant management paradigm: Has the pendulum swung too far?
- If selective management is chosen, what are the essential diagnostic modalities required for optimal evaluation?

Anatomy

There are very few anatomic regions of the body that have as many vital organs as the neck. Almost every major vital system, including respiratory, vascular, digestive, endocrine, and neurologic organs, is represented. Expert knowledge of the anatomy is essential to the optimal management of penetrating neck trauma. The platysma muscle is enclosed in superficial fascia, a thin layer of connective tissue, and it is the anatomic landmark that is most often cited when determining whether a penetrating neck wound is superficial or deep, and whether operative or selective management should be considered. There is a deep cervical fascia, which is subdivided into investing, pretracheal, and prevertebral tissue layers. The investing layer envelops many neck structures, including the sternocleidomastoid and trapezius muscles. The pretracheal layer extends into the thoracic cavity and blends with the endothoracic and mediastinal fascia. This fascial layer also envelops the thyroid and binds it to the larynx. The prevertebral layer encompasses the prevertebral muscles, including the scalenus anterior, scalenus medius, longus capitis, longus cervicis, levator scapulae, and splenius capitis. The axillary sheath, which surrounds the subclavian artery, is an extension of the prevertebral layer. The three layers of the deep cervical fascia form the carotid sheath. This tight fascial matrix provides a natural tamponade effect in case of vascular injuries. In a small, enclosed space, this effect can result in extrinsic compression of the airway and subsequent obstruction.

There are three anatomic zones of the neck that are important in the management of penetrating cervical injuries (Fig. 16-1). Zone I is the horizontal area between the clavicles and the cricoid cartilage that encompasses the thoracic outlet vasculature, along with the vertebral and proximal carotid arteries, the lung, trachea, esophagus, spinal cord, thoracic duct, and major cervical nerve trunks. Zone II is the area between the cricoid cartilage and the angle of the mandible. The jugular veins, vertebral and common carotid arteries, and external and internal branches of the carotid are located in this zone. The trachea, esophagus, spinal cord, and larynx also pass through this area. Zone III, the most cephalad area, lies between the angle of the mandible and the base of the skull. The pharynx is located in this zone, along with the jugular veins, vertebral arteries, and the distal internal carotid arteries. Unlike zones I and III, the central neck area (zone II) can be accessed expeditiously should an injury necessitate operative intervention. Injuries in zone I might require a clavicle resection or median sternotomy for exposure, while exposure of zone III might necessitate disarticulation of the mandible or resection of the base of the skull.

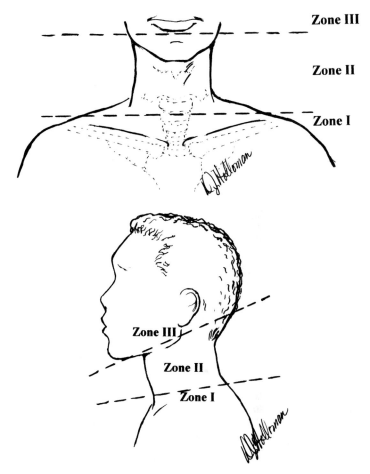

FIG. 16-1. Anatomic zones of the neck. Top: Anterior view. Bottom: Lateral view.

Evaluation

Initial evaluation and management of a patient with penetrating neck trauma is the same as with any other injury. The Advanced Trauma Life Support (ATLS)–directed primary survey, with its mandatory emphasis on the ABCDEs (airway, breathing, circulation, disability, environment/exposure), resuscitative efforts, and secondary survey, are all imperative in the optimal management of penetrating neck injuries. Expeditious airway management is the top priority. A definitive airway, such as a translaryngeal endotracheal intubation, should be performed to establish a secure airway in the patient who has sustained penetrating neck injuries and has a compromised airway. If a translaryngeal airway cannot be established, a surgical airway should be established. For most situations, a cricothyroidotomy would be the surgical

airway of choice; however, expeditious intubation of a tracheotomy site created by a penetrating neck injury may be a life-saving procedure in some circumstances. Depending on the object and the trajectory, pleural space entry is
a possibility with penetrating neck injuries. Life-threatening complications,
such as pneumothorax, hemothorax, or a tension pneumothorax, can be associated with penetrating neck injuries, necessitating prompt recognition and
pleural space decompression. Circulatory assessment and stabilization are
required after appropriate airway and ventilatory management. Significant
bleeding at the wound site should be managed by application of direct pressure. At no time should blind clamping, a tourniquet, or pressure dressing be
applied. These lifesaving measures can all be done simultaneously.

With respect to the mechanism of injury, penetrating neck trauma is most
commonly a result of stabbing and gunshot wounds (characteristically, stab
wounds cause less-severe injuries than neck wounds sustained from missile
injuries). There is a greater negative exploration rate for stab wounds as compared to firearm injuries. With a gunshot wound, the amount of kinetic energy
($K = MV^2/2$) generated and dissipated in the tissue is an important factor in
determining the morbidity and mortality of the injury, and unlike a stab wound
it has an unpredictable trajectory. Some knowledge of projectile ballistics is
crucial in the planning of the diagnostic and management strategies. For example, missiles from high-powered rifles attain a velocity that results in generation
of 60 times more energy than missiles from handguns. This difference accounts
for the overwhelming mortality from high-velocity injuries compared to that of
low-velocity handgun wounds. Injuries can also be sustained from multiple
projectiles, as is often seen with shotgun blasts. These are usually low-velocity
missiles, primarily pellets. The severity of the wound is determined by several
factors, including the distance between weapon and victim, weapon type, choke
setting, and the type of shot (birdshot or buckshot). A high-velocity type injury
can be sustained when a shotgun is fired at close range.

After ensuring an adequate airway, appropriate ventilation, hemodynamic
stability, and cervical spine stabilization, the surgeon should conduct a
detailed and systematic physical examination. Although the focus should be
on the entire neck, thorough examinations of the head, chest, and upper
extremities are important because of the close proximity of these areas.
Attention should be directed toward the entrance and possible exit site(s) of
the neck injury. A firm rule is that neck wound(s) should not be probed or
locally explored in the emergency department because of the possibility of
dislodging a clot and causing uncontrollable bleeding. Signs and symptoms
consistent with damage to the vital structures of the neck may be subtle or
quite obvious (Table 16-1). Subcutaneous emphysema, stridor, dysphonia,
hemoptysis, and pneumomediastinum are consistent with respiratory damage.
A digestive tract injury should be considered when dysphagia, crepitation,
retropharyngeal air, or pneumomediastinum is present. If persistent bleeding,
hypotension, pulse deficit, hematoma, bruit, or neurologic deficit is present, a
vascular injury should be suspected.

Diagnostic studies are often needed in the evaluation of penetrating neck
injuries. The specific study needed is dependent on the mechanism and location of injury. However, patients with hemodynamic lability, rapidly
expanding cervical hematomas, or uncontrollable bleeding require expeditious operative intervention, and supercede the need for any diagnostic study.
In a hemodynamically stable patient with a penetrating neck injury, there is a
variety of diagnostic modalities that may be helpful in determining the indi-

TABLE 16-1 Clinical Findings Consistent with Significant Injury in Cervical Neck Injuries

Active external bleeding from the wound
Neck bruit (or thrill)
Dysphagia
Hoarseness
Subcutaneous emphysema
Large, expanding, or pulsatile hematoma
Oropharyngeal bleeding
Sucking neck wound
Neurologic deficit

cation for surgery and the specific operative approach that may be required (Table 16-2).

Management and Ongoing Controversies

Although not universally accepted, many surgeons would endorse performing neck exploration in those patients who present with findings consistent with injury to a vital structure (see Table 16-1). There is little if any controversy about the need for immediate exploration in patients who present with hemodynamic lability, exsanguinating hemorrhage, an expanding or pulsatile hematoma, air-bubbling wound, or stridor. A more selective approach is taken for zones I and III because of the inherent difficulty in examining and operatively exposing these areas.

The main controversy centers on those patients who present hemodynamically stable, with penetrating neck wounds in zone II and no findings suggestive of injury to a vital structure. While many factors must be considered and each case should be individualized, there is an ongoing debate over how this subset of patients should be managed. There are two main schools of thought for treating penetrating zone II injuries: (1) mandatory operative intervention for any injury that penetrates the platysma, and (2) selective management that involves panendoscopy (laryngoscopy/tracheoscopy/bronchoscopy and esophagoscopy), esophagography, and arteriography. With selective management, a neck exploration is performed only if a vital structure is noted to be injured. Of greatest concern are the esophagus and carotid arteries, where an overlooked injury can lead to catastrophic results.

Because of a relatively high negative exploration rate, over the last decade mandatory exploration has lost widespread support. Many surgeons have adopted a more selective approach for this subset of patients. Selective management has the advantage of necessitating fewer nontherapeutic explorations and results in no surgical scar. It is the approach of choice in most tertiary medical centers. There is an emerging camp that has challenged the necessity

TABLE 16-2 Diagnostic Modalities Used in Selective Management

Arteriography
Doppler studies
Laryngoscopy
Bronchoscopy
Esophagoscopy
Esophagography
Computed tomography

of various diagnostic modalities used in selective management. Alteberry and colleagues have advocated a strictly nondiagnostic and nonoperative approach for zone II penetrating injuries when there is no "hard clinical finding" of a vascular injury. Even though some of the preliminary data from Alteberry and colleagues are encouraging, this expectant management scheme in which no diagnostic modalities are utilized should be cautiously examined. Under no circumstances should a high-velocity missile wound be managed nonoperatively in the viable patient. Close-range shotgun blasts can cause significant tissue destruction and should be managed similarly to a high-velocity missile injury. Figure 16-2 offers some guidance in the management of penetrating neck injuries.

Operative Approach

Operative exposure of zone I injuries may necessitate a supraclavicular incision, with removal of the head of the clavicle or a median sternotomy.

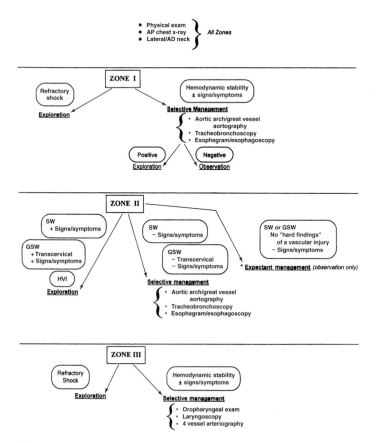

FIG. 16-2. Management guidelines for penetrating neck injuries. GSW = gunshot wound; SW = stab wound; HVI = high-velocity injury. *Controversial.

Optimal exposure of zone III injuries may necessitate cephalad extension of the incision at the anterior border of the sternocleidomastoid muscle and possible disarticulation or partial resection of the mandible or craniotomy. For most penetrating zone II injuries that require operative intervention, an incision at the anterior border of the sternocleidomastoid muscle is the approach of choice. If there is suspicion or evidence that the projectile has traversed the cervical region, a collar incision might provide adequate access to both the left and right neck, therefore obviating the need for bilateral neck incision. Either incision can be expeditiously extended into the chest should a sternotomy be required for better exposure and vascular control.

SUMMARY

Although the definitive management of penetrating and blunt neck trauma continues to be debated, the basic principles are well highlighted in the algorithm in Fig. 16-2. The resounding admonition should always be that having the occasional success with a certain novel approach does not make it an acceptable protocol. Outcome analysis in a tertiary setting should be done for all unproven management paradigms.

ADDITIONAL READINGS

Alteberry LR, Dennis JW, Menawalt SS, et al: Physical examination alone is safe and accurate for evaluation of vascular injuries in penetrating zone II neck trauma. *J Am Coll Surg* 179:657, 1994.

Bishara RA, Pasch AR, Douglas DD, et al: The necessity of mandatory exploration of penetrating zone II neck injuries. *Surgery* 100:655, 1986.

Demetriades D, Theodorou D, Cornwell E: Penetrating injuries of the neck in patients in stable condition. *Arch Surg* 130:971, 1995.

Golueke PJ, Goldstein AS, Sclafani SJA, et al: Routine versus selective exploration of penetrating neck injuries: A randomized prospective study. *J Trauma* 24:1010, 1987.

Wood J, Fabian TC, Mangianate EC: Penetrating neck injuries: Recommendations for selective management. *J Trauma* 25:819, 1985.

Injury to the Vertebrae and Spinal Cord

EPIDEMIOLOGY

In the United States the incidence of spinal cord injuries is estimated to be 28 to 50 per million population, or 8000 to 10,000 injuries per year. More than two-thirds of spinal cord injuries occur in those younger than 40 years of age, and 75 percent are male. In adults, cord injuries are most often the result of motor vehicle crashes (40 percent), falls (20 percent), and gunshot wounds (14 percent). In children the most common causes are motor vehicle crashes (39 to 52 percent) and sports (20 percent). For those older than 65 years, falls account for 53 percent of spinal cord injuries. In the population as a whole, 25 percent of spinal cord injuries are related to alcohol or other illicit drug use. The most common level of spinal cord injury is cervical (55 percent), with thoracic injuries accounting for 30 percent and lumbar injuries for 15 percent. Eighty percent of spinal cord injuries occur in victims of multiple trauma. Approximately 45 percent of spinal cord injuries are complete, defined as a total loss of sensory and motor function below the level of the injury. The mortality from spinal cord injuries ranges from 2 to 16 times greater than that from other injuries, with most deaths occurring in the first 24 hours after injury. The average length of stay in the intensive care unit is 1 week, and the average length of acute care hospitalization ranges from 2 to 4 weeks. The overall economic burden of spinal cord injury on the federal government is estimated to be 4 to 5.6 billion dollars annually, and the average direct costs for hospitalization and home modification are in excess of $100,000 per patient. Lifetime costs for paraplegic individuals who are 35 years of age at the time of injury exceed $500,000, and for quadriplegic individuals is at least twice that amount.

PATHOGENESIS

Neurologic disability resulting from injury to the spine is a result of mechanical deformation of the vertebrae, the ligaments that stabilize the vertebrae, and the spinal cord itself. While most of this damage usually occurs at the time of the initial trauma, failure to recognize and/or protect the unstable spine early after injury also can cause or worsen spinal cord injury. Several physiologic and molecular abnormalities that are initiated by trauma can cause secondary spinal cord injury, and this secondary injury is thought by some to significantly contribute to the ultimate neurologic disability. Laboratory and clinical research is focused on identifying the most important molecular intermediates of secondary spinal cord injury, and identifying and testing therapies that effectively limit the toxicity of those intermediates. During the past several years laboratory investigations have identified lipid peroxidation as an important intermediate of secondary injury, and high doses of methylprednisolone as an effective treatment. Subsequent multicenter clinical trials found that early treatment with this drug improved neurologic outcomes. Preclinical studies have also suggested an important role of hypoperfusion of the damaged cord as well as excess levels of excitatory amino acids, intracellular calcium, and endogenous opioids. To date, however, clinical trials of therapies aimed at treating these abnormalities (e.g., naloxone, GM I ganglioside) have not demonstrated their efficacy.

Clinical instability describes the loss of the spine's ability to maintain segmental alignment under physiologic loads so as to prevent spinal cord injury.

The clinical recognition of instability is simplified by dividing the spine into several distinct biomechanical columns. A commonly used three-column model divides the spine into the anterior longitudinal ligament and anterior two-thirds of the vertebral body, the posterior third of the body and posterior longitudinal ligament, and the remaining posterior elements. Injury to any two or all three columns produces instability. In addition, limits of normal motion in various segments of the spinal column are known, and motion exceeding those limits is considered to indicate instability (Table 17-1).

CLASSIFICATION OF INJURIES

The most basic classification of spinal cord injuries differentiates between partial and complete loss of function at a given level. A complete injury is defined as total loss of sensory and voluntary motor function below the level of injury and persisting for more than 48 hours. Anatomic continuity of the cord is usually preserved. If the injury is above T6, autonomic nervous function also may be lost, resulting in peripheral vasodilation, hypotension, and bradycardia (spinal shock). If there is some preservation of sensation or voluntary motor function three or more segments below the level of the spinal cord lesion, the injury is referred to as incomplete, and prognosis for some recovery is much better. In older individuals with preexisting degenerative spinal stenosis, relatively mild trauma to the cervical spine can cause two unique injury syndromes: the anterior cord syndrome, characterized by a loss of corticospinal and spinothalamic pathways and preservation of dorsal column function and resulting in motor weakness and diminished pain and temperature sensation below the level of the lesion, with preservation of vibratory and joint position sense; and the central cord syndrome, which results from damage to the centrally located fibers that control upper limb motor and sensory functions. Sensation and strength in the hands and arms are diminished but lower limb function is preserved. Bowel and bladder function often is impaired. In cases of penetrating spine injuries in which there is damage to the sagittal half of the cord, motor, proprioceptive, and vibratory functions on the side of the lesion and pain and temperature sensation on the side opposite the lesion may be lost, and this finding is referred to as the Brown-Sequard syndrome. Damage to the vertebrae or ligaments also can injure individual nerve roots as they exit the neural foramina, causing radiculopathies (motor and sensory deficits) specific to that nerve root.

Injuries to the structural elements of the spine can be classified by the distinct regions of the spine in which they occur, as well as by the nature of the

TABLE 17-1 Normal Motion and Relationships Between Vertebrae

Segment of spine	Normal motion or relationship
Occiput-C1	Axial rotation <9°
C1–C2	Axial rotation <57°
Overhang of lateral masses of C1 on C2	<8 mm total (right + left sides)
Atlantodental interval	<4–5 mm
Lower cervical vertebrae (C2–C7)	<3.5 mm subluxation between vertebrae <11° angulation between vertebrae
Thoracic vertebrae	<2.5 mm subluxation between vertebrae <5° angulation between vertebrae
Lumbar vertebrae	<4.5 mm subluxation between vertebrae <22° angulation between vertebrae

forces that cause them. In the upper cervical spine (occiput to C2) the most common injuries are Jefferson fractures, hangman's fractures, and odontoid fractures. Jefferson fractures usually result from an extreme axial load and are fractures through the anterior and posterior arches of C1 associated with outward displacement of the lateral masses (>7 mm total overhang of the lateral masses of C1 on C2 when viewed on an open-mouth odontoid x-ray). Hangman's fractures are bilateral fractures through the pedicles of C2 and are usually the result of a hyperextension injury. Odontoid fractures are subclassified into 3 types: type I refers to a fracture through the tip of the dens, type II is a fracture through the base of the dens, and type III is an oblique fracture through the anterior body of the C2 vertebrae. Injuries in the lower cervical spine (C3 to C7) vary depending on the mechanism. Flexion with axial loading can cause compression fractures of the vertebral bodies with possible displacement of fracture fragments into the spinal canal. Extreme flexion injuries may disrupt the posterior ligamentous elements, leading to subluxation and jumped facets. Rotational injuries may cause a unilateral jumped facet with little or no subluxation, a condition that is easily missed on plain x-rays of the cervical spine.

The most common injuries in the thoracic and lumbar spine are compression fractures, usually the result of hyperflexion. Severe fractures associated with retropulsion of fracture fragments into the spinal canal are referred to as burst fractures, and are frequently associated with paraplegia if they occur above the conus medullaris (L1). Subluxation is much less common in the thoracic and lumbar spine than in the cervical spine. Chance fractures are transverse fractures through the vertebral body, pedicles, and lamina. Before the advent of shoulder restraints, these injuries were typically seen at the thoracolumbar junction following high-speed motor vehicle crashes in which the occupant was wearing only a lap belt.

PREHOSPITAL AND EMERGENCY DEPARTMENT MANAGEMENT

Spine injury can occur or become worsened during extrication, resuscitation, immobilization, or transport of the trauma patient if proper procedure is not followed. The cervical spine should usually be immobilized in a properly fitting rigid plastic collar even if the trauma patient is ambulatory, and should remain immobilized until evaluation at the trauma center. Most trauma patients, and particularly those who are obtunded or who complain of neck or back pain, should be transported to the trauma center on a long spine board. When necessary, intubation should be done with a second person providing in-line cervical traction. At the trauma center, evaluation for spine injury should only be done after cardiopulmonary resuscitation is accomplished and all life-threatening injuries are attended to. Ventilatory function must be closely monitored in patients with cervical spine injuries because it may acutely deteriorate from ascending spinal cord swelling or hemorrhage. Cervical and thoracic spine injuries can cause chest and abdominal anesthesia, complicating the clinical assessment for life-threatening injuries in these cavities. The following variables have been associated with an increased risk for spinal cord injury:

- Fall of greater than 10 feet
- Subjective numbness
- Sensory loss
- Motor loss

- Neck spasm
- Neck tenderness
- Weakness or loss of anal sphincter tone

Neurologic Assessment

A thorough motor and sensory evaluation is essential and should be carefully documented for comparison with subsequent examinations in order to detect improvement or deterioration. Perineal sensation as well as rectal sphincter tone and contraction also must be assessed. Strength in all major muscle groups of the upper and lower extremities is graded according to the five-point Medical Research Council grading system (Table 17-2). The extremities, chest, and abdomen are tested for sensory loss; the finding of a level on the chest or abdomen below which the patient is anesthetic is pathognomonic for a spinal cord injury. For comatose patients a reliable sensory and motor examination is not possible, though extremity movement, either spontaneously or with painful stimuli, should be noted.

Radiologic Assessment

For those patients who are alert, awake, have no neurologic deficits, no midline neck tenderness or pain on full range of motion of the neck, and are not intoxicated, cervical spine radiographs are not necessary to clear the cervical spine and remove the collar. For all others, lateral, anteroposterior, and open-mouth odontoid radiographs are recommended. Thin-slice axial CT images from the occiput through C2 of suspicious areas identified on the plain radiographs, and through the lower cervical spine if not well imaged on the plain films, also are obtained. In comatose patients with normal plain radiographs and CT images, ligamentous instability of the cervical spine may be detected with flexion/extension lateral fluoroscopy or MRI. Flexion/extension lateral radiographs are recommend for awake patients with normal static images who have neck pain, and MRI is recommended if there are neurologic deficits referable to a spinal cord injury. Injuries of the thoracic and lumbar spine are usually detected with anteroposterior and lateral plain radiographs. The most common reasons for missed spine injuries are poor quality or inadequate radiographs, or improper interpretation of the studies obtained.

TREATMENT

The definitive management of spine injury is aimed at preventing or limiting secondary and iatrogenic injury, and providing long-term biomechanical stability of the spinal column. Unfortunately, there still are no medical or surgical

TABLE 17-2 The Medical Research Council Grading System for Motor Strength

Grade	Description
0	No contraction
1	Flicker or trace contraction, unable to move across a joint
2	Able to move across a joint with gravity eliminated
3	Able to move against gravity but not with resistance
4	Movement against some resistance but detectable weakness
5	Normal strength

Source: Medical Research Council: *Aids to the Examination of the Peripheral Nervous System.* Philadelphia, Bailliere Tindall, 1986, p 1.

treatments that will effectively repair the damaged spinal cord and restore lost neurologic function.

During the initial phase of acute care, the priorities are to protect the damaged segment of the spine and reduce secondary injury. This is accomplished by ensuring adequate perfusion and oxygenation of the spinal cord, aggressively treating fever, keeping the cervical spine collar in place (for cervical spine injuries), and using proper log-rolling techniques when moving patients with thoracic or lumbar injuries. Use of a long spine board for more than 2 to 4 hours is not recommended because it can cause pressure sores, particularly in paraplegic or quadriplegic patients. Intravascular volume should be kept normal and hypotension avoided. There is evidence that the early administration of high doses of methylprednisolone also may help limit secondary injury, and to some extent at least, improve neurologic recovery. Based on several reports of the National Acute Spinal Cord Injury Study, the following is suggested for those who are seen within 8 hours of injury (methylprednisolone has not been found to be beneficial if administered after 8 hours):

- Intravenous infusion of 30 mg/kg over 45 minutes
- If treatment is begun within 3 hours of injury, give an additional 5.4 mg/kg/h for 24 hours
- If treatment is begun at 3 to 8 hours, give an additional 5.4 mg/kg/h for 48 hours

Early restoration of normal anatomic alignment of the spinal column is also recommended for those with fracture dislocations. In the cervical spine, this can be accomplished either with closed reduction using axial traction, or with surgical reduction. If closed reduction is used, Gardner-Wells tongs or a similar C-clamp device is applied to the skull and inline traction gradually increased at 2.5- to 5-pound increments, with frequent lateral radiographs obtained to detect reduction of the subluxation as soon as it occurs. Frequent x-rays also are important to be sure there is not overdistraction and separation of the involved vertebrae as may occur with severe ligamentous disruption. Benzodiazepines and narcotics are usually administered to provide muscle relaxation and analgesia. For thoracic and lumbar fracture dislocation, closed reduction is usually not possible.

The two treatment options for ensuring long-term stability of spine injuries are rigid external orthoses and internal (surgical) fixation. If the fracture is considered stable and unlikely to cause injury to the spinal cord with normal patient activity, an external orthosis is usually recommended. Such fractures include injuries that involve only one of the three columns as previously defined, such as most compression fractures of the cervical, thoracic, and lumbar spine, in which there is less than 30 to 40 percent collapse of the body and no disruption of the posterior vertebral elements. Jefferson fractures of the upper cervical spine, most nondisplaced hangman's fractures, and most type III odontoid fractures also are treated with either a rigid cervical collar or halo brace. In most cases the external orthoses should be used for 10 to 12 weeks. Smoking and diabetes are significant risk factors for nonunion of spine fractures.

If there is disruption of two or three columns of the spine (anterior and posterior elements), there is a significant risk for new or worsening dislocation of the vertebrae and damage to the spinal cord even with external braces. For these patients internal fixation is recommended. The surgical approach taken depends on the nature of the injury, and adequate fixation of the spine can usually be achieved through posterior, anterior, or lateral approaches. Thus if the primary injury is a fracture dislocation with little or no damage to the vertebral body, a posterior approach is often used, and internal reduction of the subluxation accomplished by exposing the jumped facets, restoring their normal relationship, and fusing the involved vertebrae with bone and metal instrumentation. If the primary injury is a burst fracture with retropulsion of fracture fragments into the spinal canal, an anterior approach will allow for a corpectomy, removal of the fragments, and fusion of the two adjacent vertebrae with a strut graft, often buttressed by a metal plate fixed to those bodies.

Treatment of penetrating spine injuries is generally conservative. Gunshot wounds typically damage the cord either by direct penetration or as a result of pressure waves transmitted as the bullet penetrates tissues adjacent to the cord. However, they rarely cause biomechanical instability of the vertebral column. Extraction of a bullet lodged in the spinal canal is not likely to improve neurologic outcome. Indeed, because the bullet often has an irregular contour caused by impact with bone and is typically intertwined with neural elements, surgical extraction is likely to worsen damage to the spinal cord. Knife wounds also do not typically destabilize the spinal column. High-dose methylprednisolone has not been shown to benefit victims of penetrating spine injuries. Because these patients are at increased risk for infection, steroids are not recommended.

CHRONIC CARE

Patients with quadriplegia and paraplegia are at risk for a variety of delayed neurologic and medical problems. Painful spasticity is common during the first several months after injury and is usually managed with oral or intrathecal baclofen. Decubitus ulcers over the sacrum and heels are also common and are best avoided with proper padding and frequent movement. The leading cause of death in these patients is respiratory complications, particularly pneumonia. Aggressive pulmonary toilet is essential, especially for ventilator-dependent patients. Deep venous thrombosis and pulmonary emboli are another common source of respiratory embarrassment. As soon as possible after injury the patient should receive prophylaxis for deep venous thrombosis, and anticoagulant therapy is recommended for at least 3 to 6 months after injury. Complete spinal cord injuries also cause bowel and bladder dysfunction. Stool softeners are administered and a Foley catheter is used acutely. Significant infections and other complications are associated with both chronic indwelling and intermittent catheterization. Fortunately, most patients are eventually able to learn techniques that allow them to void intermittently without the need for catheterization.

PROGNOSIS

Survival and recovery from spinal cord injury are related to several factors, including the level and severity of injury, associated injuries, premorbid health, age, and the availability of comprehensive rehabilitation facilities. The overall first-year mortality rate for patients with an isolated spinal cord injury is 5 to 7 percent. The 12-year survival rate for patients under 25 years of age who have an incomplete spinal cord injury is 95 percent, in contrast to an 18 percent 12-year survival rate for individuals over the age of 50 years who have a complete spinal cord injury. Among children with incomplete injuries, 74 percent have significant improvement and 59 percent recover completely. Unfortunately, most children with complete injuries do not improve.

ADDITIONAL READING

American Spinal Injury Association and International Medical Society of Paraplegia (ASIA/IMSOP): International Standards for Neurological and Functional Classification of Spinal Cord Injury.

Bracken MB, Shepard MJ, Holford TR, et al: Methylprednisolone or tirlazad mesylate administration after acute spinal cord injury: 1-year follow up. Results of the Third National Acute Spinal Cord Injury Randomized Controlled Trial. *J Neurosurg* 89:699, 1998.

Marion DW, Pryzbylski G: Injury to the vertebrae and spinal cord, in Mattox KL, Feliciano V, Moore EE (eds): *Trauma*. New York, McGraw-Hill, 2000, pp 451–471.

Pasquale M, Marion DW, Domeier R, et al: Practice management guidelines for trauma; identifying cervical spine instability after trauma. *J Trauma* 44:945, 1998.

Tator CH: Spinal cord syndromes: physiologic and anatomic correlations, in Menezes AH, Sonntag VKH (eds): *Principles of Spinal Surgery*. New York, McGraw-Hill, 1995.

18 | Indications for Thoracotomy

HISTORIC PERSPECTIVE

One of the earliest references to thoracic injury is a report of penetrating trauma to the sternum noted in the *Edwin Smith Surgical Papyrus,* printed in 3000 BC and probably authored by Imhotep, the builder of the step pyramid. Open chest injuries during the time of the Greeks and Romans were considered fatal injuries. Galen reported attempting to treat gladiators with chest injury with open packing. In North America, the first written thoracic operative record appeared in the diary of Cabeza de Vaca in 1635.

Thoracic injury directly accounts for 20 to 25 percent of deaths due to trauma. It is estimated that approximately 16,000 deaths per year in the United States are attributable to chest trauma. Despite the emphasis on massive injuries, the most common thoracic injury is injury to the chest wall itself.

PHILOSOPHY

The evaluation and management of patients with thoracic injuries can be philosophically different depending on mechanism, timing, and associated injuries. For vehicular trauma, conferring with emergency medical services (EMS) providers to determine the mechanism of injury, condition of the vehicle, and direction of impact, will help direct physicians to possible injuries. Other vehicular issues such as rollover, difficult extrication, and signs of significant energy transfer such as high-speed deceleration can give clues to initiate further studies (Table 18-1). While the majority of penetrating trauma to the chest can be managed with tube thoracostomy, the use of mediastinal surgery is evolving. Emergency center thoracotomy historically has been reserved for patients who suffer penetrating trauma and present with signs of life. The patients who benefit most from emergency center thoracotomy are those with penetrating injury to the chest who have short transport times and have undergone endotracheal intubation. These injuries are likely to be limited to a single organ system that can be readily controlled. Emergency center thoracotomy for blunt trauma has had very limited success.

EMERGENCY CENTER ISSUES

Patients with thoracic trauma are evaluated with the standard Advanced Trauma Life Support (ATLS) protocols. The primary survey in the ATLS course concentrates on life-threatening injuries related to the chest and the airway. Endotracheal intubation in the field is one of the few procedures that have been shown to be efficacious in the trauma patient. The patient should be carefully examined for all penetrating injuries, and attempts should be made to reconstruct the path of a missile. It must be remembered, however, that bullets may not always travel in straight lines, and this is a significant pitfall. Tension pneumothorax is a clinical diagnosis that does not require x-ray to diagnose. The presence of a hematoma, particularly at the thoracic outlet, should arouse suspicion of a thoracic vascular injury.

The chest x-ray is a fundamental examination in the evaluation of the patient with chest trauma. Wounds should be identified with radiopaque markers to assist in assessing injury patterns. The chest x-ray should routinely be evaluated for position of the tracheobronchial tree, the lung parenchyma, the mediastinal silhouette, the silhouette of the vascular structure/aortic knob, and the pleural cavities. Specifically, the presence of tubes, hemopneumothorax,

161

TABLE 18-1 Historical Factors from EMS Providers

Mechanism of injury
Condition of vehicle
Direction of impact
Rollover
Difficult extrication
Other injuries/deaths
Signs of significant energy transfer

pneumomediastinum, rib fractures, spinal or other skeletal fractures, foreign bodies, and great vessel injuries should be sought.

The most common therapeutic activity in treating a patient with chest trauma is observation with judicious fluid administration to prevent overre-suscitation. With both penetrating and blunt injury to the chest, contusion of the lung parenchyma absorbs excess fluid. One of the key elements in managing these patients is to limit fluid administration to below 1 L/d if possible. For penetrating trauma, survival has been shown to be increased when crystalloid resuscitation has been delayed until operation.

TUBE THORACOSTOMY

Tube thoracostomy is one of the most underrated procedures performed in the patient with chest injury. It is the only invasive procedure that 85 percent of patients with chest trauma will require. One pitfall of tube thoracostomy relates to the use of trocar chest tubes, which contain a sharp metal rod that can produce injury to both upper abdominal and intrathoracic organs. Because 15 percent of the population have some element of pleural symphysis, blind insertion of a trocar chest tube often results in lung injury with subsequent air leakage. In adolescents and adults, the chest tube should be at least 36 F or larger and have more that 4 to 6 distal holes in the tube.

The majority of systems have a suction control chamber or device. The amount of suction applied to the chest tube is approximately 20 cm H_2O of negative pressure. If the patient's arterial saturation decreases and the physician is unable to ventilate the patient because of a large air leak, bronchopleural fistula should be suspected and the patient should be removed from suction and left to underwater seal. The patient may then be taken to the operating room for definitive repair. There is seldom an indication in trauma to clamp a chest tube, because a patient with significant air leak may rapidly develop an iatrogenic tension pneumothorax.

The decision for chest tube removal should be based on the absence of an air leak and a steady decrease in the amount of fluid removed from the chest, assuming the tube remains functional. Examining the water seal area for fluctuation with respiration can give the surgeon an indication of whether the tube continues to function. After a pulmonary resection or with a lung injury in which there has been a significant air leak, a trial of water seal may be helpful to avoid having to replace a tube.

ACUTE INDICATIONS FOR THORACOTOMY

Thoracotomy may be indicated for acute or chronic conditions. Tables 18-2 and 18-3 list acute and nonacute indications for thoracotomy.

Indications for thoracotomy in acute thoracic injury are based on physical findings, evidence on chest x-ray and contrast studies, and the clinical course

TABLE 18-2 Acute Indications for Thoracotomy

Cardiac tamponade
Acute hemodynamic deterioration/cardiac arrest in the trauma center
Patients with penetrating truncal trauma (resuscitative thoracotomy)
Vascular injury at the thoracic outlet
Traumatic thoracotomy (loss of chest wall substance)
Massive air leak from the chest tube
Endoscopic or radiographic demonstration of tracheal or bronchial injury
Endoscopic or radiographic evidence of esophageal injury
Radiographic evidence of great vessel injury
Mediastinal traverse with a penetrating object
Significant missile embolism to the heart or pulmonary artery
Transcardiac placement of inferior vena cava shunt for hepatic vascular wounds

of the patient. One clinical presentation, pericardial tamponade, is recognized with the classic physical findings of hypotension, narrow pulse pressure, and muffled heart sounds. These findings combined with proximity of the wound to vital structures are appropriate indications for operation. Unfortunately, from a practical standpoint, the presentation often is not that straightforward. Pulsus paradoxus or simply the loss of the radial pulse when the patient takes a deep breath may be suggestive of tamponade. Acute or hypovolemic cardiac arrest in the patient with penetrating trauma suggests the need for resuscitative thoracotomy. Widening of the upper mediastinum on routine chest x-ray is suggestive of vascular injury to the thoracic outlet, which should be confirmed by angiography, if possible, to help plan incisions and operative approach. Tracheal, bronchial, and esophageal injuries are diagnosed by endoscopy or contrast studies and require thoracotomy for repair and prevention of postinjury complications. The presence of cervical, mediastinal, and pleural air may be a significant clue to an injury of intrathoracic structures. Massive air leaks via tube thoracostomy are also indicative of major injury to the airway.

Blunt great-vessel injury, particularly to the descending thoracic aorta, is highly lethal. Angiography continues to be the diagnostic procedure of choice for diagnosis. Computed tomography (CT) and transesophageal echocardiography have limitations, but may have selected indications in multiply injured patients to assist in triage. The high-resolution helical dynamic CT shows promise for the screening of patients with blunt aortic injury, due to its ability to resolve subtle injuries as well as its short scan time.

Another indication for acute thoracotomy is often based on chest tube output. The amount of blood evacuated prior to thoracotomy has recently increased from an immediate output of 1 L to 1500 mL as being sufficient indication for thoracotomy. However, the trend is probably more important.

Table 18-3 Nonacute Indications for Thoracotomy

Nonevacuated clotted hemothorax
Chronic traumatic diaphragmatic hernia
Traumatic cardiac septal or valvular lesions
Chronic traumatic thoracic aortic pseudoaneurysms
Nonclosing thoracic duct fistula
Chronic (or neglected) posttraumatic empyema
Infected intrapulmonary hematoma (traumatic lung abscess)
Missed tracheal or bronchial injury
Tracheoesophageal fistula

Many patients present late after injury, and if 1500 mL of blood is evacuated, the lung is reexpanded, and no further output occurs, the patient can be observed for continuing bleeding or recurrence of hemothorax. If bleeding persists with a steady trend of over 250 mL/h, thoracotomy is likely indicated.

Mediastinal traverse continues to be controversial. In the unstable patient, immediate thoracotomy is indicated. The incision is typically made in the hemithorax with the most obvious injury or blood loss. Simultaneous antero-lateral thoracotomies (with or without trans-sternal extension) may be chosen if the patient is unstable and it is unclear which side should be entered first. There have been recent data, however, to challenge routine thoracotomy for mediastinal traverse. If the patient is stable and no injury is detected on bronchoscopy, esophagoscopy, aortography, or CT scanning, close observation (without thoracotomy) might be considered.

A missile embolus to the right side of the heart commonly requires removal unless it is small (i.e., smaller than a BB). Missile emboli can present an extremely confusing presentation, again emphasizing the inability to draw straight lines from injury to the final resting place of the projectile. Careful examination of all peripheral pulses can lead to the diagnosis of missile embolus to the iliac arteries with an absent femoral pulse or to the innominate or carotid arteries with absent radial or carotid pulse.

Subacute conditions related to previous trauma that may require thoracotomy are often secondary to unrecognized or incompletely treated acute injuries. Historically, the most common chronic postinjury condition that leads to formal thoracotomy is an unevacuated clotted hemothorax. Recently, this condition has also been very successfully treated using video-assisted thoracoscopy.

Several clinical conditions that have soft indications for thoracotomy for which treatment should be individualized include flail chest or fractured sternum, fibrothorax, posttraumatic pulmonary embolism, and selected vascular injuries for proximal vascular control. Thoracotomy is contraindicated for the conditions noted in Table 18-4, unless there is other evidence to suggest injury.

At times a thoracic incision must be made to treat an abdominal injury, such as for transcardiac placement of an inferior vena cava shunt for retrohepatic vena cava injury or for proximal control of a supraceliac aortic injury.

Thoracoabdominal injury was cited during World War II as an indication for thoracotomy. Thoracoabdominal wounds are typically an indication for laparotomy, but not necessarily formal thoracotomy. Unfortunately, the algorithms for the chest and the algorithms for the abdomen are often difficult to integrate. It is not uncommon for the wrong cavity to be entered initially. The majority of thoracoabdominal injuries are managed with tube thoracostomy and laparotomy. Thus in patients with both thoracic and abdominal wounds, extremely close surveillance and increased sensitivity to potential injuries is essential. An algorithm for determining the need for thoracotomy is presented in Fig. 18-1.

TABLE 18-4 Contraindications to Thoracotomy
_____
Suspicion of bullet in proximity to major structure
Simple bullet removal
Minimal hemothorax
Pneumomediastinum not associated with tracheal/bronchial or esophageal injury
Wide mediastinum
_____

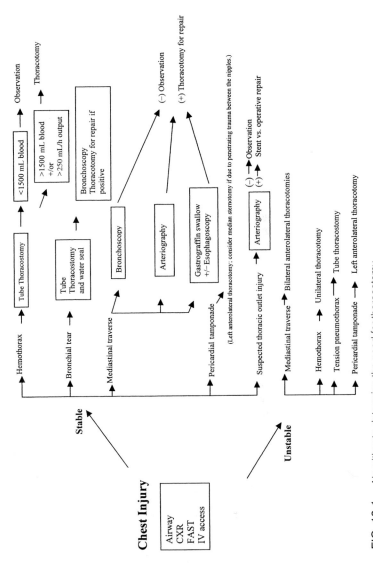

FIG. 18-1. Algorithm to determine the need for thoracotomy.

OPERATIVE ISSUES

Incisions

The incision chosen for a trauma patient who requires operation for chest injury is often an educated guess dictated by the diagnosis and anticipated injuries. While in the abdomen the midline laparotomy is the basic incision in trauma, there are many basic incisions available for thoracic trauma (Fig. 18-2). The left anterolateral thoracotomy is the most useful incision for resuscitation under circumstances of acute deterioration or cardiac arrest. This

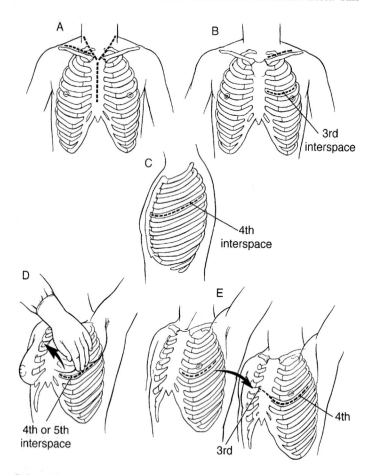

FIG. 18-2.   Thoracic incisions for trauma. A. Median sternotomy with cervical or supraclavicular extensions. B. Third interspace anterolateral thoracotomy with separate supraclavicular incision. C. Posterolateral thoracotomy. D. Anterolateral thoracotomy (in females, the left breast should be retracted prior to making the incision). E. Extension of an anterolateral thoracotomy across the sternum should be directed superiorly into the third interspace. *(Reproduced with permission of Baylor College of Medicine.)*

incision allows exposure for opening the pericardium, open cardiac massage, clamping of the descending thoracic aorta, and treatment of a large percentage of cardiac and left lung injuries. Injury to the right side of the heart commonly requires trans-sternal extension for full visualization and repair. The right anterolateral incision alone provides limited exposure to the heart and has limited use in trauma. To determine whether a large amount of blood is present in the opposite chest, a finger can be placed immediately anterior to the pericardium entering the opposite pleural space.

The left posterolateral thoracotomy incision provides excellent exposure of the posterior mediastinum, left lung, hilum, and descending thoracic aorta. This incision provides some access to the heart for cardiac massage and management of cardiac injuries on the posterior left side, as well as good exposure of the proximal left subclavian artery and some access to the proximal left common carotid artery. A right posterolateral thoracotomy incision provides good exposure for managing pulmonary, tracheal, and proximal esophageal injuries. Although this incision provides some exposure of the heart for management of right atrial and some left atrial injuries, this exposure is suboptimal for the management of cardiac injuries. This incision also provides good exposure to the superior and inferior vena cavae and the azygos vein, and limited exposure of the right subclavian artery. Its primary use, however, is for pulmonary, esophageal, or tracheal injuries.

The "book" or "trap-door" incision has been advocated for exposure of left-sided thoracic outlet injuries. It has the advantage of providing exposure of a long segment of the left common carotid and left subclavian artery. Difficulties with the book incision include stretching of the brachial plexus and upper posterior costal junctions, which can result in long-term neurologic and upper back pain syndromes that can be quite disabling. Thus this incision is typically only used when absolutely necessary for control and repair. At our center, the current approach for the management of left subclavian artery injuries is to gain proximal control via anterolateral thoracotomy in the left third interspace combined with a separate clavicular incision for definitive repair.

The median sternotomy incision, while the most common elective cardiac incision, has limited usefulness in trauma. It provides excellent exposure for isolated anterior cardiac and great vessel injuries, but provides no access to the esophagus and posterior thorax, and is very difficult to use to cross-clamp the descending thoracic aorta.

The subxiphoid pericardiotomy is an abdominal approach to a suspected cardiac wound that provides less than ideal exposure. Should an injury be present, it can convert tamponade into exsanguination.

DAMAGE CONTROL

Damage control in the abdomen has consisted of limiting the operative procedure to controlling injuries, such as vascular injuries that result in immediate death, followed by planned reoperation after the patient's condition has stabilized. Damage control approaches in the chest include pulmonary tractotomy with selective vascular ligation to avoid formal resection, en masse resection of a lobe of the lung with a stapling device, packing of the limits of the chest, massive drainage of esophageal injuries, stapling of heart injuries, and rapid closure techniques. Many of the thoracotomy incisions involve cutting large muscles that continue to bleed. Thus en masse closure with a single suture may be a more efficacious technique. Damage control techniques in the chest are designed not so much with planned reoperation in mind, but rather offer a simpler procedure to accomplish hemostasis than the more lengthy classical approach.

OTHER CONSIDERATIONS

Digital Thoracotomy

Valuable information may be obtained by a digital thoracotomy, particularly for the left chest. The pleural space is entered by the surgeon's finger rather than a sharp instrument or trocar. Digital exploration is performed to examine for the conditions noted in Table 18-5, which if present, indicate the need for further diagnostic and therapeutic measures.

Thoracoscopy

Thoracoscopy has been used to remove clotted blood, evaluate the diaphragm, look for hemopericardium, remove foreign bodies, control chest wall or mammary artery bleeding, or examine for hemomediastinum or hematomas around the great vessels. These video systems technically make the procedure much more user friendly for the entire operative team. Thoracoscopy has had its greatest application in chest trauma for evacuating clotted hemothorax.

Extracorporeal Support Devices

The intra-aortic balloon pump has been used post-cardiac surgery to support a failing heart, and it has also been used in a small number of patients with post-traumatic myocardial dysfunction. Unfortunately, many trauma patients have tachycardia and significant dysrhythmias such that the intra-aortic balloon pump is unable to track their rhythm and provide adequate counterpulsation. This device is most efficacious in posttraumatic cardiac failure caused by direct cardiac injury, such as unrevascularizable coronary artery injury or bridge support of an exacerbation of preexisting congestive heart failure. More applications in trauma and use of similar devices are anticipated.

Cardiopulmonary Bypass

Cardiopulmonary bypass may be indicated for proximal coronary artery injuries, posttraumatic massive pulmonary embolism, acute valvular and septal lesions that are hemodynamically unstable, and myocardial or ascending aortic rupture. Recent work using heparin-bonded circuits and heparinless cardiopulmonary bypass showed a few survivors in patients with massive trauma. However, this requires a significant commitment of resources per patient. Acute cardiopulmonary bypass is likely best reserved for high proximal left anterior descending coronary artery lesions, ascending aortic and arch injuries, or refractory intracardiac injuries.

Focused Abdominal Sonography for Trauma (FAST) Examination

The surgeon-performed ultrasound exam of the pericardium and abdomen has been a significant advance in the care of the trauma patient. The initial view is

TABLE 18-5 Positive Findings During Digital Thoracotomy

Tense pericardium without cardiac pulsation suggesting a hemopericardium
Pleural symphysis from previous trauma or disease
Palpable holes in the pericardium or diaphragm
Palpable abdominal organs herniated through a tear in the diaphragm

a subxiphoid window visualizing the liver, heart, and pericardium, and is anticipated to become the standard of care for diagnosing pericardial tamponade. By avoiding the use of ionizing radiation, this test can also be repeated as many times as needed to follow a patient. The FAST exam can be used prior to laparotomy for thoracoabdominal trauma, thus virtually eliminating the need for subxiphoid pericardiotomy and pericardiocentesis.

SUMMARY

Thoracic injury accounts for a significant amount of the morbidity and mortality of the trauma patient. The majority of thoracic injuries can be managed conservatively or with tube thoracostomy alone; however, the more unstable presentations require significant diagnostic and therapeutic decisions. Acute and subacute indications for thoracotomy have been discussed, including the particular pitfall of dealing with the thoracoabdominal injury for which no specific integrated algorithm currently exists. The choice of incision is guided by clinical road maps provided by arteriography or the surgeon's best guess of the anticipated pathology. New technology, such as extracorporeal support devices, thoracoscopy, helical CT, transesophageal echocardiography, and ultrasound technology, may affect the approach to the patient with thoracic injuries. The FAST exam is likely to become the standard of care in diagnosing pericardial tamponade. Limitation of fluid resuscitation while managing penetrating thoracic injuries is emphasized.

ADDITIONAL READING

Bricker DL, Noon GP, Beall AC Jr, et al: Vascular injuries of the thoracic outlet. *J Trauma* 10:1, 1970.

Durham LA, Richardson R, Wall MJ Jr, et al: Emergency center thoracotomy: Impact of prehospital resuscitation. *J Trauma* 32:775, 1992.

Grover FL, Ellestad C, Arom KV, et al: Diagnosis and management of major tracheobronchial injuries. *Ann Thorac Surg* 28:384, 1979.

Hirshberg A, Mattox KL, Wall MJ Jr: Double jeopardy: Thoracoabdominal injuries requiring surgery in both chest and abdomen. *J Trauma* 39:1, 1995.

Ledgerwood AM, Kazmers M, Lucas CE: The role of thoracic aortic occlusion for massive hemoperitoneum. *J Trauma* 16:610, 1976.

Milfield DJ, Mattox KL, Beall AC Jr: Early evacuation of clotted hemothorax. *Am J Surg* 136:686, 1978.

Reul GJ, Beall AC Jr, Jordan GL Jr, et al: The early operative management of injuries to the great vessels. *Surgery* 74:862, 1973.

Rozycki GS, Ochsner MG, Jaffin JH, et al: Prospective evaluation of surgeons' use of ultrasound in the evaluation of trauma patients. *J Trauma* 34:516, 1993.

Wall MJ Jr, Mattox KL, Chen C, et al: Acute management of complex cardiac injuries. *J Trauma* 42:905, 1997.

19 | Injury to the Chest Wall

INTRODUCTION

Chest injuries are responsible for up to 25 percent of all annual trauma deaths in the United States, and significant long-term disability is common after major chest wall injury. Associated injuries must be expected since trauma is isolated to the chest wall in only 16 percent of patients.

PATHOPHYSIOLOGY

Penetrating mechanisms cause direct injury to structures encountered by a sharp object or missile, and indirect injury occurs due to dissipation of the energy imparted by a missile to adjacent tissues. The extent of internal injuries cannot be judged by the appearance of a skin entry wound, and deep penetration should be assumed. Blunt forces applied to the chest wall cause injury by three mechanisms: rapid deceleration (motor vehicle crashes and falls); direct impact (from blunt objects); and compression (due to crush injury or traumatic asphyxia).

Massive blunt injury to the chest wall may comprise elements of deceleration, direct impact, and compression, to yield multiple adjacent rib fractures in more than one location. In this setting, a free-floating segment of the chest wall can move paradoxically with respiration, causing abnormalities of ventilation, oxygenation, and compliance. Large flail chest segments may disrupt the normal bellows-like action of the thorax. Pain and muscular splinting restrict chest wall expansion, leading to abnormal respiratory mechanics. However, most of the pulmonary dysfunction observed after severe blunt chest wall trauma is probably secondary to underlying pulmonary contusion.

An algorithm for the diagnosis and treatment of chest wall trauma is outlined in Fig. 19-1.

INITIAL MANAGEMENT

The highest priorities in the management of patients with significant chest wall trauma are:

- Assurance or establishment of a patent airway
- Initiation or support of adequate ventilation and administration of oxygen
- Treatment of shock

Some specific caveats in the prehospital management of chest wall injuries are:

- Penetrating wounds of the thoracic cage should not be probed or explored.
- Sucking chest wounds should not be totally covered; a three-sided occlusive petrolatum dressing may improve ventilation.
- The rib cage should not be circumferentially taped.
- External stabilization of a flail segment with sandbags is not effective.

DIAGNOSIS

History

- Mechanism of injury
- Onset and progression of symptoms
- Past medical history, pulmonary illnesses, past surgical history
- Tobacco use

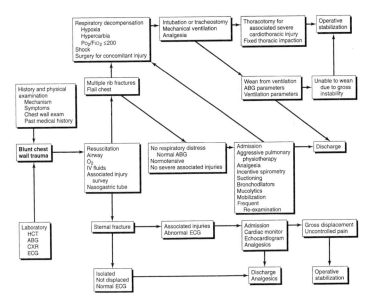

FIG. 19-1. Algorithm for diagnosis and treatment of chest wall trauma.

Physical Examination

The entire skin surface area must be inspected for wounds, lacerations, contusions, abrasions, or other external evidence of trauma. The chest wall should be observed during several full respiratory cycles for differential ventilation, splinting, paradoxical motion of a chest wall segment, or obvious bony deformity. Palpation of the entire chest wall may reveal fractures of the ribs or clavicles; flail segments, point tenderness, or subcutaneous emphysema. Pulses and blood pressure should be measured in each upper extremity to investigate the possibility of great vessel disruption. Careful neurologic examination of the per extremities may disclose potential trauma of the brachial plexus. Finally, the chest must be examined serially to detect progressive changes in function. Pneumothorax may develop several hours after injury and a small hemothorax may continue to increase in size over a period of several hours. A flail segment missed on initial examination may become obvious 1 to 10 days after an injury.

Laboratory and Radiographic Data

Arterial blood gas determination may gauge the severity of an injury as well as the results of resuscitation. The ratio of arterial oxygen tension to the fraction of inspired oxygen ($PaO_2:FIO_2$ ratio) yields an estimate of the extent of intrapulmonary shunt and may be used as a parameter to determine the need for mechanical ventilation in patients with pulmonary contusion and flail chest. Pulse oximetry can also be used as a continuous indicator of the degree of injury and response to treatment.

Chest x-ray should be taken early in the evaluation of patients with chest wall injury. Serial chest x-rays are very useful for identifying conditions of delayed onset as well as for recognition of intercurrent pulmonary complications.

All patients with penetrating chest wounds below the fourth intercostal space should undergo diagnostic peritoneal lavage for the identification of associated diaphragmatic and intra-abdominal injury.

All patients with sternal fractures should have a baseline 12-lead electrocardiogram.

INJURY CLASSIFICATION

Traumatic Asphyxia

Traumatic asphyxia is a rare syndrome of craniocervical cyanosis, facial edema, petechiae, subconjunctival hemorrhage, and occasional neurologic symptoms that results from a severe crush injury to the thorax by a very heavy object. The pathophysiology involves a marked increase in thoracic and superior vena cava pressure from chest compression and concurrent closure of the glottis.

Treatment

Careful neurologic assessment should be performed repeatedly and other causes of neurologic compromise must be excluded. Supportive care should consist of airway and ventilation maintenance and oxygen administration.

Outcome

Despite the strikingly moribund appearance of patients with this syndrome, mortality is low and is related to the duration of asphyxia and severity of associated injuries. Neurologic sequelae are uncommon.

Penetrating Wounds of the Chest Wall

Penetrating thoracic wounds most frequently involve the anterior chest. Up to 80 percent of these wounds can be managed nonoperatively or by simple techniques such as tube thoracostomy. Indications for urgent thoracotomy include:

• Pericardial tamponade
• Need for significant ongoing chest tube drainage
• Hypovolemic shock

Furthermore, urgent laparotomy is indicated for patients with low anterior or posterior chest wounds with unequivocal abdominal signs of trauma or a positive result from peritoneal lavage.

Indications for observation of penetrating chest wall wounds are:

• Stable vital signs
• Normal results on physical examination
• Normal initial chest x-ray

Patients should be observed in a monitored unit and have a repeat examination and repeat chest x-ray 6 hours after admission. Asymptomatic patients with continuously stable vital signs and a normal repeat chest x-ray may be discharged. Specific wound management should consist of cleansing, debridement, and open wound care. Tetanus prophylaxis should be administered. Prophylactic antibiotic administration has not been shown to be necessary or effective.

Large Open Chest Wall Defects

These are often the result of close-range shotgun blasts, explosions, or degloving injuries. Techniques of primary closure to improve pulmonary function include the use of myocutaneous flaps, transposition of the diaphragm, or the use of prosthetic material.

Lung Herniation

This can occur through defects caused by penetrating or blunt mechanisms. Clinical manifestations include pain and a localized bulge, which may change in size with respiration. The diagnosis is confirmed by chest x-ray or thoracic CT scan. Although small defects may be managed nonoperatively, large lung hernias or those in which incarceration is evident mandate surgical reduction and repair by using direct suture techniques or the placement of a prosthetic patch.

Chest Wall Hemorrhage

Hemorrhage may be associated with stab and gunshot wounds, or with severe blunt thoracic trauma. Sites of hemorrhage include muscular, intercostal, and internal mammary arteries. Although continued hemorrhage from these chest wall vessels usually requires open thoracotomy for control, video thoracoscopic procedures have been successfully employed in selected hemodynamically stable patients.

Scapular Fractures

Considerable direct force is required to cause a fracture of this sturdy, well-protected bone. Recognition of a scapular fracture should prompt careful examination for thoracic, neurologic, vascular, and abdominal injury. Treatment consists of simple shoulder immobilization with a sling followed by early active range-of-motion exercises. Open procedures for internal fixation are rarely necessary. Most fractures of the body and neck of the scapula heal without sequelae.

Scapulothoracic Dissociation

Scapulothoracic dissociation is a rare condition caused by blunt trauma in which violent lateral or rotational displacement of the shoulder girdle results in severe soft tissue injury. The spectrum of injury includes musculoskeletal, vascular, and neurologic structures. Physical signs include shoulder instability, tenderness, palpable hematomas or swelling, rapid pulse, and neurologic deficits. Chest and shoulder x-rays reveal lateral displacement of the scapula and acromioclavicular disruption, sternoclavicular disruption, or a distracted fracture of the clavicle. Limited functional recovery of the involved extremity occurs in only 17 percent of patients. In patients with complete brachial plexus disruption and a flail extremity, early above-elbow amputation and prosthesis fitting is most appropriate.

Clavicular Fractures

Nearly 80 percent of these fractures occur in the middle third of the bone, following a fall or blow with lateral force applied to the shoulder. Injuries to the underlying subclavian artery have been reported with displaced clavicle fractures. Clinical signs of clavicle fracture are tenderness, crepitus, and palpable deformity. The vast majority of clavicle fractures can be successfully managed by immobilization with a figure-of-eight dressing. Open procedures are reserved for widely displaced fractures and selected injuries of the distal third of the bone.

Sternoclavicular Joint Dislocation

The sternoclavicular joint is the only articulation between the torso and the upper extremity. Anterior dislocation of the sternoclavicular joint is most frequent. The affected shoulder may appear shortened and thrust forward. With anterior dislocation, the medial end of the clavicle is prominent on observation and palpation, and closed reduction is often successful with local anesthesia. With posterior dislocation, a hollow may be palpable or visible along the edge of the sternum; closed reduction usually requires general anesthesia.

Sternal Fractures

These usually result from direct impact of the sternum against a hard object such as the steering column of an automobile. The incidence of clinically significant myocardial injury is very low in patients with isolated sternal fractures. It is most prudent to remain clinically suspicious of myocardial trauma in those patients with multiple injuries or high-energy mechanisms of injury. The clinical manifestations of sternal fracture include anterior chest pain, tenderness, ecchymosis, swelling, and palpable deformity. Patients with isolated sternal fractures and normal hemodynamic, radiologic, and electrocardiographic evaluations do not require hospital admission. Specific management of a sternal fracture consists of analgesics. Open reduction and internal fixation of sternal fractures is indicated for severe pain and gross deformity.

First and Second Rib Fractures

Because of the considerable force necessary to cause a fracture of the first and second ribs, associated injuries are relatively common. Isolated, nondisplaced fractures are associated with a low incidence of vascular injury. Indications for arteriography for patients with first or second rib fractures should include:

- Multiple thoracic injuries
- Clinical evidence of distal vascular insufficiency
- X-ray evidence of mediastinal widening or additional signs of potential aortic injury
- Large apical hematoma or hemothorax
- Concomitant brachial plexus injury
- Significant displacement of the first or second rib fracture

Rib Fractures

Rib fractures have been identified in approximately 10 percent of patients admitted after blunt trauma. Compression of the chest by anteroposterior forces may cause ribs to fracture in an outward direction at midshaft; intrapleural damage is uncommon. A direct blow applied to the chest wall may also result in rib fractures at the point of impact. In this case, the ribs at the site of fracture may be driven into the underlying pleural and lung parenchyma, causing significant injury. Fractures of the ninth through twelfth ribs may entail liver, spleen, or kidney trauma. The absence of rib fractures does not preclude the possibility of serious injury to intrathoracic or intra-abdominal organs, especially in children. Special rib views may help visualize fractures of the first and second ribs, or be used to document cases of suspected child abuse. Adequate analgesia may prevent muscular splinting, hypoventilation, and the accumulation of secretions that would otherwise result in atelectasis, pneumonia, and respiratory compromise. Elderly patients and individuals with preexisting pulmonary disease are particularly vulnerable to these complications; hospitalization is often necessary. Relief of pain caused by rib fractures can be achieved with the following techniques:

- Oral, intramuscular, or intravenous narcotic administration
- Repetitive intercostal nerve blocks
- Administration of a local anesthetic via intrapleural catheter
- Administration of a local anesthetic via an extrapleural catheter
- Continuous narcotic epidural analgesia

Significant chest wall deformity and thoracic cage pain may be observed months or years after multiple adjacent rib fractures.

Flail Chest

In flail chest, an unstable segment of the normally rigid chest wall moves separately and in an opposite direction from the rest of the thoracic cage during the respiratory cycle. Separation of the sternum from surrounding costochondral joints or adjacent broken ribs is termed *sternal flail chest.* Flail chest usually results from direct impact. In pediatric patients, severe pulmonary contusion is possible without fractured ribs. In contrast, elderly patients with osteopenic bones may develop flail chest without underlying contusion after simple, low-energy falls.

The diagnosis of flail chest injury is made by physical examination. Observation from each direction for several respiratory cycles and during coughing or deep inspiration may be necessary to detect a chest segment with paradoxical motion. Computed tomography is more accurate than plain films in evaluating the presence of underlying injury to the lung parenchyma.

Treatment

Treatment for flail chest includes aggressive pulmonary physiotherapy, effective analgesia, selective use of endotracheal intubation and ventilation, and close observation for respiratory decompensation. Operative stabilization of multiple rib fractures may be useful in selected patients. Treatment is directed more toward improving abnormalities in gas exchange than reversing the chest wall instability, on the principle that the severity of the underlying parenchymal injury plays a greater role than paradoxical motion in compromising pulmonary function. Specific indications for endotracheal intubation and mechanical ventilation depend on objective evidence of respiratory failure manifested by one or more of the following criteria:

- Clinical signs of progressive fatigue
- Respiratory rate >35/min or <8/min
- PaO_2 <60 mm Hg at FIO_2 >0.5
- $PaCO_2$ >55 mm Hg at FIO_2 >0.5
- PaO_2:FIO_2 ratio <200

- Clinical evidence of severe shock
- Associated severe head injury with lack of airway control or need to ventilate
- Severe associated injury requiring surgery

Tracheostomy should be considered in patients who present with massive craniofacial injury and in those intubated patients in whom duration of ventilatory support is expected to exceed 7 to 10 days. Weaning from ventilation is based on measured pulmonary mechanics and arterial blood gas determinations rather than on resolution of the flail chest.

Orthopedic fixation of flail chest with struts, wires, or plates is indicated in patients undergoing thoracotomy for other reasons, especially if massive chest wall instability is apparent. Other relative indications for the surgical stabilization of flail chest injuries include a fixed thoracic impaction and failure to wean from mechanical ventilation because of prolonged, gross chest wall instability.

Patients without respiratory impairment do not require intubation or mechanical ventilation. Attentive observation in an intensive care unit and aggressive pulmonary physiotherapy are essential to prevent deterioration. Treatment should include:

- Supplemental oxygen to maintain O_2 saturation >90 percent
- Humidification of inspired air
- Active physical therapy, early mobilization
- Incentive spirometry
- Nutritional support
- Analgesia: oral, intramuscular, or intravenous narcotic administration; non-steroidal anti-inflammatory drug (NSAID) administration; repetitive intercostal nerve blocks; administration of local anesthetic via intrapleural catheter; administration of local anesthetic via extrapleural catheter; continuous narcotic epidural analgesia
- Upper airway and endobronchial suctioning
- Continuous reassessment

Outcome and Complications

Early

Hospital-acquired pneumonia, acute respiratory distress syndrome (ARDS), barotrauma, or major atelectasis occur in half of flail chest patients. Mortality ranges from 6 to 30 percent and depends upon associated injuries (especially head injuries), presence of shock, injury severity score (ISS), concomitant pulmonary contusion, and age.

Late

Impairment of pulmonary function can be documented in the majority of long-term flail chest survivors. Measured decreases in lung volume correlate with size of associated pulmonary contusion rather than residual chest wall deformity.

ADDITIONAL READINGS

Brookes JG, Dunn RJ, Rogers IR: Sternal fractures: a retrospective analysis of 272 cases. *J Trauma* 35:46, 1993.

Kishikawa M, Yoshioka T, Shimazu T, et al: Pulmonary contusion causes long-term respiratory dysfunction with decreased functional residual capacity. *J Trauma* 31:1203, 1991.

Landercasper J, Cogbill TH, Lindesmith LA: Long-term disability after flail chest injury. *J Trauma* 24:410, 1984.

Mackersie RC, Karagianes TG, Hoyt DB, et al: Prospective evaluation of epidural and intravenous administration of fentanyl for pain control and restoration of ventilatory function following multiple rib fractures. *J Trauma* 31:443, 1991.

Richardson JD, Adams L, Flint LM: Selective management of flail chest and pulmonary contusion. *Ann Surg* 196:481, 1982.

Tanaka H, Maemura T, Yukioka T, et al: Surgical stabilization or external pneumatic stabilization? An evaluation study of management of severe flail chest patients. *J Trauma* 41:200, 1996.

ESOPHAGEAL TRAUMA

Injury to the esophagus, although relatively rare, poses difficult challenges due to the complexity of the presentation, work-up, and various treatment options. Even in this era of superior surgical technique, advanced diagnostic modalities, and antibiotics, the morbidity and mortality associated with esophageal injury remain high. Perforation along the length of the esophagus can be one of the most lethal injuries of any site in the gastrointestinal tract and presents a great therapeutic challenge. Controversy over the diagnosis and management of esophageal injuries evokes strong opinions. While most injuries today are iatrogenic or endoluminal, we will concentrate on injury specifically related to external trauma (i.e., to penetrating injury and blunt esophageal rupture).

Surgical Anatomy

- The esophagus and trachea are unprotected
- Membranous portion of the trachea is in intimate contact, thus simultaneous injury to both structures is common
- No serosal covering
- Surrounded by loose areolar tissue
- Planes of paraesophageal and prevertebral spaces communicate freely with the mediastinum
- Blood supply is segmental, with little collateralization

Incidence and Pathophysiology (Table 20-1)

Penetrating Injuries

- Majority of injuries are due to penetrating trauma
- Injury is most common in the cervical portion but may occur at any location

Blunt Injuries

- Blunt esophageal trauma is uncommon
- Usually result from a direct blow to the organ
- May result from increased intraluminal pressures against a closed glottis
- Almost exclusively in the neck

Clinical Presentation

Clinical signs or symptoms are present in 60 to 80 percent of injuries.

- Odynophagia
- Dysphagia
- Hematemesis
- Oropharyngeal blood
- Cervical crepitus
- Pain and tenderness in the neck or chest
- Resistance to passive motion
- Dyspnea
- Hoarseness
- Bleeding

TABLE 20-1 Incidence of Various Injuries Associated with Esophageal Trauma

Site	Percentage of total injuries
Trachea	15–64
Thyroid	5–18
Spinal cord	8–16
Vocal cord or recurrent nerve	5–10
Vascular	26–43
Carotid	4–25
Major venous	8–17
Lung	5–37
Thoracic duct	4–5
Heart	10
Diaphragm	9–20
Great vessels	5–10

- Cough
- Stridor
- Mediastinal-crunching sounds (Hamman's sign)

Evaluation

Plain Radiographs of the Neck or Chest

- Abnormal in up to 82 percent of perforations
- Pneumothorax
- Hydrothorax
- Pneumomediastinum
- Mediastinal widening
- Air dissecting in retropharyngeal tissues or subcutaneous cervical air

Contrast Esophagography

- Cineradiography with two-dimensional views is best
- Sensitivity of 62 to 100 percent and specificity of 94 to 100 percent

Water-Soluble Agents (e.g., Gastrografin™)

- Use as first agent
- Nontoxic if extravasated into mediastinum
- May cause chemical pneumonitis if aspirated
- Less radiodense and may not satisfactorily demonstrate small leaks or perforations

Barium Sulfate

- After a negative Gastrografin study
- Higher density
- May better delineate an occult injury
- Intense mediastinal reactions if extravasated

Endoscopy

- A small but definite (0.1 to 1 percent) risk of further esophageal injury
- The experience of the endoscopist affects accuracy and safety
- Cervical injuries are the most difficult to see

Surgical exploration of potential esophageal injuries is advocated in some instances.

The diagnostic algorithm for evaluating potential penetrating trauma to the esophagus is based on the missile trajectory and path. For penetrating injuries near the organ without other indications for operation, one is obligated to prove that the esophagus is uninjured, either by direct exploration of the wound that demonstrates a path inconsistent with esophageal injury, or by exploring the esophagus and finding no injury. Otherwise, proof must be obtained with a variety of diagnostic tests. For blunt trauma, determining which victims need further study is a vexing task. The patient who has pneumomediastinum, which is extensive or associated with any of the symptoms of esophageal injury (odynophagia or blood in the esophagus), should have the organ evaluated. Simple pneumomediastinum rarely warrants an evaluation of the esophagus. Injury to the thoracic esophagus from blunt trauma is so unusual in comparison to the other causes of simple pneumomediastinum, one needs only to evaluate for esophageal injury in the presence of other suggestive conditions, such as pleural effusion, free air, or mediastinitis.

Treatment

Cervical Esophagus The cervical esophagus may be repaired via a collar incision or an incision along the anterior border of the sternocleidomastoid muscle. The recurrent laryngeal nerves must be identified and protected. Many esophageal wounds can be repaired by direct suture. More complex wounds may require a resection of the esophagus with or without a combined repair of the trachea. Prophylactic antibiotics effective against oral and skin flora should be initiated at the time of diagnosis. It is advisable to place muscle (sternohyoid, sternothyroid, or sternocleidomastoid) between the esophagus and an associated tracheal injury, and a closed suction drain exiting through a separate stab wound is routine.

Thoracic Esophagus Injuries to the thoracic esophagus due to external trauma are less common and more often fatal than those to the cervical esophagus. Trauma to the thoracic esophagus is almost exclusively caused by gunshot wounds, because the organ's location in the chest protects it from most stab wounds. Frequently, these injuries are also associated with injury to the surrounding structures, such as the lungs, heart, diaphragm, and great vessels, which makes the incident more likely to be fatal. Care of the associated injuries to major airways and vascular structures takes precedence in the management scheme. Guidelines for the evaluation of transmediastinal penetrating wounds are shown in Fig. 20-1. Surgical repair entails local debridement, wide drainage, primary repair of the perforation, and buttressing with a pedicle flap of viable muscle. Primary repair can usually be accomplished when the perforation is operated on within 24 hours. Various tissue flaps have been used to buttress the repair. Free pericardium, pleura, intercostal muscles, diaphragm, rhomboid muscle, lung, and the gastric fundus (as in a Thal patch) have all been used with variable success. While each has its own set of advantages, the use of any viable flap is associated with improved anastomotic outcome. Richardson has described primary muscle flap coverage alone of large esophageal defects, including repair for loss of up to 75 percent of the circumference. As the injury progresses, mediastinal and pleural inflammation becomes severe and the patient may develop signs of systemic sepsis, which make primary repair difficult and dangerous. If primary repair is not feasible, there are several techniques available: esophageal diversion, total esophageal exclusion as described by Urschel,

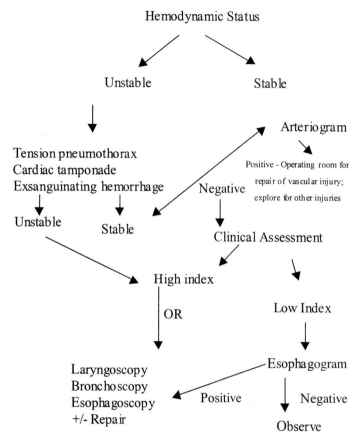

FIG. 20-1.   Algorithm for the evaluation and management of transmediastinal penetrating wounds.

esophagectomy as described by Orringer, and T-tube drainage as described by Abbott. Most experience with these delayed repairs has been acquired in patients with perforations due to instrumentation or for emetogenic esophageal rupture, and these situations are not entirely analogous to the injuries seen with external trauma. Late perforations or leaks seen following trauma are much more likely to respond to wide local drainage and creation of a controlled fistula than those due to other causes. Since there is usually no underlying esophageal or gastric pathology, or forceful distribution of mediastinal sepsis, these fistulas will commonly heal without resection, diversion, or replacement of the esophagus.

Complications after esophageal repair include: esophageal leaks and fistulas, wound infections, mediastinitis, empyema, sepsis, and pneumonia. Long-term complications such as esophageal stricture are also possible, but are more common following iatrogenic perforation of an already diseased esophagus. Worthy of special mention is the fact that esophageal anastomotic leak is the most common complication associated with repair of perforations. This occurs in 10 to 28 percent of repairs. Potential reasons for such leakage are typically technical and include: inadequate debridement, devascularization, closure under tension, and the presence of associated infection. Treatment is usually successful with adequate drainage, limiting oral intake, supplemental parenteral nutrition, and antibiotics.

INJURY TO THE TRACHEA AND BRONCHUS

For most of history, acute tracheobronchial injuries have been considered uniformly fatal. In 1874, Winslow observed the healing potential of a canvasback duck that survived some time after rupture of the left main bronchus, until finally being shot for sport. In 1927, Krinitzki reported autopsy findings of a 31-year-old woman, who had been injured at age 10 years when a keg of wine fell on her chest, suggesting that humans with tracheobronchial disruption might have the same healing potential as the canvasback duck. She suffered several broken ribs and recurrent bouts of pleurisy until autopsy demonstrated a completely occluded right main stem bronchus. Repair of such injuries probably was not attempted until 1945, when Sanger performed the first successful suture repair of a bronchial laceration; in 1949, Griffith successfully repaired a rupture of the tracheobronchial tree. Although tracheobronchial injuries are still lethal, many patients are surviving to reach emergency care. A high index of suspicion is required to make a timely diagnosis and to provide a timely intervention, both of which are essential if the patient is to have the best opportunity for recovery.

Surgical Anatomy

The anatomy and function of the trachea and bronchial tree contribute greatly to the perilous outcome after injury to the chest.

The anterior two-thirds of the trachea is protected by 18 to 22 U-shaped cartilage rings. The posterior wall of the trachea is membranous and in intimate contact with the esophagus. The recurrent laryngeal nerve lies in the tracheoesophageal groove. The blood flow to the trachea is supplied laterally and segmentally. When dissecting and mobilizing the trachea, one should avoid the lateral pedicles and mobilize only one tracheal ring circumferentially in order to maintain adequate vascular supply. One may resect a substantial length (up to 4 or 5 cm or half) of trachea and still perform primary repair.

Incidence

Injury to the tracheobronchial tree is a rare but well-recognized complication of both penetrating and blunt chest trauma. Most victims die prior to emergency care, from associated injuries to vital structures, hemorrhage, tension pneumothorax, and respiratory insufficiency due to the lack of an adequate airway. Overall, the reported incidence of injury to the trachea or bronchus varies from 0.2 to 8 percent. Greater than 80 percent of tracheobronchial ruptures occur within 2.5 cm of the carina. Main stem bronchi are injured in 86 percent of patients and distal bronchi in only 9.3 percent; complex injuries are seen in 8 percent. Tracheobronchial injuries appear to be slightly more common on the right side, perhaps because the heart and aortic arch protect the left main stem bronchus or because concomitant injury has led to early fatality.

Pathophysiology

Penetrating Injury

Penetrating injuries consist of the hole created by the path of a knife or projectile. Knife wounds occur almost exclusively in the cervical trachea, but gunshot wounds can occur at any point along the tracheobronchial tree.

Blunt Injury

Blunt trauma can be caused by a direct blow or "clothesline"-type injury. Shear forces on the trachea create damage at its relatively fixed points, the cricoid and the carina. Burst injury can also occur, usually within 2.5 cm of the carina. A combination effect of these mechanisms is probably responsible for producing the injury.

While concomitant injury is the rule rather than the exception, patterns of associated injuries vary widely. Major vascular, cardiac, pulmonary, esophageal, bony thoracic (ribs, clavicles, sternum, spine), and neurologic injuries are common and reflect the site, magnitude, and mechanism of the trauma. The mechanisms of injury can aid in searching for the sites of injury. Transcervical and transmediastinal penetrating injuries pose particular danger to the structures that they traverse (Fig. 20-2).

Presentation

Signs and Symptoms of Tracheobronchial Injury

- Stridor
- Severe respiratory distress
- Hoarseness
- Hemoptysis
- Cervical subcutaneous emphysema
- Pneumothorax: "Fallen lung" sign—lung falling away from the hilum, laterally and posteriorly, in contrast to the usual simple pneumothorax, which collapses toward the hilum; may persist despite placement of a thoracostomy tube; continuous air leak is suggestive of tracheobronchial injury and bronchopleural fistula; dyspnea may actually worsen after insertion of the chest tube due to the siphoning off of inspired air
- Pneumomediastinum

As many as two-thirds of tracheobronchial tears will go unrecognized longer than 24 hours. Up to 10 percent of tears will not produce any initial clinical or radiological signs and are recognized months later after stricture occurs. Following tracheobronchial transection, the peribronchial connective tissues may remain intact and allow continued ventilation of the distal lung analogous to the way perfusion is maintained after traumatic aortic transection. If unrecognized and not primarily repaired, this injury heals with scarring and granulation tissue and may create bronchial obstruction such as in the duck reported by Krinitzi. Distal to the obstruction, pneumonia, bronchiectasis, abscesses, and even empyema can result.

Evaluation

- Suspicion raised by mechanism of injury
- Plain radiographs
- Possible intervention (i.e., chest tube) after x-ray

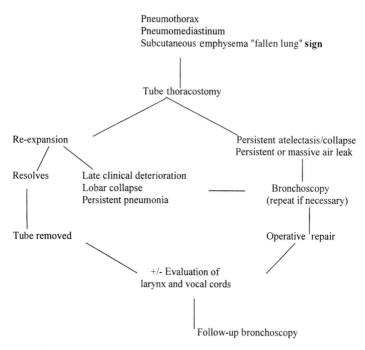

Pneumothorax
Pneumomediastinum
Subcutaneous emphysema "fallen lung" **sign**

Tube thoracostomy

Re-expansion

Persistent atelectasis/collapse
Persistent or massive air leak

Resolves

Late clinical deterioration
Lobar collapse
Persistent pneumonia

Bronchoscopy
(repeat if necessary)

Tube removed

Operative repair

+/- Evaluation of
larynx and vocal cords

Follow-up bronchoscopy

FIG. 20-2.   Algorithm for evaluation of suspected tracheobronchial injury.

- CT scan rarely conclusive
- Bronchoscopy is the most reliable means of establishing a diagnosis
- Rigid bronchoscopy: requires general anesthesia to perform; requires a stable ligamentous and bony cervical spine; allows direct visualization; ability to provide ventilation
- Flexible bronchoscopy: performed without general anesthesia; allows controlled intubation while maintaining cervical stabilization; the entire larynx and trachea can be visualized, as can the major lobar bronchi
- Repeat bronchoscopy should be liberally performed

Work-up can be completed after other life-threatening injuries are stabilized. Careless handling or mishandling of the airway can rapidly lead to disaster in these trauma patients. Inadvertently placing an endotracheal tube through a transected or ruptured airway into the soft tissue is disastrous, and may compound the injury. Emergency tracheostomies performed in the emergency department are difficult and not gratifying. Blind endotracheal intubation is fraught with the uncertainty of not knowing the path of the tube distal to the larynx and losing the lumen or creating a false passage. Intubation over a flexible bronchoscope allows visualization of the tube as it passes beyond the site of injury, and therefore alleviates some of the dangers of blind intubations. However, this usually entails some degree of sedation, and if the patient is oversedated he or she may lose his or her extant airway. Paralytic medications should generally be avoided for the same reason. Tube thoracostomies should be appropriately placed at this time and connected to suction, even though dyspnea may worsen. If dyspnea worsens the suction must be removed from the chest tube collection device. After the airway is controlled, there is time for an orderly identification of concurrent injuries, esophagoscopy, arteriography, transport to definitive care areas, and celiotomy, if necessary, to treat more urgent priorities. Otherwise, control of the airway is best obtained in the operating room.

Management (Fig. 20-3)

Intraoperative Airway Management

- Care should be coordinated with anesthesiologist
- Sterile anesthesia circuit should be available
- May need to intubate distal airway lumen in operative field
- Consideration for a double lumen endotracheal tube
- Selective ventilation through either tube: larger size of double lumen tube may worsen injury; independent lung ventilation is possible
- Extracorporeal membrane oxygenation (ECMO): uses only low-dose anticoagulation; allows complete visualization of injury without obstruction from endotracheal tube
- Tracheostomy: proximally 2 to 3 rings above the injured segment; place through incision separate from wound; may use distal tracheostomy for complex proximal injuries

Postoperative Airway Management

- Maintain low airway pressures: allows immediate extubation and spontaneous breathing; use sedation to avoid tube trauma; use high-frequency ventilation if needed; use ECMO as an adjunct for oxygenation and ventilation
- Endotracheal tube may cross repair as a stent
- Proximal tracheostomy above repair probably not necessary

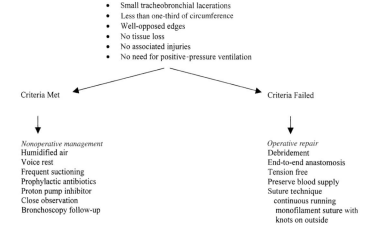

FIG. 20-3.   Management of tracheobronchial injury.

Nonoperative Management

- Reserved for selected patients with small tracheobronchial tears
- No loss or devitalization of tracheal tissue
- Involve less than one-third the circumference of the tracheobronchial tree
- Consider endobronchial stent
- Tube thoracostomy must fully re-expand the lung and air leaks should stop soon after insertion
- No associated injuries and no need for positive-pressure ventilation
- Prophylactic antibiotics
- Humidified oxygen
- Voice rest
- Frequent suctioning
- Close observation for sepsis and airway obstruction is required.
- Bronchoscopy should be liberally repeated

Surgical Approach

Extrathoracic airway injuries best reached through a transverse collar incision. Intrathoracic tracheal injury, right bronchial injury, and injuries to the proximal left main stem bronchus are best repaired through a right posterolateral thoracotomy at the fourth or fifth intercostal space. Distal left bronchial injuries greater than 3 cm from the carina are approached through a left posterolateral thoracotomy in the fifth intercostal space. Debridement of devitalized tissue, including cartilage, should be done. Primary mucosa-to-mucosa, end-to-end anastomosis of the clean tracheal or bronchial ends is performed. Avoid anastomotic tension, mobilizing the trachea anteriorly or posteriorly, and preserve the lateral blood supply. Maintain cervical flexion postoperatively by securing the chin to the chest with a suture. A running continuous absorbable monofilament suture offers a secure repair and better visibility. Tying the suture knots on the outside of the lumen helps prevent suture granuloma formation and subsequent stricture. To prevent subsequent leak and fistula formation, reinforce suture line with a patch of pericardium, a vascularized pedicle from the pleura, intercostal muscle, strap muscles, or omentum.

If there is a delay in diagnosis, repair should proceed as soon as the diagnosis is made or when practical after treatment of other life-threatening injuries. Total bronchial disruption often leads to complete occlusion and sterile atelectasis and may be amenable to repair years later. The stenotic segment is resected and repaired in a manner similar to that of the acute injury or as one would treat a benign stenosis. Although useful for late repair, techniques of bronchial sleeve resections, lobectomy, and pneumonectomy are rarely acutely required for more extensive or distal injuries to lobar or segmental bronchi. Although bronchial rupture can be treated successfully in the acute or the delayed phase, early diagnosis and treatment minimizes the risk of infection and resection and shortens the patient's hospital stay.

OUTCOME

Despite persistent early mortality in the older published reports, today more than 90 percent of patients reaching the hospital alive should have acceptable outcomes. Most of the early mortality is due to lack of control of airway injuries and to multiple associated injuries, especially the vascular and esophageal injuries. Patients who require pulmonary resection for treatment have poorer outcomes. Pneumonectomy has an associated mortality rate as high as 30 percent from acute pulmonary hypertension and right heart failure. Early diagnosis with primary repair of these injuries leads to the fewest complications and to the best long-term results, and is the procedure of choice. Excellent anatomical and functional results should be expected with normal pulmonary function and voice characteristics after early repair. Early repair also results in fewer tracheal revisions to correct stenosis.

ADDITIONAL READINGS

Defore WW, Mattox KL, Hansen HA, et al: Surgical management of penetrating injuries of the esophagus. *Am J Surg* 134:734, 1997.

Feliciano DV, Bitondo CG, Mattox KL, et al: Combined tracheoesophageal injuries. *Am J Surg* 150:710, 1985.

Mathisen DJ, Grillo H: Laryngotracheal trauma. *Ann Thorac Surg* 43:254, 1987.

Mills SA, Johnston FR, Hudspeth AS, et al: Clinical spectrum of blunt tracheobronchial disruption illustrated by seven cases. *J Thorac Cardiovasc Surg* 84:49, 1982.

Pate JW: Thoracic trauma: Tracheobronchial and esophageal injuries. *Surg Clin North Am* 69:1, 111, 1989.

Richardson JD, Tobin GR: Closure of esophageal defects with muscle flaps. *Arch Surg* 129:541, 1994.

21 | Injury to the Lung and Pleura

Approximately 25 percent of all trauma-related deaths are attributed to thoracic injuries. The majority of injuries to the lung and pleura may be treated with a simple tube thoracostomy. There is a major difference in the mechanism of injury, pathophysiology, and treatment of penetrating and blunt injuries to the lungs and pleura.

BLUNT INJURY

Etiology and Pathophysiology

Immediately life-threatening thoracic injuries include cardiac tamponade, hemothorax, and tension pneumothorax. Other injuries, such as diaphragmatic disruption or an aortic transaction, can lead to early death if not promptly recognized. Most lung and pleural injuries cause physiologic problems through one of three mechanisms: (1) pleural space problems that interfere with lung function; (2) hemorrhage from the chest wall or lung; and (3) pulmonary parenchymal problems that impair ability to ventilate and oxygenate.

Pleural space problems can be divided into pneumothorax, hemothorax, and rarely chylothorax. Most cases of traumatic pneumothorax have associated bleeding that may not be apparent on the initial chest x-ray. Hemothorax may cause problems because it compresses the lung and interferes with lung function. Massive hemothorax may also lead to shock and death from hemorrhage. Pulmonary parenchymal injuries resulting from blunt trauma typically occur in the form of pulmonary contusion, although intrapulmonary hematoma may occur. The radiologic findings of pulmonary contusion lag behind the clinical findings, making its diagnosis more difficult.

Approach to the Patient with Blunt Chest Trauma

The airway must be secured and the patient must be rapidly and adequately resuscitated. If the patient has signs of tamponade, the possibility of blunt cardiac injury must be considered. Tension pneumothorax may produce many of the same signs as tamponade. After lifesaving measures have been instituted, a rapid physical examination should be performed. A rapid examination of the neck in search of distended neck veins, hematoma, and crepitance should be done. Chest excursion should be observed and breath sounds ascertained. If there is no air movement on one side, an emergency tube thoracostomy should be placed. If the breath sounds are slightly diminished and the patient is stable, a chest x-ray should be obtained. A careful physical examination and a good-quality chest radiograph can diagnose most thoracic injuries. (Table 21-1). Early computed tomography (CT) scan of the chest may be useful in some patients. The therapeutic approach to the most common injuries can then be carried out in a systematic manner (Fig. 21-1).

Pneumothorax

The most common intrathoracic injury following blunt trauma is a pneumothorax, which is caused by trapping of air within the pleural space. The degree of pneumothorax is usually expressed as a percentage, but this can be misleading as it does not represent a three-dimensional view. The standard treatment is tube thoracostomy. If a tension pneumothorax is suspected, it should be treated expeditiously.

TABLE 21-1 Important Features and Their Suspected Diagnosis in Patients with Blunt Chest Trauma

X-ray finding	Diagnostic abnormality
Air or fluid in pleural space	Pneumothorax, hemothorax
Widened or abnormal mediastinum	Aortic or major branch injury
Fluid density in lung field	Pulmonary contusion
Obscure diaphragm	Ruptured diaphragm
Rib fracture	Flail chest
Soft tissue air	Pneumothorax
Position of tubes	Malposition

Following placement, the tube should be connected to an underwater seal with negative suction of 20 cm H_2O. A follow-up x-ray should be taken for ensure adequate lung expansion. Treatment without a tube is reserved for patients who have isolated small pneumothoraces and are essentially asymptomatic. Treatment without a tube is not indicated for patients requiring general anesthetic or positive-pressure ventilation, those with bilateral injuries, or those who may soon be transferred. If observation alone is used, a follow-up x-ray should be done at 6 and 24 hours. The indications for prophylactic chest tube placement include multiple rib fractures in a patient who requires general anesthesia. Although supportive data are controversial, antibiotics are usually administered while the tube is in place.

Hemothorax Following Blunt Trauma

It is uncommon to have massive bleeding initially from a chest tube following blunt injury. Continuous bleeding or delayed hemorrhage is a much more common indication for thoracotomy. Pulmonary or pleural bleeding that requires surgery is the result of three factors: (1) rib fractures that lacerate the intercostal vessels, (2) displaced rib fractures that lacerate the lung, and (3) adhesions between the pulmonary parenchyma and the chest wall that tear. The treatment for acute hemothorax is tube thoracostomy. A large, posteriorly directed chest tube should be placed. Continuous bleeding from the chest tube at a volume of 200 to 300 mL/h for several hours will probably

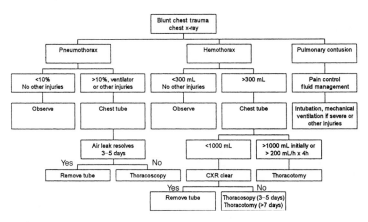

FIG. 21-1. Algorithm for the therapeutic approach to blunt chest trauma.

require thoracotomy. Delayed hemothorax is a particular problem following blunt chest trauma. Because patients with blunt trauma have multiple sources for haziness on a chest x-ray, the diagnosis may be unclear. A chest CT scan will differentiate between a parenchymal and a pleural process. A retained hemothorax is best dealt with early in the patient's course because thoracoscopic surgery is more likely to be successful.

Pulmonary Contusion

Pulmonary contusion is a direct bruise of the lung followed by alveolar hemorrhage and edema from the injury. Tissue perfusion should be restored, and adequate urine output must be maintained. If major resuscitation is needed, the use of a pulmonary artery catheter may be indicated. In patients with mild to moderate pulmonary contusions, judicious fluid management and aggressive pain control are the mainstays of treatment. Initial pain control of associated rib fractures can be rapidly achieved with rib blocks using local anesthesia. An epidural catheter can be placed for prolonged pain management. In severe pulmonary contusions, proper ventilator management is critical. The risk of barotrauma should be reduced by use of lower tidal volumes (5 to 7 mL/kg), although positive end-expiratory pressure may be required to prevent alveolar collapse. Occasionally, patients with severe unilateral pulmonary contusions may develop refractory hypoxemia on conventional volume ventilation. In these situations, switching to a pressure-control mode may improve gas distribution and oxygenation.

PENETRATING INJURIES TO THE LUNG AND PLEURA

Proper prioritization of care is especially important for patients with penetrating chest injuries. Early management requires attention to the principles of primary survey and resuscitation as outlined in the *Advanced Trauma Life Support (ATLS) Manual.* Early assessment and establishment of a patent airway, the insertion of large-bore intravenous catheters, administration of intravenous fluids, maintenance of cardiac output, and evaluation of the chest for hemothorax, tension pneumothorax, or an open sucking chest wound are the immediate objectives. The indications for early operation are:

- Continued shock with bleeding,
- Large air leak with inability to oxygenate and/or ventilate, and
- Suspected associated injuries to the heart, great vessels, esophagus, diaphragm, or intra-abdominal organs.

In evaluating patients with penetrating injuries of the chest, one must always be suspicious of these injuries.

Tube Thoracostomy

The positioning and management of tube thoracostomy are basic to the care of penetrating chest injuries. A large-bore (38 to 40 French) chest tube should be used in the majority of patients. The tube should be placed in the midaxillary line in the fourth to sixth intercostal space. The index finger should be inserted into the pleural space to confirm entry. A chest tube should never be blindly placed with a trocar. The tube is advanced in a posterior and superior direction. The chest tube should then be connected to an underwater seal with suction. The tube should be well secured to the skin of the chest wall, and a sterile dressing should be applied. The chest tube is left in place until there is no air leak from the lung and less than 100 to 150 mL/day of fluid drains through the tube. It is important to obtain a chest x-ray immediately after placement and removal of the tube. The inability to completely evacuate blood from the pleural space is one of the indications for early surgical intervention.

For open, sucking chest wounds, an inclusive dressing should be applied over the wound and taped on three sides. One side should be left open so that interpleural air can be expelled. All patients with open, sucking chest wounds require placement of a chest tube, which should never be placed through the original wound itself. Although tube thoracostomy insertion is often a lifesaving procedure and is relatively straightforward, the complication rate is 20 percent. Early chest tube insertion in a tension pneumothorax can be lifesaving, even if done imperfectly, and most of these complications can be treated.

Hemothorax

Hemothorax, defined as blood in the pleural space, is common in penetrating chest trauma. The source of the blood can be the lung, chest wall (including the intercostal or internal mammary arteries), heart, great vessels, diaphragm, or intra-abdominal organs, especially the liver or spleen. A massive hemothorax is ≥ 1500 mL of blood in the chest. Usually 200 to 300 mL of fluid must collect in the pleural space before a hemothorax can be detected on x-ray. If the x-ray is done with the patient in the supine position, the hemothorax can be harder to detect because the fluid flows out along the entire posterior portion of the hemothorax.

The treatment of hemothorax basically involves two principles: (1) drainage of blood from the pleural space, and (2) control of the bleeding. Overall, 10 to 20 percent of patients with penetrating chest injuries require thoracotomy, depending on the mechanism of the injury. Once a chest tube has been placed, it is imperative to perform a chest x-ray afterward. If the pleural space still appears to contain blood, a second chest tube should be placed. If the pleural space cannot be evacuated adequately, a thoracotomy or thoracoscopy is indicated. Immediate removal of more than 1000 mL of blood from the pleural cavity should quickly alert the clinician to the need for a thoracotomy. Continued bleeding from the chest tube is another indication for thoracotomy. A general guideline for thoracotomy is a chest tube output of 200 mL/h for 4 hours. Collection and reinfusion of pleural blood can be done for large hemothoraces if the collection apparatus is available.

Pneumothorax

Pneumothorax is extremely common in patients with penetrating injuries to the chest. A large pneumothorax is easily diagnosed on physical examination. All patients with penetrating injuries who have a pneumothorax should have a chest tube inserted. The chest tube should be left in place with an underwater seal and suction until there is no air leakage for 12 to 24 hours and the fluid output is less than 100 to 150 mL per 24 hours. Patients with stab wounds to the chest who are hemodynamically stable, do not appear to have any major cardiac or great vessel injuries, and have a normal chest x-ray must be observed for a short time because they remain at risk for pneumothorax. If the follow-up chest x-ray is normal, the patient can be safely discharged, but should be seen in the outpatient clinic a few days after discharge.

Tension Pneumothorax

In tension pneumothorax, air is trapped in the pleural space and gathers under pressure. As the pneumothorax enlarges, it causes collapse of the involved lung and shifts in the mediastinal structures. This decreases blood return to the right heart and causes hemodynamic instability. The diagnosis should be suspected in any patient with a penetrating chest injury who has hemodynamic instability. Venous distension may be present in the neck. Treatment involves immediate decompression, which is best done with a large-bore chest tube. If a chest tube is not immediately available or the patient is in the prehospital setting, insertion of a large-bore needle into the pleural space is indicated, through the second intercostal space and in the midclavicular line.

Repair of Pulmonary Parenchymal Lacerations

Most parenchymal lacerations will present as pneumothorax and can be managed with a chest tube. A small percentage will require thoracotomy. The goal of treatment for pulmonary parenchymal lacerations should be to stop bleeding or air leakage, or to remove clearly or potentially devitalized lung tissue. This should be accomplished by the simplest method possible. An anatomic resection, such as a lobectomy or formal segmental resection, is usually unnecessary. We have found the use of a stapling device to be the most effective means for controlling air leaks and hemorrhage from the lung. A lobectomy following chest trauma may be required in some circumstances. Occasionally, injury to a main stem bronchus is such that repair is not feasible. In such cases, treatment is best accomplished by resecting the involved lobe. In the occasional patient who requires a lobectomy and has other lung injuries, the use of positive-pressure ventilation, particularly with positive end-expiratory pressure, will often result in bronchopleural fistula. In this circumstance, the use of a pleural or muscle flap may prevent a secondary fistula or aid healing if a fistula occurs.

Pneumonectomy

Patients who require pneumonectomy following chest injury present a particular problem. Our experience with pneumonectomy for major hilar wounds in patients who are in shock has been dismal. These patients frequently die of right heart failure in the operating room or within the first few postoperative days. The heart does not tolerate the combination of significant peripheral vascular resistance due to shock, coupled with a sudden increase in pulmonary vascular resistance following pneumonectomy. If pneumonectomy is needed, it should be done expeditiously to prevent continued blood loss, and resuscitation should be kept to a minimum. Simultaneous stapling of the bronchus and vasculature may help deal with these injuries.

DELAYED PROBLEMS OR COMPLICATIONS

Clotted Hemothorax

Clotted hemothorax is a particular problem for patients with thoracic injuries. Many hemothoraces may fail to drain, with trapping of significant portions of the lung and resultant fibrothorax. The clotted hemothorax represents an ideal nidus for secondary infection and empyema. If a tube thoracotomy is not draining the pleural space, we advocate early surgery for the removal of clotted hemothorax. Thoracoscopy in this setting is advantageous. If done early, video-assisted thoracoscopy permits the complete evacuation of a hemothorax without thoracotomy. Late thoracoscopy, after 1 week, has usually been less successful, and conversion to a thoracotomy is often necessary. The standard indications for operative intervention have included (1) a clotted hemothorax with ≥25 percent loss of the lung volume, (2) signs of infection of the hemothorax, such as fever and leukocytosis, or an air-fluid level. The use of CT as a diagnostic refinement over standard chest radiography has been very helpful.

Persistent Air Leak and Bronchopleural Fistulas

While air leaks are very common following chest trauma, they rarely require specific treatment other than tube thoracotomy. Large air leaks may occur in any of several circumstances, including bronchial injury, unexpanded lung, underlying lung disease, and a defect in the chest tube system.

Treatment of a persistent air leak requires bronchoscopy to ensure that injury to a main airway has not occurred. If bronchoscopy demonstrates a proximal bronchial injury, surgical repair is required. If a patient continues to have an air leak after 4 to 5 days, a thoracoscopic approach may solve the problem. A pulmonary parenchymal injury may be stapled through the thoracoscope, or a mini-thoracotomy can be done to correct a parenchymal leak.

Empyema

Posttraumatic empyema is a significant problem in chest trauma. Potential etiologies of posttraumatic empyema include:

- Iatrogenic infection of the pleural space as a result of tube thoracostomy
- Direct infection of the pleural space resulting from penetrating injuries
- Secondary infection of the pleural space from injury to intra-abdominal organs with diaphragmatic disruption
- Secondary infection of a clotted hemothorax
- Hematogenous or transdiaphragmatic lymphatic spread
- Postpneumonic empyema secondary to posttraumatic pneumonia, pulmonary contusion, or adult respiratory distress syndrome

We have found CT to be particularly valuable. It is especially helpful in the evaluation of residual fluid collections following blunt trauma in the patient who has pneumonia. The treatment of empyema depends on several factors, including the etiologic agent, the ease of drainage with tube thoracostomy, and the persistence of signs of infection. Occasionally, a well-placed chest tube will drain the pleural space properly, and in combination with appropriate antibiotics, may resolve an empyema. If this treatment fails, thoracotomy is the next logical step. There is a big difference between draining early fluid collections with a thoracoscope and treating a well-established empyema. In the latter situation, a standard thoracotomy is needed. It is not uncommon for the chest film to look worse for the first few postoperative days. However, if good drainage has been established, the patient will usually begin to improve within several days. Vigorous pulmonary toilet must be used to keep the lung expanded after thoracotomy. Culture-specific antibiotics should be used for organisms cultured from the pleura or sputum.

ADDITIONAL READING

Etoch SW, Bar-Natan UT, Miller FB, et al: Tube thoracostomy: Factors related to complications. *Arch Surg* 130:521, 1995.

O'Brien J, Cohen M, Solit R, et al: Thorascopic drainage and decortication as definitive treatment for empyema thoracis following penetrating chest injury. *J Trauma* 36:536, 1994.

Richardson JD, Adams L, Flint LM: Selective management of flail chest and pulmonary contusion. *Ann Surg* 196:481, 1982.

Richardson JD, Miller FB, Carrillo EH, et al: Complex thoracic injuries. *Surg Clin North Am* 76:725, 1996.

Wagner JW, Obeid FN, Kanny-Jones RC, et al: Trauma pneumonectomy revisited: The role of simultaneously stapled pneumonectomy. *J Trauma* 40:590, 1996.

22 | The Injured Heart

PENETRATING CARDIAC INJURY

Historic Perspective

While Theodore Billroth (1883), Boerhave (1709), and Paget (1896) considered heart surgeryto be futile, Rehn carried out the first successful human cardiorrhaphy in 1896. Hill performed the first cardiorrhaphy in the United States in 1902 and ushered in the modern treatment of the wounded heart. In 1943, he recommended a nonoperative approach with repeated pericardiocentesis.

Etiology

Penetrating cardiac injuries are commonly caused by knives, guns, and rarely by other sharp objects such as a fractured sternum or rib. Iatrogenic penetrating wounds of the heart result from intracardiac injections, central venous catheters, and during percutaneous dilatation of coronary arteries.

Pathophysiology

The right ventricle, with its maximal anterior exposure, is at greatest risk of injury. In a 20-year experience with 711 cardiac injuries, Wall and colleagues found right ventricular involvement in 40 percent and left ventricular injury in 40 percent of patients they examined. The right atrium (24 percent) and left atrium (3 percent) were much less frequently involved. Sixty complex injuries were seen, including 39 to the coronary arteries.

Of those presenting with stab wounds, 80 to 90 percent present with tamponade. As little as 60 to 100 mL of blood and clots in the pericardium may produce the clinical picture of tamponade. In contrast to stab wounds, gunshot wounds of the pericardium and cardiac chambers often are large and produce massive hemorrhage.

Tachycardia, an increase in ventricular filling pressure, and enhanced myocardial contractility from endogenous catecholamines result in augmentation of right ventricular diastolic filling. Pulsus paradoxus (exaggerated fall in systolic blood pressure during inspiration) may be seen. However, as the limits of distensibility of the pericardium are reached, further accumulation of even a small amount of blood causes a significant impairment of cardiac contractility. Left ventricular filling and stroke volume are severely impaired by septal shift, cardiac output falls precipitously, and a sudden and profound systemic hypotension ensues.

Diagnosis

Cardiac injury may be present without the so-called "classic" Beck's triad of pericardial tamponade (distended neck veins, muffled heart sounds, and hypotension) or pulsus paradoxus. Chest radiographs are misleading. The most helpful findings are hemodynamic instability and a penetrating wound in the precordium, epigastrium, or superior mediastinum. Pericardiocentesis has no role in the diagnosis of cardiac tamponade, since false positives and false negatives are common.

In a small subset of patients with compensated cardiac tamponade, FAST (focused abdominal sonography for trauma) is currently the most widely used test. Rozycki and coworkers presented a multicenter experience with FAST in large series of 209 patients with precordial or transthoracic wounds. True positive examinations were found in 21 patients, all of whom had cardiac injuries. Sonography, performed by properly trained and credentialed surgeons, had a sensitivity of 100 percent and a specificity of 97.3 percent for pericardial fluid.

Subxiphoid Pericardial Window

Use of this technique is best reserved for patients already in the operating room undergoing other procedures. Under general anesthesia, a vertical midline incision is made over the xiphoid process and upper epigastrium. The xiphoid is elevated or excised, bringing into view the pericardiophrenic membrane. An incision between two stay sutures into this area creates a window in the pericardial sac for inspection. With confirmation of a cardiac injury, the incision can be extended as a median sternotomy for a cardiorrhaphy. Since direct visualization of the pericardial sac is possible, the technique is consistently accurate.

Thoracoscopy

In patients with a preexisting thoracostomy for hemo- or pneumothorax and other indications for thoracoscopy, this is a versatile test to detect hemopericardium, assess and control intrathoracic bleeding, and evacuate clotted hemothorax. In a series from Colombia, Morales and associates recently published a large series of 108 patients who had a thoracoscopic pericardial window to rule out hemopericardium. It was positive for hemopericardium in 30.6 percent of patients. The procedure was well tolerated, accurate in 97 percent, and did not lead to any complications.

TREATMENT OF CARDIAC INJURIES

Prehospital Management

Mattox and Feliciano found no survivors when they analyzed 100 traumatized patients who had external cardiac compression for more than 3 minutes in the prehospital period. In an analysis of the impact of prehospital resuscitation on survival after emergency room thoracotomy (ERT), Durham and associates analyzed 207 patients who arrived with cardiopulmonary resuscitation (CPR) in progress. The average time of prehospital CPR for survivors was 5.1 minutes (compared to 9.1 minutes for nonsurvivors). These authors also noted that prehospital endotracheal intubation significantly increased the duration of tolerance of CPR (9.4 minutes in survivors compared to 4.2 minutes for nonintubated survivors). These data argue for prompt transport of patients with truncal penetrating wounds to the emergency center.

Emergency Center Management

The ABCs (*A*irway, *B*reathing, and *C*irculation) of the initial survey are clearly the highest priority. The subsequent management of these patients is determined by their hemodynamic stability, as outlined in the algorithm (Fig. 22-1). A rapid FAST, if available, confirms pericardial fluid, and these patients are immediately transported to the operating room for sternotomy or thoracotomy. Borderline stability or instability is an indication for pericardiocentesis and/or thoracotomy in the emergency room, depending upon whether there are surgical capabilities in the emergency department.

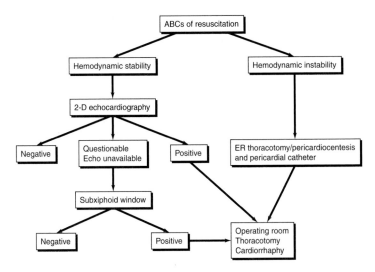

FIG. 22-1. Algorithm for management of cardiac trauma. Pericardiocentesis is used for therapeutic purposes if emergency room thoracotomy cannot be performed.

Pericardiocentesis may have a role in the initial stabilization of the patient, especially in centers which are not equipped to perform major operations in the receiving area of the hospital. An indwelling catheter in the pericardial sac and repeated aspirations may provide hemodynamic stability prior to thoracotomy. Pericardiocentesis is performed by a subxiphoid approach and the needle is advanced under electrocardiographic monitoring. In one method, the needle is advanced at a 45 degree angle to the frontal plane and advanced towards the right shoulder. In this orientation the needle is parallel, rather than at right angles, to the apex of the ventricle and the possibility of myocardial injury is decreased.

DEFINITIVE TREATMENT OF CARDIAC INJURIES

The definitive treatment of cardiac injuries is cardiorrhaphy through a thoracotomy or sternotomy. The surgical relief of tamponade and repair of cardiac lacerations should be performed as expeditiously as possible, while attempts are made to do volume expansion, partial correction of acidosis, maintenance of coronary perfusion by effective massage of the heart, and avoidance of hypothermia.

A left anterior or fifth space anterolateral thoracotomy is the incision of choice for emergency room thoracotomy (ERT). Further exposure, if necessary, is obtained by transsternal extension into the right chest. Median sternotomy is a versatile incision and provides superb exposure of the heart, the great vessels, and the pulmonary hila. Extension into the abdomen as a midline laparotomy incision provides superb access to the dome of the liver and other upper abdominal organs. Extension into the neck provides access to the major vascular structures at the inlet and the neck.

Once exposure is achieved, a distended, discolored, and often tense pericardial sac confirms cardiac injury. The pericardium is opened anterior to the phrenic nerve and the tamponade is relieved. The bleeding heart is controlled by digital occlusion and the laceration is sutured by mattress sutures of 3-0 Tevdek over Teflon pledgets. Strips of pericardium make suitable substitutes for the pledgets, if pledgets are unavailable. For larger wounds, temporary closure to control the hemorrhage may be achieved by insertion of a Foley catheter with the balloon inflated into the wound. Gentle traction on the catheter will tamponade the laceration against the balloon. For lacerations in proximity to the coronary vessels, horizontal mattress sutures placed underneath the vessels avoid obstruction of coronary flow. Wall and associates described the management of 60 complex injuries. Thirty-nine of the injuries involved the coronary arteries. Most of these injuries were treated by ligation, and emergency coronary bypass was employed only twice. These authors also detailed the intraoperative assessment of intracardiac injuries. Useful techniques include careful palpation of the chambers for a thrill, detection of murmurs with an esophageal stethoscope, a sterile stethoscope applied to the surface of the heart, and transesophageal echocardiography. Once detected, the lesions are usually addressed in more detail postoperatively.

INJURY SEVERITY

Using the cardiovascular and respiratory elements of the Trauma Score (TS) on admission, Asensio and colleagues recently published their prospective series of 105 patients with penetrating cardiac injuries, the largest yet reported. In their experience, mortality was 94 percent when the TS was between zero and 3 and a 31 percent mortality when the score was between 4 and 11.

The Organ Injury Scaling Committee of the American Association for the Surgery of Trauma has recently defined criteria for injury severity for the heart as well as other thoracic organs and this scheme is summarized in Table 22-1. It is recommended that future reports follow the AAST scale to standardize the definition of injury severity.

RESULTS OF TREATMENT IN PENETRATING CARDIAC TRAUMA

The prognosis for patients with stab wounds to the heart who can be transported to the operating room for a thoracotomy and cardiorrhaphy is excellent, with a survival of 97 percent for stab wounds and 71 percent for gunshot wounds in patients who are stable enough to be transported to the operating room without a preliminary ERT. In a collective series of 2253 patients who had ERT for penetrating cardiac trauma, 315 (14 percent) survived, and this number included 55 of 706 (7.8 percent) who arrived at the hospital without vital signs. Ninety-eight patients had no vital signs either in the field or on arrival at the hospital, with only 2 (2 percent) survivors. One of these patients was a neurologic invalid. In the recent 20-year experience reported by Wall and associates, the overall mortality was 47 percent. Among the 314 patients requiring ERT, 82.8 percent died.

PROGNOSTIC FACTORS IN PENETRATING CARDIAC TRAUMA

Single-chamber injuries, stab wounds, absence of significant intracardiac defects, hemodynamic stability on arrival and/or rapid stabilization by initial resuscitation resulting in transportation to the operating room for a thoracotomy are all associated with a significantly higher survival rate. The pres-

TABLE 22-1 AAST Organ Injury Scale for the Heart

Grade*	Description of Injury
I	Blunt injury with minor ECG abnormalities; blunt or penetrating pericardial wound without cardiac injury, tamponade, or herniation.
II	Blunt cardiac injury with heart block or ischemic changes without heart failure; penetrating tangential myocardial wound to but not extending through the endocardium without tamponade
III	Blunt cardiac injury with sustained (>5 beats/min) or multifocal ventricular contractions; blunt or penetrating injury with septal rupture, pulmonary or tricuspid valvular incompetence, papillary muscle dysfunction, or distal coronary arterial occlusion *without* cardiac failure; blunt pericardial laceration with cardiac herniation; blunt cardiac injury with cardiac failure; penetrating tangential myocardial wound up to but not extending through the endocardium, with tamponade
IV	Blunt or penetrating injury with septal rupture, pulmonary or tricuspid valvular incompetence, papillary muscle dysfunction, or distal coronary arterial occlusion *with* cardiac failure; blunt or penetrating injury with aortic or mitral valve incompetence; blunt or penetrating injury of the right ventricle, right atrium, or left atrium
V	Blunt or penetrating injury with proximal coronary artery occlusion; blunt or penetrating perforation of the left ventricle; stellate wound with <50% tissue loss of the right ventricle, right atrium, or left atrium
VI	Blunt avulsion of the heart; penetrating wound producing >50% tissue loss of a chamber

*Advance one grade for multiple penetrating wounds to a single chamber or multiple-chamber involvement.

ence of significant associated injuries, gunshot wounds, coronary vessel lacerations, multiple-chamber injuries, as well as delayed diagnosis and treatment are unfavorable prognostic factors. The presence of sinus rhythm on opening the pericardium, gunshot wounds, exsanguination, and the restoration of blood pressure were found to be the most significant predictors of mortality in the prospective studies from Demetriades.

POSTOPERATIVE COMPLICATIONS

Survivors of penetrating cardiac trauma may have a number of intracardiac complications in the remote postoperative period. However, the need for reoperation for intracardiac defects is quite rare. The Ben Taub experience estimates this at 2 percent of all patients. The postpericardiotomy syndrome, manifested by fever, chest pain, pericardial effusion, pericardial rub, and ECG abnormalities, is the most frequent sequela after pericardiotomy for trauma. Its exact etiology is not known. Suggested mechanisms include hypersensitivity of injured epicardium, inflammatory reaction to intrapericardial blood, and viral or bacterial infection. These patients exhibit a moderate fever and complain of precordial or retrosternal pain with extension to the neck or back. The diagnosis is made by exclusion of other causes of the fever. The disease is self-limited and treatment consists of aspirin, indomethacin, and occasionally steroids.

BLUNT TRAUMA TO THE HEART

Blunt trauma to the heart ranges from minor injury to frank rupture. The minor injury is a nonspecific condition variously termed *cardiac contusion, cardiac concussion,* or *myocardial contusion.* More specific abnormalities that are demonstrable and consistent include injury to the pericardium, cardiac valves, papillary muscles, chordae tendinae, septal wall, and coronary vessels. The other extreme of the spectrum of blunt cardiac trauma is the dramatic, often fatal condition of cardiac rupture.

Nonpenetrating injury to the heart may cause rupture of the valves, especially in patients with preexisting disease of these structures. Parmley and associates, in a series of 546 cases of blunt cardiac trauma, reported a 9 percent incidence of injury to the valves. The aortic, mitral, and tricuspid valves were involved in decreasing order of frequency.

New onset of a harsh holosystolic murmur of mitral regurgitation signifies a papillary muscle rupture. New loud musical murmurs may indicate valvular lesions. When severe acute left ventricular failure ensues as a consequence of these lesions, early operative intervention is indicated. Septal rupture should be suspected in all patients with abnormal murmurs and should be investigated by Doppler echocardiography and cardiac catheterization if necessary. Treatment of these lesions should be individualized. Small septal defects and those that are associated with small shunts and mild symptoms may be managed with medical therapy. A number of them may close spontaneously. Larger defects with left-to-right shunts with a Qp:Qs ratio of 2:1 or greater need operative correction.

Cardiac rupture in blunt trauma usually results from severe injury to the chest from high-speed motor vehicle crashes or, less commonly, from falls from a height. In a recent report from Tokyo, 30 were due to falls, 26 from motor vehicle crashes, and 6 were due to a crush injury of the chest.

The presenting symptoms are those of cardiac tamponade or severe hemorrhage. "Bruit de moulin," a precordial murmur that sounds like a splashing waterwheel, may be heard. The presence of associated injuries and multisys-

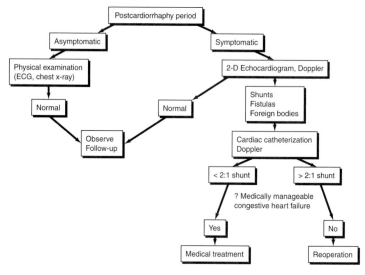

FIG. 22-2. Algorithm for postoperative evaluation of the patient with cardiac injury.

tem involvement in these patients makes the diagnosis difficult unless a high index of suspicion is maintained. The majority of patients present without vital signs on admission. In patients who arrive stable, delayed diagnosis is common. Electrocardiography may suggest bundle branch block or, in cases of cardiac herniation, axis deviation. The recent series from Tokyo by Kato and associates showed that ultrasonography is a reliable test to demonstrate pericardial fluid.

The principles of treatment of blunt rupture of the heart are the same as for penetrating trauma. Approximately 10 percent of patients with blunt cardiac rupture benefit from cardiopulmonary bypass, which facilitates a proper evaluation and treatment of a quiet heart. An intra-aortic balloon pump is a valuable adjunct in patients with significant myocardial contusion and depression. Associated injuries to the pelvis and abdomen should be considered and investigated by peritoneal lavage or ultrasonography once the cardiac rupture is controlled.

ADDDITIONAL READINGS

Asensio JA, Stewart BM, Murray J et al: Penetrating cardiac injuries: a complex challenge. *Injury* 32:533, 2001.

Fulda G, Braithwaite CEM, Rodriguez A, et al: Blunt traumatic rupture of the heart and pericardium: a ten year experience. *J Trauma* 31:167, 1991.

Ivatury RR, Nallathambi M, Rohman M, et al: Penetrating cardiac trauma: Quantifying anatomic and physiologic injury severity. *Ann Surg* 205:61, 1987.

Kato K, Henmi H, Mashiko K, et al: Blunt traumatic rupture of the heart: an experience in Tokyo. *J Trauma* 35:165, 1993.

Mattox KL, Feliciano DV: Role of external cardiac compression in truncal trauma. *J Trauma* 22:934, 1982.

Milham FH, Grindlinger GA: Survival determinants in patients undergoing emergency room thoracotomy for penetrating chest injury. *J Trauma* 34:332, 1993.

Rozycki GS, Schmidt JA, Ochsner MG, et al: The role of surgeon-performed ultrasound in patients with possible penetrating cardiac wounds. A prospective multicenter study. *J Trauma* 45:190, 1998.

Wall MJ, Mattox KL, Baldwin JC: Acute management of complex cardiac injuries. *J Trauma* 42:905, 1997.

23 | Injury to the Thoracic Great Vessels

Injuries to the thoracic great vessels—the aorta and its brachiocephalic branches, the pulmonary arteries and veins, the superior and intrathoracic inferior vena cava, and the innominate and azygos veins—occur following both blunt and penetrating trauma. Exsanguinating hemorrhage, the primary acute manifestation, also occurs in the chronic setting when the injured great vessel forms a fistula involving an adjacent structure or when a posttraumatic aneurysm or pseudoaneurysm ruptures.

PATHOPHYSIOLOGY

More than 90 percent of thoracic great vessel injuries are due to penetrating trauma: gunshot, shrapnel, and stab wounds, or therapeutic misadventures. Iatrogenic lacerations of various thoracic great vessels, including the arch of the aorta, are frequently reported complications of percutaneous central venous catheter placement. The percutaneous placement of trocar chest tubes has caused injuries to the intercostal arteries and major pulmonary and medi-astinal vessels. Intra-aortic counterpulsation balloons can produce injury to the thoracic aorta. During emergency center resuscitative thoracotomy, the aorta may be injured during cross clamping if a crushing (nonvascular) clamp is used. Overinflation of the Swan-Ganz balloon has produced iatrogenic injuries to pulmonary artery branches with resultant fatal hemoptysis. Self-expanding metal stents have produced perforations of the aorta and innominate artery following placement into the esophagus and trachea, respectively.

The great vessels particularly susceptible to injury from blunt trauma include the innominate artery, pulmonary veins, vena cava, and most commonly, the thoracic aorta. Aortic injuries have caused or contributed to 10 to 15 percent of deaths following motor vehicle accidents for nearly 30 years. These injuries usually involve the proximal descending aorta (54 to 65 percent of cases), but often involve other segments [i.e., the ascending aorta or transverse aortic arch (10 to 14 percent) and the mid or distal descending thoracic aorta (12 percent)], or multiple sites (13 to 18 percent). The postulated mechanisms of blunt great vessel injury include (1) shear forces caused by relative mobility of a portion of the vessel adjacent to a fixed portion, (2) compression of the vessel between bony structures, and (3) profound intraluminal hypertension during deceleration. The atrial attachments of the pulmonary veins and vena cava and the fixation of the descending thoracic aorta at the ligamentum arteriosum and diaphragm enhance their susceptibility to blunt rupture by the first mechanism. At its origin, the innominate artery may be pinched between the sternum and the vertebrae during anterior sternal impact.

Blunt aortic injuries may be partial thickness—histologically similar to the initial tear in aortic dissection—or full thickness and therefore equivalent to a ruptured aortic aneurysm that is contained by surrounding tissues. The histopathologic similarities between aortic injuries and nontraumatic aortic catastrophes mandate that similar therapeutic approaches be employed. Therefore, in hemodynamically stable patients, the concepts of permissive hypovolemia and aggressive minimization of dP/dT—which are widely accepted in the treatment of aortic dissection and aneurysm rupture—should be considered in patients with blunt aortic injuries.

True traumatic aortic dissection, with a longitudinal separation of the media extending along the length of the aorta, is extremely rare. The use of the term *dissection* in the setting of aortic trauma should be equally rare, being used only in appropriate cases. Similarly, the terms *aortic transection* and *blunt aortic rupture* should be used only when describing specific injuries, i.e., full-thickness lacerations involving either the entire or partial circumference, respectively.

INITIAL EVALUATION AND MANAGEMENT

History

In cases of penetrating thoracic trauma, information regarding the length of the knife blade, the firearm type and number of rounds fired, and the patient's distance from the firearm, although not always reliable, are important to obtain from the patient or witnesses.

Although the head-on automobile collision is often considered the typical mechanism for blunt aortic injury, recent epidemiologic data reveal that up to 50 percent of cases occur following side-impact collisions. Blunt aortic injuries have also been reported following equestrian accidents, blast injuries, auto-pedestrian accidents, crush injuries, and falls from heights of 30 feet or more.

Physical Examination

Upon arrival at the emergency department, each patient should be given a rapid, thorough examination. External signs of penetrating or blunt trauma are noted. With an intrapericardial vascular injury, the classic signs of pericardial tamponade (distended neck veins, pulsus paradoxus, muffled heart sounds, and elevated central venous pressure) may be present. Clinical findings associated with thoracic great vessel injury include:

- Hypotension
- Upper extremity hypertension
- Unequal blood pressures or pulses in the extremities (upper extremity from innominate or subclavian injury, or lower extremity from pseudocoarctation syndrome)
- External evidence of major chest trauma (e.g., steering wheel imprint on chest)
- Expanding hematoma at the thoracic outlet
- Intrascapular murmur
- Palpable fracture of the sternum
- Palpable fracture of the thoracic spine
- Left flail chest

Chest Radiography

Upon arrival, a supine anteroposterior 36-inch chest radiograph should be performed, ideally in the emergency department. Emergency physicians, radiologists, and surgeons should develop diagnostic experience viewing supine radiographs made with portable chest x-ray devices because many trauma patients are hemodynamically unstable or have suspected spinal injuries, making an upright 72-inch posteroanterior chest radiograph unsafe. In many cases of great vessel injury, the radiologic findings are sufficient to warrant immediate arteriography or (rarely) direct transport to the operating room.

Several radiographic findings have been associated with blunt injuries of the descending thoracic aorta. The most reliable of these signs is the loss of the aortic knob contour, creating what Richardson and Miller describe as a "funny looking mediastinum." Mediastinal widening at the thoracic outlet and leftward tracheal deviation are suggestive of innominate artery injury.

INITIAL TREATMENT

Tube Thoracostomy

When the chest radiograph indicates a significant hemothorax, the chest tube should be connected to a repository for autotransfusion. An initial gushing flow of a large volume of blood (>1500 mL) or significant ongoing hemorrhage (>200 to 250 mL/h) may indicate great vessel injury, and are considered indications for urgent thoracotomy. Trocar chest tubes should NOT be used.

Intravenous Access and Fluid Administration

As a general rule, patients with suspected injuries to the major thoracic venous branches should have large-bore intravenous access established in the lower extremities whenever possible. If a subclavian venous catheter is required in a patient with a suspected subclavian vascular injury, the contralateral side should be used.

The treatment of severe shock should include blood transfusion. However, rapid infusions of excessive volumes of either blood or crystalloid solutions prior to operation may increase the blood pressure to a point that a protective soft perivascular clot is "blown out" and fatal exsanguinating hemorrhage ensues. The principles of permitting moderate hypotension (systolic blood pressure of 60 to 90 mm Hg) and limiting fluid administration until operative control of bleeding is achieved are cornerstones in the management of rupturing abdominal aortic aneurysms and *must* equally apply to acute thoracic great vessel injury. Aggressive preoperative fluid resuscitation increases postoperative respiratory complications and may contribute to an increased mortality when compared to fluid restriction. With both penetrating and blunt chest trauma, associated pulmonary contusions are common and provide additional rationale for limiting the infusion of preoperative crystalloid solutions.

Beta-Blockade

Some centers routinely begin beta-blockade therapy as soon as an aortic injury is suspected (prior to obtaining diagnostic studies) to reduce the risk of fatal rupture during the interval between presentation and confirmation of the diagnosis. Current protocols include intensive hemodynamic monitoring, intravenous beta-blockade titrated to heart rate, and selective use of nitroprusside infusion to further control blood pressure when necessary.

It is currently difficult to make substantiated recommendations regarding the use of beta-blockers in patients with suspected or proven blunt aortic injury. While retrospective studies suggest that it is safe, no prospective studies have demonstrated either the safety or efficacy of such treatment.

DIAGNOSTIC STUDIES

Catheter Arteriography

In penetrating thoracic trauma, catheter angiography is indicated for suspected innominate, carotid, or subclavian arterial injuries. Different thoracic incisions are required for proximal and distal control of each of the brachio-cephalic vessels. Therefore arteriography is essential for localizing the injury and planning the appropriate incision. Proximity of a missile trajectory to the brachiocephalic vessels, even without any physical findings of vascular injury, is an indication for arteriography. Although aortography may also be useful in hemodynamically stable patients with suspected penetrating aortic injuries, its limitations in this setting must be recognized. A negative aor-togram may convey a false sense of security if the laceration has temporarily sealed or if the column of aortic contrast overlies a small area of extravasa-tion. Therefore an effort must be made to obtain views tangential to possible injuries.

Following blunt trauma, the potential for thoracic great vessel injury—and therefore the need to proceed with aortography—is determined based on (1) the mechanism of injury, (2) physical examination, and (3) the standard chest radiograph. As each of these factors has inherent limitations, all three must be considered in concert. Traumatic aortic ruptures following seemingly innocu-ous mechanisms, including low-speed automobile crashes (less than 10 mph) with airbag deployment, and intrascapular back blows used to dislodge an esophageal foreign body, have been reported.

Additionally, 50 percent of patients with thoracic vascular injuries from blunt trauma present without any external physical signs of injury, and 7 per-cent of patients with blunt injury to the aorta and brachiocephalic arteries have a normal-appearing mediastinum on the admission chest radiograph. Therefore, aortography should be performed if either physical signs *or* radio-graphic findings are suggestive of potential thoracic great vessel injury. In a patient with suggestive physical signs, a high level of suspicion must be main-tained and the need for timely arteriography cannot be overemphasized, even if the chest x-ray appears normal. Similarly, if the chest x-ray is consistent with a thoracic vascular injury, aortography should be performed, even if the physical examination is unremarkable. In the hemodynamically stable patient who presents following a significant mechanism of injury, but who has a nor-mal chest radiograph and no clinical signs of great vessel injury, interval chest x-rays (at 4 to 6 hours and again at 24 hours) to detect the development of sug-gestive signs should be considered.

Catheter aortography remains the gold standard imaging study for evalua-tion of suspected blunt aortic injuries. It is currently widely available in trauma centers, allows precise localization of the injury, and provides infor-mation regarding vascular anomalies and other factors which profoundly influence operative strategy. Other diagnostic techniques currently under investigation will need to match its accuracy and availability before replacing it as the imaging study of choice.

Computed Tomography and Magnetic Resonance Imaging

Conventional computed tomography (CT) can demonstrate hemomedi-astinum and other suggestive signs, but has not demonstrated the diagnostic capability of standard aortography. Therefore, we have reserved CT for patients who have a normal-appearing mediastinum on chest x-ray and require a CT for other reasons, such as a concomitant head injury. If a medi-astinal hematoma is visualized on CT, formal aortography is still performed to specifically determine the sites of the injury and to identify any vascular anomalies that require modifications in the operative approach. Because surgeons are very reticent to operate on a major thoracic vascular injury on the basis of conventional CT scan alone, in most instances this test is merely an expensive duplication of the initial chest x-ray and delays aortography.

Transesophageal Echocardiography

For patients with suspected blunt aortic injury, transesophageal echocardiography (TEE) offers several attractive advantages over other diagnostic studies: It is fast, does not require intravenous contrast, provides concomitant evaluation of cardiac function, and can be performed in the emergency center, operating room, or intensive care unit. However, transesophageal echocardiography is contraindicated in patients with potential airway problems or suspected cervical spinal injuries, both of which are extremely common in these patients. Furthermore, the presence of atheromatous disease or pneumomediastinum interfere with TEE's ability to detect an aortic injury. Blunt aortic injuries involve the proximal aorta (ascending aorta and transverse aortic arch) in 10 to 15 percent of cases and commonly involve the brachiocephalic branches, two areas that are poorly visualized by TEE. Reports describing false-negative TEE studies in patients with great vessel injuries raise concerns regarding its accuracy in this setting. A recent review of the literature reported respective sensitivities and specificities of 85.7 percent and 92.0 percent for TEE compared to 89.0 percent and 100 percent for catheter aortography. The diagnostic limitations and unproven accuracy currently prohibit the routine use of TEE in the evaluation of blunt thoracic trauma.

TREATMENT OPTIONS

Nonoperative Management

Nonoperative management of blunt aortic injuries should be considered in patients who are unlikely to benefit from an immediate repair, such as cases with severe head injury, risk factors for infection (major burns, sepsis, or heavily contaminated wounds), and severe multisystem trauma with hemodynamic instability and/or poor physiologic reserve.

In such instances, nonoperative management is actually a purposeful delay in operation that attempts to achieve physiologic optimization and improve the outcome of repair. Nonoperative management has also been used successfully in cases of "nonthreatening" aortic lesions (e.g., minor intimal defects and small pseudoaneurysms). Close observation without operation is similarly reasonable for small intimal flaps involving the brachiocephalic arteries in asymptomatic patients, as many such lesions will heal spontaneously.

Although apparent minor vascular injuries may resolve or stabilize, their long-term natural history remains uncertain. Life-threatening complications of great vessel injuries—including rupture and fistulization with severe hemorrhage—occurring more than 20 years after injury are not uncommon. Therefore, careful follow-up, including serial imaging studies, is a critical component of nonoperative management. Avoiding hypertension and use of beta-blocking agents are also recommended when patients with aortic injuries are treated nonoperatively.

Endovascular Stenting

A less-invasive means of repairing major vascular injuries is particularly attractive for patients with severe concomitant injuries who are unlikely to tolerate operative repair. Data regarding endovascular graft repairs in trauma patients, however, are limited. Until studies specifically analyzing its use in the trauma setting demonstrate an advantage over surgical treatment, stent graft repair of thoracic great vessel injuries must continue to be considered an experimental option best suited for patients who are too unstable to undergo operation.

SURGICAL REPAIR

Indications for urgent transfer to the operating room for thoracotomy include hemodynamic instability, significant hemorrhage from chest tubes, and radiographic evidence of a rapidly expanding mediastinal hematoma.

Preoperative Considerations

Whenever possible, patients and their families must be made aware of the potential for neurologic complications, such as paraplegia, stroke, and brachial plexus injuries, following surgical reconstruction of thoracic great vessels. Careful documentation of preoperative neurologic status is critical.

With any suspicion of vascular injury, prophylactic antibiotics are administered preoperatively. In hemodynamically stable patients, fluid administration is limited until vascular control is achieved in the operating room. During the induction of anesthesia, wide swings in blood pressure must be avoided; while profound hypotension is clearly undesirable, hypertensive episodes can have equally catastrophic consequences.

The operative approach to great vessel injury depends on both the overall patient assessment and the specific injury. The initial steps of patient positioning and incision selection are particularly important in surgery for great vessel injuries, as adequate exposure is mandatory for proximal and distal control. Prepping and draping of the patient should provide access from the neck to the knees to allow management of all contingencies. For the hypotensive patient with an undiagnosed injury, the mainstay of thoracic trauma surgery is the left anterolateral thoracotomy with the patient in the supine position. In stable patients, preoperative arteriography may dictate an operative approach by another incision.

ARTERIAL INJURIES

Ascending Aorta

Patients with blunt ascending aortic injuries rarely survive transportation to the hospital. Operative repair usually requires use of total cardiopulmonary bypass (CPB) and insertion of a Dacron graft. Penetrating injuries involving the ascending aorta are uncommon. Survival rates approach 50 percent for patients having stable vital signs on arrival at a trauma center. Although primary repair of anterior lacerations can be accomplished without adjuncts, CPB may be required if there is an additional posterior injury. The possibility of a peripheral bullet embolus must always be considered in these patients.

Transverse Aortic Arch

When approaching an injury to the transverse aortic arch, extension of the median sternotomy to the neck is important to obtain complete exposure of the arch and brachiocephalic branches. If necessary, exposure can be further enhanced by division of the innominate vein. Simple lacerations may be repaired by lateral aortorrhaphy. With difficult lesions such as posterior lacerations, or those with concomitant pulmonary artery injuries, CPB is recommended. As with injuries to the ascending thoracic aorta, survival rates approaching 50 percent are possible.

Innominate Artery

Median sternotomy is employed for management of innominate artery injuries. A right cervical extension can be used when necessary. Blunt injuries typically involve the proximal innominate artery, and therefore actually represent aortic injuries, and require obtaining proximal control at the transverse aortic arch. In contrast, penetrating injuries of the innominate artery may occur throughout its course. Division of the innominate vein enhances exposure.

In selected patients with only partial tears, a running lateral arteriorrhaphy using 4-0 polypropylene suture is occasionally possible. More often, injuries to the innominate artery require repair via the bypass exclusion technique. Bypass grafting is performed from the ascending aorta to the distal innominate artery (immediately proximal to the bifurcation of the subclavian and right carotid arteries) using a Dacron tube graft. The area of injury is avoided until the areas for bypass insertion are exposed. A vascular clamp is placed proximal to the bifurcation of the innominate artery to allow collateral flow to the brain via the right subclavian and carotid arteries. Neither hypothermia, systemic anticoagulation, nor shunting is required. After the bypass is completed, the area of hematoma is entered, and the injury identified (usually at the origin of the innominate artery) and repaired. If concomitantly injured or previously divided, the innominate vein may be ligated with impunity. If the vein remains intact, a pedicled pericardial flap can be positioned between the vein and overlying graft to prevent erosion.

Descending Thoracic Aorta

Prehospital mortality is 85 percent for patients with blunt injury to the descending thoracic aorta. In patients who arrive at the hospital alive, the majority of blunt aortic injuries are located at the isthmus. Patients presenting with an injury in the mid-descending thoracic aorta or distally near the diaphragm are far less common. Multiple blunt aortic injuries are rare.

Injury to the descending thoracic aorta is often accompanied by other organ injuries. If the patient has a stable thoracic hematoma and concomitant abdominal injury, laparotomy should be the initial procedure. For the patient with a rapidly expanding hematoma, however, repair of the thoracic injury should be the primary therapeutic goal.

The current standard technique of repair involves *clamping and direct reconstruction.* Three commonly employed adjuncts to this approach are (1) pharmacologic agents, (2) temporary passive bypass shunts, and (3) pump-assisted atriofemoral bypass. In the latter approach, two options exist: traditional pump bypass, which requires heparin, and use of centrifugal (heparinless) pump circuits. All three of these adjunctive approaches to the clamp-and-repair principle should be in the armamentarium of the surgeon, who must choose the approach most appropriate to the specific clinical situation.

Injury to the descending thoracic aorta is approached via a posterolateral thoracotomy through the fourth intercostal space. The injury usually originates at the medial aspect of the aorta at the level of the ligamentum arteriosum; however, one must take care to avoid missing a second injury (usually at the level of the diaphragm).

Vascular clamps are applied to three locations: proximal aorta, distal aorta, and left subclavian artery. Close communication between anesthesiologist and surgeon is essential to maintain stability of hemodynamic parameters before, during, and after clamping. The use of vasodilators (nitroprusside) prevents cardiac strain during clamping. The hematoma is entered and back bleeding from intercostal arteries is controlled. Care is taken to avoid indiscriminate ligation of intercostal vessels. Only those required for adequate repair of the aorta should be ligated. The proximal and distal ends of the aorta are completely transected and dissected away from the esophagus; this maneuver allows full-thickness suturing while minimizing the risk of a secondary aortoesophageal fistula. The injury is then repaired by either end-to-end anastomosis or graft interposition. Graft interposition is utilized in more than 85 percent of reported cases.

For patients undergoing repair of blunt descending thoracic aortic injury, the reported mortality ranges from 5 to 25 percent. As expected in these victims of major blunt trauma, mortality is primarily associated with multisystem trauma, and is ultimately due to head injury, infection, respiratory insufficiency, and renal insufficiency.

The most feared complication of great vessel injury is paraplegia. Utilization of protective adjuncts when repairing descending thoracic aortic injuries remains a topic of considerable debate. There have been proponents of the use of passive shunts and cardiopulmonary bypass, with and without heparinization. The use of bypass systems, however, is not without complications. In the trauma patient, difficulty inserting cannulas may occur due to patient position, the presence of periaortic hematoma, and time constraints imposed by an expanding, pulsatile, uncontrolled hematoma. Intraoperative and postoperative complications include bleeding at the cannulation sites and false aneurysm formation. Regardless of the technique used, paraplegia occurs in approximately 8 percent of these patients. While recent sizable series report no postoperative paralysis, others report paraplegia rates in excess of 30 percent. No prospective, randomized trial has identified the superiority of any single method. Therefore, the choice of operative technique does not imply legal liability when paraplegia occurs.

Subclavian Artery

Subclavian vascular injuries can involve any combination of the following regions: intrathoracic, thoracic outlet, cervical (zone 1), and upper extremity. Preoperative arteriography allows for planning appropriate incision(s) to obtain adequate exposure and control.

A cervical extension of the median sternotomy is employed for exposure of right-sided subclavian injuries. For left subclavian artery injuries, proximal control is obtained through an anterolateral thoracotomy (above the nipple, third or fourth intercostal space), while a separate supraclavicular incision provides distal control. Although these incisions can be connected to create a formal thoracotomy, this results in a high incidence of postoperative "causalgia"-type neurologic complications, and its use should be limited to highly selected left-sided subclavian artery injuries. In obtaining exposure, it is imperative to avoid injuring the phrenic nerve (anterior to the scalenus anticus muscle). In subclavian vascular trauma, a high associated rate of brachial plexus injury is seen; thus, documentation of preoperative neurologic status is important.

In most instances, repair requires either lateral arteriorrhaphy or graft inter-position. It is unusual that an end-to-end anastomosis can be employed. Associated injuries to the lung should be managed with stapled wedge resec-tion or pulmonary tractotomy. One pitfall in subclavian injuries is failure to anticipate the exposure necessary for proximal control. When approaching the subclavian artery via the deltopectoral groove without proximal control, exsanguination may occur. Resection of the clavicle may aid in proximal con-trol. Combination supra- and infraclavicular incisions may be used to avoid the morbidity of clavicular resection.

Left Carotid Artery

The operative approach for injuries of the left carotid artery mirrors that used for an innominate artery injury: a median sternotomy with a left cervical extension added when necessary. As with other great vessel injuries, neither shunts nor pumps are employed. With transection at the left carotid origin, bypass graft repair is preferred over end-to-end anastomosis.

Pulmonary Artery

The intrapericardial pulmonary arteries are approached via median ster-notomy. Minimal dissection is needed to expose the main and proximal left pulmonary arteries. Exposure of the intrapericardial right pulmonary artery is achieved by dissecting between the superior vena cava and ascending aorta. Although anterior injuries can be repaired primarily without adjuncts, repair of a posterior injury usually requires cardiopulmonary bypass. Mortality rates for injury to the central pulmonary arteries or veins are greater than 70 percent.

Distal pulmonary artery injuries present with massive hemothorax and are repaired through an ipsilateral posterolateral thoracotomy. When there is a major hilar injury, rapid pneumonectomy may rarely be a lifesaving maneu-ver. The use of a large tamponading balloon catheter may control exsan-guinating hemorrhage.

Internal Mammary Artery

The internal mammary artery in a young patient is capable of flows in excess of 300 mL/min. Injuries to this artery can produce extensive hemothorax or even pericardial tamponade, simulating a cardiac injury. Such injuries are usually serendipitously discovered at the time of thoracotomy for suspected great vessel or heart injury.

Intercostal Arteries

Persistent hemothorax can be caused by simple lacerations of the intercostal arteries. Because of difficulty in exposure, precise ligature can be difficult. At times, control must be achieved by circumferential ligatures around the rib on either side of the intercostal vessel injury.

VENOUS INJURIES

Thoracic Vena Cava

Isolated injury to the suprahepatic or superior vena cava is infrequently reported. Injury at either location has a high incidence of associated organ trauma and carries a mortality rate greater than 60 percent. Intrathoracic inferior vena cava injury produces hemopericardium and cardiac tamponade. Exposure of the thoracic inferior vena cava is extremely difficult unless the patient is placed on total cardiopulmonary bypass, with the inferior cannula inserted via the groin in the abdominal inferior vena cava. Repair is enhanced by a right atriotomy and intracaval balloon occlusion to prevent air entering the cannula and massive blood return to the heart except via the hepatic veins. Repair is achieved from inside the cava via the right atrium. Superior vena cava injuries are repaired by lateral venorrhaphy. At times, an intracaval shunt is necessary. For complex injuries, a Teflon patch or Dacron interposition tube graft can be used safely and is more expedient than the time-consuming construction of saphenous vein panel grafts.

Pulmonary Veins

Injury to the pulmonary veins is difficult to manage through an anterior incision. With major hemorrhage, temporary occlusion of the entire hilum may be necessary. If a pulmonary vein must be ligated, the appropriate lobe needs to be resected. Pulmonary vein injuries are often associated with concomitant injuries to the heart, pulmonary artery, aorta, and esophagus.

Subclavian Veins

The operative exposure of the subclavian veins parallels that described for subclavian artery injuries: median sternotomy with cervical extension for right-sided injuries and left anterolateral thoracotomy with a separate supraclavicular incision for left-sided injuries. In most instances, repair requires either lateral venorrhaphy or ligation.

Azygos Vein

The azygos vein is not usually classified as a thoracic great vessel, but because of its size and high flow, azygos vein injuries must be considered potentially fatal. Penetrating wounds of the thoracic outlet can produce combinations of injuries involving the azygos vein, innominate artery, trachea or bronchus, and superior vena cava. These complex injuries are particularly difficult to control if approached through a median sternotomy. Combined incisions and approaches are frequently needed for successful repair. When injured, the azygos vein is best managed by suture ligature of both sides of the injury.

POSTOPERATIVE MANAGEMENT

A significant portion of the in-hospital mortality associated with great vessel injury is secondary to the nature of the multisystem trauma in this group of patients. The operating surgeon is best qualified to direct the patient's postoperative management. Careful hemodynamic monitoring, with avoidance of both hypertension and hypotension, is critical. While urinary output is generally a good indicator of cardiac function, for the patient with massive injuries, Swan-Ganz monitoring is often necessary to optimize hemodynamic parameters and manage fluids, pressors, and vasodilators.

Various pulmonary problems—including atelectasis, respiratory insufficiency, pneumonia, and acute respiratory distress syndrome (ARDS)—represent the primary postoperative complications in this group of patients. The presence of pulmonary contusions and the potential for development of ARDS mandate that fluid administration be carefully monitored. Positive end-expiratory pressure should be provided to hemodynamically stable intubated patients in order to minimize atelectasis. Patient mobility is imperative, and adequate medication for pain relief results in fewer pulmonary complications. For the management of pain related to a thoracotomy or multiple rib fractures, postoperative thoracic epidural anesthesia should be considered in stable patients without spinal injuries; alternatively, intercostal nerve blocks can be performed intraoperatively and repeated in the intensive care unit.

Postoperative hemorrhage may be due to a technical problem, but is often the result of coagulopathy related to hypothermia, acidosis, and massive blood transfusion. Coagulation studies must be carefully monitored and corrected with administration of appropriate blood products. Blood drained via chest tubes can be collected and autotransfused.

The presence of a prosthetic vascular graft requires special attention aimed at avoiding bacteremia. During the initial resuscitation of these critically injured patients, various intravascular lines are often rapidly placed at the expense of strict sterile technique; all such lines should be replaced after the patient has stabilized in the intensive care unit. Antibiotic therapy should be continued into the postoperative period until potential sources of infection are eliminated. Patients are counseled regarding the necessity of antibiotic prophylaxis during invasive procedures, including dental manipulations.

Most late complications are related to infections or sequelae from other injuries. Long-term complications specifically related to the vascular repair—including stenosis, thrombosis, arteriovenous fistula, graft infection, and pseudoaneurysm formation—are uncommon.

ADDITIONAL READING

Bickell WH, Wall MJ, Pepe PE, et al: Immediate versus delayed fluid resuscitation for hypotensive patients with penetrating torso injuries. *N Engl J Med* 331:1105, 1994.

Feliciano DV, Mattox KL, Graham JM, et al: Major complications of percutaneous subclavian catheters. *Am J Surg* 138:969, 1979.

Fisher RG, Oria RA, Mattox KL, et al: Conservative management of aortic lacerations due to blunt trauma. *J Trauma* 30:1562, 1990.

Graham JM, Feliciano DV, Mattox KL, et al: Management of subclavian vascular injuries. *J Trauma* 20:537, 1980.

Graham JM, Feliciano DV, Mattox KL: Innominate vascular injury. *J Trauma* 22:647, 1982.

Johnston RH Jr, Wall MJ, Mattox KL: Innominate artery trauma: a thirty-year experience. *J Vasc Surg* 17:134, 1993.

Mattox KL: Fact and fiction about management of aortic transection (editorial). *Ann Thorac Surg* 48:1, 1989.

Mattox KL: Prehospital management of thoracic injury. *Surg Clin North Am* 69:21, 1989.

Mattox KL: Red River anthology. *J Trauma* 42:353, 1997.

Mattox KL, Bickell W, Pepe P, et al: Prospective MAST study in 911 patients. *J Trauma* 29:1104, 1989.

Mattox KL, Feliciano DV: Role of external cardiac compression in truncal trauma. *J Trauma* 22:934, 1982.

Mattox KL, Feliciano DV, Beall AC Jr, et al: Five thousand seven hundred sixty cardiovascular injuries in 4459 patients: epidemiologic evolution 1958–1988. *Ann Surg* 209:698, 1989.

Pate JW, Cole FH, Walker WA, et al: Penetrating injuries of the aortic arch and its branches. *Ann Thorac Surg* 55:586, 1993.

Pate JW, Fabian TC, Walker WA: Traumatic rupture of the aortic isthmus: an emergency? *World J Surg* 19:119, 1995.

Pickard LR, Mattox KL, Espada R: Transection of the descending thoracic aorta secondary to blunt trauma. *J Trauma* 17:749, 1977.

Sweeney MS, Young DJ, Frazier OH, et al: Traumatic aortic transections: eight-year experience with the "clamp-sew" technique. *Ann Thorac Surg* 64:384, 1997.

24 | Indications for Celiotomy

Abdominal trauma is a source of significant morbidity and mortality with both penetrating and blunt mechanisms of injury. Its rapid diagnosis is essential in order to minimize morbidity. Diagnostic approaches to abdominal trauma differ according to the mechanism of injury. Penetrating injuries are more straightforward in their presentation, and the work-up in such cases is consequently somewhat easier. The penetrating wound itself immediately draws attention to the high probability of intra-abdominal injury. Blunt abdominal trauma, on the other hand, usually occurs in association with multisystem injury, making its diagnosis more complex and challenging. Physical examination of the abdomen in the presence of central nervous system (CNS) injury or dysfunction is quite unreliable. Adequate examination requires application of the multiple diagnostic modalities now available. The major diagnostic modalities beyond physical examination include diagnostic peritoneal lavage (DPL), computed tomography (CT), ultrasonography, and diagnostic laparoscopy (Table 24-1).

OVERVIEW OF DIAGNOSTIC MODALITIES

Physical Examination

Physical examination remains the most important means of detecting the need for urgent laparotomy. In the mentally and neurologically intact patient with unequivocal signs and symptoms of abdominal injury, including pain, tenderness, and guarding, the standard approach has been to perform urgent laparotomy without further diagnostic measures. This remains the case for penetrating wounds. Likewise, emergent laparotomy is dictated for the patient with blunt injury and hemodynamic instability when physical examination indicates significant pathology. However, the emergency of nonoperative management of injuries identified by CT represents somewhat of a modification of this traditional approach to blunt abdominal trauma when the patient is not unstable. The issue then becomes one of ascertaining the meaning of "relative" tenderness and "degree" of stability. Many patients with solid organ injuries who are successfully managed nonoperatively will have a fair amount of intra-abdominal blood that produces varying degrees of peritoneal irritation. Furthermore, associated injuries, especially skeletal fractures, contribute to blood loss, and many patients with blood loss and associated injuries of the liver or spleen are marginally stable. Mild to moderate hypotension will respond to intravenous fluids, but the blood pressure sometimes drifts back down. In such cases it is important to determine whether the patient's condition is attributable to ongoing intra-abdominal hemorrhage or to incompletely explained bleeding from associated injuries. A good deal of clinical judgment is required in such cases.

The greatest compromise to physical examination is the presence of neurologic dysfunction. Such dysfunction can be secondary either to neurologic injury or to substance abuse. Referral centers will find variable degrees of altered mental status in patients admitted for trauma, with closed head injuries being present in 25 percent or more of their blunt injury population. This either compromises or negates the reliability of physical examination. Spinal cord injuries occur in about 2 percent of our admissions for blunt trauma. These injuries also render physical examination of no value, and often create further confusion by producing hypotension via sympathetic collapse (cervical cord injuries). Unfortunately, most trauma centers find

TABLE 24-1 Diagnostic Modalities

	Pro	Con
Physical exam	Easy	Distracting injuries
	Accurate when positive	Altered mental status
Peritoneal lavage	Sensitive	Too sensitive
	Hollow organ injuries	Invasive
		Retroperitoneal injuries missed
CT abdomen	Most useful information	Requires transport
		Not for unstable patients
Ultrasound	Rapid noninvasive	Not specific
	Sensitive	Operator dependent
	Portable	
	Serial exams	
Laparoscopy	Identifying peritoneal	Anesthesia
	penetration	Not reliable for blunt trauma

that nearly 50 percent of their patients have an altered mental status from the influence of alcohol or illicit drugs, which thus constitute another source of compromise of the physical examination. All of these limitations of physical examination have provided the impetus for the development of more objective measurements of intra-abdominal injury.

Diagnostic Peritoneal Lavage

Sampling the abdominal cavity for blood by paracentesis with a four-quadrant tap was reported nearly 40 years ago to increase the accuracy of diagnosis of abdominal injuries. However, a false-negative rate of 36 percent was reported for this technique. DPL was the first well-established, reliably objective method of diagnosis for such injuries. This technique was introduced clinically by Root and colleagues in 1965. While it is primarily helpful for diagnosing hemoperitoneum, it can also reveal a hollow viscus injury with enteric contamination. There are three techniques for performing DPL: open, closed, or semi-open. All are used after gastric and urinary bladder decompression. The open technique is done by longitudinally incising the periumbilical tissues (above in the case of a pelvic fracture, below in its absence) down to the peritoneum, which is visualized and incised for direct peritoneal insertion of the dialysis catheter. The closed method employs the Seldinger technique. The skin is incised, and intra-abdominal puncture is done with a 21-gauge needle through which a guidewire is inserted; a dilator is then placed over the guidewire and the catheter is inserted. The semi-open technique is performed by incising skin and/or fascia and then blindly advancing the dialysis catheter into the peritoneal cavity. Most centers seem to have gravitated toward either the closed or open techniques in recent years. There has been substantial clinical experience with both techniques. Proponents of the open technique argue that it is safer, whereas those who prefer the closed technique find that it is more quickly performed and equally safe. Prospective comparisons of the two methods have reported that closed lavage could be done 14 minutes faster (19 ± 9 versus 5 ± 31 minutes). Practically speaking, at institutions in which a high number of these procedures are performed, there is probably little to distinguish the various techniques for DPL once proficiency is acquired with a particular protocol. On the other hand, occasional reliance on DPL may make the surgeon more comfortable with direct visualization via the open technique.

Following catheter insertion, aspiration is attempted, and if no blood is obtained, 1 L of crystalloid solution is instilled into the adult peritoneal cavity. Criteria for a positive result of DPL in blunt trauma include 10 mL or more of gross blood with initial aspiration, a red blood cell (RBC) count of 100,000/mm^3 or more, or a white blood cell (WBC) count of 500/mm^3 or more after the instillation of 1 L of crystalloid, or the presence of bile or fibers.

DPL remained the benchmark against which other diagnostic approaches to abdominal injury were compared for two decades after its introduction. In recent years, however, it has been relegated to a role other than the routine screening for which it has been used for many years. Over time, it became apparent that problems existed in routine screening with DPL. A relatively minor issue is that of invasiveness. Complications including vascular and bowel injury associated with trocar insertion have been noted, although these occurred in less than 1 percent of 10,358 cases in a collective review. The current major concerns with DPL are its oversensitivity and nonspecificity. Only about 30 mL of blood in the peritoneal cavity are needed to produce a microscopically positive lavage. In the years before the nonsurgical management of solid organ injuries, it was thought that practically every damaged spleen required extirpation and that nearly every injured liver required hemostasis and drainage. As it became apparent that a significant proportion of these procedures were nontherapeutic, and that nonoperative management in selected cases of abdominal injury is indeed safe, the role of DPL has been redefined. Currently, it is used most widely for two purposes: rapid screening in the hemodynamically unstable patient with an equivocal ultrasound and evaluation for hollow viscus injuries. In patients who are hemodynamically unstable or marginally stable but have multiple injuries that may contribute to instability, a grossly positive lavage will dictate emergent laparotomy in lieu of further work-up. Many institutions are adopting this approach. Even in the face of a grossly positive study, approximately 30% of patients will still be found to have insignificant injuries. DPL also remains valuable in those instances in which gastrointestinal injury cannot be ruled out. CT scanning has been widely reported to have a relatively low diagnostic sensitivity for such injury, with missed bowel injuries occurring in from 1 to 5 percent of scans. DPL can be beneficial in those situations in which CT is equivocal, especially when fluid is noted without associated solid organ injury. Likewise, tenderness beyond normal expectations in association with a known solid viscus injury (that is being managed nonoperatively) should prompt a further evaluation in which DPL can be quite helpful. Bowel injury, especially when associated with neurologic injury, remains problematic. Unless one is extremely liberal with DPL in screening for such injury, it is inevitable that it will occasionally be initially missed, only to be picked up with the onset of peritoneal sepsis. It should also be noted that bowel injuries can also be missed if DPL is performed within a few hours after injury, presumably because the degree of inflammation is insufficient to produce the peritoneal leukosequestration required for a microscopically positive DPL (500 WBC/mm^3). This has prompted the suggestion of leaving the lavage catheter in place for a repeat study a few hours later in cases in which there remains a significant index of suspicion.

Computed Tomography of the Abdomen

Over the past decade, computed tomography of the abdomen (CTA) seems to be gradually replacing DPL as the routine method of screening for blunt abdominal trauma. Reports of retrospective analyses of CTA in the early to mid-1980s began suggesting its utility. Purported ancillary advantages of CTA beyond those of abdominal evaluation have included the ability to simultaneously evaluate associated injuries, most notably vertebral and pelvic fractures. Subsequent prospective studies found CTA to be as sensitive as DPL for abdominal injury. However, reservations remained because of the greater costs associated with CTA, as well as the greater amount of time required for its use. These concerns have significantly diminished with the recent ascent of nonoperative management of a high proportion of abdominal injuries. Ultimately, the issue of specificity is what has altered the diagnostic evaluation of blunt trauma. DPL can only reveal the presence of hemorrhage, while CTA can usually also reveal the source of hemorrhage. Additionally, many retroperitoneal injuries go undetected with DPL, whereas CTA provides good, although not perfect, information for evaluation of the pancreas, duodenum, and genitourinary system. In blunt trauma, CTA has in some centers supplanted intravenous pyelography for the evaluation of hematuria. With it, renal artery injuries are being detected more frequently and earlier than in the past. This is because many of these injuries are associated with minimal or absent microscopic hematuria, and are consequently picked up incidentally during CTA. More widespread use of CTA may ultimately reveal many renal artery injuries at a relatively early stage. Current drawbacks to CTA include its marginal sensitivity for the diagnosis of diaphragmatic, pancreatic, and bowel injuries, and the requirement for intravenous contrast administration. If performed early after pancreatic injury, before the development of fluid sequestration and hematoma, CTA can miss up to 50 percent of cases of such injury. Although they are rare, serious reactions to ionic intravenous contrast agents occur in one per 1000 patients (and less frequently with nonionic contrast agents), and fatal reactions occur in 0.9 per 100,000 patients.

The technique for using CTA for identifying abdominal trauma has become fairly standardized. Beginning at the lower chest, 1- to 2-cm cuts are taken down through the pelvis. Both nonenhanced and contrast-enhanced scans may be performed. The noncontrast studies demonstrate intraparenchymal hematomas that can be missed if only contrast scans are performed. However, it has been argued that the nonenhanced study adds 5.5 minutes to the scan time, and that the information it provides is rather trivial. Enhancement with 250 to 400 mL of 1 percent diatrizoate, administered orally or via a nasogastric tube, delineates the location and integrity of the upper gastrointestinal tract. Intravenous contrast medium is administered to define organ injury and evaluate vascular supply, and occasionally to demonstrate active bleeding. For this purpose 100 to 150 mL of a contrast agent is administered just prior to initiation of the scan.

The most recent generation of volumetric CT scanners, which scan in a helical or spiral manner, has added substantially to the value of CTA. The enhanced hardware and software permit more rapid scanning with greater resolution. Previously, abdominal scanning required approximately 30 minutes, prompting some to forgo non–contrast-enhanced studies. The new scanners can complete both enhanced and nonenhanced studies in approximately 5 minutes. The time for transfer of the patient with vascular, nasogastric, bladder, and airway catheters from the stretcher to the CT table and back generally equals or exceeds the time required for the scan. The greater resolution provides a better definition of solid organ injury than was possible with earlier technology. This same capacity also provides for reasonably good imaging of blood vessels, and may in the future prove to be an important adjunct for diagnosing aortic, carotid, and other vascular injuries. Further software advances should improve the CT images. Although cost remains a concern with CTA, it will likely be of less impact as changes in the financing of health care progress. Most of the costs associated with CTA are fixed costs. Instruments in the recent generation of helical/spiral scanners cost approximately $1.5 million each. Once the scanner is purchased and technicians are employed to run it, the true costs for its use change minimally, whether 5 or 50 scans are performed per unit of time. There is no place in the United States where major trauma care now can be provided in the absence of CT.

Abdominal Ultrasonography

While abdominal ultrasonography (US) has been utilized by European and Japanese surgeons for more than a decade, it has only recently been aggressively used in the United States. No longer is US strictly performed by radiology; rather, surgeons are now integrating US into the residency training programs, as is done in Europe. Advantages of US include its relatively low cost, rapidity, portability, noninvasiveness, and sensitivity. Examinations are rapid and can be performed in the resuscitation area shortly after admission. The subphrenic spaces, subhepatic space, paracolic gutters, pelvis, and pericardium may easily be evaluated for fluid. Most investigators have reported sensitivities of 80 to 95 percent for detection of intra-abdominal hemorrhage. The examination is technically compromised by obesity, subcutaneous emphysema, and significant bowel distention with air.

Drawbacks of US include its relatively low specificity for individual organ injury and operator dependency. In general, US is currently used primarily for detecting hemorrhage and has been shown to be highly accurate. In this sense, it is similar to DPL, with the distinct advantages of rapidity, noninvasiveness, and practicality of serial examinations. US will likely relegate DPL to a historical role, as has been suggested. Some organ-specific injuries may be reported from centers with significant experience with US, but likely do not represent its use in most trauma centers. In fact, recent reports suggest 25 percent of solid organ injuries may be missed. It is unlikely that US will replace CT, because CT enables better organ definition and evaluation of the retroperitoneum. Further technical improvements in US will likely enable quantitation of solid organ injury, and may reduce the role of CT as a screening exam. The issue of operator dependency has diminished as more trauma centers are implementing training programs for the surgeons. There remains a learning curve for the effective application of US, and it has been suggested that 200 examinations are necessary for competency. The occasional ultrasonographer/surgeon will not likely become proficient. It is important for trauma centers to have dedicated programs for internal certification so that surgeons will remain proficient. In addition, US is more cost effective, because it can identify significant injuries requiring operation and replace costlier CT scanning in selected patients.

Diagnostic Laparoscopy

Laparoscopy has taken center stage in general surgery in recent years, initially because of its clear superiority to open surgery for routine cholecystectomy. It has spread rapidly into related surgical therapeutic and diagnostic applications. In reality, however, laparoscopy for diagnostic use in trauma represents a rediscovery. An early report in the surgical literature supported the efficacy of diagnostic laparoscopy (DL). Recently, DL has been used with increasing frequency with trauma patients. A theoretical advantage of DL is its facilitation of direct examination of the intraperitoneal structures. Disadvantages include its invasiveness, unproven accuracy, and cost.

Although there has been some experience with DL done under local anesthesia, most reports have described its use with general anesthesia. A 5- or 10-mm trocar is usually placed below the umbilicus, and a laparoscope of the appropriate diameter is introduced. Most surgeons utilize videolaparoscopy, with a camera attached to the laparoscope. The operating table is liberally rotated to optimize visualization of the upper abdomen and pelvis. Some surgeons have found angled laparoscopes to be useful, in addition to subcostal insertion of the laparoscope for enhanced visualization of the diaphragm and subphrenic regions. Ancillary trocars are placed for the insertion of graspers, clamps, and retractors to facilitate evaluation of the bowel and retroperitoneum.

A cautionary note has been sounded about the accuracy of DL for bowel injury with penetrating trauma. Ivatury and associates reported a sensitivity of only 18 percent for DL in diagnosing hollow viscus injury. Most investigators who have applied DL have remained conservative in their indications for its use as opposed to laparotomy, with peritoneal penetration generally dictating the latter technique. With this approach, approximately 20 percent of laparotomies have been nontherapeutic. As individual experience grows and skill is gained in bowel evaluation, many of these non-therapeutic explorations can be avoided. As laparoscopic techniques advance, there is likely to be a trend toward their use in treating some injuries, including diaphragm lacerations and perhaps some bowel injuries.

It is questionable whether DL will have a significant diagnostic impact in cases of blunt abdominal trauma. The retroperitoneum is and is likely to remain a relatively difficult area to visualize during DL. Another significant problem is that while DL permits direct visualization of liver and some splenic injuries, one cannot use it to visualize the extent and depth of injury. CT offers more information in this regard, and eliminates the need for patient transfer to the operating room, which would be required for a thorough DL evaluation in this setting.

The invasiveness of DL carries several potential problems. There is a risk of trocar injury to underlying structures. Although this has been reported with laparoscopy in general, the incidence of such injury is low and becomes rare with experience. Potential complications of DL for trauma include gas embolization and tension pneumothorax. Embolization might occur in conjunction with venous injury associated with either liver injury or a nonparenchymal venous conduit. However, there has been no documented gas embolization in the recent literature. Two cases of tension pneumothorax with DL have been reported among a total of 47 reported diaphragmatic injuries. Both were quickly recognized and promptly resolved with tube thoracostomy. When DL is used, the lower thorax should be prepared and draped in the surgical field, and appropriate hemodynamic and gas-exchange monitoring (oximetry and end-tidal carbon dioxide [CO_2] measurement) should always be done in order to ensure immediate diagnosis. A technique that can avoid the complications of embolization and pneumothorax is that of gasless laparoscopy. Favorable results with this technique have been reported in a preliminary series of 27 patients; conventional instrumentation was used to repair four bowel injuries and two diaphragm lacerations. This cannot be done with the insufflation technique because of the loss of pneumoperitoneum, which eliminates the visualization and exposure of injuries. Because a major expense of laparoscopy is the cost of trocars and highly specialized instrumentation, the gasless technique may be considerably cheaper, and may allow the practical use of DL for some therapeutic applications in stable patients.

Although DL has real drawbacks, as do both CT and US, technologic advances will certainly enhance its applicability. Research into and development of the technique are prominent because of the huge market currently associated with minimally invasive surgical techniques. Miniature optics will permit DL to be done more easily under local anesthesia in the hospital receiving area, an advance that will substantially reduce its cost below that in the operating room. Higher resolution optics and imaging will also make DL more practical for therapeutic applications in hemodynamically stable patients.

BLUNT ABDOMINAL TRAUMA

With the variety of diagnostic modalities now available, it can be difficult to choose the proper one for initial assessment of the trauma patient. No single technique is applicable to all patients, with their differing mechanisms of injury, because each technique has its own weaknesses. The following section will discuss the patient with blunt abdominal trauma. The diagnostic schemes described are based on the hemodynamic stability of the patient.

Hemodynamically Unstable and Marginally Stable Patients

As stressed in the Advanced Trauma Life Support (ATLS) Program for Physicians, sponsored by the American College of Surgeons Committee on Trauma (ACSCOT), a rapid primary survey of the trauma patient must be performed to identify life-threatening injuries. This consists of the ABCs of trauma care: airway maintenance with cervical spine control, breathing and ventilation, circulation with control of hemorrhage; assessment of disability, and exposure. The majority of patients can be quickly resuscitated from hemorrhagic shock. The etiology of the hemorrhage may be obvious (i.e., an external wound with active blood loss). If external blood loss is not the obvious source of hemorrhage, the internal cavities must be considered. The most common internal sites of exsanguinating hemorrhage are the pleural cavities, abdominal cavity (including the pelvis), and thighs. Immediate chest radiography can reveal whether or not the pleural cavity contains a significant amount of blood. Physical examination can reveal the presence or absence of a femoral fracture, which is often an underappreciated source of blood loss. Because the thigh is analogous to a cylinder or truncated cone, its volume is proportional to the square of its radius. Thus, small changes in the radius produce large changes in volume. Once the chest and thigh have been quickly ruled out as sites of exsanguinating hemorrhage, attention must turn to the abdomen.

Diagnostic modalities for evaluating the abdomen of a hemodynamically unstable patient are somewhat limited. CTA is not practical in this situation because patient transport to the CT suite and performance of the scan are too time-consuming. DL is likewise impractical in the unstable patient because of the need for special equipment, inability to do a rapid assessment of the abdominal cavity, and capacity of pneumoperitoneum to compromise the patient's already tenuous hemodynamic status. In the case of the unstable patient, the most important determination the surgeon must make is whether or not the patient is exsanguinating into the abdominal cavity, rather than the specific organ that is injured. This can be done with only two diagnostic modalities: DPL and US.

In North America, DPL is probably the most commonly used method of assessment following abdominal trauma. It can define the presence of hemo-peritoneum but not the source. Consequently, because the surgeon's main concern is whether or not there is significant intraperitoneal hemorrhage, DPL is an ideal procedure for determining this in the unstable patient. In this scenario, however, only a grossly positive lavage (aspiration of >10 mL of blood) should be considered diagnostic. In patients with a microscopically positive lavage, an exsanguinating abdominal hemorrhage is extremely unlikely. In the unstable patient, therefore, a grossly positive DPL is a rapid indicator of significant abdominal bleeding.

Evaluation of the marginally stable patient is not quite as straightforward. Frequently, the pelvic radiograph will reveal a fracture, perhaps involving the sacrum and posterior elements. Because of the marginal hemodynamic stability of the patient, CTA is not feasible. Yet, DPL in these patients has been associated with significant false-positive rates. Recently, a false-positive rate of 1 percent for DPL was reported by Mendez and associates. Their technique was to perform an infraumbilical incision for open DPL. If a preperitoneal hematoma was encountered, a supraumbilical DPL was performed. Decreasing the frequency of unnecessary abdominal exploration is important in this patient population, because it has been shown to create significant morbidity and mortality.

The second method for rapidly ascertaining the existence of intra-abdominal hemorrhage is US. As previously mentioned, it is rapid, accurate, noninvasive, and unlike DPL, is virtually without complications. It can be repeated without difficulty at various time intervals to identify ongoing hemorrhage. The drawback of operator dependency is diminishing as more trauma centers are implementing training programs for surgeons. The effectiveness of training multiple surgeons was demonstrated by Rozycki and colleagues. After training, four attending surgeons, four fellows, and 25 surgical residents (PGY-4) demonstrated a 79 percent sensitivity and 96 percent specificity with US. Thomas and colleagues evaluated an eight-hour trauma US course for six attending surgeons and two fellows. They reported a sensitivity of 81 percent, specificity of 99 percent, and accuracy of 98 percent. Similar rates were reported by Healey and associates, who had trauma surgeons interpret the examination performed by US technicians. Ultimately (and in most urban academic centers already), US will likely replace DPL as the primary diagnostic method for detecting significant abdominal hemorrhage.

Hemodynamically Stable Patients

As in the case of the hemodynamically unstable patient, the initial treatment priorities of airway, breathing, circulation, disability, and exposure apply to the hemodynamically stable patient. Once the airway is secured (which may or may not necessitate tracheal intubation) and appropriate vascular access is obtained, the secondary survey is performed. Evaluation of the abdomen can be difficult in the patient with multisystem injury. As mentioned previously, an altered sensorium from head injury, alcohol, or other intoxicants makes physical examination inaccurate. This has led to the use of multiple diagnostic modalities for evaluation of the abdomen in trauma, and the options for using these are greater in the hemodynamically stable than in the unstable patient. The following section deals specifically with the diagnostic methods described earlier as they relate to the hemodynamically stable patient with blunt trauma, with a brief discussion of more specialized tests.

Diagnostic Peritoneal Lavage/Ultrasound

As mentioned previously, the primary advantages of DPL are its simplicity, safety, low cost, and accuracy. The only absolute contraindication to its use is an indication for laparotomy; relative contraindications include the presence of previous midline incisions, significant obesity, and pregnancy. In the face of hemodynamic stability, however, the role of DPL is diminishing. Perhaps US alone is all that is necessary in stable, alert patients. However, US may initially miss blunt hollow viscus injuries. Root and colleagues described the migration of white cells following hollow viscus injury, but this phenomenon does not occur immediately. In most clinical studies, a WBC count of $500/mm^3$ in the fluid from DPL is associated with a hollow viscus injury, but agreement about this is not uniform. Repeat lavage after 4 to 6 hours, with an analysis of white cells, may be beneficial.

Computed Tomography

In the stable patient with an unevaluable abdomen, CTA will provide the most information about intra-abdominal pathology. If the patient is not cooperative, CT is either precluded or, more likely, the patient is sedated. A quality CT scan may require tracheal intubation and pharmacologic paralysis of the patient. Whether CT is as accurate as DPL for diagnosing abdominal injury has been debated in the literature. Peitzman and colleagues prospectively evaluated CTA as an adjunct to physical examination in the initial assessment of blunt abdominal trauma. They found that it had an accuracy of 98 percent, with only one missed pancreatic injury. Another prospective trial involved a comparison of CTA and DPL in 91 patients with blunt trauma. The diagnostic accuracy with CTA ranged from 91 percent for initial interpretation to 97 percent for review by an attending radiologist, as compared to 98 percent for DPL. Other investigators have confirmed an accuracy rate of greater than 95 percent for CTA. The two techniques should be considered as complementary rather than mutually exclusive, and one must recognize the inherent limitations of each.

Abdominal Ultrasonography

There are few indications for US in the stable patient when CTA is available. One of these is when nonoperative management of an organ injury is not possible because of a lack of availability of local resources. In this instance, US can identify peritoneal blood with a high degree of certainty. It can also be used by surgeons in the resuscitation area. Another indication involves the pregnant patient. The routine use of US by obstetricians is well established and should be used liberally, because trauma remains one of the leading causes of nonobstetric mortality in pregnant patients.

Diagnostic Laparoscopy

Despite the relative strengths of DPL, CTA, and US, none of these modalities is particularly helpful for evaluating a patient with potential diaphragmatic rupture. In this scenario it is possible to visualize the diaphragm with DL, and to differentiate between rupture and eventration. For other abdominal injuries, DL offers no advantages over other diagnostic modalities.

Other Modalities

Other diagnostic modalities can be used to evaluate the patient with blunt trauma. Angiography has been used as a screening tool in the past, but is not currently practical in this regard. Its main indication is to identify and embolize pelvic arterial bleeding in patients with hemorrhage from pelvic fractures. Another use of angiography is to delineate a blunt renal artery injury, which is usually identified when the affected kidney fails to take up contrast medium in an abdominal CT scan. CTA has replaced scanning of the liver and spleen with radioisotopes. Hepatic iminodiacetic acid (HIDA) scanning can help in detecting bile leaks either postoperatively or during the observation of a liver injury. Magnetic resonance imaging (MRI) is valuable for evaluating abdominal pathology, but is not practical in the multiply injured trauma patient. In the acute setting, the spine of the trauma patient is usually immobilized, and the patient may be mechanically ventilated, precluding the use of MRI. However, MRI can be useful later in the course of hospitalization of patients with spinal fractures.

PENETRATING ABDOMINAL TRAUMA

A basic principle in managing penetrating abdominal trauma (PAT) is that any wound from the nipple line to the gluteal crease has the potential for peritoneal or retroperitoneal injury. In fact, a gunshot wound anywhere on the trunk should be considered to potentially damage internal structures, because the trajectory of a bullet is very difficult to predict. Most civilian wounds are caused by low-velocity bullets, which usually change course when striking bone or even soft tissue. This makes it extremely risky to trace straight lines between bullet entry and exit sites, because these missiles usually do not take the shortest path between these two points. Two thirds of low-velocity missiles striking the torso do not exit the body. In addition to the course of a missile in the body, the position of the victim when struck is often unknown. A bullet may enter the supraclavicular fossa or upper thorax and travel inferiorly through the diaphragm. Stab wounds tend to be slightly more predictable, but caution must be taken in probing any wound. Sometimes the penetration is not directly below the skin wound. A sharp object may travel parallel to the abdominal wall for several centimeters before penetrating the peritoneum.

Torso wounds associated with clear signs of peritoneal irritation on physical examination require urgent celiotomy. Many wounds are not so clear cut. If liberal policies are followed in exploring stab wounds of the torso that have the potential for penetration but are unaccompanied by evidence of peritonitis, approximately two-thirds of laparotomies will yield negative results. Even with gunshot wounds, the potential for negative laparotomy in equivocal wounds is not trivial. Approximately 20 percent of gunshot wounds of the torso in which there is a potential for intra-abdominal injury but no clear evidence of peritonitis will produce negative laparotomies.

There are currently four basic approaches to managing PAT in the stable patient with equivocal abdominal findings: observation, local wound exploration, diagnostic peritoneal lavage, and diagnostic laparoscopy. The following sections, dealing with stab and gunshot wounds, will consider these four approaches.

STAB WOUNDS

The high rate of negative explorations associated with policies requiring the exploration for stab wounds made this an early area of focus on selective management. In one retrospective analysis, an overall complication rate of 4.9 percent was reported for 160 patients in whom laparotomy was negative. Most of the complications were pulmonary, and the average length of hospitalization for patients with a negative laparotomy was 6 days. A similar evaluation of 129 patients with negative laparotomies and no other injuries following stab wounds noted that 22 percent had complications, including a 3 percent rate of small bowel obstruction. The average hospitalization in this study was 5 days. However, a prospective analysis found unnecessary laparotomy to be associated with an even higher morbidity. In this latter evaluation of 254 unnecessary laparotomies, complications occurred in 41 percent of cases, including atelectasis in 15 percent, postoperative hypertension requiring treatment in 11 percent, pleural effusion in 9.8 percent, pneumothorax in 5.1 percent, prolonged ileus in 4.1 percent, pneumonia in 3.9 percent, wound infection in 3.2 percent, small-bowel obstruction in 2.4 percent, and urinary tract infection in 1.9 percent. Another practical concern with negative laparotomy in urban trauma centers with a large patient volume is resource utilization. It is common to have multiple victims of penetrating wounds admitted during a single day, which can tax the utilization of operating room facilities and personnel. Reducing the incidence of unnecessary laparotomies will promote more efficient utilization of these critical resources.

Observation and Local Wound Exploration

Shaftan was the first to support a policy of observation with repeated examination for both equivocal civilian stab and gunshot wounds. Nance, at the Charity Hospital in New Orleans, was a leader in proving the safety and practicality of observation of stable patients with abdominal stab wounds. His experience with 393 patients demonstrated that this policy reduced the rate of negative laparotomy from 53 to 11 percent and of all complications from 14 to 8 percent, and the duration of hospitalization from 7.8 to 5.5 days. When observation is utilized, the diagnosis of some injuries will be delayed. An experience with 176 stab wound patients undergoing observation found three with initially missed injuries, of whom one had a small bowel injury, one a gallbladder injury, and one colon and pancreas injuries. A series of 651 patients with stab wounds was reported by Demetriades and Rabinowitz. Fifty-three percent required emergent laparotomy, and the remaining 306 (47 percent) were observed. The observed patients included 26 with omental or intestinal evisceration, 18 with air under the diaphragm, 12 with blood on paracentesis, and 18 with shock on admission (requiring 23 total units of blood). This nonconventional management scheme should be reserved for study protocols until further data are available. Only nine patients (2.9 percent) required subsequent surgery for missed injuries, three of which were in the colon, two in the stomach, two in the liver, and two in the kidney. The overall incidence of negative laparotomy was 5 percent. Some delayed diagnoses will not add significantly to morbidity, but missed bowel wounds will occasionally produce major septic complications.

There are four groups of stab wounds to be addressed in relation to selective management: anterior, flank, posterior, and lower thoracic wounds. Anterior wounds are those ventral to the midaxillary lines and from the subcostal region to the inguinal ligaments. Flank wounds are those located between the anterior and posterior axillary lines. With wounds in these regions, the peritoneum is relatively superficial in the average-sized individual. Policies of local exploration of wounds in these areas have been utilized to determine whether the peritoneum has been penetrated. If the posterior fascia is unequivocally intact, the patient can be discharged. When the anterior fascia is penetrated it can be very difficult to locally explore more deeply in order to assess for peritoneal penetration. Many patients with abdominal stab wounds are young and muscular, and some are obese, both of which make accurate exploration beyond the anterior fascia difficult. In one study, however, a policy of mandatory exploration following the discovery of anterior fascial penetration led to a 50 percent negative laparotomy rate, which parallels our own experience. Consequently, adjunctive techniques have been applied when fascial penetration has been found. These have included DPL and most recently diagnostic laparoscopy (DL).

Posterior stab wounds are different because of the extremely thick groups of paraspinal muscles around the vertebral column. It is difficult to penetrate these muscles, which in the average adult male are approximately 10 to 15 cm thick. DPL has been applied in this situation. However, because there is a small risk of retroperitoneal injury to the large vascular structures, upper genitourinary system, and colon, a low threshold should be maintained for diagnostic work-up beyond observation, and DPL is unlikely to reveal a retroperitoneal injury. Double-contrast CT with the additional rectal instillation of barium has been suggested for detecting such injury. Intravenous pyelography (IVP) has also been supported, as a means for revealing both genitourinary injury and ureteral deviation associated with retroperitoneal hematoma. Demetriades and colleagues, describing a series of 223 patients with stab wounds to the back, supported a policy of observation for stable patients. Five (2.2 percent) patients required delayed surgery without serious morbidity, of whom one had a pancreatic injury, one a retroperitoneal hematoma, one an injury to the small bowel, one an injury to the colon, and one a renal aneurysm (requiring partial nephrectomy).

The basic concern with thoracoabdominal stab wounds is that the diaphragm can be injured in thoracic penetration, with subsequent intra-abdominal injury. Patients with such injury can be more difficult to evaluate and follow because of the discomfort they experience with tube thoracostomy. DPL and DL have both been utilized in this circumstance. Diagnostic thoracoscopy has recently also been reported as a means of evaluating diaphragmatic integrity.

Diagnostic Peritoneal Lavage

DPL was introduced for the evaluation of stab wounds in order to expedite management beyond observation and to minimize the rate of missed injury. A problem has been establishing an RBC count that is appropriately positive for injury. In contrast to the situation with blunt injury, significant injuries, particularly to the intestines, can occur in association with minimal blood loss in penetrating wounds of the abdomen. Accordingly, some false-negative rate might be expected if standard microscopic criteria for RBC counts are utilized. As previously noted, approximately 30 mL of intraperitoneal blood are required for an RBC of 100,000/mm^3 on DPL, and some bowel lacerations are associated with a smaller volume of intraperitoneal blood. Diaphragmatic as well as intestinal injuries are also frequently associated with false-negative DPL studies, just as they are among the most frequent injuries associated with false-negative DPL results in blunt abdominal trauma. To improve upon these results, some surgeons have reduced the criteria for positivity in DPL. However, since only a few milliliters of blood can produce a positive tap with reduced RBC criteria, an enhanced sensitivity to injury may well be expected to be accompanied by a reduced specificity. The sensitivity of the technique varies from 80 to 95 percent when high RBC counts are used (>100,000/mm^3) as opposed to low RBC counts (>10,000/mm^3); the specificities based on these limits range from 100 to 67 percent. DPL continues to be widely used in urban trauma centers for the evaluation of equivocal stab wounds in patients with positive findings on local wound exploration, but awareness should be maintained of the issue of sensitivity and specificity when interpreting microscopic results.

Diagnostic Laparoscopy

DL has the potential to permit the immediate evaluation of peritoneal penetration and evaluation of injury. This could provide an advantage over a policy of observation, by eliminating the 24 to 48 hours of hospitalization required for patients who turn out to have no injury and also by eliminating the complications associated with delayed diagnosis in those with injuries. Two recent studies have had an experience of reasonable magnitude with DL in patients with stab wounds. One of these, involving 65 patients, found a 34 percent incidence of negative laparoscopy and a 46 percent incidence of laparoscopy positive for significant pathology, with the remaining 20 percent of patients undergoing laparotomy for insignificant pathology. The other study involved 99 patients, with a 50 percent rate of negative laparoscopy, 31 percent rate of significant positive laparoscopy, and 19 percent rate of laparotomy for insignificant injuries. These two studies demonstrate that a high percentage of patients can undergo DL as outpatients, thus reducing hospital bed occupancy and associated costs. However, the 20 percent collective rate of non-therapeutic laparotomy in the two studies illustrates that in its present state, DL will not be 100 percent specific as an indicator of the need for laparotomy. Operator confidence, combined with improved optics and instrumentation, may permit greater confidence in the ability to rule out significant pathology with DL in those cases in which the peritoneum has been violated. There does need to be awareness of the 5 percent rate of pneumothorax that will occur with methods involving gas insufflation, owing to associated diaphragmatic injury. Financial analysis has demonstrated that for patients who have anterior fascial penetration, policies of mandatory local wound exploration will essentially entail the same overall cost as DL. A cost analysis of policies of observation versus DL would undoubtedly find the former to be less costly if disposable DL instrumentation were used. However, nondisposable instrumentation would probably eliminate the difference because of the savings associated with decreased hospitalization.

Ultrasound

Probably the best utility of US following penetrating truncal trauma is its evaluation of the pericardium. In a series of 247 patients with penetrating injury, 10 were identified as having cardiac injury, with 100 percent accuracy. US is more cost effective than operative pericardial window, and the results may influence the incision or order of exploration. Certainly, more clinical trials are necessary to further define the role of US in patients with penetrating trauma.

GUNSHOT WOUNDS

The considerations for the diagnostic evaluation of patients with gunshot wounds and equivocal abdominal examinations are essentially the same as those for stab wounds. The differences are primarily due to the much higher percentage of gunshot wounds of the torso that will produce significant abdominal pathology. As opposed to approximately one-third of stab wounds being associated with significant injury, approximately 80 percent of gunshot wounds cause significant injury. This is because gunshot wounds are associated with a greater degree of energy transmission than stab wounds and because bullets travel through greater distances within the body and thus increase the probability of injury. In addition to gunshot wounds having an increased likelihood of producing injury, the degree of injury as measured by the abdominal trauma index is characteristically higher than with stab wounds. This higher degree of injury also tends to render the physical examination less equivocal in the face of peritoneal penetration. In those patients with gunshot wounds who have clear evidence of peritoneal irritation, little work-up is required. In addition to routine laboratory work and the typing and cross-matching of blood, a scout x-ray of the abdomen can be somewhat helpful in patients from whom a bullet has not exited. Absence of the bullet may suggest associated thoracic injury or the rare but important event of missile embolism in the circulation. The presence of hematuria will indicate the need for a single IVP to both indicate the likely area of injury and at least as importantly to demonstrate the presence of a functioning kidney on the contralateral side, should nephrectomy become imminent at the time of exploration. Time should not be spent in making radiographs if the patient is hemodynamically unstable.

Observation

Policies of observation for gunshot wounds have been slower to develop than those for stab wounds. This is because of the recognition that much fewer gunshot wounds yield negative results with noninvasive examination and because the injuries involved in gunshot wounds are generally more significant. Nonetheless, it has become apparent that some gunshot wounds are tangential in the abdominal and lower chest walls.

A recent study of 146 patients with abdominal gunshot wounds found 41 (28 percent) with minimal findings, who were then observed. Seven of these 41 (17 percent) required subsequent exploration, of whom three had colon wounds, three had wounds of the small bowel, and one had a wound in the liver. It would appear that with proper case selection, the results of observation for gunshot wounds may mirror those for stab wounds. However, a cautionary note should be sounded about policies of observation of gunshot wounds, since little experience in this area has thus far been reported. In circumstances in which repeated examination every 4 to 6 hours is not feasible, policies of observation will probably not be practical. Exploratory laparatomy, DPL, or DL should be considered.

Diagnostic Peritoneal Lavage

DPL has been used to evaluate for abdominal injury in gunshot wounds. Reports including gunshot with stab wounds have recommended lower RBC counts as criteria for positivity than those describing only stab wounds. In a prospective study of 168 patients with abdominal gunshot wounds, 109 patients (65 percent) were stable and underwent DPL. Fifteen (24 percent) of these had a false-negative result, and of these 15, had RBC counts below 1000/mm^3. The investigators concluded that DPL was not safe for use in gunshot wounds and recommended exploratory laparotomy.

Diagnostic Laparoscopy

The results of DL have been reported for 66 patients at our institution with abdominal gunshot wounds and equivocal abdominal examinations. Sixty-two percent had negative findings on laparoscopy, 29 percent underwent a therapeutic laparotomy, and 9 percent had nontherapeutic laparotomies. In another report documented peritoneal penetration was found in 14 of 35 patients (40 percent) with gunshot wounds. Five of these 14 patients had intestinal injuries, but only one was visualized on laparoscopy. DL can be quite helpful in reducing rates of negative laparotomy in patients with gunshot wounds, but a low threshold for laparotomy should be maintained.

SHOTGUN WOUNDS

Shotgun wounds have traditionally been associated with hunting accidents, in connection with the rural roots of North America. However, there has been a recent change in the use of shotguns. In the surge of societal violence associated with illegal drugs and urban gang warfare, the fire-power associated with these activities has escalated, and the shotgun has become a favored weapon in this setting because of its close-range accuracy and destructive capacity. At close range, the shotgun behaves basically as a high-velocity weapon because of the great energy imparted to its load, while at intermediate and far ranges the injuries caused by shotgun pellets are more akin to those caused by multiple low-velocity missiles.

Practically speaking, pellets the size of birdshot (roughly No. 8 or greater) quickly lose energy and disperse as the distance through which they travel is increased. In contradistinction, buckshot pellets (roughly No. 3 or smaller) cause significant injury even at significant distances because of their mass. Pellets of intermediate size behave in a spectral fashion in terms of the issues of weight and distance.

Not all shotgun wounds require surgical management. The need for surgery because of a high likelihood of injury has been based on the size of the shot and the distance at which it was fired. However, the distance from which a shotgun was fired is usually difficult to document. We base our guidelines for the treatment of shotgun wounds primarily on the pattern of the pellets from a review of 63 patients with abdominal shotgun wounds. Wounds are divided into three types, with type I involving a pattern of 25 cm or more in diameter, type II a pattern of from 10 to 25 cm, and type III a pattern of less than 10 cm. Type III injuries occur at close range with obvious devastation requiring aggressive soft-tissue debridement and laparotomy; these wounds carry a 38 percent mortality. Type II wounds occur at intermediate distances and require abdominal exploration in addition to varying degrees of debridement; they are associated with a 20 percent mortality. Patients with type I wounds are explored if there are physical signs of peritoneal irritation. This occurred in 33 percent; the remaining two-thirds were observed. The use of this approach in 27 patients with type I wounds led to subsequent laparotomy for a small bowel injury that did not seal in only one of 18 patients undergoing observation, while the remaining nine patients with peritoneal irritation underwent therapeutic laparotomy.

AUTHORS' PREFERRED METHOD FOR EVALUATING BLUNT TRAUMA

An algorithm for the evaluation of patients with blunt trauma is presented in Fig. 24-1. For unstable patients, a physical examination is performed after the airway, breathing, and circulation are controlled and disability and exposure assessed. Immediate chest and pelvic radiographs are obtained in an attempt to identify major hemorrhage. After gastric and bladder intubation, DPL is performed. If more than 10 mL of blood is aspirated after catheter placement, the patient is taken to the operating room for emergent celiotomy. If the DPL effluent is negative or microscopically positive for red cells, other etiologies for shock should be strongly considered. It is extremely unlikely that anything less than an exsanguinating hemorrhage could account for a grossly positive tap. A complete DPL is important, however, so that the white cells can be evaluated to rule out blunt intestinal injury. We have little current experience with US, although this modality could easily be used in place of DPL to identify significant hemoperitoneum.

For the hemodynamically stable patient, the ABCs must be performed, followed by physical examination and chest and pelvic radiographs. In patients with either equivocal or unevaluable findings on abdominal examination, further investigation is necessary. Abdominal CT scanning with oral and intravenous contrast media provides the most information about solid organs and retroperitoneal structures. In addition, it permits some quantification of

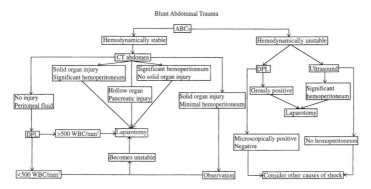

FIG. 24-1.   An algorithm for evaluation of blunt abdominal trauma.

hemoperitoneum. If there is significant solid organ injury with hemoperitoneum, or evidence of hollow organ injury, the patient should be explored. If hemoperitoneum is present but no solid organ is injured, the patient should also be explored, since a likely etiology for peritoneal blood is a mesenteric injury. If peritoneal fluid is the only finding and it is less dense than blood, DPL should be performed to rule out a hollow viscus injury. For patients with lesser grades of solid organ injury without a large amount of hemoperitoneum, nonoperative management is an option. These patients should be closely monitored in an intensive care unit (ICU). If they become unstable or require unexplained blood transfusions, they should immediately be explored. If nonoperative management is considered, each institution should have defined protocols outlining the management scheme. If local circumstances preclude reliable immediate access to an operating room and nonoperative management is inappropriate, it is prudent to perform celiotomy after a CT scan.

Patients sustaining penetrating wounds who present with peritoneal irritation should undergo urgent exploration following a single IVP if hematuria is present. Those with stab wounds and without obvious intra-abdominal penetration should have a local wound exploration. If the fascia is penetrated, diagnostic laparoscopy is performed. We believe that policies of observation or DPL are also quite acceptable, but use laparoscopy for evaluating equivocal gunshot wounds. We are reluctant to recommend either DPL or observation for such gunshot wounds until further controlled clinical trials are reported. If laparoscopy is unavailable, we continue to recommend mandatory laparotomy.

ADDITIONAL READING

Fabian TC, Croce MA, Stewart RM, et al: A prospective analysis of diagnostic laparoscopy in trauma. *Ann Surg* 217:557, 1993.

Ivatury RR, Simon RJ, Stahl WM: A critical evaluation of laparoscopy in penetrating abdominal trauma. *J Trauma* 34:822, 1993.

Liu M, Lee CH, P'eng FK: Prospective comparison of diagnostic peritoneal lavage, computed tomography scanning, and ultrasonography for the diagnosis of blunt abdominal trauma. *J Trauma* 35:267, 1993.

Root HD, Hauser CW, McKinley CR, et al: Diagnostic peritoneal lavage. *Surgery* 57:633, 1965.

Rozycki GS, Ochsner MG, Schmidt JA, et al: A prospective study of surgeon-performed ultrasound as the primary adjuvant modality for injured patient assessment. *J Trauma* 39:492, 1995.

Thompson JS, Moore EE, Van Duzer-Moore S: The evolution of abdominal stab wound management. *J Trauma* 20:478, 1980.

25 | Injury to the Diaphragm

INTRODUCTION

The diaphragm is an arched, thin, flat muscle. Responsible for our breathing, it serves as a divisory landmark and as the unknown frontier between the two largest territories of the body, the thoracic and abdominal cavities. Injuries to the diaphragm have always proven a diagnostic challenge to surgeons. Missed injuries, particularly those with associated organ herniations, can have grave consequences.

ANATOMY

The diaphragm is a dome-shaped musculoaponeurotic partition located between the pericardium and pleurae above and the peritoneal cavity below. When relaxed and viewed from below, it forms a dome-shaped roof for the abdomen. Its circumferential portion is fleshy, and the muscle fibers in this region curve upward and forward from every side to form the edges of an aponeurotic sheath called the central tendon. This tendon acts as the site of insertion for the diaphragm. The most anterior portion of the diaphragm attaches to the lowermost aspect of the sternum in the posterior aspect of the xiphisternal junction. The most posterior portion inserts in the periosteal surfaces of the first through the third lumbar vertebral bodies. The broadest portion of the diaphragmatic muscle spans laterally and attaches to the internal surfaces of the lower ribs. This lateral insertion extends from the sixth rib anteriorly to the twelfth rib posteriorly.

The crura of the diaphragm are long, tapering bundles that are fleshy above and tendinous below. The right crus arises from the lateral aspect of the border of the upper three lumbar vertebrae and the intervetebral disks; the left crus arises from the upper two lumbar vertebrae. The medial fibers of the two crura decussate in front of the commencement of the abdominal aorta; the fibers of the right crus encircle the esophagus. Both crura ascend forward and reach the posterior border of the central tendon.

The continuity of the diaphragm is interrupted by three major openings: the caval, esophageal, and aortic apertures. The inferior vena cava opening is located at the eighth thoracic vertebral level, the esophagus at the tenth, and the aorta at the twelfth. The aortic hiatus transmits the aorta, thoracic duct, and azygos vein. The esophageal hiatus transmits the esophagus and both right and left vagi, while the caval hiatus has as its only occupant the inferior vena cava.

The arterial blood supply arises superiorly from the pericardiophrenic arteries, and inferiorly from branches of the abdominal aorta, such as the phrenic artery and multiple branches from the intercostal arteries.

The right and left hemidiaphragms are innervated separately by their respective phrenic nerves. The phrenic nerves arise from the third through the fifth cervical roots. These nerves course anteriorly on the medial border of the *scalenus anticus* muscle and traverse the thoracic cavity, traveling along the posterolateral mediastinum on the pericardial surface. The phrenic nerves typically divide into branches, either at the level of the diaphragm or 1 to 2 cm immediately above. Each branch divides into four major rami: a sternal (anterior), an anterolateral, a posterolateral, and a crural (posterior) ramus (Fig. 25-1). Radial incisions in the diaphragm should be avoided because of the risk of damage to these branches that would cause paralysis of portions of the diaphragm; the use of circumferential incisions in the periphery of the

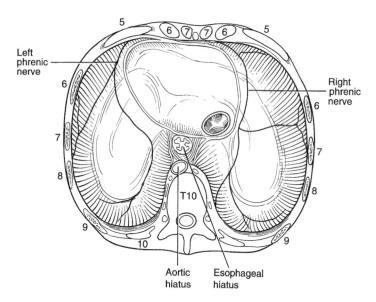

FIG. 25-1. Anatomic distribution and branching pattern of the phrenic nerves. The diaphragm may be detached along its lateral insertions, 2 cm from the costal margin, without damaging the phrenic nerves.

diaphragm which result in little if any dysfunction is instead recommended. Incisions through the central tendon almost as far medially as the entrance of the phrenic nerve, as well as lateral or transverse incisions from the midaxillary line medially, likewise result in no paralysis of the diaphragm.

PHYSIOLOGIC ASPECTS OF DIAPHRAGMATIC INJURY

The function of each hemidiaphragm in the thorax is dynamic. During exhalation, the right hemidiaphragm rises anteriorly to the level of the fourth intercostal space and the left hemidiaphragm rises to the fifth intercostal space. Posteriorly, both hemidiaphragms descend to the eighth intercostal space.

A close relationship also exists between the diaphragm and the musculature of the abdominal wall. These muscles also have both inspiratory and expiratory functions. During expiration, they contract forcing the diaphragm cephalad and into the thoracic cavity. Physiologic factors have been implicated in the genesis of diaphragmatic injury, the chief culprit being sudden and abrupt increases in the pleuroperitoneal pressure gradient. It has been postulated from these data that sudden and abrupt increases in the pleuroperitoneal pressure gradient, which can occur with the acute transfer of kinetic energy to the dome of the diaphragm (as is the case with severe abdominal trauma) will lead to diaphragmatic disruption.

In the presence of a violation of the anatomic integrity of the diaphragm by laceration, perforation, or rupture, the pleuroperitoneal gradient will encourage the transdiaphragmatic migration and herniation of intra-abdominal viscera. The pathophysiology of diaphragmatic disruption will produce immediate hemodynamic, respiratory, and gastrointestinal derangement. The disruption may act as an acute tension pneumothorax with sudden increases in intrapleural pressures, displacement of the mediastinal structures to the contralateral side, and twisting of the heart in its axis, restricting ventricular filling and thus diminishing ventricular end-diastolic volumes, thus effectively reducing the ejection fraction and cardiac output. In addition, if air escapes from the lung or from herniated hollow viscera, an even greater increase in positive intrapleural pressure will occur, collapsing the lung and further compromising its ventilatory function. All of these events result in hypoxemia, with its deleterious consequences to the patient.

INCIDENCE OF DIAPHRAGMATIC INJURIES

The incidence of diaphragmatic injuries is hard to estimate. Seven series were collected from the literature and diaphragmatic injuries occur with an average of 3 percent of all abdominal injuries (range 0.8 to 5.8 percent). The incidence of blunt diaphragmatic injuries is estimated at 0.8 percent of all trauma admissions.

It has been frequently stated that diaphragmatic hernias from penetrating injuries are considerably more common than from blunt injuries. In order to establish which mechanism of injury prevails in cases of diaphragmatic hernia, 38 series with a total of 2254 cases were reviewed, of which 1136 occurred as a result of penetrating trauma and 1102 as a result of blunt trauma, with 16 others due to other miscellaneous etiologies, but excluding all series reporting exclusively blunt injuries (Table 25-1).

ASSOCIATED INJURIES

Due to its location, certain patterns of associated injuries occur to the diaphragm, depending on the mechanism of injury. Blunt trauma generally produces a significant number of extra-abdominal and/or extrathoracic injuries, such as pelvic fractures (55 percent), head injury (42 percent), hepatic/splenic injuries (25 percent), and aortic rupture (4.8 percent). Another study reported associated intra-abdominal injuries in 122 of 163 patients (75 percent) sustained with penetrating injuries to the diaphragm. Wiencek and colleagues, in a series of 165 patients with diaphragmatic injuries of which 154 were due to penetrating wounds, reported an average of two associated injuries in patients sustaining stab wounds, and three associated injuries in patients sustaining gunshot wounds. This series reported a 50 percent incidence of hepatic injuries, a 26 percent incidence of gastric injuries, and a 12 to 18 percent incidence of pulmonary, colonic, splenic, and renal injuries.

ANATOMIC LOCATION OF INJURY

Injury to the left hemidiaphragm occurs with a greater frequency. The rarity of right-sided blunt diaphragmatic injuries has been explained in the literature by the buffering and protective effect of the liver on the right hemidiaphragm. This explains the common involvement of the left hemidiaphragm, which is

TABLE 25-1 Mechanism of Injury (38 series, 2254 patients)

Mechanism	No. patients
Blunt	1102
Penetrating	1136
Other	16

unprotected, as compared to the right. The incidence of left- versus right-sided injury in 32 series with a total of 1589 patients were identified, and among these patients 1187 (75 percent) sustained injuries to the left and 363 (23 percent) sustained injuries to the right hemidiaphragm. Thirty-nine (2 percent) had both hemidiaphragms injured. Injury to the left hemidiaphragm occurs three times more frequently than injury to the right.

DIAGNOSIS

The diagnosis of diaphragmatic injury presents a challenge. Falls from great heights, direct impact on the thoracoabdominal area from vehicles as in cases of pedestrian-vehicle incidents, or the history of a crush injury should alert the trauma surgeon to the possibility of an underlying diaphragmatic injury. The clinical presentation may range from hemodynamic stability with few or no physical findings to severe hemodynamic compromise and massive destruction of the thoracoabdominal area, as is usually the case with close-range shotgun injuries.

The presenting symptoms in cases of traumatic diaphragmatic hernia can be described as thoracic or abdominal. Dyspnea, orthopnea, and chest pain are the primary symptoms experienced. Pain may be diaphragmatic and may be referred to the scapular area, or may be related to chest wall injury or pleural violation. Physical findings can also be described as thoracic or abdominal. Thoracic findings include decreased breath sounds, multiple rib fractures, and chest wall disruption in the form of a flail chest, which can be either central with sternal disarticulation or peripheral with floating rib segments. Hemopneumothoraces are also common physical findings. Abdominal findings may include localized or diffuse severe abdominal tenderness with guarding and rebound, along with progressive distension of the abdominal cavity in cases of associated exsanguinating abdominal vascular injuries.

The initial approach to the diagnosis of a diaphragmatic injury includes chest x-ray (Fig. 25-2). The radiographic findings may range from the minimal to the dramatic. The initial chest x-rays are interpreted as normal in approximately 50 percent of patients, and the radiographic findings in the remaining 50 percent are usually limited to a small pneumothorax or hemothorax. Other findings may include an elevated diaphragm, fractured ribs with or without displacement, flail segments, and/or sternal fractures.

Occasionally, in acute rupture of the left hemidiaphragm, the nasogastric tube is found to be coiled in the left hemithoracic cavity. This is of course pathognomonic for rupture of the left hemidiaphragm. Even more rarely, the liver can be visualized in the right hemithoracic cavity. Other findings that are sometimes seen radiographically are curvilinear shadows and air-fluid levels consistent with other hollow viscera, such as the colon or small bowel.

Contrast studies have been proven valuable in cases in which the initial chest x-ray has failed to yield diagnosis of traumatic diaphragmatic injury. An upper gastrointestinal series (UGI) will often delineate the presence of the stomach within the left hemithoracic cavity. A barium enema (BE), as either a single-column or a double-contrast study, will also outline a herniated colon within the thoracic cavity.

Ultrasonography (US) may occasionally reveal a diaphragmatic rupture. Diagnostic peritoneal lavage (DPL) is diagnostically inexact in patients with diaphragmatic rupture. Perhaps the definitive procedure for excluding diaphragmatic injuries is exploratory laparotomy.

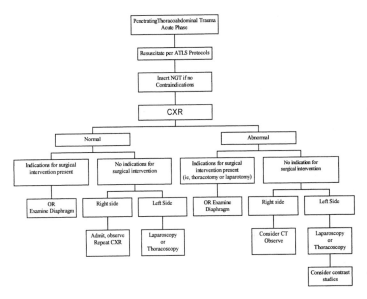

FIG. 25-2. Algorithm for penetrating thoracoabdominal trauma.

A minimally invasive technique such as laparoscopy is an excellent modality for evaluation of the intrathoracic abdomen and diaphragm. Videothoracoscopy has also proven valuable in diagnosis of diaphragmatic injuries, although it is used less frequently than laparoscopy.

A prospective study from the University of Southern California was done to evaluate laparoscopy and determine the incidence of clinically occult diaphragmatic injuries in penetrating left thoracoabdominal trauma. A group of 119 consecutive patients sustaining penetrating left thoracoabdominal injury were evaluated with clinical examination, chest x-ray, and laparoscopy. Of this group 107 were fully evaluated, 50 required emergent celiotomy, and 57 underwent laparoscopy. The overall incidence of diaphragmatic injuries was 42 percent, with a 59 percent incidence of left diaphragmatic injuries from gunshot wounds and a 32 percent incidence from stab wounds. Remarkably, among the 45 patients with diaphragmatic injuries, 31 percent had no abdominal tenderness, 40 percent had a normal chest x-ray, and 49 percent had an associated hemopneumothorax. Fifteen (26 percent) of the patients undergoing laparoscopy had occult diaphragmatic injuries. These researchers concluded that the incidence of diaphragmatic injuries in association with penetrating left thoracoabdominal trauma is high and that the clinical and radiographic findings are unreliable for detecting occult diaphragmatic injuries.

SURGICAL STRATEGIES IN THE MANAGEMENT OF DIAPHRAGMATIC INJURIES

The surgical care of diaphragmatic injuries, as well as the operative strategies employed for their definitive management, may be divided according to the phase of their clinical presentation into injuries requiring management in their acute phase and those requiring management in their chronic phase.

Acute Phase

Proven or suspected diaphragmatic injury mandates immediate exploratory laparotomy or thoracotomy. Nasogastric tubes should not be forced, because herniation of the stomach into the left hemithoracic cavity will distort the esophagogastric junction, and forceful passage may result in an iatrogenic laceration of the esophagus or stomach. Insertion of a thoracostomy tube into either of the hemithoracic cavities is contraindicated if herniated viscera are located. After initial resuscitation has been completed, the patient should be expediently transferred to the operating room and placed supine on the operating table. Most, if not all, acute diaphragmatic injuries can be approached through a laparotomy (Table 25-2). The basic principles of trauma surgery, including control of exsanguinating hemorrhage and gastrointestinal spillage, take priority; after this has been accomplished, attention should be shifted to full inspection and visualization of the diaphragm.

The right hemidiaphragm is best inspected after transection of the falciform ligament and gentle downward retraction of the liver. The left hemidiaphragm can be inspected by applying gentle downward retraction of the spleen and greater curvature of the stomach. The central tendon of the diaphragm should also be examined along with the esophageal hiatus. All herniated viscera must be carefully reduced and relocated to their original positions (Fig. 25-3).

All injuries of the diaphragm should be repaired. It is necessary to debride the edges of a laceration if devitalized tissue is found, as may happen with high-velocity missiles or close-range shotgun wounds. Hemostasis should be achieved and the most medial and lateral aspects of the laceration should be grasped with Allis clamps. The diaphragmatic laceration is then spread by applying another set of Allis clamps to the inferior and superior borders in order to inspect the ipsilateral hemithoracic cavity to assess the rate of bleeding from associated injuries within the hemithoracic cavity, and to determine the degree of cross-contamination between the abdominal and thoracic cavities. Evacuation of blood and contaminants is then done. If a chest tube has not been previously inserted, placement is recommended prior to definitive closure of the diaphragm.

Diaphragmatic lacerations less than 2 cm in size are repaired with horizontal mattress sutures of Halstead, placed approximately 1 cm from the edge of the laceration and with eversion of the diaphragmatic muscle (Fig. 25-4). We prefer 1-0 or larger monofilament sutures of nonabsorbable material (preferably polypropylene). Lacerations larger than 2 cm may in addition require a running locked or unlocked suture of the same material for reinforcement. After completion of the repair, the integrity of the suture line should be tested by increasing the intrathoracic pressure by administering a large tidal volume and assessing diaphragmatic motion. This maneuver is repeated with the field

TABLE 25-2 Surgical Approach (27 series, 1530 patients)

Surgical approach	No. patients
Laparotomy	1133
Thoracotomy	271
Thoracoabdominal	119

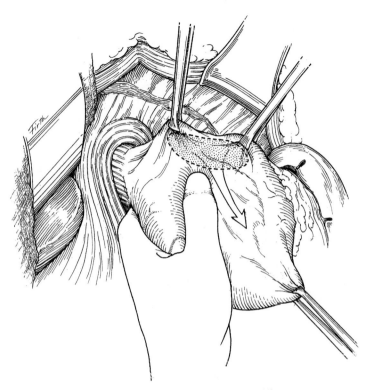

FIG. 25-3. Abdominal approach used to reduce a gastric herniation.

flooded with sterile saline to ascertain if there is escape of air or pleural fluid through the suture line.

If a diaphragmatic injury is diagnosed laparoscopically in the absence of any other injuries that mandate laparotomy or thoracotomy, laparoscopic repair should be attempted. In cases of laceration through the central tendon in which the inferior aspect of the heart is exposed, meticulous attention is given to the placement of the sutures to prevent inadvertent puncture or laceration of the myocardium (Table 25-3).

In cases in which there has been massive cross-contamination between the pleural and peritoneal cavities, we recommend performing an anterolateral thoracotomy in order to fully visualize the ipsilateral hemithoracic cavity and

TABLE 25-3 Diaphragm Organ Injury Scale*

Grade	Injury description
I	Contusion
II	Laceration ≤2 cm
III	Laceration 2–10 cm
IV	Laceration >10 cm with tissue loss ≤25 cm^2
V	Laceration with tissue loss >25 cm^2

*AAST-OIS: American Association for the Surgery of Trauma-Organ Injury Scale.

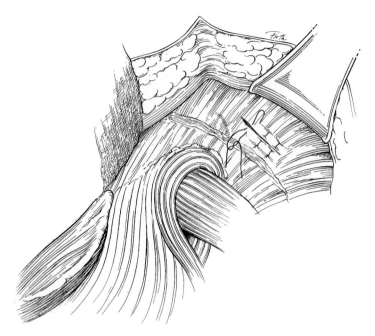

FIG. 25-4.   Repair of diaphragmatic lacerations less than 2 cm in size may be accomplished with horizontal mattress sutures of Halsted placed approximately 1 cm from the edge of the laceration, everting the diaphragmatic muscle.

evacuate all contaminating material, rather than extending the diaphragmatic laceration. This is followed by copious lavage with sterile saline and the placement of two chest tubes. One should be curved and placed in the costophrenic sulcus to avoid the formation of an empyema.

Chronic Phase

Patients who initially sustain small, undetected, and untreated diaphragmatic lacerations will experience a progressive increase in the visceral herniation of a hollow viscus, and will eventually experience symptoms and signs of cardiorespiratory compromise, obstruction, and even strangulation. Once these patients are identified, they should undergo a thorough work-up to delineate which abdominal organ has herniated through the diaphragm. The diaphragm as a muscle is quick to retract and atrophies rapidly, the effect being that tissues that could easily be approximated on the day of the injury may never be approximated after retraction and atrophy have taken place. Caution is also important with regard to adhesions, which tend to become hazardous problems in late repairs, as well as the quality of the diaphragmatic tissue in regions of atrophy, which is invariably poor and subject to a higher rate of suture line dehiscence.

Acute diaphragmatic injury should be approached through an exploratory laparotomy. For diaphragmatic injuries that are diagnosed on a delayed basis, thoracotomy appears to be a safe approach, and in some cases will facilitate the tedious dissection required to separate herniated intra-abdominal viscera from intrathoracic organs. In order to analyze the prevailing surgical approach to the repair of diaphragmatic injuries, an analysis of 27 series consisting of 1530 patients revealed that 1133 (74 percent) were repaired via laparotomy, 271 (18 percent) had their injuries repaired via thoracotomy, and 119 (8 percent) had thoracoabdominal approaches, which are defined as both thoracic and abdominal incisions, either separate or in continuity.

MORBIDITY AND MORTALITY

The morbidity incurred in diaphragmatic injuries can be subdivided into that directly related to such injury or the surgery done for it, and that related to the underlying trauma and associated injuries. The morbidity incurred in the first case includes suture line dehiscence and failure of diaphragmatic repair; hemidiaphragmatic paralysis secondary to iatrogenic phrenic nerve injuries; respiratory insufficiency; empyema and subphrenic abscess, which are generally manifested during the acute injury period; and the strangulation and perforation of herniated intra-abdominal viscera and recurrent bowel obstruction, which are generally manifested in the period remote from injury. The morbidity rates from atelectasis range from 11 to 68 percent, sepsis 2 to 28 percent, empyema 5 percent, and pneumonia 6 to 20 percent. The mortality from diaphragmatic injuries is generally due to associated injuries. The mortality rate for diaphragmatic injuries reported in 33 series varied from zero to 41 percent.

ADDITIONAL READING

Asensio JA, Rodriguez A, Demetriades D: Injury to the diaphragm, in Mattox KL, Feliciano DV, Moore EE (eds): *Trauma,* 4th ed. McGraw-Hill, New York, 2000, pp 603–632.

Fulda G, Rodriguez A, Turney SZ, et al: Blunt traumatic pericardial rupture. *J Cardiovasc Surg* 31:525, 1990.

Marchand P: A study of the forces productive of gastroesophageal regurgitation and herniation through the diaphragmatic hiatus. *Thorax* 12:189, 1957.

Merendino KA, Johnson RJ, Skinner HH, et al: The intradiaphragmatic distribution of the phrenic nerve with particular reference to the placement of diaphragmatic incisions and controlled segmental paralysis. *Surgery* 39:189, 1956.

Murray JA, Demetriades D, Cornwell EE, et al: Penetrating left thoracoabdominal trauma: The incidence and clinical presentation of diaphragm injuries. *J Trauma* 43:824, 1997.

Van Loenhout RMM, Schiphorst TJM, Wittens CHA, et al: Traumatic intrapericardial diaphragmatic hernia. *J Trauma* 26:271, 1986.

26 | Liver and Biliary Tract Trauma

DIAGNOSIS AND NONOPERATIVE MANAGEMENT OF THE PATIENT WITH BLUNT HEPATIC TRAUMA

Diagnostic Adjunctive Tests

- Diagnostic peritoneal lavage
- Computed tomographic (CT) scanning
- Ultrasonography
- Laparoscopy

Nonoperative Management of Blunt Hepatic Injuries

Inclusion criteria include (1) hemodynamic stability; (2) absence of peritoneal signs; (3) precise CT scan delineation (usually with a helical scanner) and American Association for the Surgery of Trauma (AAST) grading of the injury (Table 26-1); (4) absence of associated intra-abdominal or retroperitoneal injuries on CT scan which require operative intervention; and (5) avoidance of excessive hepatic-related blood transfusions.

Current estimates suggest that up to 80 percent of all blunt injuries may be managed nonoperatively if inclusion criteria are met (Fig. 26-1). Concerns regarding missed hollow viscus injuries seem exaggerated. The incidence of missed hollow viscus injuries in patients undergoing CT scanning for blunt abdominal trauma is low, varying from 0.22 to 3.5 percent. Specific cause for concern is the presence on the initial CT scan, after the administration of intravenous contrast, of a "blush" or pooling of contrast material within the hepatic parenchyma. This finding indicates free extravasation of blood secondary to arterial bleeding and should be managed with emergency surgery or angioembolization.

Complications and Results Associated with Nonoperative Management

The success rate with nonoperative management of blunt hepatic injuries varies from 95 to 97 percent (Table 26-2).

Postobservational CT Scanning

In patients with injuries of grades I to III, the need for postobservational CT scanning should be dictated by the patient's clinical picture. In patients with grade IV and V injuries, follow-up CT scans or sonograms will allow for image-based decisions of length of stay in the intensive care unit and hospital, and of resumption of normal activities or contact sports.

OPERATIVE MANAGEMENT OF COMPLEX HEPATIC INJURIES (GRADES III TO V)

The majority of hepatic injuries can initially be managed by compressing the injury with lap pads while hemodynamic and metabolic stability are restored by the anesthesia team. If significant hemorrhage continues to emanate from within the liver after adequate resuscitation has taken place, the portal triad should be occluded with an atraumatic vascular clamp (the Pringle maneuver). An algorithm for management of complex hepatic injuries is shown in Fig. 26-2.

Complex hepatic injuries (grades III to IV) are best managed by adhering to five crucial steps:

TABLE 26-1 Liver Injury Scale (1994 AAST Revision)

Grade*	Injury description	ICD-9†	AIS90‡
I Hematoma	Subcapsular, nonexpanding, <10 cm surface area	864.01 864.11	2
Laceration	Capsular tear, nonbleeding, <1 cm parenchymal depth	864.02 864.12	2
II Hematoma	Subcapsular, nonexpanding, 10 to 50% surface area; intraparenchymal nonexpanding <10 cm in diameter	864.01 864.11	2
Laceration	Capsular tear, active bleeding; 1–3 cm parenchymal depth, <10 cm in length	864.03 864.13	2
III Hematoma	Subcapsular, >50% surface area or expanding; ruptured subcapsular hematoma with active bleeding; intraparenchymal hematoma >10 cm or expanding		3
Laceration	>3 cm parenchymal depth	864.04 864.14	3
IV Hematoma	Ruptured intraparenchymal hematoma with active bleeding		4
Laceration	Parenchymal disruption involving 25–75% of hepatic lobe or 1–3 Couinaud's segments within a single lobe	864.04 864.14	4
V Laceration	Parenchymal disruption involving >75% of hepatic lobe or >3 Couinaud's segments within a single lobe		5
Vascular	Juxtahepatic venous injuries (i.e., retrohepatic vena cava/central major hepatic veins)		5
VI Vascular	Hepatic avulsion		6

*Advance one grade for multiple injuries, up to grade III.
†International Classification of Diseases, 9th Revision.
‡Abbreviated Injury Scale, 1990.

1. Portal triad occlusion (Pringle maneuver) for 30 to 60 minutes
2. Finger fracture of the hepatic parenchyma (hepatotomy), exposing lacerated vessels and bile ducts for direct ligation or repair
3. Debridement of nonviable hepatic tissue
4. Placement of viable omental pedicle into the site of injury
5. Closed suction drainage of grade III to V injuries

Use of Hypothermia to Extend Normothermic Ischemia to the Liver

After isolating the liver from the rest of the abdominal cavity, thorax, and mediastinum (when necessary) by the extensive use of lap pads, cooling of the hepatic parenchyma with iced Ringer's lactate is initiated until a temperature of 30° to 32°C is attained.

Hemostatic Methods in Managing Complex Hepatic Injuries

The Finger Fracture Technique in Achieving Intrahepatic Hemostasis

With portal triad occlusion achieved by an atraumatic vascular clamp, the injury is approached by finger fracturing the hepatic parenchyma in the

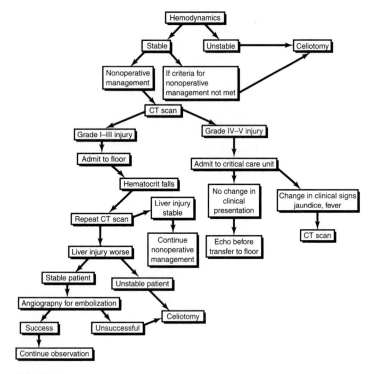

FIG. 26-1.   Algorithm for the management of adult blunt hepatic trauma.

direction of the injury. Particular care should be expended when the injury affects either Couinaud segments IVb or V. Lacerated blood vessels and bile ducts are rapidly exposed for repair or direct ligation under direct vision.

Deep Liver Suturing

The technique consists of placing multiple deep horizontal mattress or simple

TABLE 26-2 Complications Following Nonoperative Management of Adult Hepatic Injuries in 1011 Patients

Complication	Number	Percentage
Hemorrhage	33	3.3
Biloma	30	3.0
Abscess	7	0.7
Enteric injuries	3	0.3
Hepatic-related injuries	3	0.3

Sources: Croce MA, Fabian TC, Menke PG, et al: Nonoperative management of blunt hepatic trauma is the treatment of choice for hemodynamically stable patients: Results of a prospective trial. *Ann Surg* 221:744, 1995; Pachter HL, Knudson MM, Esrig B, et al: Status of nonoperative management of blunt hepatic injuries in 1995; A multicenter experience with 404 patients. *J Trauma* 40:31, 1996; and Pachter HL, Hofstetter SR: The current status of nonoperative management of adult blunt hepatic injuries. *Am J Surg* 169:442, 1995.

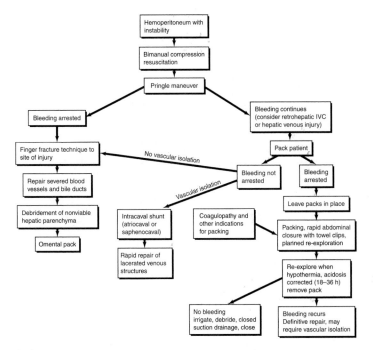

FIG. 26-2. Algorithm for the intraoperative management of complex hepatic injuries.

mass sutures through normal hepatic parenchyma to encompass the area of injury. The compressive effect that results has several major drawbacks:

1. It fails to control hemorrhage from vessels deep to the sutures.
2. This can result in intrahepatic hematoma or abscess formation.
3. Frank areas of hepatic necrosis may result from ischemic compression.

Debridement

Following debridement, the raw surface may be managed by the use of horizontal mattress sutures (2-0 chromic, blunt-nosed liver stitches) placed at least 1 cm from the free edge. The entire area may then be buttressed with a vascularized omental pedicle.

Viable Omental Pack

A vascularized pedicle of omentum used as an autologous pack will tamponade minor venous oozing, and may also stop major hepatic parenchymal bleeding while filling dead space. The liver edges are then loosely coapted around the omentum with 0 or 00 chromic, blunt-nosed liver sutures (Fig. 26-3).

The Management of Bilobar Hepatic Gunshot Wounds

One approach to treating bilobar hepatic injury has been to use intraparenchymal balloon tamponade. The balloon apparatus is constructed by ligating one

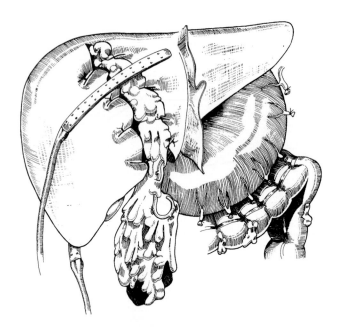

FIG. 26-3.   The omentum has been inserted into the area of the liver injury and is held in place by several interrupted liver sutures. Closed suction drainage anteriorly and posteriorly is accomplished with a pair of Jackson-Pratt drains.

end of a 1 × 12-inch Penrose drain with a 2-0 silk. A 16-inch 12 French red rubber catheter is then inserted within the Penrose drain. A second 2-0 silk ligature is then used to ligate the other end of the Penrose drain around the red rubber catheter in order to achieve a watertight seal. The balloon apparatus is then gently inserted through the entire length of the injury with 2 to 3 cm of balloon protruding on either side of the injury tract. The balloon device is then filled with a combination of saline and Gastrografin™ and slowly inflated until the bleeding ceases.

Drains

If adequate hemostasis has been achieved and no apparent bile leaks exist after repairing grade I or II injury, drainage is unnecessary. Injuries of grades III to V, on the other hand, should be drained with closed suction Jackson-Pratt drains.

Hepatic Resection

Major hepatic resection should be reserved for the following instances: (1) total destruction of the normal hepatic parenchyma; (2) the extent of the injury precludes perihepatic packing; (3) after removal of perihepatic packing, in cases in which a clean resection line lessens the likelihood of postoperative bleeding, necrosis, and subsequent abscess formation; (4) instances in which the injury has virtually performed the resection; and (5) when hepatic resection is the only way to control exsanguinating hemorrhage.

Compressive Mesh Hepatorrhaphy

Patients most likely to benefit from this approach have large, unilobar, stellate injuries.

Perihepatic Packing with Laparotomy Pads

Perihepatic packing is only used in 4 to 5 percent of operative cases. Primary indications for perihepatic packing are: (1) the onset of intraoperative coagulopathy; (2) extensive bilobar injuries in which bleeding cannot be controlled; (3) large, expanding subcapsular hematomas or ruptured hematomas; (4) the need to terminate surgery as a result of profound hypothermia; (5) failure of other maneuvers to control hemorrhage; (6) patients who require transfer to level I trauma centers; and (7) retrohepatic caval or other venous injury in selected cases.

Perihepatic packing has been associated with the development of an abdominal compartment syndrome. This syndrome is classically associated with abdominal distention, elevated peak inspiratory pressure on controlled mechanical ventilation, and oliguria as venous outflow from the kidneys becomes compromised. Clinical suspicion is confirmed by documenting an intra-abdominal pressure of 25 mm Hg. In the absence of an early abdominal compartment syndrome, perihepatic packs are usually removed 48 to 72 hours after insertion.

Selective Hepatic Artery Ligation

Selective hepatic artery ligation is used in 1 to 2 percent of operative cases, and only when there is direct injury to the extralobar or intralobar artery.

Retrohepatic Caval and Hepatic Venous Injuries

Atriocaval Shunts

Injuries to the retrohepatic vena cava or extrahepatic vein are usually recognized when the Pringle maneuver fails to significantly arrest hemorrhage from within the liver or when voluminous dark venous blood emanates from the area immediately posterior to an injured right lobe. Salvage with the shunts has been low for the following reasons: (1) delay in recognition that a juxtahepatic venous injury is present; (2) lack of personnel who are adept at insertion of the shunt; (3) delay in insertion of the shunt; and (4) blunt trauma with extensive parenchymal and venous injury. Survival with use of the atriocaval shunts ranges from 18 to 30 percent in patients who have not suffered an intraoperative cardiac arrest.

Venovenous Bypass

Venovenous bypass achieves total vascular isolation with the additional maneuvers of cross-clamping the porta hepatis and the suprarenal and suprahepatic cava. Only two cutdowns, one to the saphenous vein and the other to the axillary vein, are required for cannulation with catheters commonly available in all operating rooms (18 French, 20 French, 7-mm Gott shunt, 16 French chest tube). With the connection of the saphenous and axillary catheters to an interposed Biomedicus pump (Medtronic-Biomedicus, Inc.), unoxygenated blood from the lower extremities is circulated through the pump and returned to the axillary catheter.

Sequential Vascular Clamping

Vascular clamps are placed across the portal triad, the suprarenal vena cava, the suprahepatic vena cava, and the abdominal aorta, usually at the diaphragmatic hiatus.

Pringle Maneuver and Retrohepatic vs. Transparenchymal Approach

A direct retrohepatic approach to the vena cava or hepatic veins is predicated on prolonged portal triad occlusion and medial mobilization of the liver. Rapid finger fracture of the hepatic parenchyma to the site of the caval injury for primary repair is appropriate for large anterior wounds.

Liver Transplantation

Patients with irreparable hepatic injuries who are deemed salvagable by currently accepted criteria should always be considered as potential candidates for hepatic transplantation.

Adjunctive Hemostatic Agents

Once major hemorrhage has been controlled, topical hemostatic agents such as oxidized regenerated cellulose (Oxycel; Becton Dickinson), microfibrillar collagen hemostat (Avitene; Med Chem Products Inc.) and Instat (Johnson & Johnson) are useful adjuncts in achieving complete hemostasis.

Fibrin Glue

A commercial form of fibrin glue can be applied to the raw, oozing surfaces of the liver, where it has been extremely effective in stopping hemorrhage by acting as a biologic sealant. Intraparenchymal injection of fibrin glue should be avoided because several instances of severe reaction to fibrin glue have been reported.

Complications

Recurrent Bleeding

Postoperative hemorrhage occurring beyond the second postinjury day is uncommon after hepatic trauma and should occur in no more than 2 to 7 percent of treated patients. Currently, in the absence of hemodynamic instability, angiographic identification of the bleeding source and embolization should be the preferred initial approach.

If a repeat laparotomy is needed, persistent arterial bleeding that emanates from deep within the hepatic parenchyma may be controlled by extralobar hepatic arterial ligation. Alternatively, balloon tamponade employing Penrose and red rubber catheters can be attempted.

Hemobilia

Hemobilia, characterized by intermittent postoperative gastrointestinal bleeding without an apparent source, is best treated by embolization of the offending vessel. Surgical intervention is occasionally necessary when hemobilia is associated with a large intrahepatic cavity or angiographic access for embolization is not possible.

Intra-Abdominal Abscess

Once the diagnosis has been confirmed and localized by CT scanning, percutaneous drainage of unilocular perihepatic abscesses has a success rate approaching 95 percent. If the patient's septic picture has not significantly improved within 48 hours of percutaneous catheter drainage placement, prompt celiotomy should be undertaken.

Biliary Fistulae

Persistent postoperative bile drainage in excess of 300 to 400 mL per day occurs in 1 to 5 percent of patients. A fistulogram that identifies an injury to a major right or left duct should be followed by percutaneous transhepatic stenting, obviating the need for immediate surgery. Other therapeutic endoscopic procedures include sphincterotomy or insertion of an endostent.

EXTRAHEPATIC BILIARY TRACT

Three to five percent of all abdominal trauma victims sustain injury to the extrahepatic biliary tract. Penetrating injuries account for 85 percent of such injuries.

Diagnosis

Neither abdominal CT nor US are likely to recognize the biliary tract as the source of intraperitoneal fluid collections in the presence of free intraperitoneal blood. Radionuclide hepatobiliary scanning [technetium-99m N-2, 6-dimethylacetanilido iminodiacetic acid (HIDA)] may document the presence of a bile leak.

Classification

Gallbladder Injuries

- Disruption
- Avulsion
- Contusion
- Hemobilia

Bile Duct Injuries

Simple bile duct injuries consist of lacerations involving less than 50 percent of the ductal wall circumference, without any loss of a portion of the wall itself. *Complex bile duct injuries* include lacerations involving more than 50 percent of the ductal wall circumference, those with segmental losses of a portion of the ductal wall, or complete transections.

Treatment of Specific Injuries

Gallbladder

An injured gallbladder is usually treated with cholecystectomy and placement of a closed-suction, Jackson-Pratt drain.

Extrahepatic Bile Ducts

Meticulous dissection to preserve the blood supply to the bile ducts, reconstruction without tension (Kocher maneuver), and mucosa-to-mucosa approximation (single-layer) with fine absorbable sutures, usually 5-0 polydioxanone suture are used for the repair of simple injuries. Cholecystectomy, construction of a Roux-en-Y biliary-enteric anastomosis, and external drainage is the treatment of choice for complex bile duct injuries.

ADDITIONAL READING

Fabian TC, Croce MA, Stanford GG, et al: Factors affecting morbidity following a prospective analysis of 482 liver injuries. *Ann Surg* 213:540, 1991.

Feliciano DV: Biliary injuries as a result of blunt and penetrating trauma. *Surg Clin North Am* 74:897, 1994.

Feliciano DV, Pachter HL: Hepatic trauma revisited. *Curr Prob Surg* 26:453, 1989.

Moore EE, Shackford SR, Pachter HL, et al: Organ injury scaling: Spleen, liver and kidney. *J Trauma* 29:1664, 1989.

Pachter HL, Knudson MM, Esrig B, et al: Status of nonoperative management of blunt hepatic injuries in 1993: A multicenter experience with 404 patients. *J Trauma* 40:31, 1996.

Pachter HL, Spencer FC, Hofstetter SR, et al: Significant trends in the treatment of hepatic trauma: Experience with 411 injuries. *Ann Surg* 215:492, 1992.

27 | Injury to the Spleen

The spleen is the most commonly injured organ in blunt abdominal trauma. It is also frequently injured as a result of penetrating trauma to the left torso and upper abdomen. The management of splenic injury has continued to evolve over the past century. The trend has been increasingly toward avoiding splenectomy in favor of splenic preservation, either operatively or nonoperatively. With this shift in philosophy, minor controversies have arisen and continue to exist. These revolve around the grading of splenic injuries, the optimal patient population for operative versus nonoperative therapy, and the risk:benefit ratio of transfusion spurred by the heightened awareness of the transmissibility of bloodborne pathogens. The use of ultrasonography and interventional radiology have added to the surgical armamentarium for treating splenic injuries.

SPLENIC FUNCTION

The spleen is a critical component of the host defense system. The clearance of bloodborne bacteria occurs primarily within the spleen. In the adult, the spleen comprises 25 percent of the reticuloendothelial cell mass and is perfused with approximately 200 mL of blood per minute. Bacterial clearance is greatly facilitated by the unique circulation of the spleen. Ten percent of splenic arterial blood empties directly into the venous sinuses. The remaining 90 percent of splenic blood flow enters into the "open circulation" of the red pulp from which it is subsequently forced into the splenic sinuses. This allows a more prolonged period within the splenic microcirculation and permits splenic phagocytes to remove even poorly opsonized bacteria. The spleen is responsible for generating IgM, tuftsin, and properdin.

ANATOMY

The spleen originates from the embryonic mesoderm during fetal development. It is first seen in the fifth week of gestation as a mesodermal thickening in proximity to the tail of the pancreas. Lymphocytes are present by the fourth month of gestation. The appearance of surface immunoglobulin-bearing B and T cells is noted by the 13th week. By the sixth month, red and white pulp can be discerned. Although proportionately large at birth, the spleen remains immature and continues to enlarge until adolescence. The average adult spleen weighs approximately 100 to 250 grams.

The organ is completely covered by the peritoneum in a double layer except at the hilum. There are eight ligaments in association with the spleen. The two chief ligaments are the gastrosplenic and splenorenal ligaments. The six minor ligaments are the splenophrenic, splenocolic, presplenic fold, pancreaticosplenic, phrenicocolic, and pancreaticocolic.

The spleen is encapsulated by an external serous coat derived from the peritoneum and an internal fibroelastic coat. The parenchyma of a child's spleen appears to contain more functional smooth muscle and elastic than that of the adult. The capsule is also relatively thicker than that of the adult spleen.

The spleen receives approximately 5 percent of the cardiac output, primarily via the splenic artery. Lobar vessels from either the splenic artery or branches of the celiac axis are not uncommon. The primary branches of the splenic artery divide further within the splenic substance creating distinct anatomic segments. Each segment is supplied by a large artery and vein. The orientation of these vessels is transverse, coursing through the splenic tissue within a trabecular sheath and without anastomosis to adjacent vessels. The parenchymal architecture and vasculature of the spleen facilitate maximal interface between the reticuloendothelial system and formed elements of the blood. Blood passes through the spleen with intimate contact among plasma cells, lymphocytes, and fixed macrophages, finally draining into the venous sinusoids. In contrast to the arterial anatomy of the spleen, the veins of the organ are intricately interconnected, following no patterns of segmental anatomy.

DIAGNOSIS OF INJURY

There are no pathognomonic clinical signs and symptoms specific to splenic injury. Pertinent factors that should be taken into account in the history and clinical assessment of the patient are noted in Table 27-1. While the physical exam may have an acceptable negative predictive value for intra-abdominal injury, including the spleen, adjunctive diagnostic tests are often helpful, if not mandated. The most common adjunctive diagnostic tests, with their advantages and disadvantages, are noted in Table 27-2.

INITIAL MANAGEMENT

An algorithm for the initial management of the patient with suspected splenic trauma is provided in Fig. 27-1. In the unstable patient, after attention to airway, breathing, circulation, and assessment of disability and exposure, focused abdominal sonography for trauma (FAST) is the adjunctive diagnostic test of choice to ascribe instability to an intraperitoneal source. If free fluid is demonstrated in this setting, essentially all patients should be brought directly to the operating room for exploratory laparotomy. If the exam

TABLE 27-1 History and Assessment for Splenic Injury

Mechanism/kinematics
   Force
   Direction
   Weapon
     Type
     Distance
     Caliber
     Length
Past medical history
   Medication
     Anticoagulants
   Splenomegaly/hematologic disease
Signs and symptoms
   Hypotension/tachycardia
   Left upper quadrant
     Pain
     Tenderness
     Ecchymosis
   Left shoulder pain
   Associated injuries
     Left lower ribs
     Pelvic fracture
     Diaphragm rupture
   Base deficit (acidosis)
   Penetrating wound left torso

TABLE 27-2 Diagnostic Modalities for Splenic Injury

Physical exam
    Nonspecific
    May have acceptable negative predictive value
Ultrasonography (Focused abdominal sonography for trauma [FAST])
    Useful for both stable and unstable patients
    Portable, rapid, noninvasive
    Nonspecific—only detects presence of fluid
    Operator dependent
    No clear correlation between amount of fluid and need for laparotomy
CT scan
    Stable patients only
    Detects and defines specific solid organ injury
    Noninvasive
    Essential to nonoperative management
    Resource intensive, potential adverse effects of oral and IV contrast administration
    Requires patient transport
Diagnostic peritoneal lavage (DPL)
    Applicable to stable and unstable patients (preferentially unstable)
    Rapid, invasive, inexpensive
    Technical expertise required
    Sensitive but nonspecific for organ injury
    Objective criteria for positive test and need for laparotomy
Laparotomy
    Diagnostic test of necessity for patients with hypotension referable to intraperitoneal source
Laparoscopy
    Useful only in stable patients with penetrating injury to left upper quadrant
Angiography
    Most appropriate as adjunct to CT scan for therapy in stable patients with contrast blush
    Rare use as diagnostic test in conjunction with thoracic aortography or pelvic angiography

demonstrates a very minimal amount or no free fluid, then consideration must be given to other potential sources (particularly pelvic fracture) as the etiology of the instability. Diagnostic peritoneal lavage (DPL) may be useful to supplement a negative or equivocal FAST. DPL may also be used instead of FAST. If DPL is positive, the patient should be brought directly to the operating room for laparotomy. If negative, attempts must be made to identify other sources of the instability. In the presence of a pelvic fracture, angiography and/or external fixation of the pelvis must be entertained.

In the case of a stable patient, once again ultrasound is the test of choice to supplement a physical examination. If free fluid is demonstrated, then CT scan of the abdomen is indicated. When no free fluid is demonstrated, a CT scan is indicated if the physical exam is equivocal or if the patient will be lost to follow-up for a significant period of time. In patients with a negative physical exam, repeat ultrasound or further clinical observation is the standard practice.

If CT scan of the abdomen reveals splenic injury with or without other significant visceral injury, then the appropriate operative or nonoperative management should be undertaken. In the case of an isolated splenic injury, grade I and grade II injuries are generally managed nonoperatively. If the patient

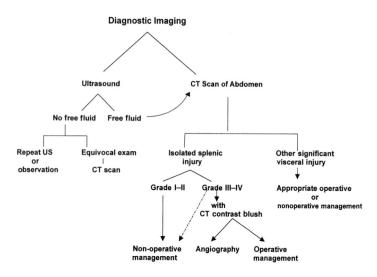

FIG. 27-1.   Algorithm for blunt abdominal trauma and suspected splenic injury.

demonstrates grade II, III, IV, or V splenic injuries and/or the presence of a contrast blush, nonoperative management may still be considered, but angiography and/or operative management is more likely indicated. Description of the injury grades applied to the spleen as laid out in the American Association for the Surgery of Trauma splenic injury scale is noted in Table 27-3.

For penetrating injury to the left upper quadrant or left flank, the same general principles of assessment apply. In the unstable patient, exploratory laparotomy is indicated without need for further diagnostic testing. In stable patients, FAST is the initial diagnostic test of choice. If this demonstrates fluid, exploratory laparotomy is indicated in most cases. When FAST is negative, local wound exploration followed by DPL if fascial penetration is demonstrated is common practice. Cell counts defining a positive DPL in penetrating trauma vary from one institution to another. Greater than 10,000 RBCs/mm^3 is considered positive in our practice. Penetrating wounds to the flank are more commonly evaluated using triple-contrast CT scan in stable patients. Laparoscopy, while more invasive and resource-intensive, is commonly used to demonstrate peritoneal penetration and organ injury in penetrating trauma. It has, however, been shown to be of little value in relation to the other diagnostic modalities in the case of blunt trauma.

MANAGEMENT OF SPLENIC INJURY

Two options are available: operative, involving splenectomy or splenorrhaphy; or nonoperative. Many issues factor into appropriate patient selection for either type of management. These caveats apply: Unstable patients are not candidates for nonoperative management; patients with significant multiple intra- or extraperitoneal injuries are not candidates for splenorrhaphy; patients selected for nonoperative management need close monitoring initially and the

TABLE 27-3 AAST Spleen Injury Scale (1994 Revision)

Grade*		Injury description	ICD-9	AIS90
I	Hematoma	Subcapsular, nonexpanding, <10% surface area	865.01 865.11	2
	Laceration	Capsular tear, nonbleeding, <1 cm parenchymal depth	865.02 865.12	2
II	Hematoma	Subcapsular, nonexpanding, 10–50% surface area; intra-parenchymal, nonexpanding, <5 cm in diameter	865.01 865.11	2
	Laceration	Capsular tear, active bleeding; 1–3 cm parenchymal depth which does not involve a trabecular vessel	865.02 865.12	2
III	Hematoma	Subcapsular, >50% surface area of expanding; ruptured subcapsular hematoma with active bleeding; intraparenchymal hematoma >5 cm or expanding		3
	Laceration	>3 cm Parenchymal depth or involving trabecular vessels	865.03 865.13	3
IV	Hematoma	Ruptured intraparenchymal hematoma with active bleeding		4
	Laceration	Laceration involving segmental or hilar vessels producing major devascularization (>25% of spleen)	865.04 865.14	4
V	Laceration	Completely shattered spleen	865.04 865.14	5
	Hematoma	Hilar vascular injury which devascularizes spleen		5

*Advance one grade for multiple injuries up to Grade III.
Source: Reproduced with permission, from Moore EE, Cogbill TH, Jurkovich GJ, et al: Organ injury scaling: Spleen and liver. *J Trauma* 38:323, 1995.

ready availability of resources to initiate operative or interventional radiologic management.

OPERATIVE MANAGEMENT

Splenectomy

Splenectomy is performed through a midline incision in acute trauma patients. Mobilization is carried out through incision of the peritoneal attachments and ligaments. Short gastric vessels should be identified and individually ligated. The hilar vessels should likewise be individually dissected and ligated. Attention to the avoidance of iatrogenic pancreatic tail injury should be maintained. Placement of drains is rarely if ever indicated, except in the case of pancreatic injury. Reoperation for splenic bed bleeding is reported in less than 2 percent of cases.

SPLENORRHAPHY

Mobilization of the spleen is also required for most splenorrhaphies to be successful. The actual technique of splenorrhaphy includes cauterization, application of topical hemostatic agents, suture repair, hemisplenectomy, omental patch, and mesh wrap. Some of these may be used in combination.

Undue persistence at attempts to perform splenorrhaphy at the expense of increased blood loss, transfusion requirement, and operative time are inadvisable, particularly in the adult patient. Rebleeding after splenorrhaphy which requires reoperation is reported at under 3 percent.

Other complications of operative management in addition to rebleeding include atelectasis, pneumonia, splenic cysts, pseudoaneurysms, iatrogenic splenic injury, and intra-abdominal abscess. Thrombocytosis may also be seen in the splenectomized patient. The rate of serious infection in patients undergoing splenic surgery is approximately 8 percent. Of particular concern is overwhelming post-splenectomy sepsis (OPSI). The most common etiologic agents include *Streptococcus pneumoniae,* meningococcus, *E. coli, Haemophilus influenzae,* and *Staphylococcus aureus.* Children are most at risk for OPSI due to their greater longevity post-splenectomy. Occurrence of this entity has been reported in up to 2 percent of splenectomized patients. The overall mortality from OPSI in post-splenectomy patients is approximately 0.6 percent. Case fatality rates for OPSI are higher, reported at upwards of 50 percent. Post-splenectomy vaccination with polyvalent pneumococcal, meningococcal, and *H. influenzae* type B (HIB) vaccines is the standard of care. Timing of vaccination remains controversial, but a standard protocol to avoid inadvertent omission is advisable. Splenectomized patients should also receive repeat pneumococcal vaccination every 6 years. Antibiotic prophylaxis should be administered prior to procedures with the potential to induce bacteremia. Patients and their physicians should be alerted to these needs.

NONOPERATIVE MANAGEMENT

A number of factors are considered in selecting patients for nonoperative management as well as use of adjunctive angiography and conversion to operative management. Some of these are noted in Table 27-4. In general nonoperative management involves bedrest, NPO status, and IV hydration. Close hemodynamic monitoring for 24 to 48 hours in conjunction with serial clinical exams and hemoglobin and hematocrit determinations are routine. At least one report advocates routine repeat CT scan at 24 to 48 hours. The patient's

TABLE 27-4 General Considerations for Operative versus Nonoperative Management

Patient factors
Age
Hemodynamic state
Stable clinical exam
Serial hemoglobin and hematocrit
Splenic injury grade
Resource factors
Appropriate patient monitoring
Immediately available surgical support
Transfusion services
Availability of interventional radiology
Risk: benefit factors
Risk of missed injury/delayed diagnosis
Risk of transfusion
Risk of a splenic state and post-splenectomy sepsis
Risk of nontherapeutic laparotomy
Probability of splenic salvage with immediate versus delayed operation

activity and diet are gradually advanced over several days to the point of regular diet and ambulation. The patient is discharged when a sufficient period of stability has passed and any other trauma issues have been addressed. Periods of initial intense observation and subsequent hospitalization are influenced by severity of splenic injury grade.

There are no universally accepted or defined criteria for transfusion, subsequent imaging while hospitalized, or conversion to operative management (i.e., failure of nonoperative management). However, if the patient's clinical course deteriorates, repeat imaging if the patient can safely tolerate it, and appropriate intervention including transfusion, angiography, and/or operation are indicated.

It is reported that about 60 percent of splenic injuries are initially managed nonoperatively. Success rates are generally better than 90 to 95 percent in children but only 70 to 80 percent in adults. For this reason, preference for splenectomy in patients over 55, and for those with higher-grade injuries has been the trend. Recent evidence does show the use of adjunctive angiography with embolization of acute bleeds and pseudoaneurysms increases the success rate of nonoperative management, particularly in patients at high risk for failure.

Postdischarge care of patients managed nonoperatively also varies with regard to mode (ultrasound versus CT scan) and timing of follow-up imaging. Another issue is the period of time needed before returning to vigorous activity which may cause splenic reinjury. The general practice at this institution involves CT scan at time of discharge, followed by CT scan prior to return to vigorous activity, unless symptoms referable to splenic cyst, late rupture, or other complications ensue. The interval of limited activity is clinician-dependent, ranging from several months to 1 year, and again is influenced by the degree of parenchymal disruption.

ADDITIONAL READING

Bee TK, Croce MA, Miller PR, et al: Failure of splenic nonoperative management: Is the glass half empty or half full. *J Trauma* 50:230, 2001.

Esposito TJ, Gamelli RL: Injuries to the spleen, in Mattox KL, Moore EE, Feliciano DV, (eds): *Trauma,* 4th ed. Appleton & Lange, Norwalk, CT, 1999.

Peitzman AB, Heil B, Rivera L, et al: Blunt splenic injury in adults: Multi-institutional study. *J Trauma* 49:177, 2000.

Shackford SR, Molin M: Management of splenic injuries. *Surg Clin North Am* 70:595, 1990.

28 | Stomach and Small Bowel Injuries

Injuries to the stomach and small bowel are common in cases of penetrating injury. Although much less common than after penetrating injury, blunt injuries to the stomach and small bowel are increasing in frequency and can present difficult diagnostic dilemmas.

ANATOMY, PHYSIOLOGY, AND MICROBIOLOGY

Because of high intraluminal acidity, the stomach is relatively free of bacteria. However, if gastric physiology is altered by preexisting disease, the risk of peritoneal contamination is increased. Leakage of acidic gastric juice into the peritoneal cavity often results in profound chemical peritonitis.

Because of the increase in bacterial load from the proximal to the distal end of the small bowel, the likelihood of infection is greater when there is a perforation in the distal bowel. The ileum is critical for the absorption of vitamin B_{12} and the reabsorption of bile salts.

MECHANISM OF INJURY/PATHOPHYSIOLOGY

Most blunt gastric injuries are "blow-out" injuries on the anterior surface or greater curvature of the stomach. Associated injuries are almost universal. The small bowel is the most commonly injured intra-abdominal viscus in cases of penetrating trauma.

Blunt injury to the small bowel is increasing in frequency. During rapid deceleration in motor vehicle crashes, lap belts compress the viscera and closed loops of bowel are created. Ecchymoses of the anterior abdominal wall in the distribution of the belt are sometimes seen. Significant blunt injury to the mesentery is also possible.

Patients with blunt injury to the small bowel can have a variety of associated injuries, but about one-fifth have isolated intestinal injuries. Approximately 25 percent of patients have more than one such injury, which emphasizes the need to fully inspect the entire bowel. Chance fractures are a particularly important indicator of the possible presence of such injury.

DIAGNOSIS

Patients with penetrating gastric trauma usually present with an injury to the abdominal wall. Bloody nasogastric aspirate or free air on x-ray may be a sign of occult gastric injury, but neither is very sensitive or specific.

Blunt small bowel injury can be a diagnostic dilemma. The physical examination of awake and alert patients will usually reveal peritoneal signs. In patients with any condition that makes an abdominal examination unreliable, diagnostic peritoneal lavage (DPL) is sensitive to blunt small bowel injuries.

Computed tomography (CT) is less reliable for making the diagnosis of blow-out of the small bowel, particularly when done in the early postinjury period. The use of oral contrast does not appreciably increase the sensitivity of CT scanning. When CT scans are positive for blunt small bowel injury, they may reveal only free fluid in the peritoneal cavity that is not explainable by a solid organ injury. Other findings may include free intraperitoneal air, thickening or enhancement of the bowel wall, and thickening of the mesentery. Ultrasound, a relatively new technique in the United States for the diagnosis of intra-abdominal pathology, is proving to have some of the same disadvantages as CT for the diagnosis of blunt intestinal injury.

Isolated injuries to the small bowel are not life-threatening if the diagnosis is made expeditiously. If the delay in diagnosis lasts for an extended period of time, a missed small bowel injury can result in serious morbidity and even mortality.

OPERATIVE MANAGEMENT

Lesions should be addressed operatively in the order of their potential lethality. Injuries to major blood vessels should be dealt with first. Major hemorrhage from solid abdominal viscera is the next priority. Too much early focus on the stomach or small bowel to the exclusion of a thorough examination of the rest of the peritoneal cavity is a mistake. An algorithm for operative assessment of potential gastric or small bowel injury is presented in Fig. 28-1.

Exposure of gastric injuries is generally easier if a nasogastric tube is in place and is facilitated by extending the midline laparotomy incision to the left of the xiphoid process. The gastroesophageal junction can be approached following division of the left triangular ligament and mobilization of the lateral segment of the left hepatic lobe.

When the stomach has been injured, the diaphragm should be closely inspected because of the potential for contamination of the pleural cavity. If necessary, segments of the gastrocolic or gastrohepatic ligaments should be divided to provide better exposure of the gastric curvatures. Exploration of the lesser sac exposes injuries to the posterior wall of the stomach. If the presence or extent of gastric injury is unclear, another diagnostic adjunct is to have the anesthesiologist fill the stomach with saline. The gastroesophageal junction and pyloric outlet are occluded and the stomach is squeezed. Leakage of fluid from the stomach localizes any missed injuries.

It is sometimes emphasized that in cases of penetrating injury to hollow abdominal viscera there should be an even number of bowel holes. Tangential wounds may produce a single long, continuous hole rather than two discrete ones. A hollow viscus as large as the stomach may be injured on one wall but not the other. A danger of the "even number of holes" rule is that the surgeon will settle for an even number of wounds when there is an additional missed injury.

We close the stomach with two layers of sutures: an inner layer of running, absorbable sutures for hemostasis and an outer layer of interrupted silk Lembert sutures. If the pylorus has been seriously damaged, a pyloroplasty should be incorporated into the repair.

The key to rapid mesenteric inspection is complete evisceration of the small bowel. If serious ongoing bleeding is discovered, it should be controlled with clamps or with rapid, shallow whip-stitching of the edge of the mesenteric rent. Once bleeding and bowel leakage have been controlled, the bowel should be carefully inspected. No injuries should be definitively repaired until the entire length of the bowel has been inspected. Injuries to the most proximal portion of the jejunum are particularly easy to miss if they are small. Mobilization of the right colon and root of the mesentery improves exposure of this area.

Mesenteric bleeding should be definitively controlled by suture ligation of large bleeding points and closure of any defects with a running suture. Mesenteric hematomas that follow penetrating trauma should be explored and active sites of bleeding controlled.

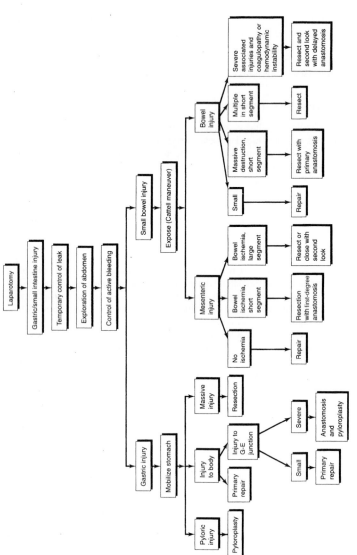

FIG. 28-1.   Algorithm for operative decisionmaking following gastric or small bowel injuries.

Large serosal tears should be closed. A single layer of interrupted silk Lembert sutures is used for this. Small serosal tears that do not appear to be either very deep or very long do not require closure.

After debridement of devitalized tissue, closure of holes in the small bowel is relatively simple. The closure should generally be done in two layers and all wounds should be closed transversely so that the gut lumen is not compromised. Injuries to more than 50 percent of the circumference of the small bowel should be resected. In the case of injuries in close proximity to one another, it is often easiest to connect the wounds and close the combined defect. When a large number of holes exist in a short segment of bowel, the segment should be resected. Mesenteric injuries severe enough to cause vascular compromise and ischemia of a segment of bowel are another circumstance in which resection is sometimes necessary.

When small bowel resection is necessary, either stapling or suturing can be used. If suturing is chosen, a side-by-side, functional end-to-end anastomosis should be created if there is a major size discrepancy between the two ends of bowel.

Mesenteric hematomas after blunt trauma, unlike those following penetrating trauma, do not always require exploration. Only large, pulsatile, or obviously expanding hematomas should be explored. In the rare instance of a very large tear in which an entire segment of bowel has been stripped of serosa, that segment of bowel should be resected.

Adjunctive techniques for determining bowel viability are somewhat useful, but interpretation of their results is subjective and dependent upon experience. The accuracy of such tests and the consequences of a misjudgment are such that the time-honored practice of obligatory reoperation at 24 hours in cases of questionably viable bowel should generally be followed.

On rare occasions involving extremely unstable patients, it is best to simply resect badly damaged bowel and defer bowel anastomosis.

POSTOPERATIVE MANAGEMENT

The postoperative care of patients with gastric and small bowel injuries is usually straightforward, and most decisions about postoperative care are based on considerations relating to associated injuries. Parenteral nutrition is not needed in most patients with isolated gastric or small bowel trauma, but may prove necessary because of associated injuries. Enteral nutrition is preferred when feasible.

The postoperative use of nasogastric tubes in patients who have undergone small bowel surgery is controversial. We usually place a nasogastric tube if there is a full-thickness injury to the stomach or small bowel, particularly if there are severe associated injuries.

Several postoperative doses of antibiotics are all that is necessary after gastric or small bowel injury. We close the skin primarily if there has been minimal evidence of contamination. If there is significant contamination, delayed primary closure is performed.

COMPLICATIONS

Postoperative complications after gastric and small bowel injury are rare; complications related to associated injuries are more common. Bleeding from a repair is unusual, but may occur either into the peritoneal cavity or the gut lumen. The risk of wound infection and abscess formation after small bowel injury is related not only to the amount of spillage, but also to the location of the injury.

The combination of diaphragm and stomach injuries can result in empyema formation. Early postoperative video-assisted thoracic surgery (VATS) to remove residual blood and fluid from the left chest may decrease the likelihood of subsequent empyema development.

Breakdown of a repair with leakage or fistula formation is another rare complication of surgery for gastric or small bowel injury. Postoperative intra-abdominal abscess has one of several etiologies, including the persistence of intraperitoneal contamination from the original injury, a missed injury, or the breakdown of a repair.

Possible causes of postoperative bowel obstruction after small bowel injury include a technical error in anastomosis, longitudinal repair of traumatic enterotomies, and excessive inversion of a primary repair.

Short-gut syndromes and associated complications may be a problem postoperatively if large portions of the small bowel require resection. A minimum of 50 to 60 cm of small bowel are necessary to allow for oral nutrition, assuming the colon is intact. The clinical manifestations of vitamin B_{12} deficiency after ileal resection are delayed and are treated with injections of the vitamin every 2 to 3 months. Most of the treatment for short-gut syndrome is medical, involving the administration of special diets and drugs. Surgical options for its treatment are limited and reserved for recalcitrant cases.

ADDITIONAL READING

Blaisdell FW, Trunkey DD (eds): *Abdominal Trauma,* 2nd ed. New York, Thieme Medical Publications, 1993, p 59.

Dellinger EP: Antibiotic prophylaxis in trauma: Penetrating abdominal injuries and open fractures. *Rev Infect Dis* 13:S847, 1991.

Durham RM: Management of gastric injuries. *Surg Clin North Am* 70:517, 1990.

Guarino J, Hassett JM, Luchette FA: Small bowel injuries: Mechanisms, patterns, and outcome. *J Trauma* 39:1076, 1995.

Nghiem HV, Jeffrey RB, Mindelzun RE: CT of blunt trauma to the bowel and mesentery. *Semin Ultrasound CT MR* 16:82, 1995.

Wisner DH, Chun Y, Blaisdell FW: Blunt intestinal injury: Keys to diagnosis and management. *Arch Surg* 125:1319, 1990.

29 | Duodenum and Pancreas Injuries

INTRODUCTION

Duodenal and pancreatic injuries incur complication rates ranging from 30 to 60 percent and mortality ranging from 6 to 34 percent. Delays in diagnosis are common and contribute to this high morbidity and mortality. This is an overview of the management principles that need to be considered when faced with these difficult injuries.

DUODENAL INJURIES

Penetrating wounds are the cause of about 75 percent of duodenal injuries. Blunt duodenal injuries result from a direct blow to the epigastrium, which in adults is usually from impact with a steering wheel, and in children is the result of impact with a bicycle handlebar or similar mechanism. The initial presentation is often insidious, adding to the diagnostic difficulty and delays in management. A high index of suspicion is essential.

Diagnosis

In blunt trauma patients with possible injury to the pancreas or duodenum, a serum amylase should be obtained. Although a single elevated serum amylase value is unreliable for diagnosing either duodenal or pancreatic injuries, a persistently increased or rising amylase mandates further evaluation or operative exploration. An early suspicion of retroperitoneal duodenal rupture is best confirmed or excluded by either an abdominal computed tomographic (CT) scan with both oral and intravenous contrast or an upper gastrointestinal series. Contrast must be visible at some time within all portions of the duodenum, and it must pass without any extravasation. Nonetheless, false-negative exams are known to occur. While diagnostic peritoneal lavage (DPL) is unreliable in detecting *isolated* duodenal (and other retroperitoneal) injuries, DPL is often helpful since approximately 40 percent of patients with a duodenal injury have associated intra-abdominal injuries that will result in a positive peritoneal lavage. The findings of amylase or bile in the lavage effluent (greater than serum levels) are more specific indicators of possible duodenal injury. At celiotomy, the presence of any central upper abdominal retroperitoneal hematoma, bile staining, or air mandates visualization and a thorough examination of the duodenum. Penetrating abdominal trauma is generally managed by exploratory celiotomy, and direct inspection of the entire path of the offending agent should diagnose any duodenal injury.

Treatment

Approximately 80 percent of duodenal wounds can be safely repaired primarily. Approximately 20 percent are severe injuries that require more complex procedures. Duodenal injury severity has been classified by the American Association for the Surgery of Trauma (AAST) Organ Injury Scaling Committee (Table 29-1). For patients with complete transection of the duodenum, debridement of mucosal edges and primary repair should be accomplished in all but those with injury involving the region of the ampulla. If adequate mobilization of the two ends of the duodenum is impossible, or if the injury is very near the ampulla and mobilization risks common bile duct

TABLE 29-1   AAST Duodenal Organ Injury Scale

Grade	Injury description
I	Hematoma: Involving single portion of duodenum
	Laceration: Partial thickness, no perforation
II	Hematoma: Involving more than one portion
	Laceration/disruption <50% of circumference
III	Laceration/disruption >50% of circumference

injury, a Roux-en-Y jejunal limb anastomosis to the proximal duodenal injury and oversewing of the distal injury is a reasonable option. Pancreatoduodenectomy may be required for duodenal injuries if uncontrollable pancreatic hemorrhage or combined duodenal and distal common bile duct or pancreatic duct injury is present.

Protection of a tenuous duodenal repair may be aided by several techniques. Buttressing the repair can be accomplished with omentum (our preference) or a "serosal patch" from a loop of jejunum. Diversion of gastric contents is another option, most commonly accomplished by the Vaughan/Jordan pyloric exclusion technique (Fig. 29-1). While no prospective, randomized trial has proven the true benefit derived from gastric diversion, several reports suggest that pyloric exclusion and gastrojejunostomy is helpful in severe duodenal injuries, or in cases of delayed diagnosis. Nonetheless, the additional operating time and the extra anastomosis highlight the need for some selectivity regarding the use of pyloric exclusion.

An alternative or addition to gastric diversion is duodenal decompression via retrograde jejunostomy (preferred) or lateral tube duodenostomy. Stone and Fabian report a fistula rate of less than 0.5 percent for duodenal injuries treated by retrograde jejunostomy tube drainage, in contrast to a 19.3 percent incidence of duodenal complications when decompression was not utilized.

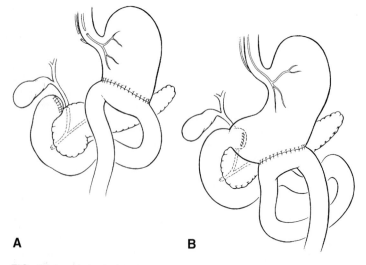

A   B

FIG. 29-1.   Methods for diversion of gastric flow used in selected patients with duodenal or combined pancreaticoduodenal injuries. A. Duodenal diverticulization. B. Pyloric exclusion.

Direct drainage with a tube through the suture line gave an even higher dehiscence or fistula rate of 23 percent. These observations are supported by a recent review of the literature demonstrating an overall mortality of 19.4 percent and a fistula rate of 11.8 percent without decompression, compared to 9 percent mortality and 2.3 percent fistula rate with decompression. These authors concluded that tube drainage should be performed either via stomach or retrograde jejunostomy, because these methods had a lower fistula rate and less overall mortality than lateral tube duodenostomy. Unfortunately, as is the case for pyloric exclusion for gastric diversion, there has been no prospective, randomized analysis of the efficacy of tube duodenal drainage techniques, and the controversy continues.

Duodenal Hematoma

Duodenal hematoma can occur in adults following motor vehicle accidents, but it is usually considered an injury of childhood play or abuse. Nearly one-third of the patients present with obstruction of insidious onset at least 48 hours after injury, presumably the result of fluid shift into the hyperosmotic duodenal hematoma. The diagnosis is usually made by findings on an abdominal CT scan. Although the initial treatment is nonoperative, associated injuries should be excluded, with particular attention directed at the potential for pancreatic injuries, which occur in 20 percent of patients. Continuous nasogastric suction should be employed and total parenteral nutrition begun. The patient should be re-evaluated with upper gastrointestinal contrast studies at 5- to 7-day intervals if signs of obstruction do not spontaneously abate. Operative exploration and evacuation of the hematoma may be considered after 2 weeks of conservative therapy, to rule out stricture, duodenal perforation, or injury to the head of the pancreas as factors that might be contributing to the obstruction. If a duodenal hematoma is incidentally found at celiotomy, a thorough inspection must ensue to exclude perforation. This will require an extended Kocher maneuver, which usually successfully drains the subserosal hematoma. It is unclear whether the serosa of the duodenum should intentionally be incised along its extent to evacuate the hematoma, or whether this increases the likelihood of converting a partial duodenal wall tear into a complete perforation. A feeding jejunostomy should be placed, because an extended period of gastric decompression will likely be required.

PANCREATIC INJURIES

Diagnosis

The single most important determinant of outcome following pancreatic injury is the status of the main pancreatic duct. However, the early morbidity and mortality is primarily the result of associated vascular and gastrointestinal tract injury. Therefore, initial priority is given to controlling hemorrhage and containing bacterial contamination. Recognition and precise identification of the pancreatic injury should follow and cannot be overlooked. Resection distal to a major ductal injury, as opposed to drainage alone, has been shown to decrease mortality rates from 19 to 3 percent. Furthermore, the use of intraoperative pancreatography for accurate determination of the status of the pancreatic duct resulted in a decrease in complications from 55 to 15 percent in one series.

Evaluating a patient for a possible pancreatic injury depends on the mechanism of injury, indications for laparotomy, and time interval following the initial abdominal insult. Patients with clear indications for laparotomy (e.g., gunshot wound to the abdomen) need no preoperative evaluation directed at identifying a possible pancreatic injury, as the diagnosis of pancreatic injury is made intraoperatively. However, patients without clear indications for laparotomy require more extensive assessment. Early identification of a pancreatic injury requires a high index of suspicion. Soft-tissue contusion in the upper abdomen and disruption of the lower ribs or costal cartilage indicate that a significant force has been dissipated in this area. Epigastric pain out of proportion to the findings of abdominal examination is often a clue to a retroperitoneal injury. Unfortunately, hyperamylasemia is not a reliable indicator of pancreatic trauma. The sensitivity of serum amylase in detecting blunt pancreatic trauma varies from 48 to 85 percent, and the specificity varies from zero to 81 percent. Sensitivity and positive predictive value may improve if serum amylase is assayed more than 3 hours after injury or if hyperamylasemia persists or worsens. While an elevated serum or peritoneal lavage effluent amylase does not necessarily confirm the presence of a pancreatic injury, it does mandate further evaluation.

Asymptomatic patients with elevated serum pancreatic isoamylase warrant observation and repeat amylase determination. Patients with hyperamylasemia and a potential abdominal injury who present with a reliable, benign abdominal examination are carefully observed and serial amylase is remeasured after several hours. Persistent elevation or the development of abdominal symptoms is grounds for further evaluation, either by abdominal CT scan, endoscopic retrograde cholangiopancreatography (ERCP), or surgical exploration. If the abdominal examination is initially equivocal or unreliable, hemodynamically stable patients with hyperamylasemia should undergo a dual-contrast abdominal CT scan. If the patient subsequently develops abdominal symptoms or the amylase fails to normalize, consideration must be given to a more careful and directed evaluation of the pancreas, which can be done with dual-contrast CT, ERCP, or surgical exploration. Abdominal CT scans have a reported sensitivity and specificity as high as 80 percent in diagnosing pancreatic injury. Some of the CT signs of pancreatic injury may not yet be apparent if the patient is examined immediately after injury, perhaps attributing to reports of false-negative CT scans in up to 40 percent of patients with significant pancreatic injuries. However, this is not grounds for delaying a CT evaluation, but is an argument for repeating a CT scan if symptoms persist.

Intraoperative Evaluation

Classification of pancreatic injuries is based on the status of the pancreatic duct and the site of injury relative to the neck of the pancreas (Table 29-2). Clues suggesting potential pancreatic injury include the presence of upper abdominal wall contusion or abrasion, and concomitant lower thoracic spine fractures. The presence of a central retroperitoneal hematoma, edema about the pancreatic gland and lesser sac, and retroperitoneal bile staining mandate thorough pancreatic inspection.

Evaluation of the pancreas requires complete exposure of the gland. Exposure of the anterior surface and the superior and inferior borders of the body and tail is obtained by opening the lesser sac through the gastrocolic ligament. Adequate visualization of the pancreatic head and uncinate process requires mobilization of the duodenum via the Kocher maneuver. In addition, mobilization of the hepatic flexure of the colon (a frequently overlooked

TABLE 29-2 AAST Pancreatic Organ Injury Scale

Grade	Injury description
I	Hematoma: Minor contusion without duct injury
	Laceration: Superficial laceration without duct injury
II	Hematoma: Major contusion without duct injury or tissue loss
	Laceration: Major laceration without duct injury or tissue loss
III	Laceration: Distal transection or parenchymal injury with duct injury
IV	Laceration: Proximal (to right of superior mesenteric vein) transection or parenchymal injury
V	Massive disruption of pancreatic head

maneuver) greatly facilitates visualization and bimanual examination of the head and neck. If injury involves the tail of the pancreas, mobilization is achieved first by division of the peritoneal attachments lateral to the spleen and colon. The colon, spleen, and body and tail of the pancreas are then mobilized forward and medially by creating a plane between the kidney and the pancreas with blunt finger dissection. This maneuver permits bimanual palpation of the pancreas and inspection of its posterior surface.

Injuries to the major duct occur in 15 percent of pancreatic trauma cases and are usually the result of penetrating wounds. The majority of these injuries can be diagnosed by careful inspection. Any penetrating wound that goes near the substance of the pancreas requires exposure and careful inspection of the entire path of the injury as well as the contiguous pancreatic gland. Intravenous injection of cholecystokinin pancreatozymin may stimulate pancreatic secretions enough to localize an otherwise unrecognized major duct injury. The remaining few injuries may require the more elaborate investigative techniques, including pancreatography. Blunt force to the pancreas in the area overlying the spine is the cause of blunt transections. Remarkably, transection of the major duct can occur without complete transection of the gland, emphasizing the point that pancreatic gland contusions in this region must be carefully examined.

Routine performance of intraoperative pancreatography when proximal duct injury was suspected decreased the postoperative morbidity rate from 55 to 15 percent at our institution. A variety of techniques exist for intraoperative pancreatography. The simplest technique is a needle cholecystocholangiogram. Water-soluble contrast (60 to 100 mL) is injected into the gallbladder under fluoroscopic visualization. In our experience, a pancreatogram will be obtained with the cholangiogram in about 60 to 70 percent of cases. Alternatively, duodenotomy and cannulation of the ampulla of Vater, or a very distal pancreatic resection and distal duct cannulation, can be performed to gain access to the pancreatic duct, although these two techniques carry their own morbidity. Direct cannulation of the pancreatic duct is performed with a small pediatric feeding tube (5 French) or cholangiocatheter and 2 to 5 mL of water-soluble contrast under low pressure is instilled. Intraoperative ERCP is another alternative, one that requires the cooperation of a skilled endoscopist.

Treatment of Pancreatic Injuries

Contusions and Lacerations Without Duct Injury

AAST grade I and II injuries (60 percent of pancreatic injuries) require only hemostasis and adequate external closed suction drainage. No attempt should be made to repair capsular lacerations, because closure may result in a pancreatic pseudocyst, whereas a controlled pancreatic fistula is usually self-limiting. If the amylase concentration in the drain is less than that of serum, the drains are removed after 24 to 48 hours. Some surgeons prefer to leave the drains in place until oral feedings are tolerated without increasing drain output. If the effluent amylase concentration persists above that of serum, the drain is left in until there is no evidence of pancreatic leak. Eighty percent of pancreatic fistulas spontaneously resolve with a mean time to resolution of 30 days. Nutrition can be provided via the oral or gastric route as soon as possible, although prolonged gastric ileus and pancreatic complications may preclude standard gastric feeding for long periods in many patients with more severe injuries.

Distal Transection and Distal Parenchymal Injury With Duct Disruption

The anatomic distinction between the proximal and distal pancreas is generally defined by the superior mesenteric vessels passing behind the pancreas at the junction of the pancreatic head and body. Since most blunt trauma pancreatic injuries occur at the spine, which is just to the patient's left of the portal vein as it crosses behind the pancreas, a "distal pancreatectomy" in this circumstance is on average a 56 percent gland resection. Although reports of normal endocrine and exocrine function after 90 percent pancreatectomy do occur, every effort should be made to leave at least 20 percent residual pancreatic tissue to minimize postoperative complications.

Distal parenchymal transections, particularly with disruption of the main pancreatic duct, accounts for about 30 percent of pancreatic injuries, and are best treated by distal pancreatectomy. If there is any concern regarding the status of the remaining proximal main pancreatic duct, intraoperative proximal pancreatography should be performed through the open end of the proximal duct. If the remaining proximal duct is normal, the transected duct should be closed with a direct suture ligature either as a U-shaped stitch or a figure-of-eight stitch with nonabsorbable monofilament suture. The parenchyma is controlled with mattress sutures placed through the full thickness of the pancreatic gland from the anterior to posterior capsule to minimize leakage from the transected parenchyma. A small omental patch can be used to buttress the surface and a drain should be left near the transection line. Stapling devices have also been advocated for closure of the pancreatic parenchyma, although they may compress the glandular tissue. If possible, the duct itself should be identified and individually ligated. Adequate external drainage should also be established.

Concern for the possibility of postsplenectomy sepsis may prompt attempted splenic preservation while performing distal pancreatectomy. The increased operative time and potential blood loss incurred while performing pancreatectomy without splenectomy must be balanced against the slight risk of overwhelming postsplenectomy sepsis. The balance would seem to favor splenic salvage only when the patient is completely hemodynamically stable and normothermic and the pancreatic injury is isolated or present with only minor associated injuries.

Proximal Transection or Injury With Probable Duct Disruption

Injuries to the pancreatic head represent the most challenging management dilemmas, and fortunately are uncommon, perhaps 5 to 10 percent of all pancreatic injuries. It is essential that the surgeon define the pancreatic duct anatomy. Injuries to the head and neck of the pancreas that spare the major pancreatic duct are best managed by adequate external drainage. If duct injury cannot be excluded by direct inspection, and intraoperative pancreatography is unhelpful or not an option, wide external drainage with numerous closed suction drains and postoperative ERCP should be performed. Magnetic resonance imaging of the pancreatic duct is a new and largely untested option in trauma. In the critically injured and hemodynamically unstable patient in whom time to evaluate the status of the pancreatic duct can not be afforded, wide external drainage should be performed, with postoperative evaluation of the duct either with ERCP or perhaps MR imaging.

If the proximal duct is known to be injured, but the ampulla and duodenum are spared (rare), the surgeon has several options. We would recommend extended distal pancreatectomy, resulting in subtotal removal of the gland, generally without pyloric exclusion, although others advocate its use in this circumstance. If there is concern that the residual proximal pancreatic tissue is inadequate to provide endocrine or exocrine function, preservation of the pancreatic tail distal to the injury using a Roux-en-Y pancreaticojejunostomy is an option, but risks an additional two anastomoses. Simply completing the gland transection (if needed), and ligating the distal pancreatic duct has also been proposed, but has a high morbidity. Provisions should be made for early enteral nutritional support in all patients with major pancreatic injury. The surgeon's foresight in placing a jejunal feeding tube at the time of initial celiotomy is rewarded by a simplified and potentially advantageous enteral nutrition regimen.

Combined Pancreatic–Duodenal Injuries

Severe combined pancreatic head and duodenal injuries are fortunately rare. These injuries are most commonly caused by penetrating wounds and occur in association with other multiple intra-abdominal injuries. The best treatment option is predicated on the integrity of the distal common bile duct and ampulla, as well as the severity of the duodenal injury. For that reason, any patient with a combined pancreatic–duodenal injury requires a cholangiogram, a pancreatogram, and evaluation of the ampulla. When the common bile duct and ampulla are intact, the duodenum can be closed primarily and the pancreatic injury treated as previously described. If the status of the pancreatic duct cannot be determined intraoperatively, wide external drainage of the pancreatic head with closed suction drains should be performed rather than a total pancreatectomy. If there is concern about the integrity of the duodenal closure, decompression via a side duodenostomy or three-tube system (gastrostomy, retrograde tube jejunostomy for duodenal decompression, and antegrade tube jejunostomy for feeding) may assist by reducing tension at the suture line. With severe injury to the duodenum in association with pancreatic head injury, it may be advisable to divert gastric contents away from the duodenal repair. This is most commonly accomplished with a pyloric exclusion procedure.

In very massive injuries of the proximal duodenum and head of the pancreas, destruction of the ampulla and proximal pancreatic duct or distal common bile duct may preclude reconstruction. In this situation, a pancreatoduodenectomy (Whipple procedure) is required. We advocate a staged Whipple procedure for patients who are hemodynamically unstable or hypothermic and coagulopathic. In this situation, an initial damage control procedure should seek to control hemorrhage and complete the limited resection, followed by definitive reconstruction at a second operation after a period of additional resuscitation and correction of coagulopathy.

Complications

Complication related to the pancreatic injury following surgical intervention are seen in 20 to 40 percent of patients. Although the majority of complications related to pancreatic injury are self-limiting or treatable, the development of sepsis and multisystem organ failure result in nearly 30 percent of the deaths in pancreatic trauma.

Fistula

This is the most common complication following pancreatic injury, with an incidence of 7 to 20 percent, rising to 26 to 35 percent after combined pancreaticoduodenal injury. The vast majority of these are minor (less than 200 mL/day) and spontaneously resolve within 2 weeks of injury, providing adequate external drainage has been provided. High-output fistulae (greater than 700 mL/day) generally require longer periods of external drainage or surgical intervention for resolution. If a high-output fistula fails to progressively decrease in volume or persists more than 10 days, ERCP is indicated to establish the cause of the persistent fistula and plan further therapy. A somatostatin analogue (octreotide) has shown promise in treating prolonged, high-output pancreatic fistulae, but only after eradicating any infection and in the absence of pancreatic duct obstruction or stricture. Octreotide as an adjuvant to standard fistula management probably diminishes fistula output, but improvement of the time to fistula closure remains to be proven.

Abscesses

The incidence of abscess formation after pancreatic trauma ranges from 10 to 25 percent, depending on the number and type of associated injuries. Early operative or percutaneous decompression or evacuation is critical, although the mortality rate in this group of patients remains about 25 percent. The intraabdominal abscess is most often subfascial or peripancreatic, resulting from inadequate debridement of dead tissue or inadequate initial drainage. True pancreatic abscesses are often not amenable or responsive to percutaneous drainage, and prompt surgical debridement and drainage is required. Percutaneous decompression may be helpful in distinguishing between abscess and pseudocyst.

Pancreatitis

Transient abdominal pain and elevation of the serum amylase concentration may be anticipated in 8 to 18 percent of postoperative patients. This type of pancreatitis is treated with nasogastric decompression, bowel rest, and nutritional support and can be expected to resolve spontaneously. A much more infrequent but deadly complication is hemorrhagic pancreatitis. The first sign of this complication may be bloody pancreatic drainage or a fall in the serum hemoglobin concentration. It is fortunate that this complication occurs in less than 2 percent of operative pancreatic trauma patients, since mortality may approach 80 percent.

Pseudocysts

Overlooked significant blunt pancreatic injuries managed nonoperatively often result in the formation of a pseudocyst. The major determinant of outcome, and indicator of preferred treatment, is the status of the pancreatic duct. If the pancreatic duct is intact, percutaneous drainage of the pseudocyst is likely to be effective. ERCP should therefore precede any percutaneous drainage. If pancreatic duct stenosis or injury is demonstrated, treatment options include (1) re-exploration and partial gland resection (preferred), (2) distal gland internal Roux-en-Y drainage, or (3) endoscopic transpapillary stenting of the pancreatic duct.

ADDITIONAL READING

Asensio J, Feliciano D, Britt L, et al: Management of duodenal injuries. *Curr Prob Surg* 11:1021, 1993.

Bulger EM, Jurkovich GJ: Pancreas: Diagnosis, drainage/debridement, repair and resection. *Operative Techniques Gen Surg* 2:221, 2000.

Cogbill T, Moore E, Morris JJ, et al: Distal pancreatectomy for trauma: A multicenter experience. *J Trauma* 31:1600, 1991.

Patton JH Jr, Lyden SP, Croce MA, et al: Pancreatic trauma: a simplified management guideline, *J Trauma* 43:234, 1997.

Smego D, Richardson J, Flint L: Determinants of outcome in pancreatic trauma. *J Trauma* 25:771, 1985.

Takishima T, Sugimoto K, Hirata M, et al: Serum amylase level on admission in the diagnosis of blunt injury to the pancreas: its significance and limitations. *Ann Surg* 226:70, 1997.

30 | Injury to the Colon and Rectum

COLONIC INJURIES

Diagnosis

Colonic injuries are readily diagnosed at the time of laparotomy. For the occasional patient with a penetrating wound of the flank in whom there is no clear evidence of intraperitoneal injury, a soluble-contrast enema or triple-contrast computed tomography exam (CT) may be helpful. In contrast to penetrating injuries, colonic injuries caused by blunt trauma are rarely subtle.

Treatment

There are three therapeutic options for the treatment of colonic injuries: primary repair, colostomy, and exteriorized repair. Primary repair can be accomplished by the suturing of perforations or by the resection of the damaged colon with reconstruction by ileocolostomy or colocolostomy. Several types of colostomies have been employed to treat colonic injuries. The injured portion of the colon can be exteriorized on the abdominal wall. Advantages of this procedure include avoidance of resection, elimination of fecal contamination from the peritoneal cavity, and speed of construction. The disadvantages of exteriorization are the inability (or undesirability) of exteriorizing particular portions of the colon (e.g., the ascending and descending colons and the cecum). A loop colostomy can be performed proximal to a suture repair or anastomosis. However this does not provide complete protection against dehiscence of the intraperitoneal repair. Today resection of the damaged colon and creation of an end colostomy or (rarely) ileostomy is the most commonly employed stomal technique. End ileostomy is seldom necessary because ileocolostomy anastomosis has an excellent track record. Furthermore, ileostomy can significantly complicate fluid and electrolyte management.

An exteriorized repair is a primary repair which is temporarily suspended on the abdominal wall like a loop colostomy. If the suture line doesn't leak by 10 days, it is returned to the peritoneal cavity. If it does leak, it becomes a loop colostomy. Unfortunately, all patients treated with exteriorized repair require a second operation, either to return the healing suture line within the peritoneal cavity or to close a colostomy. For those reasons, exteriorized repair has largely been abandoned.

Primary repair is now established as the optimal and most common procedure at virtually all major trauma centers. It remains to be determined, however, how often and when it can be safely employed. Many studies have addressed this issue and risk factors and scoring systems have been developed. Unfortunately, they are predictive of bad outcomes regardless of treatment. There have been four comparable prospective randomized studies in recent years, comparing primary repair with colostomy (Table 30-1). The results are similar to those of previous prospective and retrospective studies, which indicated an increase in septic complications with the use of colostomy. These studies have clearly demonstrated that primary repairs are as safe or safer than routine diversion.

The only contemporary study that attempted to determine how often primary repairs can be safely accomplished was published by George and

TABLE 30-1 Prospective Randomized Studies Comparing Colostomy and Primary Repair

Author	Year	Repair			Colostomy		
		No. patients	Fistula	Abscess	No. patients	Fistula	Abscess
Chappuis et al.	1991	26	0	3	28	0	4
Falcone et al.	1992	9	0	1	11	0	1
Sasaki et al.	1995	43	0	1	28	0	5
Gonzalez et al.	1996	56	0	7	53	1	8
Totals		134	0	12(9.0%)	120	1	18(15%)

associates in 1989. In the first half of the study, colonic injuries that required resection due to the extent of injury were treated with colostomy, whereas all others were treated with primary repair. In the second half of the study, all patients were treated with either suture repair or resection and anastomosis. This approach resulted in an unprecedented 95 of 102 patients (93 percent) treated by primary repairs with only a single suture line failure. However, 4 years later, this same group of surgeons recognized a subgroup of patients with colonic injuries requiring resection who were at excessive risk for suture line failure. These included patients who received massive transfusions or had serious associated medical conditions. Patients with both these risk factors had a 42 percent incidence of anastomotic failure. This author agrees with the surgeons from Memphis that massive hemorrhage, especially when it leads to damage control procedures, is a relative contraindication to anastomosis. The visceral edema that invariably occurs in this setting renders the placement of and tension on sutures uncertain and results in unpredictable healing. Colostomies should be considered for colonic injuries when such patients undergo reoperation (Fig. 30-1).

The need for resection is determined by the local extent of the injury and ischemia. Somewhat less obvious is the need for resection based on the extent of damage to the colonic wall. Injuries of between 50 and 100 percent of the diameter of the colon or multiple closely spaced perforations require careful consideration. For injuries requiring resection in the right colon proximal to the middle colonic artery, there should be no hesitation to resect the entire right colon and perform an ileocolostomy. More extensive resections of the right colon to the left of the middle colonic artery are ill-advised in trauma patients because of the additional insult to the patient, the excessive time required, and the complexity of the reconstruction. In the left colon resection and colocolostomy is indicated if optimal conditions exist.

When resection is necessary and local conditions or the patient's overall condition is less than optimal, an end colostomy should be performed (Fig. 30-1). The surgeon must ensure that the same precautions are adhered to as with an end-to-end anastomosis (i.e., an adequate blood supply, no tension, and technical precision). The clamped end of the colon must lay in a relaxed condition on the abdominal wall with at least 2 to 3 cm of healthy-appearing colon proximal to the clamp. Prior to closure of the fascial layer of the abdomen, the colon is transected a centimeter or two above the level of the skin to visualize the bleeding from the submucosa. If a question remains regarding tension or blood supply, additional colon is mobilized and/or the stoma relocated as necessary to meet these criteria. The distal colon in a patient with an end colostomy is best managed as in Hartmann's procedure.

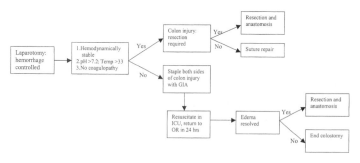

FIG. 30-1. Algorithm for determining whether colon resection is required after trauma. GIA, gastrointestinal anastomosis; ICU, intensive care unit; OR, operating room.

This is preferable to a mucous fistula, because the latter is associated with the potential complications of a second stoma, but has no possible benefit.

For primary repairs, single-layer continuous monofilament suture lines and anastomoses have many potential and real advantages: they are faster, cost less, the suture material is nonabrasive, and a single-layer anastomosis is less likely to decrease the size of the lumen. The technique for creating single-layer suture lines varies between surgeons. For the suturing of perforations, the author employs a transverse closure that begins and ends a few millimeters beyond the edges of the defect to ensure that the corners are properly sealed. A running Lembert technique with 3-0 polypropylene or absorbable monofilament suture is used. For an anastomosis, the suture line is started at the mesenteric border. Little or no mesentery is cleared from the cut edge of the bowel. A double-armed 3-0 polypropylene suture is used. Sutures are placed 3 to 4 mm from the cut edge of the bowel and include all layers except the mucosa. The first stitch is tied on the outside and each arm of the suture is advanced continuously in 3- to 4-mm increments. The arms of the suture are tied at the antimesenteric border.

Results

By far the most common cause of death in patients with colonic injuries is exsanguination; however, this is virtually never due to the colonic injury. The second most common cause of death is sepsis and multiple-organ failure, which may well be related to the colonic injury or its treatment. Deaths from sepsis and multiple-organ failure are well below 5 percent in contemporary series.

Infectious complications are common. Intra-abdominal abscess is the most frequent septic complication and occurs in 5 to 15 percent of patients. Suture line failures or fecal fistulas can occur with any method of treatment. Fistulas occur in 1 to 2 percent of primary repairs, but are rare in patients treated with colostomies. Wound infections should not be considered complications related to treatment of the colonic injury, since leaving the skin and subcutaneous tissues open can prevent almost all infections.

Missile or stab wound tract infections can occur and should be considered in the differential diagnoses of a febrile patient once the usual sources of infection have been eliminated. It is appropriate to remove bullets or wadding that have passed through the colon and are embedded in the patient, provided a hazardous or extensive dissection is not required.

Stomal complications include necrosis, obstruction, peristomal evisceration, and peristomal abscess. The incidence of these complications in aggregate is approximately 5 percent. The majority of stomal complications require operative repair.

Many septic complications can be managed nonoperatively. Intra-abdominal abscesses can often be treated with percutaneous drainage guided by computed tomography. Following drainage of an abscess, a fistula may be discovered. If the patient is not septic, the fistula can also be managed nonoperatively. Treatment consists of serial fistulograms until the associated abscess cavity has been obliterated; once this has occurred, the catheter is slowly withdrawn.

RECTAL INJURIES

In many respects, injuries of the rectum are similar to those of the colon. However, there are important anatomic differences between the two organs that force the surgeon to take an indirect approach to rectal injuries. First, approximately two-thirds of the rectum is extraperitoneal and cannot be mobilized into the peritoneal cavity. Second, much of the rectum is surrounded by the rigid bony pelvis, which makes direct access to extraperitoneal injuries difficult. Third, the rectum is readily accessible via the anus. This fact has both etiologic and diagnostic implications. Because of these anatomic realities, wounds of the extraperitoneal rectum cannot be easily treated by primary repair, and the surgeon must rely on resection or proximal diversion, with or without drainage.

In recent series from urban trauma centers, firearms have been responsible for approximately 80 percent of all rectal injuries. Blunt trauma accounts for about 10 percent of rectal injuries. Transanal injuries account for approximately 6 percent of rectal injuries.

Diagnosis

All patients with gunshot wounds of the trunk, buttocks, perineum, and upper thighs should be suspected of having a rectal injury. Stab wounds or impalements of the buttocks, perineum, and lower abdomen should also be suspect. Any patient with a history of anal manipulation, regardless of etiology, who complains of lower abdominal or pelvic pain should be evaluated for a rectal injury.

All patients suspected of having a rectal injury should undergo digital examination of the rectum. The presence of blood or a positive guaiac test is suggestive of a rectal injury and should trigger the need for further evaluation. It is important to note that a negative result does not rule out a rectal injury. Occasionally, a defect will be palpated on digital examination.

If a rectal injury is suspected, rigid proctoscopy should be performed. This examination may be difficult due to an uncooperative patient and the presence of blood or feces in the rectum. If the patient requires an operation regardless of the findings on digital examination, proctoscopy can be facilitated by the induction of anesthesia. In hemodynamically unstable patients, preoperative proctoscopy may not be possible. In these instances, a rectal injury may be suspected after the hemorrhage has been controlled. It may be desirable in this instance to temporarily close the abdomen and reposition the patient so that

proctoscopy can be performed. While the combination of digital rectal examination and proctoscopy enhances diagnostic accuracy, missed injuries may
still be present in spite of normal findings on both examinations. Although
seldom used, water-soluble contrast enemas are an attractive alternative in
equivocal cases.

Treatment

Colostomy and drainage, and to a lesser extent rectal irrigation have been
embraced by civilian trauma surgeons as the foundation for treatment of rectal injuries. However, because civilian rectal injuries are uncommon, there
remain considerable differences of opinion regarding the optimal type of
colostomy, the method of drainage, the role of irrigation, and the necessity for
repair of the rectal wound.

Regardless of which type of colostomy is performed, there is universal
agreement that it must completely divert the fecal stream. Loop colostomy
can provide complete diversion provided the following technical details are
adhered to: (1) maintaining the spur (the common wall between the afferent
and efferent limbs) above the level of the skin, (2) a longitudinal colotomy,
and (3) immediate maturation of the stoma by suturing the cut edge of the
colon to the skin. The advantages of a loop colostomy are the rapidity of its
construction and its ease of closure.

Hartmann's procedure is ideally suited for extensive rectal injuries. When
a significant portion of the rectal wall has been destroyed and the repair will
be tenuous or complex, the rectum should be divided at the level of the injury,
the distal rectal lumen should be closed, and an end-sigmoid colostomy
should be performed. The rectum can be divided and closed to within a few
centimeters of the anal verge, and reconstruction can still be accomplished
without undue difficulty.

The need for drainage of extraperitoneal rectal injuries has been reasonably
well established. Ideally, the drains should be placed in proximity to the
injury, but not in direct contact with suture lines. Intraperitoneal perforations
do not require drainage.

The optimal style of drain (e.g., Penrose, closed suction, etc) has not been
established. Most authors use Penrose drains because they are comfortable for
the patient, provide dependent drainage when placed through a retroanal incision, and are inexpensive. Closed suction drains have also been used successfully. Drains are usually removed when the drainage becomes serous and the
volume minimal. This usually occurs between the fourth and seventh postoperative days.

All intraperitoneal perforations and extraperitoneal perforations that are
inadvertently uncovered during dissection of adjacent structures must be
repaired. The author prefers a single-layer continuous closure with 3-0
polypropylene sutures. Extraperitoneal perforations that have not been disturbed may or may not require closure, depending on the circumstances.
Experience with civilian penetrating injuries has demonstrated that most
extraperitoneal perforations do not require suture closure. If a large defect in
the rectal wall which the surgeon feels must be closed is encountered, the rectum should probably be divided at the level of the injury and a Hartmann's
procedure performed.

There is no conclusive evidence that irrigation of the distal rectal lumen is
essential, nor is there any contemporary consensus as to whether it is needed.

In creating a plan of treatment for a particular patient, it is appropriate to tailor the operation according to the extent of the injury. Low-energy injuries of the intraperitoneal rectum can be managed by suture closure without a proximal colostomy. High-energy injuries of the intraperitoneal rectum with significant loss of the rectal wall are best treated by Hartmann's procedure. Drainage is not necessary for isolated intraperitoneal injuries. Wounds of the extraperitoneal rectum with little or no loss of the rectal wall can be treated with colostomy and drainage alone. Extraperitoneal injuries of greater magnitude can be treated with mobilization of the rectum, debridement of devascularized tissue, repair of the wounds if accessible, colostomy, and transperineal drainage. If the rectal injury cannot be easily approached because of its distal location, no exhaustive efforts to do so should be made. In this instance, it is important that drains are properly positioned as outlined above. Rectal irrigation may also be helpful in this situation. With very high-energy extraperitoneal rectal injuries and those associated with significant loss of rectal wall, it is prudent to employ Hartmann's procedure. Transperineal drainage is not essential if all perforations are resected and all devitalized tissue has been debrided. In rare instances in which the distal rectum or anal sphincter has been destroyed or if necrosis of the distal rectum occurs postoperatively, an abdominoperineal resection may be necessary.

Table 30-2 lists the mortality and complications related to rectal injuries from recent series.

TABLE 30-2 Results of Treatment of Rectal Injuries in Recent Series

Author	Year	No. patients	% Abscess	% Rectal fistula	% Death from sepsis or MOF
Shannon et al.	1988	26	27	15	4
Burch et al.	1989	100	4	3	4
Thomas et al.	1990	52	2	0	0
Ivatury et al.	1991	54	6	2	0
Renz et al.	1993	30	3	NA	0

MOF, multiple-organ failure, NA, not applicable.

ADDITIONAL READING

Burch JM, Martin RR, Richardson RJ, et al: Evolution of the treatment of injured colon in the 1980s. *Arch Surg* 126:979, 1991.

Franko ER, Ivatury RR, Schwalb DM: Combined penetrating rectal and genitourinary injuries: A challenge in management. *J Trauma* 34:347, 1993.

Shannon FL, Moore EE, Moore FA, McCroskey BL: Value of distal colon washout in civilian rectal trauma—Reducing gut bacterial translocation. *J Trauma* 28:989, 1988.

Stewart RM, Fabian TC, Croce MA, et al: Is resection with primary anastomosis following destructive colon wounds always safe? *Am J Surg* 168:316, 1994.

Velmahos GC, Degiannis E, Wells M, et al: Early closure of colostomies in trauma patients—A prospective randomized trial. Surgery 118:815, 1995.

31 | Abdominal Vascular Injury

Although any vessel in the abdomen can bleed, the term *abdominal vascular injury* generally refers to injury to vessels located in zone 1, midline retroperitoneum; zone 2, upper lateral retroperitoneum; zone 3, pelvic retroperitoneum; and the portal–retrohepatic area of the right upper quadrant, as described below:

- Zone 1—midline retroperitoneum
  Supramesocolic area—suprarenal abdominal aorta, celiac axis, proximal superior mesenteric artery, proximal renal artery, and superior mesenteric vein (either supramesocolic or retromesocolic)
  Inframesocolic area—infrarenal abdominal aorta, infrahepatic inferior vena cava
- Zone 2—upper lateral retroperitoneum
  Renal artery, renal vein
- Zone 3—pelvic retroperitoneum
  Iliac artery, iliac vein
- Portal–retrohepatic area
  Portal vein, hepatic artery, retrohepatic vena cava

The significantly higher number of abdominal vascular injuries treated in civilian as opposed to military practice reflects the modest wounding capacity of many handguns and the short prehospital transit times in most urban areas of the United States.

At present, the incidence of injury to major abdominal vessels in patients sustaining blunt abdominal trauma is estimated to be about 5 to 10 percent. Patients with penetrating stab wounds to the abdomen will sustain a major abdominal vascular injury 10 percent of the time. Patients with gunshot wounds to the abdomen will have injury to a major vessel 25 percent of the time.

PATHOPHYSIOLOGY

The blunt trauma associated with rapid deceleration in motor vehicle crashes causes two different types of vascular injury in the abdomen. The first is avulsion of small branches from the major vessels. Another type of vascular problem seen with blunt deceleration injury is the intimal tear with secondary thrombosis of the lumen, such as is seen in patients with renal artery thrombosis.

Blunt injuries associated with a direct anterior crush (lap seat belt) or posterior blow to the spine also cause two different types of vascular injury. The first is an intimal tear or flap with secondary thrombosis of a vessel such as the superior mesenteric artery, infrarenal abdominal aorta, or iliac artery. Direct blows can also completely disrupt exposed vessels, such as the left renal vein over the aorta or the superior mesenteric artery or vein at the base of the mesentery, leading to massive intraperitoneal hemorrhage, or even partly disrupt the infrarenal abdominal aorta, leading to a false aneurysm.

Penetrating injuries, in contrast, create the same kinds of abdominal vascular injuries as are seen in the vessels of the extremities, producing blast effects with intimal flaps and secondary thrombosis, lateral-wall defects with free-bleeding or pulsatile hematomas (early false aneurysms), or complete transection with either free bleeding or thrombosis.

Iatrogenic injuries to major abdominal vessels are an uncommon but persistent problem. Reported iatrogenic causes of abdominal vascular injury have included diagnostic procedures (angiography, cardiac catheterization, laparoscopy), abdominal operations (pelvic and retroperitoneal procedures), spinal operations (removal of a herniated disk), and adjuncts to cardiac surgery (cardiopulmonary bypass, intra-aortic balloon assist).

DIAGNOSIS

On physical examination, the findings in patients with abdominal vascular injury will obviously depend on whether a contained hematoma or active hemorrhage is present. Patients with contained hematomas in the retroperitoneum, base of the mesentery, or hepatoduodenal ligament, particularly those with injuries to abdominal veins, may be hypotensive in transit but will respond rapidly to the infusion of fluids. They may remain remarkably stable, with modest peritoneal signs on examination, until the hematoma is opened at the time of celiotomy. Other patients will have a distended abdomen and hypotension related to intraperitoneal hemorrhage from the injured vessel. The other major physical finding that may be noted in patients with abdominal vascular injury is loss of the pulse in the femoral artery in one lower extremity when the ipsilateral common or external iliac artery has been transected or is thrombosed.

In patients with blunt abdominal trauma, hematuria, and modest to moderate hypotension in the emergency department, a preoperative one-shot intravenous pyelogram (IVP) during resuscitation has been useful for documenting the presence of an intact kidney. If the kidney is mostly intact without extravasation of the dye, the surgeon will not have to open a perirenal hematoma at the subsequent laparotomy. Any stable patient with blunt trauma who does not require an immediate laparotomy and who has significant hematuria may best be served by an immediate abdominal CT scan without a preliminary one-shot IVP.

Preoperative abdominal aortography is not commonly used to document intra-abdominal vascular injuries after penetrating wounds. In patients with blunt trauma, aortography is used to diagnose and treat deep pelvic arterial bleeding associated with fractures and to diagnose unusual injuries such as the previously mentioned intimal tears with thrombosis in the infrarenal aorta, iliac artery, or renal artery. An algorithm for treatment of abdominal vascular injury is presented in Fig. 31-1.

INITIAL MANAGEMENT

Resuscitation in the field in patients with possible blunt or penetrating abdominal vascular injuries should be restricted to basic airway maneuvers, intubation, or cricothyroidotomy and decompression of a tension pneumothorax at the scene. Insertion of intravenous lines for infusing crystalloid solutions is best attempted during transport to the hospital.

In the emergency department, the extent of resuscitation clearly depends on the patient's condition at the time of arrival. In the agonal patient with a distended abdomen, emergency department thoracotomy with cross-clamping of the descending thoracic aorta may be necessary to maintain cerebral and coronary flow if the trauma operating room is geographically distant from the emergency department. Although all trauma surgeons agree that performing a thoracotomy in this setting will complicate the patient's intraoperative course,

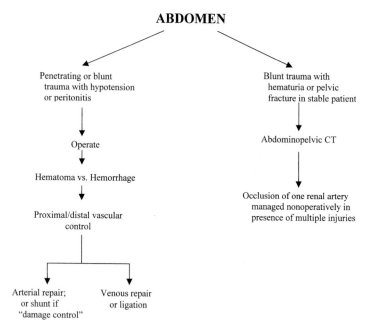

FIG. 31-1. Algorithm for the treatment of abdominal vascular injury.

the thoracotomy and cross-clamping are sometimes the only way to prevent irreversible ischemic changes to the patient's brain and heart until a celiotomy with vascular control can be performed.

If the patient arrives in the emergency department with marked abdominal distention under a pneumatic antishock garment (PASG), it is appropriate to leave the garment inflated during the period of transit to the operating room. The garment is removed only when the anesthesiologist and surgeons have completed the usual preparations for celiotomy.

In the usual patient arriving with abdominal distention and hypotension, *a time limit of less than 5 minutes in the emergency department is mandatory.* An identification bracelet is applied, while multiple, large-bore intravenous catheters should be inserted in the upper extremities or, if necessary, into the central veins at the thoracic inlet in the operating room. Blood samples for typing and cross-matching, and other basic studies are obtained on insertion of the first catheter and are immediately sent to the laboratory.

Measures in the emergency department that will diminish the hypothermia of resuscitation include the use of prewarmed (37 to 40° C) crystalloid solutions, passage of all crystalloids and blood through high-flow warmers, and covering the patient with prewarmed blankets or heating units.

OPERATION

Draping and Incisions

In the operating room, the entire trunk from the chin to the middle thighs is prepared and draped in the usual manner.

Maneuvers to Prevent or Decrease Hypothermia

In addition to the maneuvers previously described for preventing hypothermia in the emergency department, operative maneuvers with the same purpose include warming the operating room; covering the patient's head; covering the upper and lower extremities with a heating unit (Bair Hugger, Augustine Medical, Inc., Eden Prairie, Minnesota); the irrigation of nasogastric tubes, thoracostomy tubes, and open body cavities with warm saline; and the use of a heating cascade on the anesthesia machine.

General Principles

A preliminary operating room thoracotomy with cross-clamping of the descending thoracic aorta is used in some centers when the patient's blood pressure on arrival is less than 70 mm Hg. This maneuver will maintain coronary and cerebrovascular flow if the heart is still beating, but has little effect on intra-abdominal vascular injuries because of persistent bleeding from backflow.

A midline abdominal incision is made, and all clots and free blood are manually evacuated or removed with suction. A rapid inspection is then done for contained hematomas or areas of hemorrhage. One intra-abdominal physical finding that may be of benefit to the surgeon is the "black bowel," which has been seen in patients with total transection or thrombosis of the proximal superior mesenteric artery.

If there is active hemorrhage, it will have to be controlled before any other intraoperative maneuvers are undertaken. Hemorrhage from solid organs is controlled by packing, while standard techniques of vascular control are used to control the active hemorrhage from major intra-abdominal vessels. Finger pressure, compression with laparotomy pads, or formal proximal and distal control will be needed to control any actively hemorrhaging major abdominal artery. Options for control of bleeding from major veins such as the inferior vena cava, superior mesenteric vein, renal veins, or iliac veins include finger pressure, compression with laparotomy pads or spongesticks, or the application of vascular clamps. Once hemorrhage from the vascular injuries is controlled in patients with penetrating wounds, it may be worthwhile to rapidly apply Babcock clamps, Allis clamps, or noncrushing intestinal clamps to as many large gastrointestinal perforations as possible to avoid further contamination of the abdomen during the period of vascular repair. If only a few holes are present in the gastrointestinal tract, rapid one-layer closure using 3-0 polypropylene suture may be performed. The vascular repair is then performed, a soft-tissue cover is applied over the repair, and the remainder of the operation is directed toward repair of injuries to solid organs.

If the patient has a contained retroperitoneal hematoma at the time of celiotomy, the surgeon occasionally has time to first perform necessary gastrointestinal repairs in the free peritoneal cavity, change gloves, and irrigate with saline solution and antibiotics. The surgeon can then open the retroperitoneum to expose the abdominal vascular injury causing the hematoma.

Hematomas or hemorrhage associated with abdominal vascular injuries generally occur in zone 1, midline retroperitoneum; zone 2, upper lateral retroperitoneum; zone 3, pelvic retroperitoneum; or in the portal–retrohepatic area of the right upper gradient, as previously described. The magnitude of injury is best described using the Organ Injury Scale of the American Association for the Surgery of Trauma (AAST).

Injuries in Zone 1—Midline Supramesocolic Area

When a hematoma is present, as it frequently is with aortic wounds in the hiatus, the surgeon usually has time to reflect all left-sided intra-abdominal viscera, including the colon, kidney, spleen, tail of the pancreas, and fundus of the stomach to the midline (medial mobilization maneuver) (Fig. 31-2).

Because of the dense nature of the celiac plexus of nerves connecting the right and left celiac ganglia and the lymphatics that surround the supraceliac aorta, it is frequently helpful to transect the left crus of the diaphragm at the two o'clock position to allow for exposure of the distal descending thoracic aorta above the hiatus. With the distal descending thoracic aorta or abdominal aorta in the hiatus exposed, the supraceliac aortic clamp can be applied without difficulty.

If active hemorrhage is coming from this area, the surgeon may attempt to control it manually or with one of the aortic compression devices. An alternative approach is to divide the lesser omentum manually, retract the stomach and esophagus to the left, and digitally separate the muscle fibers of the crura from the supraceliac aorta to obtain the same exposure as described for the left-sided medial mobilization maneuver, but more quickly. Distal aortic control may require ligation and division of the celiac axis.

With small perforating wounds to the aorta at this level, lateral aortorrhaphy with 3-0 or 4-0 polypropylene suture is preferred. If two small perforations are adjacent to one another, they should be connected and the defect closed in a transverse fashion with the polypropylene suture. When closure of the perforation(s) results in significant narrowing, or if a portion of the aortic wall is missing, patch aortoplasty with polytetrafluoroethylene (PTFE) is indicated. The

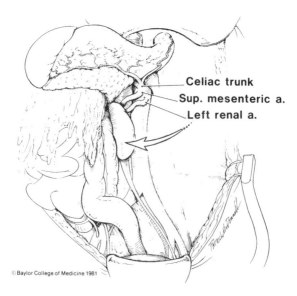

Celiac trunk
Sup. mesenteric a.
Left renal a.

© Baylor College of Medicine 1981

FIG. 31-2. Medial mobilization of all left-sided intra-abdominal viscera allows for visualization of the entire abdominal aorta from the hiatus to the aortic bifurcation. *(Reproduced, with permission, from Baylor College of Medicine.)*

other option is to resect a short segment of the injured aorta and perform an end-to-end anastomosis. This can be difficult because of the limited mobility of both ends of the aorta at this level. On rare occasions, patients with extensive injuries to diaphragmatic or supraceliac aorta will require insertion of a synthetic vascular conduit or spiral graft after resection of the area of injury.

As previously noted, repairs of the intestine and the aorta should not be performed simultaneously. Once the perforated bowel has been packed away and the surgeon has changed gloves, the aortic prosthesis is sewn in place with 3-0 or 4-0 polypropylene suture. After appropriate flushing of both ends of the aorta and removal of the distal aortic clamp, the proximal aortic clamp should be removed very slowly as the anesthesiologist rapidly infuses fluids. If a long aortic clamp time has been necessary, the prophylactic administration of intravenous bicarbonate is indicated to reverse the "washout" acidosis from the previously ischemic lower extremities. The retroperitoneum is then copiously irrigated with an antibiotic solution and closed in a water-tight fashion with an absorbable suture. The survival rate of patients with injuries to the suprarenal abdominal aorta is approximately 35 percent.

When branches of the celiac axis are injured, they are often difficult to repair because of the dense neural and lymphatic tissue in this area and the small size of the vessels in a patient in shock with secondary vasoconstriction. There is clearly no good reason to fix major injuries to either the left gastric or proximal splenic artery in the patient with trauma to this area. In both instances, these vessels should be ligated.

If an injury to the superior mesenteric artery is beneath the pancreas (Fullen zone I), the pancreas may on rare occasions have to be transected between Glassman or Dennis intestinal clamps to control the bleeding point. Because the superior mesenteric artery has few branches at this level, proximal and distal vascular control is relatively easy to obtain once the overlying pancreas has been divided. Another option is to perform medial rotation of the left-sided intra-abdominal viscera, as previously described, and apply a clamp directly to the proximal superior mesenteric artery at its origin from the left side of the aorta. In this instance, the left kidney may be left in the retroperitoneum as the medial rotation is performed.

Injuries to the superior mesenteric artery also occur beyond the pancreas at the base of the transverse mesocolon (Fullen zone II, between the pancreaticoduodenal and middle colic branches of the artery). Although there is certainly more space in which to work in this area, the proximity of the pancreas and the potential for pancreatic leaks near the arterial repair make injuries in this location almost as difficult to handle as the more proximal injuries.

In the patient with hypothermia, acidosis, and a coagulopathy, the insertion of a temporary intraluminal shunt into the debrided ends of the superior mesenteric artery in zone I or II is most appropriate and fits the definition of *damage control*. If replacement of the proximal superior mesenteric artery is necessary in a more stable patient, it is safest to place a saphenous vein or prosthetic graft on the distal infrarenal aorta, away from the pancreas and other upper abdominal injuries.

The survival rate among patients with penetrating injuries to the superior mesenteric artery is approximately 58 percent. This decreases to 22 percent when any form of repair more complex than lateral arteriorrhaphy is necessary.

Injuries to the proximal renal arteries may also present with a supramesocolic hematoma or with hemorrhage in this area. The medial mobilization maneuver described earlier allows visualization of much of the posterior left renal artery from the aorta to the kidney. This maneuver does not, however, allow for visualization of the proximal right renal artery. The proximal vessel is best approached through the base of the mesocolon beneath the left renal vein and between the infrarenal abdominal aorta and inferior vena cava. Options for repair of either the proximal or distal renal arteries are described later in this chapter.

One other major abdominal vessel, the proximal superior mesenteric vein, lying to the right of the superior mesenteric artery, may be injured at the base of the mesocolon. For proximal exposure, the pancreas may have to be transected between noncrushing vascular or intestinal clamps to gain access to a perforation.

When multiple vascular and visceral injuries are present in the upper abdomen and the superior mesenteric vein has been severely injured, ligation can be performed in the young trauma patient. The survival rate among patients with injuries to the superior mesenteric vein is approximately 72%.

Injuries in Zone 1—Midline Inframesocolic Area

In this location, injuries occur to either the infrarenal aorta or inferior vena cava. Exposure of an inframesocolic injury to the aorta is obtained by duplicating the maneuvers used to gain proximal aortic control during the elective resection of an abdominal aortic aneurysm. The transverse mesocolon is pulled up toward the head, the small bowel is eviscerated toward the right (surgeon's) side of the table, and the midline retroperitoneum is opened until the left renal vein is exposed. A proximal aortic clamp should then be placed immediately inferior to the left renal vein. Exposure to allow for application of the distal vascular clamp is obtained by dividing the midline retroperitoneum down to the aortic bifurcation, carefully avoiding the left-sided origin of the inferior mesenteric artery. However, this vessel may be sacrificed whenever necessary for exposure.

As with injuries to the suprarenal aorta, injuries in the infrarenal abdominal aorta are repaired primarily with 3-0 or 4-0 polypropylene suture or by patch aortoplasty, end-to-end anastomosis, or insertion of a woven Dacron graft, albumin-coated Dacron graft, or a PTFE graft—none of which require pre-clotting.

The survival rate among patients with injuries to the infrarenal abdominal aorta is approximately 46 percent.

If the aorta is intact and an inframesocolic hematoma appears to be more extensive on the right side of the abdomen than on the left, or if there is active hemorrhage coming through the base of the mesentery of the ascending colon or hepatic flexure of the colon, injury to the inferior vena cava below the liver should be suspected. Although it is possible to visualize the vena cava through the midline retroperitoneal incision previously described, most trauma surgeons are more comfortable with visualizing the vena cava by mobilizing the right half of the colon and C-loop of the duodenum, and leaving the right kidney in situ (right medial mobilization maneuver) (Fig. 31-3). This permits the entire vena caval system from the confluence of the iliac veins to the suprarenal vena cava below the liver to be visualized.

If active hemorrhage appears to be coming from the anterior surface of the vena cava, a Satinsky-type vascular clamp should be applied directly to the perforation as it is elevated by a pair of vascular forceps or an Allis clamp. When the vena cava has been extensively lacerated and partial occlusion

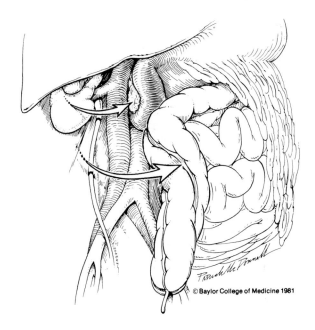

FIG. 31-3.   Medial mobilization of right-sided intra-abdominal viscera except the kidney allows for visualization of the entire infrahepatic inferior vena cava. *(Reproduced, with permission, from Baylor College of Medicine.)*

cannot be performed, it is often helpful to compress the proximal and distal vena cava around the partial transection or extensive laceration, using gauze sponges placed in straight spongesticks. Because of backbleeding from lumbar veins, it may be necessary to use large DeBakey aortic clamps and completely occlude the vena cava above and below some injuries. This maneuver carries a risk in the already hypotensive patient, since venous return to the right side of the heart is essentially interrupted. For this reason, the infrarenal abdominal aorta should be clamped simultaneously.

One interesting approach to wounds at the confluence of the common iliac veins is temporary division of the overlying right common iliac artery with mobilization of the aortic bifurcation to the left. This will improve the surgeon's view of the venous injuries, which can be repaired in the usual fashion. The right common iliac artery is then reconstituted by an end-to-end anastomosis. When the perforation occurs at the junction of the renal veins and the inferior vena cava, it should be directly compressed with either spongesticks or the fingers. An assistant then clamps or compresses the infrarenal vena cava and the suprarenal infrahepatic vena cava, and loops both renal veins individually with vascular tapes to allow for the direct application of angled vascular clamps. One other useful technique for controlling hemorrhage from the inferior vena cava in all locations is to use a Foley balloon catheter for tamponade.

Anterior perforations of the inferior vena cava are best repaired in a transverse fashion using running sutures of 4-0 or 5-0 polypropylene, frequently in a two-layer fashion, to buttress the repair. In the unstable patient who has developed a coagulopathy, no further attempt should be made to enlarge a narrowed repair. In the stable patient, there may be some justification for applying a large venous patch taken either from the resected inferior mesenteric vein or ovarian vein, or a PTFE patch.

In the case of a young patient who is exsanguinating and in whom extensive repair of the infrarenal inferior vena cava appears to be necessary, ligation of this vessel is usually well tolerated as long as certain precautions are taken. The first of these is to perform bilateral below-knee four-compartment fasciotomies at the first operation, depending on the patient's hemodynamic status. Bilateral thigh fasciotomies may be necessary as well, within the first 48 hours after ligation. The second is to maintain circulating volume in the postoperative period through infusion of the appropriate fluids. The third is to apply elastic compression wraps to both lower extremities and keep them continuously elevated for approximately 5 to 7 days after operation.

Survival rates for patients with injuries to the inferior vena cava obviously depend on the location of injury. If one eliminates suprahepatic and retrohepatic vena caval injuries from seven series, the average survival for 515 patients with injuries to the infrahepatic vena cava was 72.2 percent. When injuries to the infrarenal vena cava alone are included, the average survival for 318 patients was 76.1 percent.

Injuries in Zone 2—Upper Lateral Retroperitoneum

In patients who have suffered blunt abdominal trauma and have a normal preoperative IVP, renal arteriogram, or CT of the kidneys, there is no justification for exploring the kidney through its perirenal hematoma.

In highly selected patients with penetrating wounds to the flank, CT has been used to document an isolated minor renal injury and operation has been avoided. All other patients found to have a perirenal hematoma at the time of exploration for a penetrating abdominal wound should have unroofing of the hematoma and exploration of the wound track. If the hematoma is not rapidly expanding and there is no free intra-abdominal bleeding, most surgeons will loop the ipsilateral renal artery with a vascular tape in the midline at the base of the mesocolon. If there is active bleeding from the kidney through Gerota's fascia or from the retroperitoneum overlying the renal vessels, no central renovascular control is necessary. The surgeon should simply open the retroperitoneum lateral to the injured kidney and manually elevate the kidney directly into the wound. A large vascular clamp can be applied proximal to the hilum either at the midline on the left or just lateral to the inferior vena cava on the right to control any further bleeding.

In patients with multiple intra-abdominal injuries or a long preoperative period of ischemia, nephrectomy is an appropriate choice, as long as intraoperative palpation has confirmed a normal contralateral kidney. The survival rate for patients with injuries to the renal arteries from penetrating trauma is approximately 87 percent, with renal salvage in only 30 to 40 percent.

As previously noted, the nonvisualization of one kidney on an IVP typically prompts an immediate abdominal CT scan with contrast enhancement rather than a renal arteriogram in many trauma centers. If either study documents occlusion of a renal artery, many surgeons choose to observe this injury without operation—as long as the other kidney is intact.

Lateral venorrhaphy remains the preferred technique of repair for injuries of the renal vein. If ligation of the right renal vein is necessary to control hemorrhage, nephrectomy should be performed. The medial left renal vein can be ligated as long as the left adrenal and gonadal veins are intact. The survival rate for patients with penetrating injuries to the renal veins has ranged from 42 to 88 percent in the recent literature, with the difference presumably due to the magnitude and number of associated visceral and vascular injuries.

Injuries in Zone 3—Pelvic Retroperitoneum

If a hematoma or hemorrhage is present after penetrating trauma, compression with a laparotomy pad or finger should be maintained as proximal and distal vascular control is attained. The proximal common iliac arteries are exposed by eviscerating the small bowel to the right and dividing the midline retroperitoneum over the aortic bifurcation. In young trauma patients, there is usually no adherence between the common iliac artery and vein in this location, and vascular tapes can be passed rapidly around the proximal arteries. Distal vascular control is obtained at the point at which the external iliac artery comes out of the pelvis proximal to the inguinal ligament. The artery is readily palpable under the retroperitoneum and can be rapidly elevated into the field of view with a vascular tape. The major problem in this area is continued backbleeding from the internal iliac artery. This artery can be exposed by further opening the retroperitoneum on the side of the pelvis, elevating the vascular tapes on the proximal common iliac and distal external iliac arteries, and looking for the large branch of the iliac artery that descends into the pelvis.

Injuries to the common or external iliac artery should be repaired if at all possible. Ligation of either vessel will lead to progressive ischemia of the lower extremity and the need for an above-knee amputation in the later postoperative course in many hypotensive trauma patients. In patients with severe shock, insertion of an intraluminal shunt is a better choice for damage control. In contrast, an injured internal iliac artery can be ligated with impunity even with injuries that occur bilaterally.

Extensive injuries to the common or external iliac artery in the presence of *significant* enteric or fecal contamination in the pelvis remain a serious problem for the trauma surgeon. Both end-to-end repairs and vascular conduits in this location have suffered late postoperative blowouts secondary to pelvic infection from the original intestinal contamination. In recent years, we have occasionally avoided end-to-end anastomosis or the insertion of a saphenous vein or PTFE graft in either the common or external iliac artery in such a situation. Rather, the artery is divided just proximal to the injury, closed with a double running row of 4-0 or 5-0 polypropylene sutures, and covered with noninjured retroperitoneum. If the patient's lower extremity on the side of the ligation appears to be in jeopardy at the completion of the abdominal operation, an extra-anatomic femorofemoral crossover graft should be performed to return arterial inflow to the extremity. If the surgeon chooses not to perform a femorofemoral crossover graft until the patient's condition has been stabilized in the surgical intensive care unit, an ipsilateral four-compartment below-knee fasciotomy should be performed, since ischemic edema below the knee will often lead to a compartment syndrome.

The survival rate among patients with injuries to the iliac arteries will vary with the number of associated injuries to the iliac vein, aorta, and vena cava, but was approximately 61 percent in 189 patients reviewed in four large series. When patients with other vascular injuries, especially to the iliac vein, were eliminated, the survival rate among 57 patients in three series was 81 percent. If the injury is large and free bleeding from the iliac artery into the peritoneal cavity has occurred during the preoperative period, the survival rate will be only 45 percent.

Injuries to the iliac veins are exposed through a technique similar to that described for injuries to the iliac arteries. It is not usually necessary to pass vascular tapes around these vessels, however, because they are readily compressible with either spongesticks or fingers. As previously noted, the somewhat inaccessible location of the right common iliac vein has led to the suggested transection of the right common iliac artery in order to improve exposure at this location. Similarly, transection and ligation of the internal iliac artery on the side of the pelvis will allow improved exposure of an injured ipsilateral internal iliac vein.

Injuries to the iliac veins are best treated either with lateral repair using 4-0 or 5-0 polypropylene suture or with ligation. Ligation in the young patient has been well tolerated in our experience and that of others if the same precautions used after ligation of the inferior vena cava are applied; however, some centers strongly recommend repair rather than ligation for injuries of the iliac veins. The survival rate of patients with injuries to the iliac veins is variable, but was approximately 70 percent in 404 patients reviewed in five large series. When patients with other vascular injuries, especially to the iliac artery, were eliminated, the survival rate among 137 patients in three series was 90 percent.

Injuries in the Porta Hepatis

When a hematoma is present in the porta hepatis, the proximal hepatoduodenal ligament should be looped with a vascular tape, or a noncrushing vascular clamp should be applied (the Pringle maneuver) before the hematoma is entered. If hemorrhage is occurring, finger compression of the bleeding vessels will suffice until the vascular clamp is in place. Because of the short length of the porta in many patients, it may be impossible to place a distal vascular clamp right at the edge of the liver. In such patients, manual compression with forceps may allow distal vascular control until the area of injury can be isolated. Because of the proximity of the common bile duct, no sutures should be placed into the porta until the vascular injury is precisely defined.

Ligation of the hepatic artery appears to be well tolerated in the young trauma patient, even when performed beyond the origin of the gastroduodenal artery, owing to the extensive collateral arterial flow to the liver. If an associated hepatic injury is present, however, there will be increased necrosis of parenchyma underneath mattress sutures. Selective ligation of the hepatic artery and portal vein to one lobe of the liver will obviously lead to necrosis of the lobe and mandates hepatectomy, whereas selective ligation of the right hepatic artery alone should be followed by a cholecystectomy.

Injuries to the portal vein in the hepatoduodenal ligament are isolated in much the same fashion as injuries to the hepatic artery. The posterior position of the vein, however, makes the exposure of these injuries more difficult. Mobilization of the common bile duct to the left end and the cystic duct superiorly, coupled with an extensive Kocher maneuver, will usually allow for excellent visualization of any suprapancreatic injury after proximal (and, if possible, distal) vascular control has been obtained. Techniques for repair of the vein are varied, but lateral venorrhaphy with 4-0 or 5-0 polypropylene suture is preferred. More extensive maneuvers that have occasionally been used with success include resection with an end-to-end anastomosis, interposition grafting, transposition of the splenic vein down to the superior mesenteric vein, an end-to-side portacaval shunt, or a venovenous shunt from the superior mesenteric vein to the distal portal vein or inferior vena cava. Ligation of the portal vein should be performed if an extensive injury is present and the patient is hypothermic and acidotic (damage control). The surgeon must then be prepared to infuse tremendous amounts of fluids to reverse the transient peripheral hypovolemia secondary to splanchnic hypervolemia. The survival rate among 134 patients with injuries to the portal vein in six series from 1978 to 1987 was approximately 50 percent.

COMPLICATIONS

The complications of vascular repairs in the abdomen are much the same as those seen in the extremities. They include such problems as thrombosis, dehiscence of a suture line, and infection. Occlusion is not uncommon when small, vasoconstricted vessels, such as the renal artery or superior mesenteric artery, undergo lateral arteriorrhaphy. In such patients, it may be valuable to perform a second-look operation within 12 to 24 hours after the patient's temperature, coagulation abnormalities, and blood pressure have returned to normal. When this is done, correction of a vascular thrombosis may be successful.

Dehiscence of vascular suture lines in the abdomen has occurred in two locations in our experience. A substitute vascular conduit inserted in the superior mesenteric artery near a pancreatic injury may be disrupted if a small pancreatic leak occurs in the postoperative period. For this reason, the proximal anastomosis of such a graft should be on the infrarenal aorta, far away from the pancreas, as previously noted. The dehiscence of end-to-end anastomoses and conduit suture lines in the iliac arteries can be avoided by limiting the extent of repair if there is significant enteric or fecal contamination in the pelvis.

One vascular complication unique to the abdomen is the postoperative development of vascular–enteric fistulas. This will occur most commonly in patients who have anterior aortic repairs, aortic grafts, or grafts to the superior mesenteric artery from the aorta. Again, this problem can be avoided by proper coverage of suture lines on the aorta with retroperitoneal tissue or a viable omental pedicle, and on the recipient vessel with mesentery.

ADDITIONAL READING

Accola KD, Feliciano DV, Mattox KL, et al: Management of injuries to the superior mesenteric artery. *J Trauma* 26:313, 1986.

Burch JM, Richardson RJ, Martin RR, et al: Penetrating iliac vascular injuries: Experience with 233 consecutive patients. *J Trauma* 30:1450, 1990.

Feliciano DV: Injuries to great vessels of the abdomen, in Holcroft JW (ed): *Scientific American Surgery,* Trauma Section, Section 4, Chapter 9. New York, Scientific American, 1998, p 1.

Feliciano DV: Management of traumatic retroperitoneal hematoma. *Ann Surg* 211:109, 1990.

Stone HH, Fabian TC, Turkleson ML: Wounds of the portal venous system. *World J Surg* 6:335, 1982.

32 | Pelvic Fractures

INTRODUCTION

There are few injuries that represent as broad a spectrum and as significant a challenge as pelvic fractures. Many pelvic fractures are minor and require little therapy. However, pelvic fractures can be a marker of injury severity. The force required to fracture the bony pelvis is substantial, particularly in young patients. Bleeding can be torrential. Mature judgment and a multidisciplinary approach maximizes survival.

PELVIC FRACTURE ANATOMY AND CLASSIFICATION

The pelvis is formed by a ring of bone consisting of two innominate bones and the sacrum held together by extremely strong ligaments (Fig. 32-1). Three major vectors of force injure the pelvic ring. The most common is lateral compression (LC). These forces produce acute shortening of the diameter of the pelvis. They are often markers for severe torso injury, but usually do not result in pelvic ligamentous injury. LC injuries typically do not produce severe blood loss except in elderly patients.

The second most frequent vector of force is anteroposterior (AP). AP forces widen the pelvic diameter. The pelvic injury is often an open book injury with pubic symphysial diastasis and/or opening of the sacroiliac joints. These often cause substantial blood loss from arterial injury in the hypogastric distribution.

Vertical shear injuries are most frequently seen in individuals who jump or fall from a height. They usually affect only one hemipelvis, but may disrupt all ligamentous structures. The pelvic structure may be skeletally unstable, as in AP compression injuries, but blood loss is generally not quite as substantial.

There are a number of schemes to classify fractures. Perhaps the most useful method is that described by Young and Burgess, which describes both vectors of force and degree of displacement (Table 32-1). This scheme can also predict degree of hemorrhage.

DIAGNOSIS OF PELVIC FRACTURE

All patients with high-energy blunt trauma should be assumed to have a pelvic fracture. Patients usually complain of pain and/or have pelvic tenderness. However, patients may also complain of hip or lower abdominal pain. Common findings include abrasions and contusions or hematomas over the bony prominences. A perineal examination will identify scrotal or vulvar hematomas. Rectal and vaginal examinations may reveal lacerations, which strongly suggest an open pelvic fracture. Physical findings that suggest associated urethral injury are scrotal hematomas, high-riding prostate on rectal examination, or blood at the urinary meatus.

The clinician should gently compress both sides of the pelvis toward the midline and then gently externally rotate the pelvis to determine its stability. Vigorous rocking of the pelvis may exacerbate pelvic bleeding in an unstable fracture.

Patients who are awake and alert and have no symptoms or physical findings of a pelvic fracture do not require an x-ray. However, all patients with multisystem injury or an unreliable history should have a pelvic x-ray.

Additional x-ray views are often helpful. Inlet views of the pelvis are taken at a 45° angle to the pelvis from above and help to better visualize the sacrum

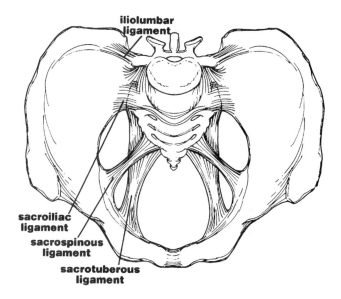

FIG. 32-1.   Ligamentous anatomy of the pelvis.

and anterior pubis bone. Outlet views are taken at a 45° angle from underneath the pelvis and aid in visualizing the sacrum and the sacroiliac joints. Judet views are AP views with the patient's body rotated 45°. These provide additional information about the acetabulum.

CT scanning can be a very valuable tool in selected cases. Using 3- to 5-mm cuts, it can determine the integrity of sacroiliac ligaments and degree of displacement. Subtle sacral fractures can also be seen. CT scanning can also image the abdomen and can help quantify retroperitoneal bleeding.

INITIAL MANAGEMENT

After airway and breathing are addressed, hemodynamic stability is the next concern. All patients with pelvic fractures are at risk for hemorrhage either from the pelvic fracture or associated injuries. All patients require large-bore IV access. All lines should be placed in the upper extremity peripheral veins or superior mediastinal veins to avoid worsening pelvic venous injury. Blood should be typed and cross-matched. Bleeding can arise from fracture fragments or adjacent small arteries and veins. Major arterial or venous injury usually occurs in the hypogastric distribution. Patients in shock require more than 5 units of blood per 24 hours, and 20 percent will require over 15 units. Fresh frozen plasma and platelets should always be available.

EVALUATING THE ABDOMEN

Differentiating intra-abdominal bleeding from pelvic fracture bleeding can be quite difficult. Physical examination is notoriously unreliable. Diagnostic peritoneal lavage (DPL) is quite reliable if performed early. In patients with pelvic fractures, DPL must be performed open in a supraumbilical location. A

TABLE 32-1   Classification of Pelvic Fractures

AP Compression	
Type I	Disruption of the public symphysis of <2.5 cm of diastasis; no significant posterior pelvic injury
Type II	Disruption of the public symphysis of >2.5 cm, with tearing of the anterior sacroiliac and sacrospinous and sacrotuberous ligaments
Type III	Complete disruption of the public symphysis and posterior ligament complexes, and hemipelvic displacement

Lateral Compression	
Type I	Posterior compression of the sacroiliac joint without ligament disruption; oblique public ramus fracture
Type II	Rupture of the posterior sacroiliac ligament; pivotal internal rotation of a hemipelvis on the anterior sacroiliac joint with a crush injury of the sacrum and an oblique pubic ramus fracture
Type III	Findings in type II injury with evidence of an AP compression injury to the contralateral hemipelvis

negative DPL rules out intra-abdominal bleeding. False positives can occur in up to one-third of patients due to diapedesis of red cells from a tense retroperitoneal hematoma into the abdomen. Thus a positive tap is relatively reliable and should prompt abdominal exploration, but a positive lavage should be viewed with some skepticism.

Focused abdominal sonography for trauma (FAST) can be extremely useful. A relatively small hemoperitoneum or blood from diapedesis of red cells will not be visualized on FAST examination. However, a clinically relevant hemoperitoneum (over 200 mL) is generally seen with FAST.

If patient stability permits, the additional information gained by abdominal CT scanning is usually beneficial. CT diagnoses retroperitoneal hemorrhage as well as associated intra-abdominal or retroperitoneal injury.

MANAGING PELVIC FRACTURE BLEEDING

One should suspect pelvic fracture bleeding in high-risk fractures such as those from AP compression or vertical shear forces, particularly those with substantial displacement. However, any pelvic fracture can produce serious hemorrhage, even with a relatively normal x-ray (Fig. 32-2).

External Compression Devices

External compression can closely realign pelvic bones, thus reducing pelvic volume (Table 32-2). This helps stop bleeding from bony fragments and acts to tamponade small vessel bleeding. No method of external compression will stop arterial blood loss.

In general, there are four expedient methods of providing external compression. A bed sheet can be placed on the stretcher before the patient arrives. The ends are then crisscrossed across the patient's abdomen, acting as a pelvic splint. This is often useful in the emergency department or during transport. Commercially available pelvic girdles serve the same purpose.

The military antishock garment (MASG) will act as a very effective pelvic splint. The MASG will stop venous bleeding by raising intra-abdominal pressure, but may also produce abdominal compartment syndrome. The MASG helps keep pelvic fractures reduced during transport.

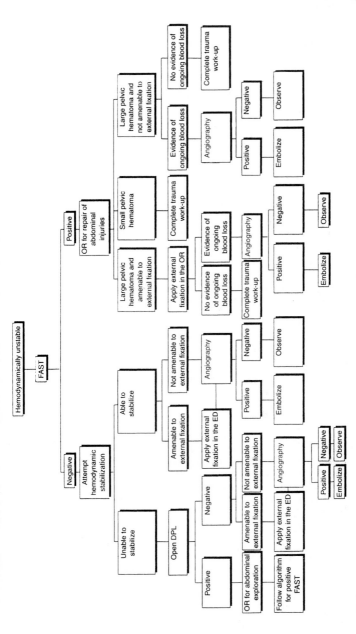

FIG. 32-2. Management algorithm for pelvic fractures in a hemodynamically unstable patient. DPL, diagnostic peritoneal lavage; FAST, focused abdominal sonography for trauma.

TABLE 32-2 Types of External Compression Devices

	Ease	Time	Fx reduction	Hemostasis
Bed sheet/pelvic girdle	+ +	Rapid	Inexact	+
C-clamp	− −	Substantial	Good posteriorly	+ +
Military antishock garment	+ +	Rapid	Inexact	+
External fixator	−	Indeterminate	Good	+ +

A variety of pelvic clamps have been designed to provide pelvic fracture stabilization. Pelvic clamps reduce and compress the posterior fragments of a pelvic fracture. While these clamps can be manipulated to facilitate CT scanning, angiography, or abdominal surgery, they have the disadvantage of potentially limiting visibility during those procedures.

An external fixator is perhaps most useful in patients with severe AP compression injuries. It can be applied quickly in some emergency departments, or it can be applied in the operating room simultaneously with laparotomy for intra-abdominal injury. External fixation is occasionally used as definitive therapy.

Selective Embolization

Angiography precisely defines bleeding sites and can be used as definitive therapy with transcatheter embolization of pelvic bleeding. Particulate Gelfoam® can be injected to produce vascular occlusion. Gelfoam is usually reabsorbed in several weeks. Stainless steel coils can be used to supplement Gelfoam in larger vessels. Multiple pelvic vascular injuries can be definitively treated by embolization of a number of Gelfoam particles or main hypogastric artery occlusion with a large stainless steel coil. The yield of angiography varies by indication (Table 32-3). With careful use, angiography should be positive 30 to 50 percent of the time.

Operative Hemostasis

Operative hemostasis is extremely difficult to accomplish with pelvic fractures. The hypogastric artery is quite short and quickly branches. Opening a pelvic hematoma risks the loss of tamponade of major venous injury, making it extremely difficult to visualize the bleeding vessels. The one circumstance amenable to operative exploration is the patient in shock with a badly displaced pelvic fracture and a unilaterally absent femoral pulse. Although rare, these patients have either common or external artery injury amenable to bypass grafting.

OPEN PELVIC FRACTURES

Open pelvic fractures can bleed not only into the pelvic retroperitoneum, but also externally. In addition, the risks of infection are significant. Principles for treatment are (1) control of hemorrhage; (2) debridement and management of concomitant soft tissue injuries; (3) recognition and treatment of associated injuries; and (4) treatment of the pelvic fracture itself. Patients with external blood loss are best treated initially with direct compression. Packing with laparotomy pads or towels can be augmented with temporary skin closure or manual pressure. More definitive hemostasis can be accomplished either by wound exploration in the operating room or with angiography and coil embolization. Laparotomy is occasionally beneficial.

TABLE 32-3 Indications for Angiography

>4 Units transfused for pelvic bleeding in <24 hours
>6 Units transfused for pelvic bleeding in <48 hours
Hemodynamic instability with a negative FAST and DPL
Large pelvic hematoma on CT
Pelvic pseudoaneurysm on helical CT
Large and/or expanding pelvic hematoma seen at the time of laparotomy

FAST, focused abdominal sonography for trauma; DPL, diagnostic peritoneal lavage.

Once hemostasis is secure, the soft tissue injury should be addressed (within the first 24 to 48 hours). A complete perineal evaluation including sigmoidoscopy and a pelvic examination is necessary. Any patient with significant perineal laceration adjacent to the rectum should undergo fecal diversion. Associated injuries such as ureteral injuries should be managed concurrently. Finally, definitive management of the pelvic fracture can be accomplished during the first several days.

ASSOCIATED INJURIES

Associated injuries are relatively common (Table 32-4). Prompt resuscitation is key in patients with traumatic brain injury (TBI) because hypotension may worsen neurologic outcome. Bleeding from long-bone fractures, when combined with pelvic bleeding, can produce voluminous hemorrhage. There is a strong association between blunt aortic injury and pelvic fractures, particularly AP compression and LC injuries. Genitourinary injuries are also common. They occur between 15 and 20 percent of the time. All patients with pelvic fractures should have lower urinary tract evaluation. Males should be imaged with retrograde urethrograms. All patients should have a cystogram.

OUTCOME

Mortality in pelvic fracture is relatively low (6 percent). Death occurs from bleeding (39 percent), TBI (31 percent), or organ failure (30 percent). Common complications include deep venous thrombosis (DVT) and pulmonary embolus. All patients with pelvic fractures should have DVT prophylaxis. Consideration should be given to caval interruption in high-risk patients.

TABLE 32-4 Associated Injuries

Closed head injury	51%
Long-bone fracture	48%
Peripheral nerve injury	26%
Thoracic injury	20%
Bladder injury	10%
Spleen injury	10%
Liver injury	7%
Gastrointestinal tract injury	7%
Kidney injury	7%
Urethral injury	6%
Mesentery injury	4%
Diaphragm injury	2%

ADDITIONAL READING

Mucha E, Farnell P: Analysis of pelvic fracture management. *J Trauma* 24:370, 1984.

Panetta T, Sclafani SJA, Goldstein AS, et al: Percutaneous transcatheter embolization for massive bleeding from pelvic fractures. *J Trauma* 25:1021, 1985.

Richardson JD, Harty J, Amin M, et al: Open pelvic fractures. *J Trauma* 22:533, 1982.

Salvino CK, Esposito TJ, Smith LD, et al: Routine pelvic x-ray studies in awake blunt trauma patients: a sensible policy? *J Trauma* 33:413, 1992.

Young JWR, Burgess AR, Brumback RJ, et al: Pelvic fractures: value of plain radiography in early assessment and management. *Radiology* 160:445, 1986.

33 | Urologic Trauma

INTRODUCTION

Traumatic injuries to the genitourinary tract represent about 10 percent of all injuries seen in the emergency department. Frequently, the urologist will be called to the ED for an emergent consult; the urgency of the patient's overall clinical condition will dictate how quickly a diagnosis must be made. As a first principle of management, careful examination of the urethral meatus for the presence of blood is essential before Foley placement, as this finding indicates urethral injury. A retrograde urethrogram must be performed to assess the extent of urethral injury prior to catheterization. The second urologic principle of management is to assess for renal injury in any major blunt or penetrating trauma to the upper abdomen, which can be accomplished with a double-dose (150 mL of renografin) IV bolus urogram performed on the trauma table if CT scan of the abdomen and pelvis cannot be performed because of hemodynamic instability. It is important that urologic consultation is obtained before laparotomy is performed.

RENAL INJURY

The kidney is the organ most commonly involved in genitourinary trauma. Microscopic or gross hematuria indicates injury to the urinary system. However, 10 to 25 percent of significant renal injuries will present without hematuria. The mechanism of renal injury can be penetrating trauma (20 percent) or blunt trauma (80 percent).

Radiographic Assessment in the Adult

Adults with gross hematuria or microhematuria and shock (systolic blood pressure <90 mm Hg) after blunt trauma should undergo urgent renal imaging if the patient's hemodynamic status improves (Fig. 33-1). Major renal injury is rarely seen in patients with microscopic hematuria and no shock after blunt trauma. However, patients with multisystem trauma from a major mechanism (e.g., deceleration injuries) should undergo urgent renal imaging to rule out renal injury or renal vascular injuries, even when there is no gross or microscopic hematuria. Patients with any degree of hematuria after penetrating trauma should undergo imaging only if hemodynamically stable, and nonoperative management is a possibility. If a retroperitoneal hematoma is discovered at laparotomy after penetrating trauma, it should be opened.

Whenever possible a double-dose intravenous pyelogram (IVP) or computed tomography (CT) scan of the abdomen and pelvis should be performed before taking the patient to surgery. In cases with radiographic evidence of unilateral renal nonfunction or vascular injury, renal arteriography is recommended.

Radiographic Assessment in Pediatric Renal Trauma

Children with more than 50 red blood cells per high-power field (RBC/hpf), gross hematuria, or evidence of multisystem trauma (regardless of the degree of hematuria) after blunt trauma should all undergo urgent renal imaging (Fig. 33-2). Hypotension is not a reliable indicator of renal injury in children. Most renal lacerations produce substantial hematuria. Conversely, major renal vascular injuries usually are associated with other organ injuries, but hematuria may be absent. Congenital anomalies (ureteropelvic junction

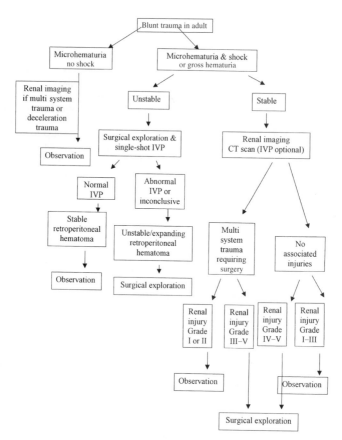

FIG. 33-1. Algorithm for treatment of renal trauma in the adult.

obstruction, hydronephrosis) must be suspected when the degree of hematuria is out of proportion to the severity of injury. Children with isolated insignificant microhematuria (<50 RBC/hpf on initial urinalysis and no evidence of substantial associated injuries) after blunt trauma have an extremely low incidence of renal injury (≤2%). Close outpatient follow-up to observe resolution of hematuria should be done, and delayed imaging should be performed when hematuria persists.

Principles of Management

Successful management of patients with renal trauma requires definition of the extent of injury and knowledge of the indications for exploration. In stable patients, CT provides detailed anatomic and functional information regarding the degree of renal injury with simultaneous delineation of associated abdominal injuries. In unstable patients (especially those requiring immediate surgical intervention for penetrating injuries), a properly performed intraoperative one-shot IVP (2 mL/kg bolus infusion of intravenous contrast and a single 10-

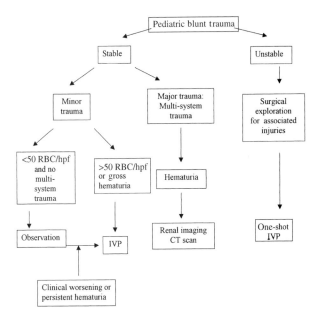

FIG. 33-2. Algorithm for treatment of renal trauma in pediatric patients.

minute film) provides important information that is useful for the genitourinary surgeon called upon to reconstruct or surgically remove the injured kidney. The classification system for renal injuries (based on CT findings) devised by the American Association for the Surgery of Trauma has proven extremely useful in standardizing the assessment and management of these patients (Table 33-1).

Indications for Surgery

In general, the decision to operate is determined by the clinical circumstances (hemodynamic stability), and guided by radiographic data. Most blunt trauma injuries do not require surgery, whereas most penetrating injuries do. This is the general rule: In cases of blunt injury, there should be compelling reasons to operate, whereas in cases of penetrating injury there should be compelling reasons *not* to operate. Minor injuries (grade I or II) do not require surgical management. Intraoperative consultation after blunt trauma to assess the significance of a retroperitoneal hematoma overlying the kidney is common. If preoperative studies have confirmed a minor injury to the kidney corresponding to the hematoma, exploration of the kidney is not necessary unless the hematoma is seen to be actively expanding. However, if it is found after a penetrating trauma, the hematoma generally should be explored, particularly if the injury is located medially, which may suggest injury to the great vessels, main renal vessels, renal pelves, ureter, or other organs.

In nonoperative cases, follow-up imaging studies should be obtained in the first 24 to 48 hours for grade III and IV renal lacerations to evaluate the size of hematoma, amount of extravasation, and to evaluate renal perfusion. Late

TABLE 33-1 Renal Injury Classification

Grade	Description of injury
I	Contusion: microscopic or gross hematuria with normal radiologic studies
II	Hematoma: subcapsular, nonexpanding, without parenchymal laceration
	Hematoma: nonexpanding perirenal, confined to retroperitoneum
III	Laceration <1 cm deep, without urinary extravasation
IV	Laceration >1 cm deep, without collecting system injury or urinary extravasation
	Laceration through renal cortex, medulla, collecting system
V	Vascular: main renal artery or vein injury, contained hemorrhage
	Laceration: shattered, destroyed kidney
	Vascular: renal artery and venous avulsion

complications may arise when injury is treated conservatively, and the urologist has to be aware of these problems to manage them properly.

URETERAL INJURY

Ureteral injuries from external trauma constitute approximately 1 percent of all genitourinary injuries. Most external ureteral injuries are from gunshot wounds that can cause significant damage from passage of the bullet near the ureter, even when the bullet does not transect the ureter.

Ureteral injury from blunt trauma is rare. It usually occurs in children and involves ureteral disruption at the level of the ureteropelvic junction (UPJ). This location is vulnerable to injury because the child's vertebral column is extremely flexible and the UPJ is relatively fixed. During rapid deceleration, excessive bending of the vertebral column causes the ureter to separate. This can occur bilaterally and is usually associated with significant spinal injuries.

Diagnosis of ureteral injury is based primarily on a high index of suspicion; there are no classic signs or symptoms. Hematuria is common, but may be absent in 20 to 30 percent of cases. Furthermore, severe ureteral contusion with delayed necrosis may not initially demonstrate urinary leakage. Any patient with penetrating abdominal trauma should be suspected of having a ureteral injury and should be appropriately evaluated. Similarly, children with significant blunt abdominal trauma who cannot be adequately examined because of associated injuries should undergo a radiographic evaluation, regardless of the findings on urinalysis. Frequently, a traumatic injury to the ureter is unrecognized at the time of presentation. Delayed manifestations arise from urinary leakage and include fever, flank pain, and fistula formation. Initial imaging can be obtained with a complete excretory urogram (2 mL contrast per kilogram body weight). This may demonstrate extravasation of contrast, delayed function, or mild ureteral dilation proximal to the injury. CT can also be used for the evaluation of ureteral injuries. Extravasation of contrast in the medial perirenal space is the most consistent finding; if complete ureteral transaction occurred, contrast will be absent in the distal ureter. If the results of the excretory urogram and CT scan are inconclusive, a retrograde ureterogram is indicated. Intraoperative recognition of injury may be facilitated by the intravenous or intraureteral injection of indigo carmine or methylene blue, although this may be unreliable if renal perfusion is decreased due to systemic hypotension or ipsilateral renal injury.

Selection of appropriate surgical management depends on the patient's condition, the site and extent of injury, and the time of diagnosis. At the time of laparotomy, the injured ureter is carefully inspected for evidence of contusion, discoloration, or lack of bleeding suggestive of ischemia. Ureteral injuries with a significant delay in diagnosis or in an unstable patient are best managed initially by percutaneous nephrostomy drainage. Once adequate healing has occurred and the acute inflammatory response has resolved, ureteral reconstruction can be performed.

General principles of ureteral reconstruction include careful debridement; creation of a tension-free, spatulated anastomosis; isolation of the anastomosis from associated injuries; and adequate ureteral and retroperitoneal drainage. Several reconstructive techniques can be used, depending on the site and grade of ureteral injury.

Radiographic evaluation (IVP or nuclear renal scan) should be obtained 6 weeks and 3 months postsurgery to assure proper healing.

BLADDER INJURY

The mechanism of injury may be either penetrating or blunt trauma, most commonly due to a motor vehicle crash, but occasionally from iatrogenic manipulation. Extraperitoneal bladder rupture is most commonly associated with pelvic fracture; approximately 85 percent of cases of blunt injury to the bladder occur in the presence of pelvic fracture, and roughly 10 to 15 percent of pelvic fractures are complicated by bladder or urethral injury. Typically, intraperitoneal bladder rupture results from lower abdominal impact in the presence of a full bladder. Combined intraperitoneal and extraperitoneal rupture may be seen in as many as 10 percent of patients. Iatrogenic bladder injury may commonly result from laparoscopic surgery (especially if adequate bladder drainage is not established), cystoscopic procedures, or intra-abdominal or vaginal surgery. Spontaneous bladder rupture may be seen when there is a history of known bladder pathology (i.e., neurogenic bladder dysfunction) or prior surgery (i.e., bladder augmentation).

The clinical presentation of a bladder injury depends on the mechanism of injury. The history and physical findings will provide information suggestive of bladder injury. The classic findings of suprapubic pain, hematuria, and inability to void are not always present. Diffuse abdominal pain or tenderness or signs of intra-abdominal or pelvic sepsis may occur, especially with delayed presentation. As in urethral trauma, the presence of blood at the urethral meatus should prompt radiographic urethral and subsequent bladder assessment. Hematuria is present in almost 100 percent of cases, with gross hematuria noted in >90 percent. In female patients, the presence of blood on urethral or vaginal examination should prompt careful bimanual pelvic and speculum examination, and occasionally cystoscopic assessment, to determine the precise anatomy of the injury.

Cystography should be performed only after urethral injury has been excluded. A plain abdominal and pelvic radiograph should be obtained before contrast material is instilled into the bladder through a urethral catheter under gravity drainage. In adults, the bladder should be filled with at least 350 mL of contrast medium, or until a bladder contraction is precipitated, and then a postvoid film should be taken. Failure to fill the bladder completely or to take a postvoid film will result in failure to diagnose approximately 20 percent of bladder injuries. In some centers a CT cystogram is performed, which yields excellent accuracy.

Extraperitoneal injuries that are limited in extent can be managed with urethral catheterization and bladder drainage alone. Intraperitoneal injuries require open repair and urinary diversion of the bladder. Lacerations should be closed from inside the bladder with 2-0 or 3-0 chromic suture. A suprapubic catheter should be left in place in most instances. Bladder healing usually is adequate for catheter removal by postoperative day 10 to 14. Healing should be confirmed by cystography before the catheter is removed.

URETHRAL TRAUMA

Most urethral injuries are secondary to blunt trauma, occur along the posterior urethra, and are associated with pelvic fractures or straddle-type injuries. Urethrography should be performed before catheter placement in any patient thought to have urethral injury. Absolute indications for urethrography include blood at the meatus, a perirenal hematoma or extensive laceration, and a high-riding prostate or large hematoma noted on rectal examination. Relative indications include a pelvic fracture, a palpable bladder, or a suprapubic hematoma.

The primary site of posterior urethral injury is the prostatomembranous junction. The prostate is sheared from the membranous urethra, which is anchored in the urogenital diaphragm. Patients present with blood at the meatus in >80 percent of cases and rectal examination may reveal a high pelvic prostate. A retrograde urethrogram will demonstrate pelvic extraperitoneal extravasation above and sometimes below the urogenital diaphragm. Management consists of suprapubic urinary diversion by open cystostomy with definitive repair in 3 to 6 months. Primary realignment may be attempted if it can be accomplished easily and without disturbing the pelvic hematoma. An associated bladder rupture occurs in 20 percent of cases and should be repaired primarily without delay. Complications include stricture, impotence, and incontinence.

Anterior urethral injuries are most often caused by a straddle fall or perineal trauma. Crushing of the bulbar urethra against the inferior margin of the symphysis pubis results in contusion or laceration. This type of injury accounts for <10 percent of all urethral injuries. Patients typically present with a bloody urethral discharge and a perineal bruise (butterfly hematoma). A retrograde urethrogram may demonstrate extravasation below the urogenital diaphragm. Management requires suprapubic drainage for 1 to 3 weeks if extravasation is noted. The catheter may be removed in 1 week if a voiding cystourethrogram (VCUG) is normal. Occasionally, an extensive perineal hematoma with urinary extravasation will require primary surgical drainage. Stricture is the most common complication.

BLUNT SCROTAL TRAUMA

Kicks and straddle injuries are the leading causes of blunt scrotal trauma, which can cause testicular rupture, hematocele, scrotal hematoma, or intratesticular hematoma. Usually, the scrotum is enlarged and painful, making clinical assessment difficult. It is important to rule out testicular torsion or epididymitis. The introduction of scrotal ultrasonography has provided an invaluable tool for the evaluation of scrotal trauma and has decreased the rate of orchiectomy, which was once as high as 45 percent. Sonographic signs of rupture include loss of the normal homogeneous echo pattern and areas of irregular hyper- or hypoechogenicity. Early aggressive imaging and surgical exploration have markedly improved the testicular salvage rate.

Hematoceles and large scrotal hematomas should be drained and complete hemostasis obtained. Testicular rupture should be managed with surgical debridement of extruded, nonviable tubules and evacuation of the hematoma. After careful hemostasis, the tunica albuginea should be closed with a running suture of 3-0 or 4-0 chromic catgut. Intratesticular hematoma should be evacuated with limited debridement of tubular parenchyma.

PENETRATING SCROTAL TRAUMA

Surgical exploration should be performed with identification of the scrotal contents and its layers. Debridement of necrotic, devitalized tissue and seminiferous tubules and primary closure of the tunica with absorbable sutures should be performed. Penrose drain placement after profuse irrigation of the wound is recommended. Finally, management of scrotal lacerations must be guided by a thorough knowledge of the tissue layers involved.

PENILE INJURIES

Penile injuries are usually the result of penetrating trauma from bullets or stab wounds, and strangulation injury from constricting rings. Fracture of the corpora cavernosa can occur from blunt trauma during a state of tumescence. The extent of injury is often readily apparent from physical examination. If Buck's fascia is intact, the hematoma will be confined to the penis, whereas disruption of Buck's fascia will allow spread of the hematoma under Colles' and Scarpa's fascia onto the perineum and abdominal wall, respectively. A retrograde urethrogram and corpus cavernosography may be necessary to localize the injury.

Penile fracture is a traumatic rupture of the corpus cavernosum that occurs most frequently during coitus, masturbation, and in other circumstances that involve an abnormally forced bending of the erect penis. A tear is produced in the tunica albuginea, usually with a transverse orientation. This lesion is usually unilateral, and there is urethral involvement in 20 percent of cases. Characteristically, the patient hears a popping or cracking sound, followed by pain and detumescence. Hematoma and deviation of the shaft to the side opposite of the injury are prominent physical findings. Associated injury to the urethra is evidenced by retention of urine, blood at the meatus, or gross hematuria. A standard retrograde urethrogram should be performed when urethral injury is suspected. The location of the hematoma, focal tenderness, and palpation of a defect can reveal the rupture site. Cavernosography, ultrasound, and magnetic resonance imaging have been used with varying levels of success.

The treatment is surgery, which involves a degloving distal circumferential incision of the penis with evacuation of hematoma and limited debridement inside the corpora to avoid unnecessary injury to the erectile sinusoids. The defect is closed with a running or interrupted watertight suture using absorbable material, such as 3-0 or 4-0 polydiaxone. Urethral injuries are best managed by immediate primary repair over a urethral catheter.

Genital Bite Injuries

Human and animal bites are considered heavily contaminated wounds and have a high potential for infection. Animal bites can transmit rabies, and human bites can transmit syphilis, hepatitis B and C, human immunodeficiency virus (HIV), tetanus, tuberculosis, actinomycosis, and herpes simplex. Human genital bites are usually related to orogenital sexual practices and most are superficial self-treated injuries. Patients seldom seek medical assistance unless complications arise. Animal bites are usually the result of accidents with domestic animals.

Management includes administration of tetanus toxoid, and profuse wound cleansing and irrigation. If the patient is in a high-risk group (e.g., diabetes, HIV, immunosuppressed, or debilitated patient) or complication (infection or necrosis) is present, the patient should be hospitalized and antibiotic treatment and wound management should be initiated. Debridement of all infected or necrotic tissue is pivotal, as is wound culture and broad-spectrum intravenous antibiotics. Primary closure of the wound is formally contraindicated. The subsequent course of the infectious process will dictate the need for repeated debridement or antibiotic changes. In the case of recent noninfected wounds, empiric outpatient antibiotic treatment is recommended.

Burn Injury

Burn injury to the genitalia requires careful monitoring because the extent of injury is often greater than is initially apparent. Management consists of debridement of devitalized tissue and topical therapy with silver sulfadiazine. A Foley catheter or suprapubic catheter should be placed in extensively burned patients.

ADDITIONAL READING

Dixon CM, McAninch JW: Traumatic Renal Injuries. Part I and 11. American Urological Association Update Vol. X, no. 35 and 36.

McAninch JW: *Traumatic and Reconstructive Urology.* Philadelphia, W.B. Saunders, 1996.

Moore EE, Cogbill TH, Jurkovich GJ, et al: Organ injury scaling III: Chest wall, abdominal vascular, ureter, bladder, and urethra. *J Trauma* 33: 337, 1992.

Moore EE, Shackford SR, Pachter HL, et al: Organ injury scaling: Spleen, liver, and kidney. *J Trauma* 29:1664, 1989.

Sagalowsky AI, Peters PC: Genitourinary trauma, in Walsh PC, Retik AP, Vaughan ED, et al (eds): *Campbell's Urology,* 7th ed. Philadelphia, W.B. Saunders, 1998.

34 | Reproductive System Trauma

As maternal deaths resulting directly from pregnancy or the complications of labor and delivery have declined sharply in recent years, trauma now accounts for an estimated 50 percent of maternal deaths. Current data suggest that 6 to 7 percent of pregnancies are complicated by trauma and 0.4 percent of all pregnant patients require hospitalization for the treatment of injuries. However, the true number of injured gravid women is most likely underestimated by these figures, as many injuries are unreported, especially those resulting from domestic violence. Thus it is essential that all trauma care professionals recognize the anatomic and physiologic changes unique to pregnancy to aid in the treatment of the injured gravid patient. Complete evaluation of these patients includes an assessment of the fetus, and the treating physician must not only be cognizant of the signs of fetal distress, but must also be able to make rapid interventions in the interest of salvaging the pregnancy. Additionally, recognition and prompt treatment of pelvic trauma in the nongravid patient will optimize preservation of her sexual and reproductive function.

ANATOMIC AND PHYSIOLOGIC CHANGES UNIQUE TO PREGNANCY

Although the initial assessment and management priorities for resuscitation of the injured pregnant patient are the same as those for other traumatized patients, the specific anatomic and physiologic changes that occur during pregnancy may alter the response to injury, and necessitate a modified approach to the resuscitation process. An understanding of these adaptations (summarized in Table 34-1) is necessary in order to provide appropriate and timely care to both mother and unborn child. Changes in the cardiovascular system can be characterized by blood volume expansion (beginning at 10 weeks' gestation, and peaking at an increase of 45 percent over pregravid levels by term), accompanied by a relatively smaller increase in red blood cell mass. This pregnancy-induced hypervolemia may create a false sense of security for the resuscitating physician because almost 35 percent of maternal blood volume may be lost before signs of maternal shock appear. Clotting factors and fibrinogen also increase, with a corresponding decrease in fibrinolytic activity, creating a hypercoagulable state that is most pronounced near term, when thromboembolic events are most likely to occur. Maternal pulse rate is normally increased by 10 to 15 beats/min during pregnancy, while blood pressure decreases. Cardiac output increases to 25 percent above normal during the first trimester and may reach values as high as 6 L/min at term.

Several changes in the maternal respiratory system occur during pregnancy to meet increased oxygen requirements, including progressive increases in tidal volume and minute ventilation, while the functional residual capacity (FRC) decreases. This results in a normal PAO_2 but a reduced PCO_2, creating a state of respiratory alkalosis that is only partially compensated for by the kidney. Renal blood flow increases by 30 percent during gestation, and both blood urea nitrogen (BUN) and serum creatinine are reduced. Hydronephrosis and hydroureter may result from uterine compression of the ureters and bladder. By the end of full-term gestation, the weight of the uterus has increased to 20 times its prepregnancy weight and uterine blood flow approaches 500 mL/min. Uterine veins may dilate up to 60 times their size to accommodate the uteroplacental blood flow. This increased vascularity carries an attendant risk of massive blood loss with pelvic injury.

TABLE 34-1 Physiologic Alterations in Pregnancy

System	Change	Potential Implication
Cardiovascular	↓ Peripheral vascular resistance, ↓ venous return, ↓ blood pressure (10–15 mm Hg)	Supine hypotensive syndrome
Blood volume	↑ Plasma volume, ↓ RBC volume, ↑ WBC (20,000 WBC/mm³)	Physiologic hypervolemia may mask hypotension secondary to blood loss
Coagulation	Hypercoagulable; ↑ fibrinogen; ↑ factors VII, VIII, IX, X, XII; ↓ fibrinolysis	↑ Venous thromboembolism
Respiratory	↑ Subcostal angle (68–103 degrees), ↑ chest circumference (5–7cm), ↑ diaphragmatic excursion (1–2 cm), elevated diaphragm, ↑ tidal volume, ↑ minute ventilation, ↓ FRC, ↓ P_{CO_2}, HCO_3^-	Alteration in FRC and lung volume, chronic compensated respiratory alkalosis
Gastrointestinal	↑ Motility, ↓ Intestinal secretion, ↓ nutrient absorption, ↓ sphincter competency (progesterone) Organ displacement	Aspiration
Hepatobiliary	↑ Gallbladder volume, ↓ gallbladder emptying, ↓ albumin, ↑↑ AP, ↑ ALT, ↓↓ bilirubin (free), ↓ GGT	Clinical examination unreliable ↑ Cholestasis, ↑ cholesterol saturation, ↑ chenodeoxycholic acid, ↑ gallstones
Renal	↑ Glomerular filtration rate, ↑ renal plasma flow, ↑ creatinine clearance, ↓ serum creatinine, BUN Dilation of collecting system ↓ Bladder/urethral muscle tone	Hydronephrosis, hydroureter
Endocrine	↑ Parathormone, ↑ calcitonin	↑ Calcium absorption
Musculoskeletal	Pelvic ligaments soften (relaxin, progesterone)	Pelvic widening, lordosis, shift in center of gravity

ALT, alanine aminotransferase; AP, alkaline phosphatase; BUN, blood urea nitrogen; FRC, functional residual capacity; GGT, gamma-glutamyl transferase.

ASSESSMENT OF THE INJURED PREGNANT PATIENT

Initial Assessment and Management: Primary Survey

The priorities for treatment of an injured pregnant patient are the same as those for the nonpregnant patient. Ensuring an adequate airway and supplying supplemental oxygen are essential for preventing maternal and fetal hypoxia (Fig. 34-1). Because the oxyhemoglobin dissociation curve for fetal blood is steep, small increments in maternal oxygen concentration improve the blood oxygen content for the fetus, even though the maternal arterial oxygen content may not change appreciably. In the supine position, the pregnant patient

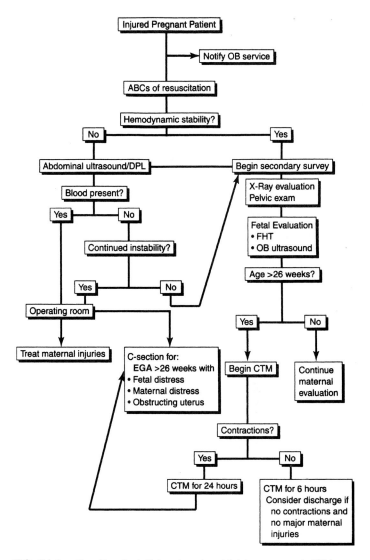

FIG. 34-1. Algorithm for initial maternal and fetal assessment. CTM, cardiotocographic monitoring; DPL, diagnostic peritoneal lavage; EGA, estimated gestational age; FHT, fetal heart tones.

may become hypotensive from the pressure of her enlarged uterus, which causes aortocaval compression. Prevention of this supine hypotensive syndrome is accomplished by placing the patient in the left lateral decubitus position, or by tilting the backboard to the left. Because physiologic hypervolemia is to be anticipated during pregnancy, the signs of shock may be delayed.

Thus vigorous crystalloid resuscitation is encouraged, even for patients who appear normotensive.

Secondary Survey: Maternal Assessment

Following the primary survey of the mother and performance of any life-saving measures, the secondary survey is initiated. This consists of obtaining a thorough history, including an obstetric history, performing a physical examination in search of all injuries, and evaluating and monitoring the fetus. The obstetric history includes the date of the last menstrual period, expected date of delivery, and date of the first perception of fetal movement, as well as any problems or complications of the current and previous pregnancies. Measurement of fundal height is a rapid method for estimating fetal age. As an easy point of reference, if the most superior part of the uterine fundus is palpated at the umbilicus, the fetal age is estimated to be 20 weeks. A discrepancy between dates and uterine size may result from a ruptured uterus or intrauterine hemorrhage. Determination of fetal age and maturity is an important factor in the decision about whether early delivery is indicated (see below). Pelvic and rectal examinations should be performed, with special attention to vaginal discharge, dilation, and fetal station. The presence of an obstetrician as part of the trauma team is strongly encouraged, particularly during the pelvic exam in late pregnancy. The presence of any of the following conditions indicates an acute status of pregnancy:

- Vaginal bleeding
- Ruptured membranes (amniotic sac)
- Bulging perineum
- Presence of contractions
- Abnormal fetal heart rate or rhythm

Fetal Assessment

Unfortunately, direct assessment of the fetus following trauma is somewhat limited. Currently, the most valuable information regarding fetal viability can be obtained by a combination of fetal heart rate (FHR) monitoring and ultrasound (US) imaging. Fetal heart tones can be detected with Doppler ultrasound by the 12th week of pregnancy. The normal FHR is between 120 and 160 beats/min. Because the fetal stroke volume is fixed, the initial response to the stress of hypoxia or hypotension is tachycardia. Severe hypoxia in the fetus, however, is associated with bradycardia (FHR <120 beats/min) and should be recognized as fetal distress, demanding immediate attention. Initial FHR monitoring of all pregnant patients with potentially viable pregnancies (i.e., those >26 weeks gestation) is indicated following even relatively minor abdominal trauma. This is best accomplished using cardiotocographic monitoring (CTM) devices that record both uterine contractions and FHR.

Blunt trauma to the abdomen can result in uterine rupture, but this event is uncommon, unlikely to be missed, and is usually rapidly fatal to the fetus. A much more common event is placental separation from the uterus as a result of the shearing forces following blunt injury. Major cases of placental abruption (i.e., >50 percent separation) are uniformly fatal to the fetus, but more minor cases may initially go undetected. CTM will detect early fetal distress, often manifested as a decelerated heart rate associated with uterine contraction. Most cases of placental abruption become evident within several hours of trauma. A minimum of 24 hours of CTM is recommended for patients with frequent uterine contractions ($\geq$6/min), abdominal or uterine tenderness, vaginal bleeding, or hypotension following injury. In the absence of these symptoms, at least 6 hours of CTM should be performed before considering discharging a patient after trauma.

High-resolution, real-time US has proven valuable for the assessment of fetal age and well-being. In the trauma setting, US is used primarily to identify acute problems that may be due to maternal events such as placental abruption, placenta previa, or cord prolapse. Additionally, it is routine to evaluate the fetus for gestational age, cardiac activity, and movement. Biophysical profile scoring rates fetal breathing movements, gross body movements, body tone, reactive heart rate, and amniotic fluid volume. An additional benefit of US is the ability to detect maternal injuries associated with pericardial, pleural, or peritoneal fluid seen on the focused abdominal sonography for trauma (FAST) examination.

Diagnostic Modalities

Following the secondary survey and the initial assessment of the fetus, appropriate diagnostic studies should be utilized to fully evaluate the extent of maternal injuries. Although there is much concern about radiation exposure during pregnancy, a diagnostic modality deemed necessary for maternal evaluation should not be withheld on the basis of its potential hazard to the fetus. There are three phases of recognized radiation damage during pregnancy, which relate to the gestational age of the fetus: fetal death (less than 3 weeks gestational age); organ damage (3 to 16 weeks); and neurologic damage or cancer (>16 weeks). It is generally accepted that x-ray exposure below 10 rads is safe for the human embryo or fetus. A direct-beam film of the abdomen or pelvis incurs a dose of 1 rad to the uterus, whereas an indirect beam (i.e., chest x-ray) incurs a dose of only 0.1 rad. The estimated absorbed dosage of radiation from abdominal CT scanning is 0.2 rad, provided that the windows are wide and not overlapped. Thus necessary radiographic examinations in the injured pregnant patient should be performed according to the following guidelines:

- Order the minimum number of films to obtain maximum information
- Shield the abdomen with a lead apron
- Use a radiation badge (dosimeter) when the patient will require many radiographs over a prolonged period of time.

Abdominal Evaluation

Evaluation of the abdomen following trauma is difficult and may be particularly challenging in the gravid patient. Because of the lack of sensitivity of physical findings, objective evaluation should be considered in patients with rib or pelvic fractures, unexplained hypotension, blood loss or base deficit, in patients with hematuria, and in patients with altered sensorium secondary to drugs, alcohol, or concomitant head injury. As mentioned above, abdominal CT scanning can be safely performed in the pregnant patient and is capable of not only detecting blood loss and its source, but can also evaluate the fetus for injuries. In unstable patients or in patients without other indications for CT scanning, the FAST ultrasound exam can be performed rapidly and repeatedly to detect abdominal fluid following trauma during pregnancy.

MANAGEMENT OF ABDOMINAL INJURIES IN PREGNANCY

Once diagnosed, the management of abdominal injuries during pregnancy differs little from the nonpregnant state. Nonoperative management of solid organ injuries has been performed successfully in the gravid state and should be considered the treatment of choice for stable patients with these injuries, thus avoiding the potential teratogenic complications of general anesthetics. On the other hand, *unstable* patients or those in whom an intestinal injury is suspected benefit from early operative treatment, as both hypotension and intra-abdominal infection can be harmful and potentially lethal to the fetus. As with any other emergency laparotomy during pregnancy, the uterus should be left intact, unless it is directly injured or it presents a mechanical limitation for treatment of maternal injuries. The management of pelvic fractures following blunt trauma may be particularly challenging during late pregnancy. Hemorrhage from massively dilated retroperitoneal vessels can rapidly cause shock. In fact, pelvic fracture is the most common injury to the mother that results in fetal death, with a fetal mortality rate as high as 25 percent. Although management of hemorrhage may include pelvic angiography and embolization of bleeding vessels, the dose of radiation associated with this approach usually exceeds the threshold considered safe during pregnancy, and these patients should be appropriately counseled.

The fetus is generally well protected from blunt forces by the pelvic bones and surrounding amniotic fluid. Occasionally, blunt trauma to the fetal-placental unit may result in fractures of the fetal skull or extremities. Severe blunt trauma occasionally causes rupture of the uterus. Manifestations of uterine rupture include severe maternal shock, a uterus small for dates, and the presence of fetal parts outside of the uterus. More commonly, however, blunt abdominal trauma cases separation of the placenta from the relatively inelastic uterine wall (placental abruption). While minor placental abruptions may be tolerated by the fetus, major abruptions are the most common cause of fetal death if the mother survives. The manifestations of placental abruption include vaginal bleeding, abdominal tenderness, and contractions. CTM is the most useful method of detecting clinically silent cases of placental separation that result in fetal distress.

In cases of penetrating trauma caused by stab wounds, these injuries rarely penetrate the thick uterine wall and usually present little risk to either the mother or her unborn child. Death of the mother after abdominal gunshot wounds is similarly uncommon, as only 20 to 30 percent have injuries outside the uterus. In contrast, gunshot wounds to the upper abdomen can result in severe maternal damage, as the abdominal organs and vasculature are compressed into this small space. Up to 70 percent of fetuses will sustain injuries following abdominal gunshot wounds and 40 to 65 percent will die. If the bullet has penetrated the uterus and the fetus is both viable and alive, cesarean section should be performed and the baby's injuries addressed surgically, if indicated.

Cesarean Section Following Injury

The American College of Obstetricians and Gynecologists developed guidelines for performing cesarean section for the mother in extremis following a medical disaster (i.e., amniotic fluid embolism, major cardiac event). These guidelines recommend cesarean section for fetuses who are ≥26 weeks gestation and who can be delivered within 5 to 10 minutes of maternal death.

Recommendations for the performance of a cesarean section following trauma are included in Fig. 34-1, and include fetal or maternal distress detected either in the operating room or during CTM monitoring.

Outcomes Following Trauma and Pregnancy

The injured pregnant mother may present considerable challenges while being treated in the intensive care unit. While a full discussion of critical care obstetrics is beyond the scope of this chapter, Table 34-2 outlines the salient points. A poor fetal outcome has generally been associated with the presence of direct uteroplacental fetal injury, maternal shock, pelvic fracture, hypoxia, or the presence of severe maternal head injury.

Trauma in the Nonpregnant Patient

The female reproductive organs are usually well protected by their location deep within the pelvis, making injuries relatively uncommon except during pregnancy or when they are pathologically enlarged. Occasionally, severe blunt trauma resulting from a motor vehicle crash may result in injuries to the female genital system, usually associated with pelvic fractures. In young girls, perineal injuries generally occur during sports activities such as gymnastics or in falls. Missed or improperly treated female genital injuries can result in hemorrhage, sepsis, and the loss of endocrine and reproductive function. Any suspicion of perineal or pelvic injury should prompt a thorough examination, which may require anesthesia. This evaluation must include the rectum and urinary tract as well. Management of perineal injuries is usually straightforward and includes debridement and primary closure. Similarly, vaginal

TABLE 34-2 Critical Care Obstetrics

Condition	Manifestations	Treatment
Pregnancy-induced hypertension	BP ≥160 mm Hg systolic BP ≥110 mm Hg diastolic Pulmonary edema Oliguria Cerebral dysfunction	Delivery if possible Magnesium sulfate Hydralazine
Amniotic fluid embolism	Dyspnea Hypotension Cardiorespiratory arrest Disseminated intravascular coagulation	Oxygenation Maintain cardiac output Support blood pressure Correct coagulopathy

Premature labor	Uterine contractions
	Cervical effacement
		Rule out abruption
		Tocolytic drugs:
		    terbutaline,
		    indomethacin,
		    calcium channel
		    blockers

Thromboembolism	Leg swelling Shortness of breath Cardiovascular collapse Sudden death	Heparin Mechanical devices Duplex scanning Cardiovascular support Removable vena cava filter?

injuries can usually be closed primarily. The most devastating perineal injuries are those associated with an open pelvic fracture, and require prompt control of hemorrhage, pelvic stabilization, multiple debridements, and often a diverting colostomy.

Injury Prevention

Three areas of injury prevention deserve specific attention during pregnancy:

- Substance abuse (drugs or alcohol)
- Interpersonal and domestic violence
- Proper use of seat belts

Every obstetrician should be trained to provide counseling in these three areas as part of prenatal care. In addition, emergency care providers need training in the recognition of domestic abuse, which can grow in severity if the cycle is not interrupted.

Prevention of perineal and pelvic injuries in the nongravid state must include pedestrian safety programs, education in child restraint devices for all parents, and redesigning sporting equipment with safety in mind. Prevention of secondary complications following the initial injury must include an organized team of trauma professionals, including trauma surgeons, orthopedic surgeons, urologists, gynecologists, and pediatricians.

ADDITIONAL READING

Kissinger DP, Rozycki GS, Morris JA Jr, et al: Trauma in pregnancy: predicting pregnancy outcome. *Arch Surg* 126:1079, 1991.

Laverly JP, State-McCormick M: Management of moderate to severe trauma in pregnancy. *Obstet Gynecol Clin North Am* 22:69, 1995.

McFarlane J, Parker B, Soeken K, et al: Assessing for abuse during pregnancy: severity and frequency of injuries and associated entry into prenatal care. *JAMA* 267:3176, 1992.

Morris JA, Rosenbower TJ, Jurkovich GJ, et al: Infant survival after cesarean section for trauma. *Ann Surg* 223:481, 1996.

Neufield JDG, Moore EE, Marx JA, et al: Trauma in pregnancy. *Emerg Clin North Am* 5:623, 1987.

Towery R, English TP, Wisner D: Evaluation of pregnant women after blunt injury. *J Trauma* 35:731, 1993.

35 | Trauma Damage Control

This chapter will describe the techniques used during "damage control" operations (as named by Rotondo and colleagues); the sequelae of an abdominal compartment syndrome; the alternate techniques for closure of a thoracic, abdominal, or extremity incision in patients with major trauma; care of the patient in the surgical intensive care unit (SICU) after a damage control operation; the approach to reoperation; and late repair of incisional hernias when the abdomen has been left open at a reoperation.

DAMAGE CONTROL OPERATIONS

Definition

Damage control operations are performed in injured patients with profound hemorrhagic shock and preoperative or intraoperative metabolic sequelae that are known to adversely affect survival. The widely accepted three stages of damage control are described as follows:

1. Limited operation for control of hemorrhage and contamination.
2. Resuscitation in the SICU.
3. Reoperation.

Intraoperative Indications to Perform Damage Control Operations

The primary indication to modify the conduct of an operation for major trauma to the chest, abdomen, or an extremity is unresolved metabolic failure despite control of hemorrhage by suture, resection, or packing. Metabolic failure is characterized by severe hypothermia despite warming maneuvers initiated in the emergency department and continuing in the operating room, persistent acidemia despite vigorous resuscitation and control of hemorrhage, and a coagulopathy (nonmechanical bleeding) not amenable to operative control (Table 35-1). *Patients are more likely to die from their intraoperative metabolic failure than from the failure to complete organ repairs.* Most have received transfusion of 1 to 2 blood volumes and are expected to have a survival of less than 50 percent when severe injuries are present.

Hypothermia

There are many causes of hypothermia in victims of major trauma. Hypovolemic shock in the preoperative period adversely affects oxygen delivery and leads to decreases in oxygen consumption and, therefore, production of heat. Should the patient be intoxicated at the time of injury, vasodilatation will further compromise the ability to produce heat. The trauma team itself may be responsible for accelerating the loss of heat from a victim in shock. Undressing the patient in a cool resuscitation room, failing to cover the patient's head with a turban and the trunk and extremities with warm blankets or the Bair Hugger Patient Warming System (Augustine Medical, Inc., Eden Prairie, MN) during resuscitation, and infusion of unheated crystalloids and packed red blood cells are all sources of heat loss in the emergency department. Paralyzing the patient, which prevents shivering, and administering anesthetic agents, which prevents vasoconstriction; failing to cover areas of the body not undergoing operation; opening one or more body cavities in a cold operating room; and irrigating body cavities with unheated crystalloid solutions are further sources of heat loss during a thoracotomy or laparotomy.

TABLE 35-1 Intraoperative Indications to Perform Damage Control Operations

Factor	Level
1. Initial body temperature	<35°C
2. Initial acid-base status	
• Arterial pH	<7.2
• Base deficit	<−15 mmol/L in patient <55 years of age or <−6 mmol/L in patient >55 years of age
• Serum lactate	>5 mmol/L
3. Onset of coagulopathy	Prothrombin time and/or partial thromboplastin time >50% of normal

Source: Modified from Brasel KJ, Ku J, Baker CC, Rutherford EJ: *New Horizons* 7:73, 1999.

The effect of hypothermia on mortality in severely injured patients is no longer controversial. If the patient's last body temperature in the operating room was less than 35°C in Cushman's review, the risk of death was nearly 40 times greater than for patients with a body temperature greater than 35°C. It would appear logical, therefore, to practice damage control and rapidly complete any trauma operation in which the patient's initial body temperature is less than 34 to 35°C or the temperature decreases below this level at any time during operation.

Acidemia

Prolonged hypovolemic shock often produces a state of persistent metabolic acidosis in the patient with major trauma. This leads to a "circle" phenomenon in which secondary decreases in cardiac output and hypotension, and an increased susceptibility to ventricular arrhythmias may be irreversible, despite adequate volume replacement. Also, acidosis may cause the uncoupling of beta-adrenergic receptors, with a secondary decrease in the patient's response to endogenous and exogenous catecholamines. While acidosis by itself is an unusual reason to terminate a laparotomy being performed for trauma, it often accompanies hypothermia and a coagulopathy. A persistent metabolic acidosis is a manifestation of anaerobic metabolism occurring during hypoperfusion.

Coagulopathy

Nonmechanical bleeding is common during emergency trauma thoraco- tomies, laparotomies, or operative procedures in patients with exsanguination from an injury to an extremity. Fresh whole warm blood is not available at the time of resuscitation, and replacement of volume losses with large amounts of crystalloid solutions and cold packed red blood cells leads to clotting abnor- malities secondary to dilution, deficiency of clotting factors, and hypother- mia. In particular, hypothermia has an adverse effect on enzymes associated with the coagulation cascade and on the function of platelets. In the major trauma patient who develops a coagulopathy characterized by a prothrombin time or partial thromboplastin time 50 percent greater than normal during a thoracotomy or laparotomy after major sources of hemorrhage have been con- trolled, damage control would include the techniques to be described.

Operative Techniques in Thoracic Trauma

Lung

Exsanguinating hemorrhage from the lung is most rapidly controlled by the application of a DeBakey aortic clamp to the hilum in the emergency department or operating room. When the site of blood loss has been a stab wound deep into the pulmonary parenchyma or a gunshot wound completely through a lobe, the technique of pulmonotomy (sometimes called non-neurosurgical "tractotomy") is used. Pulmonotomy refers to the division of pulmonary parenchyma using a linear stapling/cutting device to expose injured parenchymal vessels. After selective ligation of these, the pulmonary parenchyma is closed in the usual fashion using a continuous 2-0 absorbable suture, with staple line reinforcement material added, as needed.

Heart

Other than compression with a finger, the quickest way to control hemorrhage from a small wound or rupture of a ventricle in the emergency department or operating room is to apply 6-mm-wide skin staples (Auto Suture 35 W, United States Surgical Corporation, Norwalk, CT). Formal cardiac repair with Teflon pledgets may then be accomplished over the staples or as they are sequentially removed in the operating room.

Larger wounds or ruptures of a ventricle in patients surviving by virtue of tamponade may be controlled by the insertion of a Foley balloon catheter into the hole. With the balloon inflated and traction applied to the catheter, Teflon-pledgeted sutures can then be passed through the ventricle from side to side over the balloon. With a longitudinal perforation or rupture of a ventricle, the time-honored technique of inflow occlusion is useful in avoiding cardiopulmonary bypass.

Operative Techniques in Abdominal Trauma

Liver

The liver has a blood supply of 1500 mL/min and is the major site of synthesis of all the coagulation factors except factor VIII. Indirect control of hepatic hemorrhage may be accomplished by *extensive hepatorrhaphy,* using a continuous suture or interrupted vertical mattress sutures of absorbable material. While this technique is used much less frequently than in the past, it is appropriate for a damage control operation.

Damage control techniques in which the sources of hepatic hemorrhage are approached directly include hepatotomy with selective vascular ligation, resectional debridement with selective vascular ligation, or rapid resectional debridement. Damage control techniques in which compression or tamponade rather than a suture or metal clip is used to control hepatic hemorrhage include balloon catheter tamponade, absorbable mesh tamponade, and perihepatic packing. The insertion of perihepatic packs mandates a reoperation and remains one of the classical indications for use of the alternate closures of the midline incision to be described.

Spleen

With American Association for the Surgery of Trauma (AAST) grade III, IV, or V injuries, splenectomy remains the safest choice when damage control is necessary. Should an AAST grade I or II injury be present, rapid mobilization and direct suture may be faster than splenectomy and will avoid the creation of a denuded retroperitoneal area in the patient with a coagulopathy. With rupture of the capsule, a topical agent such as microfibrillar collagen (Avitene, MedChem Products, Inc., Woburn, MA) or fibrin glue is applied to the parenchyma. If the condition of the patient does not permit the time needed to suture absorbable mesh as a replacement capsule, a mesh sheet is compressed against the parenchyma with a laparotomy pad pack.

Gastrointestinal Tract

Near transections of the duodenum are stapled shut, while an associated injury to the head of the pancreas is packed. At the reoperation, duodenal continuity can be restored with an end-to-end anastomosis. A pyloric exclusion with polypropylene suture and an antecolic gastrojejunostomy are added in selected patients with severe duodenal contusion or narrowing or a combined pancreaticoduodenal injury.

In the patient with a limited number of enterotomies or colotomies from a penetrating wound, a rapid one-layer, full-thickness closure using a continuous suture of 3-0 or 4-0 polypropylene material is appropriate. Multiple large perforations within a short segment of the small bowel or colon are treated with segmental resection, using metallic clips for mesenteric hemostasis and staples to transect the bowel. In the unstable patient, neither an end-to-end anastomosis nor the maturation of a colostomy is performed until the reoperation in 12 to 72 hours. With shotgun wounds and multiple partial and full-thickness perforations of the jejunum, a jejunectomy is appropriate as all of its absorptive capabilities are duplicated by the ileum.

Pancreas

Parenchymal defects not involving the duct are either ignored at the damage control procedure or filled with omentum held in place by a tacking suture. The insertion of a closed suction drain is delayed until the reoperation. Ductal transections to the left of the mesenteric vessels that do not involve the splenic vessels are packed or drained, with the distal pancreatectomy and splenectomy once again delayed until the reoperation. Major parenchymal or ductal injuries in the head or neck of the pancreas are also packed or drained, once hemorrhage from the gland or underlying mesenteric–portal vessels is controlled. A needed pancreatoduodenectomy or reconstruction after a pancreatoduodenectomy caused by the original injury is obviously delayed until the reoperation, as well.

Abdominal Arteries

In any patient with multiple upper abdominal visceral and vascular injuries, a significant injury to the celiac axis is treated with ligation. An injury to the renal artery is also best treated with ligation and nephrectomy in the presence of a palpably normal contralateral kidney and multiple associated injuries. The superior mesenteric artery or common or external iliac artery is smaller in young trauma patients, and an intraluminal Argyle, Javid, or Pruitt–Inahara shunt may be rapidly inserted under proximal and distal ties to avoid the need for ligation or interposition grafting.

When life-threatening arterial hemorrhage from either a blunt pelvic fracture or a penetrating wound occurs in the deep pelvis and cannot be controlled by packing, several innovative approaches are available. The first is to insert a Fogarty balloon catheter into the internal iliac artery beyond a proximal tie on the side of the hemorrhage. The other option is for the surgical team to inject a slurry of autologous clot and various coagulation factors into the distal internal iliac artery beyond a proximal ligature.

Abdominal Veins

Ligation is the treatment of choice whenever there is a significant injury to the common or external iliac veins, infrarenal inferior vena cava, superior mesenteric vein, or portal vein in a patient with profound shock. After ligation of the infrarenal inferior vena cava, bilateral four-compartment below-knee fasciotomies should be performed immediately, depending on the patient's hemodynamic status. Bilateral thigh fasciotomies will likely be necessary, as well, within the first 48 hours after ligation. When there are large defects in the sacrum or pelvic sidewall involving numerous pelvic veins or in the paravertebral area, packing the missile track with several vaginal packs (to allow for postoperative pelvic or paravertebral arteriography), inserting fibrin glue, or placing a Foley catheter with a 30-mL balloon inflated at the site of hemorrhage have been utilized.

Intra-abdominal Packing

When severe shock, hypothermia, acidosis, and massive transfusion have led to a coagulopathy and diffuse nonmechanical bleeding, the insertion of intra-abdominal packing for tamponade is appropriate. Diffuse intra-abdominal packing has been found to be particularly useful when a coagulopathy occurs and extensive retroperitoneal or pelvic dissection has been necessary during a laparotomy for a trauma.

Operative Techniques With Vascular Trauma in an Extremity

Damage control operations on an extremity are appropriate when exsanguination has caused intraoperative metabolic failure (shotgun wound of femoral triangle); when multisystem injuries have occurred, and an emergent craniotomy, thoracotomy, or laparotomy needs to be performed in addition to the vascular repair of the extremity (occlusion of superficial femoral artery from a femur fracture); or when the instability of an open fracture precludes formal repair of the associated vascular injury (mangled extremity).

After rapid control of hemorrhage, an intraluminal Argyle or Javid shunt is inserted into the debrided ends of the injured femoral or popliteal artery and tied in place to preserve distal flow as the patient is resuscitated in the intensive care unit. The Pruitt–Inahara shunt may be used also and has inflatable balloons on either end so that tying the shunt in place will not be necessary. This shunt has a T-port, which allows for the infusion of heparin, a vasodilator such as tolazoline, or for arteriography in the postoperative period.

While ligation of major venous injuries in the extremities has been well tolerated in many stable patients, patients undergoing damage control operations often have severe sequelae. Among these are a compartment syndrome below the level of ligation in the lower extremity and excessive hemorrhage from soft-tissue injuries and fasciotomy sites. For these reasons, venous outflow after segmental resection of an injured femoral or popliteal vein should be restored with a temporary intraluminal shunt as part of a damage control operation. Short segments of thoracostomy tubes (size 24 to 28 French) are used as shunts for the popliteal, superficial femoral, or common femoral veins.

ALTERNATE CLOSURES OF INCISIONS

Indications

Intraoperative Metabolic Failure

In the previously described patients with hypothermia (temperature <35°C), persistent acidemia (pH <7.2), and/or the onset of an intraoperative coagulopathy, a damage control operation should be terminated with an alternate closure of the incision.

Reoperation

One of the fundamental principles of the damage control operation is that a reoperation will be necessary to complete repairs and resections, perform anastomoses, look for missed injuries, change thoracostomy tubes, insert drains, and attempt closure of the incision. There are also techniques utilized at first operations for trauma, whether damage control was necessary or not, that mandate an early reoperation. Patients in whom these techniques are used will also benefit from alternate forms of closure of the thoracic or abdominal incision:

- Insertion of perihepatic packing
- Insertion of intra-abdominal packing
- Second-look operation.

Closure of the Incision Cannot Be Performed or Will Cause an Abdominal Compartment Syndrome

Edema and distention of the midgut are commonly noted during prolonged laparotomies for trauma in which patients in shock have been treated with massive crystalloid resuscitation in addition to blood. Presumably, these changes are related to cellular edema from metabolic failure of the sodium pump, a "capillary leak" phenomenon with secondary interstitial edema related to the release of vasoactive substances, reperfusion injury, the development of an ileus, or some combination of these.

ABDOMINAL COMPARTMENT SYNDROME

Definition

The abdominal compartment syndrome refers to the decreased blood flow to abdominal organs and secondary pressure effects on the respiratory, cardiovascular, and central nervous systems when the intra-abdominal pressure (IAP) rises above a critical level.

Measurement of Intra-abdominal Pressure

Direct measurement of IAP is accomplished by inserting an intraperitoneal catheter attached to a manometer or transducer. In the clinical setting, indirect measurement is possible through a catheter inserted into the urinary bladder, stomach, or inferior vena cava. Table 35-2 lists clinical and laboratory manifestations of increased IAP.

Proposed Classification

The group at Denver Health Medical Center first proposed a grading system for the abdominal compartment syndrome in 1996. This grading system was slightly modified in a subsequent publication and is presented in Table 35-3.

TABLE 35-2 Clinical and Laboratory Manifestations of Increased Intra-Abdominal Pressure

ABDOMINAL
Body wall
   Decreased blood flow
Gastrointestinal tract
   Decreased mucosal blood flow and intramucosal pH
   Possible bacterial translocation
Hepatic
   Decreased portal blood flow and hepatocyte mitochondrial function
Renal
   Increased renal vein pressure
   Increased plasma renin and aldosterone
   Decreased renal blood flow, glomerular filtration rate, and urine output
THORACIC
Lung
   Increased intrathoracic pressure, peak airway pressure, peak inspiratory pressure, and intrapulmonary shunt
   Decreased dynamic compliance
Heart/cardiovascular
   Decreased venous return and cardiac output
   "False" increase of central venous pressure and pulmonary artery wedge pressure
   Increased systemic and pulmonary vascular resistance
CENTRAL NERVOUS SYSTEM
   Increased intracranial pressure secondary to decreased venous return
   Decreased cerebral perfusion pressure

OPERATIVE TECHNIQUES

Towel Clip Closure of the Skin

The simplest and most rapidly performed technique for temporary closure of a thoracic, abdominal, or groin incision in the unstable trauma or septic patient is towel clip or suture closure of only the skin. A towel clip is placed across the edges of the skin incision at one end of the incision with the points approximately 1 cm back from the skin edge on either side. This first towel clip is then lifted up and pulled toward the end of the incision to create a ridge through which the next towel clip can be applied. Towel clips are then applied approximately 1 cm apart along the entire length of the incision.

TABLE 35-3 Percentage of Patients With Respective Organ Dysfunction Per Grade of Abdominal Compartment Syndrome

Grade	UO <0.5 mL/kg/h	PAP >45	SVR >1000	DO$_2$I <600
I	0%	0%	0%	0%
II	0%	40%	20%	20%
III	65%	78%	65%	57%
IV	100%	100%	100%	100%

PAP, peak airway pressure (cm H_2O); DO$_2$I, oxygen delivery index (mL O_2/min/m^2); SVR, systemic vascular resistance (dyne/sec/cm^{-5}); UO, urine output (mL/min).

Source: Reproduced, with permission, from Meldrum DR, Moore FA, Moore EE, et al: *Am J Surg* 174:667, 1997.

Temporary Silos

In patients with extensive manipulation of the heart during repair of a perforation or rupture, closure of the median sternotomy or bilateral anterolateral thoracotomy may cause cardiac failure. An Esmarch bandage borrowed from the orthopedic surgery service should then be sewn to the skin edges as a temporary silo. When cardiac edema has resolved, the patient is returned to the operating room, the congealed serum irrigated away, and a formal closure completed.

When the extent of edema and distention of the midgut or the presence of multiple intra-abdominal packs precludes complete towel clip or suture closure of the skin of the abdominal incision, a combined towel clip or suture closure/silo closure is recommended.

Silo coverage of the open abdomen can be accomplished by use of a plastic wound drape, a 3-L plastic bag of irrigating solution used by the urology service, or Silastic® sheeting (Dow Corning Corp, Midland, MI). As an alternative approach, Bender and coworkers have described placing rayon cloth as a silo, covering the cloth with "generous" gauze packs, and tying several widely spaced retention sutures above the packs to keep the midgut below the fascial edges if at all possible. As midgut edema resolves, the patient is returned to the operating room for removal of the gauze and gradual tightening of the retention sutures until the linea alba can be closed.

Zippers, Slide Fastener, Velcro Analogue

Originally described by Leguit in 1982, the zipper closure of the abdominal wall was popularized by Stone and colleagues in their open treatment of patients with pancreatic abscesses. Either a conventional zipper is sutured to the skin or fascia with a continuous suture of 0 or 2-0 nylon or polypropylene or a commercial zipper with adhesive side pieces is applied to the skin edges. The major advantage of using the skin is that it preserves the fascia for formal wound closure at an appropriate time.

Another approach is to use plastic sheets with a locking edge (Ethizip®) or a Velcro® equivalent sewn to the fascial edges of the wound. The use of a Velcro equivalent is particularly appealing, since the two edges that overlap and adhere over the open abdomen can be progressively tailored to a smaller size as the edema and distention of the midgut resolve.

Absorbable Meshes

The primary clinical use of absorbable meshes as an alternative form of closure of the abdominal incision on the trauma service has been in patients with marked distention of the midgut and an unwillingness to use a plastic silo or the recognition that secondary closure by granulation over the midgut will be necessary. It has also been used in patients with open abdomens from septic processes in the abdominal wall or in the abdominal cavity. An incisional hernia occurs in all patients in whom the mesh is allowed to granulate, and repair is deferred until the patient has fully recovered from the original traumatic or septic event.

Permanent Meshes

The data strongly suggest that a permanent rigid prosthesis such as Marlex® mesh should not be inserted in abdominal wall defects in the presence of extensive contamination from a perforated gastrointestinal tract secondary to trauma, acute intra-abdominal sepsis, or necrotizing infection in the abdominal wall. The risk of secondary infection and damage to the underlying bowel as the prosthesis develops "wrinkles" from contraction of the wound has now been documented on numerous occasions.

INTENSIVE CARE BEFORE REOPERATION

Reversal of Metabolic Failure

Major goals upon return to the ICU are to simultaneously reverse the sequelae of metabolic failure and maintain oxygen delivery in the previously or currently shocky patient.

All of the warming maneuvers used in the emergency department and operating room are obviously duplicated in the ICU. Gentilello has also described the use of a continuous arteriovenous rewarming (CAVR) device. It should be noted that a failure to correct a patient's hypothermia after a damage control operation is a marker of inadequate resuscitation or irreversible shock.

All would agree that persistent acidemia, an abnormal base deficit, and an elevated lactate level are manifestations of the failure to restore normal oxygen delivery and consumption. It is also true that a pH <7.2 may have adverse effects on cardiac contractility and the patient's response to catecholamines as previously noted. It may also be partially responsible for the onset of diffuse intravascular coagulation in patients with profound shock.

Correction of the coagulopathy induced by massive transfusions is by reversal of hypothermia, infusion of whole blood, if available, replacement of missing components including fresh frozen plasma and occasionally, platelets. The use of an autotransfusion system for scavenging blood from thoracostomy tubes or abdominal drains is also worthwhile, as retrieved red blood cells may be further washed, concentrated, and then stored in the blood bank until needed.

Endpoints of Resuscitation

The physiologic endpoints of resuscitation during the ICU phase of damage control remain controversial. There is, however, increasing evidence that the "false" elevations of central venous pressure and pulmonary artery wedge pressure in patients with increases in intrathoracic and intra-abdominal pressure make them unreliable as indicators of volume status.

Measurements of gastric intramucosal pH (pHi) continue to be used as a marker of the success of resuscitation. Using both pHi and the gastric mucosal–arterial carbon dioxide (CO_2) gap, Miller and associates found that the ability to predict multiple organ failure and death in trauma patients was highest at a pHi less than 7.25 and at a CO_2 gap greater than 18 mm Hg.

Need for Emergency Reoperation

Failure to attain the desired endpoints of resuscitation during the ICU phase of damage control may reflect continuing hemorrhage as well. An early return to the operating room is a difficult decision because the hypothermia-related coagulopathy is often not resolved. Therefore, the surgeon must decide whether mechanical or surgical hemorrhage is occurring versus diffuse oozing from a coagulopathy in which an early reoperation may not be indicated.

Another obvious indication for an early reoperation is the development of the previously described abdominal compartment syndrome. A progressive increase in inspiratory pressures on the ventilator coupled with oliguria and a "tight" abdomen mandate a rapid measurement of intra-abdominal pressure through the bladder catheter. Reoperation is necessary when the clinical signs are accompanied by an intra-abdominal pressure greater than 25 mm Hg, as previously described.

When postoperative bleeding is not a concern, a return to the operating room is based on reversal of metabolic failure and normalizing of cardiovascular and pulmonary parameters.

REOPERATION

The Routine Reoperation

A patient who is normotensive, without a coagulopathy, and is in the diuretic phase of recovery after resuscitation from shock is an ideal candidate for reoperation. While this usually takes place within 48 to 72 hours of the damage control laparotomy, it may be delayed in patients with massive distention of the midgut so that a further diuresis may occur.

Release of the Abdominal Compartment Syndrome

It has been noted that sudden release of the abdominal compartment syndrome at the time of reoperation may lead to a reperfusion phenomenon and a cardiac arrest. In one report, it was recommended that volume loading with 2 L of a solution composed of 0.45 percent normal saline, 50 g mannitol/L, and 100 mEq sodium bicarbonate/L be performed before release of the abdominal wall.

THE OPEN WOUND AT REOPERATION

In patients with persistent distention of the midgut at reoperation, a number of techniques are currently being used for coverage of the abdominal cavity.

Repeat Application of a Silo

A Steri-Drape® or plastic silo may be reapplied at the reoperation in the distended patient as it protects the midgut, prevents evaporation, and allows for visual confirmation that the midgut is decreasing in size during the diuretic phase of recovery.

Continued attempts to decrease the size of the silo as previously described are worthwhile over the first 7 days after the reoperation. If the linea alba cannot be closed by this time, the separation of the two sides of the midline incision will usually prevent further attempts at formal closure. Should this occur, the silo is removed in the ICU and a double layer of absorbable mesh is applied over the midgut. Fine mesh gauze and a bulky pressure dressing are then used over the absorbable mesh to maintain the midgut below the level of the fascia. Split-thickness skin grafts are applied when granulation tissue completely covers the abdominal wound.

LATE CLOSURE OF THE INCISIONAL HERNIA

It is appropriate to delay closure of any stomas and the incisional hernia resulting from conversion to an "open" abdomen at the original admission for trauma 3 to 6 months later. This interval allows the patient to regain lost weight and complete the formation of adhesions and scars in the abdominal cavity and body wall.

Standard Closures

In selected patients, the narrow midline defect that remains after excision of the skin graft over the midgut can be readily closed with a continuous or interrupted suture technique using No. 1 polypropylene material. When there is excessive tension on the closure of the linea alba, either unilateral or bilateral release of the external oblique aponeurosis is performed through a pararectus skin incision. Once the external oblique aponeurosis is divided in a longitudinal direction, the pararectus skin incision is closed primarily or with a split-thickness skin graft.

When a prosthesis is needed to close the midline defect and there is complete omental coverage over the midgut, a polypropylene or Marlex mesh is used. Without omental coverage, a polytetrafluoroethylene body wall patch is appropriate.

Tissue Expanders

Tissue expanders can be placed on either side of a large incisional hernia and progressively inflated at weekly intervals for 6 weeks prior to operation. At reoperation, the skin graft covering the midgut is elevated on one side, and the dermal elements scraped off with a no. 10 blade. This "neofascia" is folded back on itself and sutured to the rectus sheath to which it is still attached. The midline defect is then closed by suturing the double-layer neofascial graft to the opposite rectus sheath. Coverage over the fascial repair is provided by removing the tissue expanders and advancing the subcutaneous tissue/skin flaps to the midline over suction drains.

Components Separation

The external oblique aponeurosis is incised just lateral to the rectus sheath. The rectus abdominis muscle is then separated from the posterior rectus sheath and the internal oblique component of the anterior rectus sheath is divided from the epigastrium to the arcuate line. The final stage involves suturing the anterior rectus sheaths in the midline, as well as approximating the medial border of the posterior rectus sheath (that near the midline) to the lateral border of the anterior rectus sheath.

ADDITIONAL READING

Burch JM, Moore EE, Moore FA, et al: The abdominal compartment syndrome. *Surg Clin North Am* 76:88, 1996.

Feliciano DV, Burch JM: Towel clips, silos, and heroic forms of wound closure, in Maull KI, Cleveland HC, Feliciano DV, et al (eds): *Advances in Trauma and Critical Care,* vol 6. Chicago, Year Book Medical Publishers, 1991, p 231.

Meldrum DR, Moore FA, Moore EE, et al: Prospective characterization and selective management of the abdominal compartment syndrome. *Am J Surg* 174:667, 1997.

Morris JA Jr, Eddy VA, Binman TA, et al: The staged celiotomy for trauma. Issues in unpacking and reconstruction. *Ann Surg* 217:576, 1993.

Rotondo MF, Schwab CW, McGonigal MD, et al: "Damage control": An approach for improved survival in exsanguinating penetrating abdominal injury. *J Trauma* 35:375, 1993.

GENERAL PRINCIPLES

Care must be taken to fully evaluate the injured patient and not only the injury to the upper extremity. The history should include the mechanism of injury; location and time of its occurrence; neck, arm, or hand positioning at the time of injury; presence of any neurologic symptoms; and any previous treatment, antibiotic use, and tetanus prophylaxis. Clothing should be removed to inspect the extremity for signs of an acute injury (abrasions, swelling, asymmetry, ecchymosis) or chronic injury (well-healed scars, abrasions, muscle wasting). Active (if possible) and passive motion is assessed. The presence of crepitus, any abnormal joint motion, deformities, and location and size of open wounds are noted. A vascular examination is performed looking for pallor, cyanosis, and the presence of digital capillary refill or peripheral pulses. Doppler ultrasonography is used to detect nonpalpable pulses. An Allen's test (assessment of capillary refill of the hand through either the radial or ulnar artery) is used to determine the relative contribution of each artery in hand perfusion. Arteriography is indicated in the presence of absent pulses associated with penetrating wounds or with fracture/dislocations associated with possible arterial injuries. Vascular repair should be performed following stabilization of the injury. The repair should ideally be performed within 6 hours of the injury. Fasciotomies should be considered following an arterial repair. A compartment syndrome must be ruled out in a tense, swollen extremity. The classic signs of pain, pallor, paresthesias, paralysis, and pulselessness may not always be present. Pain with passive stretch of the muscles in the involved compartment should be present. If a compartment syndrome is suspected, all circumferential dressings should be removed. Compartmental pressures should be measured, especially in patients with an altered state of consciousness. Abnormal compartmental pressures are generally > 30–35 mm Hg or from 10 to 30 mm Hg above the diastolic pressure. A fasciotomy of all involved compartments should be performed if a compartment syndrome is suspected. The neurologic examination includes an assessment of the brachial plexus and peripheral nerve function (Fig. 36-1, Tables 36-1 and 36-2).

FRACTURES, DISLOCATIONS, AND OPEN WOUNDS

With simple contusions, the arm may be splinted or placed in a sling for comfort. Adequate radiographs are required to fully assess a fracture or dislocation. In general, nondisplaced fractures are splinted. Displaced fractures, dislocations, or fracture-dislocations are reduced with the patient adequately sedated and immobilized. An inadequate reduction generally requires further treatment (i.e., reduction under anesthesia or open reduction with or without internal fixation). Open wounds should be quickly cleansed and covered for later definitive care (i.e., surgical debridement within 6 hours). Arterial bleeding should be initially controlled with compressive dressings. A tetanus booster or toxoid should be given as needed (see Chapter 44). Antibiotics are used as needed (see Chapter 12).

Fractures and Dislocations of the Scapula

Fractures of the scapula are relatively uncommon, high-energy injuries (3 to 5

TABLE 36-1 *continued*

Nerve	Muscle(s) innervated	Test for function	Sensory distribution
Median	Extensor pollicis brevis and longus		Volar thumb, index, long, radial half of ring finger; dorsum index, long, radial half of ring finger
	Abductor pollicis longus		
	Flexor carpi radialis	Wrist flexion	
	Pronator teres and quadratus	Forearm pronation	
	Flexor digitorum sublimis	Finger proximal interphalangeal joint flexion	
	Flexor digitorum profundus (index, long)	Finger distal interphalangeal joint flexion	
	Abductor pollicis brevis	Thumb abduction	
	Opponens pollicis	Thumb opposition	
	Flexor pollicis brevis (superficial head)	Thumb metacarpophalangeal joint flexion	
	Lumbricals (index, long)	Metacarpophalangeal joint flexion Interphalangeal joint extension	
Ulnar	Flexor carpi ulnaris	Wrist flexion	Volar and dorsum little, ulnar half of ring finger; dorsal ulnar aspect of hand
	Flexor digitorum profundus (ring, little)	Finger distal interphalangeal joint flexion	
	Abductor digiti minimi	Little finger abduction	
	Flexor digiti minimi	Little finger metacarpophalangeal joint flexion	
	Opponens digiti minimi	Little finger abduction	
	Abductor pollicis	Thumb adduction	
	Flexor pollicis brevis (deep head)	Thumb metacarpophalangeal joint flexion	
	Interossei (volar, dorsal)	Metacarpophalangeal joint flexion, interphalangeal extension	
	Lumbricals (ring, little)	Metacarpophalangeal joint flexion, interphalangeal extension	

TABLE 36-2 Cervical and Thoracic Nerve Roots and Function

Nerve root	Test for function (muscle/nerve)	Sensory distribution	Reflex
C5	Shoulder abduction (deltoid/axillary)	Lateral upper arm	Biceps
C6	Elbow flexion (biceps/ musculocutaneous) Wrist extension (extensor carpi radialis longus and brevis/radial)	Lateral forearm, thumb, index finger	Brachioradialis
C7	Elbow extension (triceps/radial) Wrist flexion (flexor carpi radialis/median; flexor carpi ulnaris/ulnar) Finger extension (extensor digitorum communis, extensor indicis proprius, extensor digiti minimi/radial)	Long finger	Triceps
C8	Finger flexion (flexor digitorum superficialis, flexor digitorum profundus/ median and ulnar)	Medial forearm, ring, little fingers	None
C9	Finger abduction and adduction (dorsal and volar interossei/ulnar)	Medial forearm	None

tions (secondary to seizures, electrical shock, fall on flexed, adducted arm) are the most commonly missed dislocations. Inferior (hyperabducted arm) and superior dislocations are rare. Table 36-7 lists the classification of glenohumeral dislocations and associated injuries. The recommended radiographs are similar to those recommended for fractures of the proximal

TABLE 36-3 Classification and Treatment of Scapular Fracture

Classification	Associated injuries	Radiographic studies
Fractures Body and spine Glenoid neck Glenoid Coracoid Acromion	Thoracic cage Pulmonary Clavicle Brachial plexus Vascular Distal extremity Cranial	Recommended views: AP of shoulder (scapular plane) Axillary lateral of glenohumeral joint Trans-scapular lateral (tangential) view
Dislocations Scapular dislocation Scapulothoracic dissociation	Spine Abdominal Pelvic	Additional views: Chest x-ray Oblique view of the glenoid Tomography or CT scan

Nonoperative treatment	Acute operative treatment	Late reconstruction
Most scapular fractures	Displaced fractures of: Glenoid Acromion Coracoid Vascular injury Open fractures	Glenohumeral post-traumatic arthritis Brachial plexus injury Vascular injury

TABLE 36-4 Classification and Treatment of Clavicular Fractures

Classification	Associated injuries	Radiographic studies

Distal third of shaft
  Extra-articular
  Intra-articular
    (acromioclavicular)
Middle third of shaft
 	
Proximal third of shaft
Extra-articular
	Head and neck
	Thoracic
	
	Mediastinum
	Scapula
	
	Brachial plexus
	Vascular
		Recommended views:
		  AP of clavicle
		
		AP of glenohumeral joint
		Axillary lateral (or trans-
		  scapular lateral) of
		  glenohumeral joint
		Additional views:
		  Chest x-ray
		  45° cephalic tilt view
		    of clavicle
		  AP or PA view of both
		    shoulders with a 10-lb.
		    weight strapped to
		    each wrist (for distal
		    clavicle fractures or
		    acromioclavicular
		    joint injuries)
		Tomography or CT scan

Nonoperative treatment	Acute operative treatment	Late reconstruction

Most clavicle fractures	Severely displaced
	  fractures with
	  compromised skin
	Some displaced distal
	  third fractures
	Posteriorly displaced
	  middle third fractures
	  compromising
	  mediastinum
	Open fractures
	Vascular injury
		Symptomatic nonunion
		
		Malunion compromising
		  brachial plexus
		
		Posttraumatic arthritis of
		  AC and SC joint

TABLE 36-5 Classification and Treatment of Clavicular Dislocations

Classification	Associated Injuries

Acromioclavicular
  Superior
  Posterior
  Inferior
Sternoclavicular
  Anterior
  Posterior
Panclavicular
	Clavicle fracture
	Coracoid fracture
	Acromial fracture
	Brachial plexus
	Vascular
	Thoracic

Nonoperative treatment	Acute operative treatment	Late reconstruction

Most AC joint
  dislocations
Some SC joint
  dislocations
	Severe AC
	  joint dislocations
	Some SC dislocations
	Posterior dislocations
	  compromising the
	  mediastinum
		Posttraumatic arthritis
		
		Severe AC joint dislocations

TABLE 36-6 Classification and Treatment of Proximal Humerus Fractures

Classification	Associated injuries	Radiographic studies
Anatomic neck	Axillary nerve	Recommended views:
Surgical neck	Brachial plexus	AP of shoulder
Greater tuberosity	Vascular	Axillary lateral of
		glenohumeral joint
Lesser tuberosity	Thoracic	Additional views:
Head splitting	Shoulder girdle	Humerus x-ray, elbow x-ray
Proximal humerus		Tomography
fracture associated		CT scan
with dislocation		
2-, 3-, or 4-part fracture		Chest x-ray

Nonoperative treatment	Acute operative treatment	Late reconstruction
Nondisplaced fractures	Displaced fractures	Posttraumatic arthritis
	Fracture-dislocations	Malunion
	Fractures associated	Nonunion
	with neurovascular	Avascular necrosis
	compromise	humeral head

humerus (Table 36-6). Most glenohumeral dislocations should undergo a closed reduction with appropriate sedation. Postreduction radiographs should be made to ensure adequacy of the reduction. The indications for the acute and late operative treatment of glenohumeral dislocations are listed in Table 36-7.

Fractures of the Shaft of the Humerus

Fractures of the humeral shaft are the result of direct trauma (e.g., fall on the arm, blows to the arm, and gunshot injuries) and indirect trauma (e.g., fall on

TABLE 36-7 Classification and Treatment of Glenohumeral Dislocations

Classification	Associated injuries
Anterior	Vascular
Subcoracoid	(axillary, thoracoacromial,
Subglenoid	subscapular, circumflex arteries)
Subclavicular	Neural
Intrathoracic	(axillary, radial, musculocutaneous,
Posterior	median, ulnar, brachial plexus)
Subacromial	Soft-tissue
Subglenoid	(glenohumeral joint capsule,
Subspinous	ligaments, rotator cuff)
Inferior	
Subglenoid	
Open (luxatio erecta)	

Nonoperative treatment	Acute operative treatment	Late reconstruction
Most dislocations	Open dislocations	Chronic dislocations
	Irreducible dislocations	Recurrent dislocations
	Dislocations with vascular injury	or subluxations
	Dislocations with displaced	Posttraumatic arthritis
	fractures or soft tissue injuries	
	(rotator cuff)	

TABLE 36-8 Classification and Treatment of Humeral Shaft Fractures

Classification	Associated injuries	Radiographic studies

Proximal third
  Above insertion of
    pectoralis major
Middle third
  Below insertion of
    pectoralis major
  Below insertion
    of deltoid
Distal third
	Neural (radial nerve)
	Vascular
		Recommended views:
		  AP of humerus
		  Lateral of humerus
		  AP of glenohumeral joint
		  Axillary (or transcapular)
		    of glenohumeral joint
		
		Additional views:
		  AP and lateral of elbow

Nonoperative treatment	Acute operative treatment	Late reconstruction

Most humeral
  shaft fractures
	Fracture associated
	  with vascular injury
	Significantly displaced fracture
	Open fracture
	Fracture associated with
	  nerve (radial) injury?
	Polytraumatized patient?
		Symptomatic nonunions
		Pathologic fractures

TABLE 36-9 Classification and Treatment of Fractures About the Elbow

Classification	Associated injuries	Radiographic studies

Fractures
  Supracondylar
  Transcondylar
  Intracondylar
  Condylar
    Capitellum
    Trochlea
  Epicondylar
    Medial
    Lateral
  Supracondylar process
  Proximal ulna
    Olecranon process
    Coronoid process
  Proximal radius
    Radial head
    Radial neck
  Essex-Lopresti fracture-dislocation
    (radial head fracture + distal radioulnar joint dislocation)
	Vascular (brachial artery)
	Neural (radial, median,
	  ulnar nerve)
		Recommended views:
		  AP of elbow
		  Lateral of elbow
		Additional views:
		  Oblique views of elbow
		  Radial head view
		  Views of other areas
		    (e.g., shoulder,
		    humerus, forearm, wrist)
		  Tomography, CT scan.

Nonoperative treatment	Acute operative treatment	Late reconstruction

Nondisplaced fractures	Fractures associated
	  with vascular injury
	Open fractures
	Significantly displaced
	  fractures
	Unstable fractures
	Fracture-dislocations
		Posttraumatic arthritis
		Nonunion
		Malunion
		Avascular necrosis
		Instability
		Elbow contracture
		Myositis ossificans
		Nerve injury

TABLE 36-10 Classification and Treatment of Elbow Dislocations

Classification	Associated injuries
Posterior	Vascular (brachial artery)
Posterior	Neural (ulnar, median, radial)
Posteromedial	
Posterolateral	
Anterior	
Medial	
Lateral	
Divergent	
Isolated radial or ulnar dislocation	
Fracture associated with dislocation	
(Monteggia fracture-dislocation:	
proximal ulnar fracture + radial	
head dislocation)	

Nonoperative treatment	Acute operative treatment	Late reconstruction
Closed, reducible dislocations	Irreducible dislocations	Posttraumatic arthritis
	Dislocations associated with vascular injuries	Chronic dislocation
	Fracture-dislocations	Malunion
	Entrapment of fracture fragments in the joint	Elbow contracture
	Open dislocations	Nerve injury

outstretched arm, violent muscle contractions). Table 36-8 lists the classification of humeral shaft fractures, associated injuries, and recommended radiographs. The indications for the acute and late operative treatment of humeral shaft fractures are listed in Table 36-8.

TABLE 36-11 Classification and Treatment of Forearm Fractures

Classification	Associated injuries	Radiographic studies
Fractures	Neural (median, ulnar, radial)	Recommended views:
Proximal third	Vascular	AP of forearm
Middle third	Proximal & distal	Lateral of forearm
Distal third	radioulnar joint	AP & lateral of elbow
Single-bone fractures		AP & lateral of wrist
with dislocation		
Monteggia (proximal ulna + proximal radioulnar joint)		
Galeazzi (distal radius + distal radioulnar joint)		
Both bones		

Nonoperative treatment	Acute operative treatment	Late reconstruction
Nondisplaced fractures	Most displaced fractures	Malunion
	Fractures associated with vascular injury	Nonunion
	Open fractures	Posttraumatic arthritis of proximal or distal radioulnar joint
	Fracture-dislocations	Radioulnar synostosis
		Nerve injury
		Soft tissue injury

TABLE 36-12 Classification and Treatment of Fractures of the Distal Radius and Ulna

Classification	Associated injuries	Radiographic studies
Distal radius fractures: Extra-articular With dorsal displacement (Colles' fracture) With volar displacement (Smith's fracture)	Nerve injury (median, ulnar) Tendon injury Carpal injury (fractures, ligaments)	Recommended views: AP of wrist Lateral of wrist AP & lateral of forearm AP & lateral of elbow Additional views: Oblique views of wrist Tomography, CT scan Wrist arthrography
Intra-articular With involvement of radiocarpal joint: Radial styloid fracture Volar or dorsal lip fracture (Barton's fracture) Lunate fossa fracture With involvement of radioulnar joint		
Distal ulnar fractures: Extra-articular Ulnar neck Intra-articular fractures Ulnar head Ulnar styloid process Fracture-Dislocations		

Nonoperative treatment	Acute operative treatment	Late reconstruction
Nondisplaced fractures	Displaced fractures failing a closed reduction Fractures associated with neurovascular injury Open fractures Carpal injuries	Posttraumatic arthritis Malunion Nonunion Carpal instability Nerve injury Tendon injury Soft tissue injury

Fractures of the Elbow

Fractures about the elbow are secondary to falls on an outstretched arm or the elbow or a direct blow. The type of fracture will vary with the amount of varus or valgus stress or degree of elbow flexion at the time of injury. Table 36-9 lists the classification of fractures about the elbow, associated injuries, and recommended radiographs. Most nondisplaced elbow fractures can be treated with immobilization. The indications for the acute and late operative treatment of elbow fractures are listed in Table 36-9.

Dislocations of the Elbow

Most dislocations of the elbow result from a fall on an outstretched hand. Posterior dislocations are the most common. The type of dislocation will vary with the amount of elbow flexion and varus or valgus stress on the joint at the time of injury. Elbow dislocations are classified according to the position of

TABLE 36-13 Classification and Treatment of Carpal Fractures

Classification	Associated injuries	Radiographic studies
Scaphoid 　Tuberosity 　Distal third 　Middle third (waist) 　Proximal third Lunate 　(Kienbock's disease) Other carpal bones	Carpal ligament injury Other fractures (distal 　radius, metacarpal) Nerve injury	Recommended views: 　PA of wrist 　Lateral of wrist 　Carpal specific view 　　(e.g., scaphoid view) Additional views: 　Oblique views 　Tomography, CT scan 　Bone scan

Nonoperative treatment	Acute operative treatment	Late reconstruction
Nondisplaced 　fractures	Displaced, unstable fractures Irreducible fracture dislocations Fracture associated with 　neurovascular injury Open fractures	Nonunion Malunion Posttraumatic arthritis

the ulna and radius relative to the humerus. Table 36-10 lists the classification of elbow dislocations and associated injuries. The recommended radiographs are similar to those for elbow fractures (Table 36-9). Most elbow dislocations can be treated with a closed reduction using adequate sedation and immobilization. Postreduction radiographs should be made to ensure adequacy of the reduction. The indications for the acute and late operative treatment of elbow dislocations are listed in Table 36-10.

Fractures of the Forearm

Fractures of the radial and ulnar shaft are usually the result of a direct blow to the forearm. Table 36-11 lists the classification of forearm fractures, asso-

TABLE 36-14 Classification and Treatment of Carpal Dislocations

Classification	Associated injuries	Radiographic studies
Radiocarpal instability Intercarpal instability 　Scapholunate ligament 　　dissociation 　Lunotriquetral ligament 　　dissociation Perilunate instability 　Lunate dislocation Midcarpal instability Instability associated 　with fractures	Nerve injury Distal radius fractures Carpal fractures	PA of wrist Lateral of wrist Additional views: 　PA radial/ulnar 　　deviation view 　Clenched fist view 　Longitudinal traction view 　Wrist arthrography

Nonoperative treatment	Acute operative treatment	Late reconstruction
Mild sprains	Most displaced carpal dislocations Irreducible dislocations Dislocations associated with 　neurovascular injury Fracture-dislocations Open dislocations	Posttraumatic arthritis Chronic dislocations Persistent carpal 　instability

TABLE 36-15 Classification and Treatment of Fractures of the Hand

Classification	Associated injuries	Radiographic studies

Metacarpal fractures
Phalangeal fractures
  Proximal
  Middle
  Distal
Fracture-dislocations
	Nerve injury
	Tendon injury
	Open joint injury
		Recommended views:
		Metacarpal fractures
		  AP of hand
		  Lateral of hand
		Phalangeal fractures
		  AP of finger
		  Lateral of finger
		Additional views:
		  Oblique views
		  Tomography, CT scan

Nonoperative treatment	Acute operative treatment	Late reconstruction

Nondisplaced fractures
Reducible, stable fractures
	Displaced fractures failing
	  a closed reduction
	Displaced intra-articular
	  fractures
	Open fractures
		Posttraumatic arthritis
		Malunion
		Nonunion
		Joint stiffness
		Soft tissue injury
		Tendon adhesions

ciated injuries, and recommended radiographs. Nondisplaced forearm fractures (not common in adults) can be treated with immobilization. The indications for the acute and late operative treatment of elbow fractures are listed in Table 36-11.

Fractures of the Distal Radius and Ulna

Fractures of the distal radius and ulna usually result from a fall on an outstretched, dorsiflexed hand. Table 36-12 lists the classification of distal radius fractures, associated injuries, and recommended radiographs. Most nondisplaced distal radius and ulna fractures can be treated with immobilization. The indications for the acute and late operative treatment of distal radius and ulna fractures are listed in Table 36-12.

Fractures of the Wrist (Carpus)

The mechanism of carpal fractures and dislocations are similar to those of the distal radius fractures. Table 36-13 lists the classification of carpal fractures, associated injuries, and recommended radiographs. The scaphoid is the most commonly fractured carpal bone. Most nondisplaced carpal fractures can be treated with immobilization. The indications for the acute and late operative treatment of carpal fractures are listed in Table 36-13.

Dislocations of the Wrist (Carpus)

Table 36-14 lists the classification of carpal dislocations, associated injuries, and recommended radiographs. The most common wrist ligament injury involves the scapholunate interosseous ligament. A closed reduction, with adequate sedation, should be performed for most carpal dislocations. The indications for the acute and late operative treatment of carpal dislocations are listed in Table 36-14.

TABLE 36-16 Classification and Treatment of Hand Dislocations

Classification
Carpometacarpal (CMC)
Metacarpophalangeal (MCP)
Interphalangeal
Proximal (PIP)
Distal (DIP)
Fracture-dislocation

Nonoperative treatment	Acute operative treatment	Late reconstruction
Reducible, stable dislocations	Irreducible dislocations Unstable dislocations Open dislocations Some fracture-dislocations	Posttraumatic arthritis Unstable dislocations secondary to ligament injury

Fractures of the Hand

Fractures of the hand are among the most common of all fractures. These fractures result from a variety of mechanisms, including direct blows and twisting injuries. Table 36-15 lists the classification of hand fractures, associated injuries, and recommended radiographs. Most hand fractures can be treated with immobilization. The indications for the acute and late operative treatment of hand fractures are listed in Table 36-15.

Dislocations of the Hand

Dislocations of the hand result from a variety of forces applied to the joints (hyperextension-hyperflexion, abduction-adduction, axial load, twisting). Table 36-16 lists the classification of hand dislocations. The associated injuries and recommended radiographs are similar to those of hand fractures (Table 36-15). Most hand dislocations can be treated with a closed reduction and immobilization. The indications for the acute and late operative treatment of hand dislocation are listed in Table 36-16.

ADDITIONAL READING

Lee, DH, Neviaser RJ: Dislocations and ligamentous injuries of the digits, in Chapman, MW (ed): *Chapman's Orthopedic Surgery,* 3rd ed. Philadelphia, Lippincott, Williams & Wilkins, 2001, pp 1265–1311.

Morrey BF (ed): *The Elbow,* 3rd ed. Philadelphia, W.B. Saunders, 2000.

Rockwood CA Jr, Green DP, Bucholz RW, et al (eds): *Fractures in Adults.* Philadelphia, Lippincott-Raven, 1996.

Rockwood CA Jr, Matsen FA III (eds): *The Shoulder,* 2nd ed. Philadelphia, W.B. Saunders, 1998.

37 | Hand Injury

DIAGNOSIS

History

The history should include the patient's age, hand dominance, and occupation. Other data to collect include the patient's past medical history, any allergies, and any medications (prescription and OTC) the patient is taking. Also note the mechanism of injury, presence of any lacerations or other obvious injuries, presence of foreign bodies, whether the wounds are clean or contaminated, any chemical exposure, and any materials present from high-pressure injection injuries.

Physical Examination

The examination should take note of the appearance of the hands, including any calluses or dirt, color (cyanosis, erythema, or paleness), edema, open wounds, muscular atrophy, and the posture of the digits, as well as any deformities (angulations, displacement, or rotation). Also perform palpation to detect any tenderness, note any crepitation or mechanical blocks, and assess active and passive range of motion. Finally, assess neurologic state by doing a neuromuscular examination and rate on a scale from 0 to 5.

Every extrinsic muscle in the hand should be evaluated for its specific function. However, several muscles require performance of specific maneuvers in order to isolate their function. The extensor pollicis longus (EPL) is tested by placing the palm side of the hand on a flat surface and having the patient raise his or her thumb from the surface. To isolate an individual flexor digitorum superficialis (FDS) tendon, the distal interphalangeal (DIP) joints of the other fingers should be held in extension. When a finger is held in full extension with proximal interphalangeal (PIP) and metacarpophalangeal (MCP) flexion prevented by the examiner, flexor digitorum profundus (FDP) integrity is checked by active DIP flexion.

The intrinsic muscles are evaluated in groups. The palmar interossei adduct all the fingers toward the middle finger, and the dorsal interossei abduct away from the middle finger. The lumbricals flex the MCP joint while they simultaneously extend the PIP and DIP joints. The thenar muscles (opponens pollicis, flexor pollicis brevis, and abductor pollicis brevis) allow opposition of the thumb.

There are several potential reasons a specific motor task cannot be performed:

- Disruption of the musculotendinous unit (i.e., lacerated tendon)
- Pain from an underlying injury (i.e., fracture)
- Joint injury that is blocking motion (i.e., dislocation)
- Nerve disruption

Perform a sensory evaluation:

- Use a cotton-tipped swab to assess light touch
- Check two-point discrimination (5 mm separation with two-thirds correct response is normal)
- Use a 256 Herpes Zoster tuning fork to check nerve integrity
- Submerge hand in water for 20 minutes (skin wrinkles with normal innervation)

Perform a vascular examination by doing an Allen's test, checking skin color and temperature, and assessing capillary refill.

Radiographic Analysis

Appropriate x-rays should include at least two views, taken 90 degrees apart, and in the presence of a fracture they should include the entire length of the fractured bone from the joint proximal to the joint distal to the fracture.

FRACTURES

Many fractures of the wrist and hand can be treated with closed reduction and immobilization. Careful consideration has to be given to reduction alignment because even the smallest amount of rotational deformity can have devastating effects on hand function. In general, cast or splint immobilization maintains osseous alignment, and provides soft tissue support to help control soft tissue edema. Alignment is maintained by three-point fixation and by immobilizing at least one joint proximal and one joint distal to the fracture. Following cast application, repeat x-rays are mandatory to ensure that proper alignment has been maintained. If the fracture is unstable and the alignment cannot be held with cast immobilization, then percutaneous pinning or open reduction with internal fixation (ORIF) is indicated.

Another goal of proper casting or splinting is to hold the hand and fingers in the position of function. In general, the position of function is with the wrist in slight extension (15 to 30 degrees), MCP joints in 80 to 90 degrees of flexion, and DIP joints in full extension.

Figure 37-1 presents an algorithm for the treatment of hand injury.

FROSTBITE

Frostbite often presents with a discrepancy between skin lesions and damage to deeper structures. The primary treatment goal is to preserve viable tissue, and if amputation is required, to achieve maximal amputation stump length. The initial management of frostbite is with rapid rewarming at 110° F and anti-inflammatory medication.

When frostbite involves the immature hand, rapid rewarming may result in normal-appearing fingers of full length. However, the epiphyses may sustain irreparable damage resulting in epiphyseal arrest and often destruction of the epiphysis itself. This leads to proximal joint incongruity and ultimately destruction of the distal articular surface. The long-term sequelae are swollen joints, angular deformities, and nail abnormalities.

CHEMICAL BURNS

The degree and extent of damage from a chemical burn is dependent on the chemical agent, quantity, concentration, time of contact with the skin, and the type of chemical reaction that the agent produces. Treatment includes immediate irrigation with copious amounts of tap water, which reduces heat and dilutes or removes the offending agent. Once wound cleansing has been accomplished, topical antimicrobial agents and debridement and wound closure or coverage are performed.

EXTENSOR TENDON INJURIES

The extensor mechanism can be injured from the fingertip to the forearm. Most extensor tendon injuries can be primarily repaired following adequate

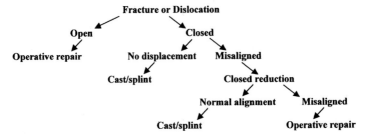

FIG. 37-1. Algorithm for the treatment of hand injury.

irrigation and debridement. Care must be taken to minimally handle the tendons during the surgical repair in order to decrease the formation of adhesions. Postoperatively, the hand should be splinted in a position that minimizes tension on the repair, but maintains functional positioning of the joints. This position is wrist in 40 degrees of extension, MCP joints in 20 to 30 degrees of flexion, and PIP and DIP joints in full extension.

Mallet Finger

A mallet finger is caused by loss of continuity of the conjoined lateral bands at the DIP joint and results in flexion deformity of the distal phalanx. Mallet fingers are classified as follows:
Type 1: Closed or blunt trauma with or without a small avulsion fracture
Type 2: Laceration at DIP joint
Type 3: Deep abrasion with loss of skin, subcutaneous tissue, and tendon substance
Type 4a. Transepiphyseal plate fracture in children
    b. Hyperflexion injury with fracture of articular surface of 20 to 50 percent
    c. Hyperextension injury with fracture of the articular surface usually greater than 50 percent and with early or late volar subluxation of the distal phalanx.

Successful treatment of type 1 injuries is with the use of a volar splint to hold the distal phalanx in neutral to slight hyperextension for 6 weeks. Fresh lacerations of the skin and extensor tendon in type 2 injuries are repaired by direct suture technique. Following repair, the DIP joint needs to be held in extension for 6 weeks. Type 3 injuries require soft tissue coverage followed by later tendon reconstruction or joint arthrodesis. Most type 4 injuries can be treated with closed reduction and extension splinting. Operative intervention has been recommended when fracture fragments involve greater than one third of the articular surface or with associated volar subluxation of the distal phalanx.

Boutonnière Deformity

Disruption of the central slip of the extensor tendon at the PIP joint with volar migration of the lateral bands will result in a boutonnière deformity, which includes loss of extension at the PIP joint and compensatory hyperextension at the DIP joint. On physical examination, the patient will have a painful and swollen PIP joint with tenderness dorsally in the region of the central slip insertion; the patient will be unable to actively extend the PIP joint from a flexed starting position.

Treatment of closed acute boutonnière injuries is dependent on restoration of the normal balance and precise length relationships between the central slip and lateral bands. This can be accomplished by splinting the PIP joint in extension, but leaving the DIP free for active motion. In a closed boutonnière deformity, operative intervention is indicated if the central slip has been avulsed with a bone fragment lying free over the PIP joint. Open injuries require copious irrigation of the joint and direct repair of the extensor apparatus, followed by splinting of the PIP joint in full extension.

FLEXOR TENDON INJURIES

All flexor tendon injuries should be surgically repaired in the operating room. The tendons can be primarily repaired within 24 hours after injury or undergo delayed primary repair, performed 3 to 4 days after the injury, when inflammation of the wound has subsided. The tendons are repaired with 3-0 braided nonabsorbable suture such as Ticron® for the core sutures. There are many suture techniques, but our preference is four core sutures using 3-0 Ticron followed by an epitendinous suture consisting of 6-0 nylon. Great care must be taken to minimize the incidence of adhesion formation, and this is achieved by limited handling of the tendons during repair.

The intricate flexor tendon system has been divided into anatomic zones for the purposes of classification, treatment, and prognosis. Zone 1 is located distal to the superficialis insertion, and only the FDP is located in this zone. Primary repair is preferred, and end-to-end reattachment is recommended. If the tendon has avulsed off the distal phalanx or the injury is near the insertion, the tendon should be advanced and reattached to the distal phalanx; it should not, however, be advanced more than 1 cm. Zone II is located within the finger flexor retinaculum, and both tendons are located in this region. Injuries in this zone are the most difficult to repair with excellent results. Zone III is defined as the region in the palm where the lumbricals take their origin from their respective FDPs. Due to the absence of retinacular structures, repairs in this zone have a relatively good prognosis. Zone IV corresponds to the area in the carpal tunnel, and at this level the flexor tendons are enclosed in synovial sheaths and held tightly within this compartment. Injuries of the flexor tendons in this zone are often associated with injuries to the main trunks of the median and ulnar nerve because of their close proximity. Zone V is located proximal to the wrist and forearm, where the prognosis is more favorable.

Postoperative care is vital to maximizing functional outcome. A dorsal splint is used to position the wrist in 30 degrees of flexion, the MCP joints in 90 degrees of flexion, and the distal joints extended. After several days, early mobilization is initiated by a certified hand therapist.

RING AVULSION INJURIES

Ring avulsion injuries occur when a ring hooks onto an object, such as a nail, as the individual is falling or jumping. Ring avulsion injuries range in severity from simple lacerations to finger devascularizations, often requiring microsurgical reconstruction or amputation. A common classification as described by Urbaniak is listed below:

Type I: Adequate circulation
Type II: Inadequate circulation
Type III: Complete degloving or complete amputation

Type I injuries require standard bone and soft tissue treatment and have the most favorable prognosis. Type II and III injuries require microvascular repair to preserve viability to the digit, and possibly other osseous or soft tissue reconstruction. For severe injuries, the decision to salvage the digit depends on two factors: the surgeon's microsurgical skill level and the understanding and compliance of the patient, who may require multiple lengthy operations and many hours of hand therapy.

AMPUTATION AND REPLANTATION

Indications for replantation include:

- All thumb amputations
- Multiple-digit amputations
- Amputation level between the palm and distal forearm
- Amputations distal to FDS insertion
- Amputation in healthy children

Relative contraindications include:

- Severely crushed or mangled parts
- Prolonged warm ischemia time
- Single-digit amputation through flexor zone II
- Severe contamination
- Age greater than 60, poor general health, or atherosclerotic disease
- Avulsion injuries
- Mental instability

In the period between injury and presentation to the health care providers, the amputated part should be properly cooled to prolong ischemic time. The upper limit for warm ischemia is 12 hours for a digit and 6 hours for a muscle-bearing part. With proper cooling at approximately 2° to 4°C these limits can be extended to 24 and 12 hours, respectively. The amputated part should be wrapped in sterile gauze moistened with Ringer's lactate solution and inserted in a plastic bag or small container that is placed on ice. The amputated part should not be placed directly on the ice. Upon arrival at the emergency department, evaluation of the injury should be performed by an experienced hand surgeon. If replantation is indicated, the amputated part should be immediately brought to the operating room to begin irrigation and debridement as well as neurovascular dissection and identification. Following adequate debridement, the order of repair is as follows:

1. Skeletal fixation (often requiring up to 1 cm of shortening to allow a tension-free repair of the neurovascular bundles)
2. Repair of extensor tendons
3. Repair of flexor tendons
4. Arterial anastomosis (although only one arterial repair is required, repair of both arteries improves survival)
5. Nerve repair
6. Vein repair
7. Loose skin closure
8. Noncompressive dressing

In healthy children, amputations at the level of the lunula of the nail can be salvaged by the "cap" technique described by Rose.

COMPARTMENT SYNDROME

Compartment syndrome is defined as a condition of increased tissue fluid pressure within a fascial muscle compartment that reduces capillary blood perfusion below the level necessary for tissue viability, and if left untreated will cause irreversible muscle and nerve damage. There are many causes for compartment syndrome.

The diagnosis of compartment syndrome is made clinically and can be confirmed by measurement of intracompartmental tissue fluid pressures. The clinical findings include: an edematous, tense compartment; pain out of proportion to that expected from the injury; sensation deficits; and motor weakness or paralysis. The most sensitive indicator of increased compartment pressure is pain associated with passive stretch of the muscles.

The initial treatment is directed toward removing any occlusive dressings or casts. If symptoms do not resolve quickly, fasciotomy is indicated. Fasciotomy of the hand requires release of all the intrinsic compartments. The intrinsic muscles can usually be decompressed through four incisions: two dorsal incisions for interosseous muscles, one radial incision for the thenar muscles, and one ulnar incision for the hypothenar muscles.

HIGH-PRESSURE INJECTION INJURIES

The extent of high-pressure injection injuries to the fingers and hands is often underestimated. The severity of injury is often quite extensive and is most directly related to the nature of the injected material. The pathophysiology of tissue damage is related to physical factors, chemical factors, and late infection. Early diagnosis is vital to tissue survival because these injuries may initially present as a small pinpoint wound accompanied by sudden swelling and digital numbness, with little immediate pain. Management of these serious injuries requires tetanus prophylaxis, broad-spectrum antibiotics, emergent surgical debridement, and possible amputation. Often, reconstructive procedures aimed at restoring motion and general hand function may be required.

FINGERTIP AMPUTATIONS

Fingertip amputations represent the most frequently encountered upper extremity amputation. The anatomy of the fingertip consists of several different tissues in a very small space. The nail plate covers the nail bed, which is composed of the germinal matrix from which the nail arises, and the sterile matrix, which adds thickness to the nail as it grows toward the fingertip. The lunula represents the transition from the germinal matrix to the sterile matrix. The nail plate is normally adherent to the underlying nail bed, but nail bed avulsion and scarring are two causes of nail plate separation. The nail plate is surrounded by the eponychium proximally, which gives the nail plate its shiny luster; the paronychium on the sides; and the hyponychium at the tip. The distal phalanx supports the nail plate, and if it is too short, the nail plate will grow around the end of the fingertip, forming a hook nail. Finally, the digital neurovascular bundle traverses the midaxial line on both sides of the digit.

Fingertip injuries can be classified by the type of defect remaining. Rossenthal classified transverse amputations into four types. Type I involves only soft tissue, type II is at the level of the proximal third of the nail plate, type III is at the eponychial fold, and type IV is proximal to the DIP joint. Oblique defects are classified as volar, lateral, and dorsal.

Several factors must be considered when selecting a method of treatment. Sensory preservation is especially important for the thumb and radial borders of the index and long fingers for the function of pinch, and for the ulnar border of the small finger for safety. In addition, the mechanism of injury, direction of amputation, and location of viable tissue are other important factors affecting treatment. Thus the type of skin coverage utilized should fulfill these criteria: maintain finger length, provide durable and sensate skin, and allow sufficient nail support.

Type I and II and oblique amputations can be treated by several different methods to attain soft tissue coverage. Healing by secondary intent with daily dressing changes is a very successful nonoperative treatment, but it takes several weeks for complete healing to occur. This is recommended for wounds less than 1 cm. When length is not a major concern for function or nail support, the bone should be shortened 2 mm below the pulp fat; otherwise, flap coverage should be considered. Surgical options include primary closure, skin grafts, local advancement flaps, and neurovascular island flaps. With a primary closure, the digital nerves are resected several millimeters from the distal wound to prevent hypersensitive neuromas. Commonly used regional flaps include cross-finger flaps and thenar flaps. Because of the lack of nail plate support in type III amputations, DIP joint disarticulation should be considered in all amputations except the thumb, where length is important for function. Type IV injuries can be considered for replantation of the amputated tip, as a composite graft has yielded excellent results.

ADDITIONAL READING

Green DP, Hotchkiss RN, Pederson WC, Lampert R: *Green's Operative Hand Surgery.* 4th ed. San Antonio, Churchill Livingstone, 1999.

Blair WF: *Techniques in Hand Surgery,* Baltimore, Williams & Wilkins, 1996.

Jupiter JB, Axelrod TS, Belsky MR: Fractures and dislocations of the hand. In Browner BD, Jupiter JB, Levine AM, Trafton PG (eds): *Skeletal Trauma.* 2nd ed. Philadelphia, WB Saunders, 1998, pp 1225–1342.

Rockwood CA Jr, Green DP, Bucholz RW, et al (eds): *Fractures in Adults.* Philadephia, Lippincott-Raven, 1996.

Rockwood CA Jr, Kasser JR, Wilkins K: *Fractures in Children.* 5th ed. Tennessee, Lippincott, Williams & Wilkins, 2001.

38 | Lower Extremity Fractures and Dislocations

INTRODUCTION

Fractures are the primary cause of more than half of all hospitalizations for trauma. The majority of these involve the lower extremities. It is important to remember that life-threatening injuries may be present together with injuries of the extremities. It is thus essential to evaluate the whole patient and not focus exclusively on an injured limb. Lower extremity trauma by itself is usually not life-threatening, but may result in long-term sequelae.

The large volume of tissue in the lower extremities, including the pelvis, increases the potential systemic effects of lower extremity injuries. Several units of blood can be lost into severely injured thighs (330 to 1300 mL from a single femur fracture). A crushing wound of the lower extremity releases intravasated debris, myoglobin, and inflammatory mediators, potentiating such problems as fat embolism, adult respiratory distress syndrome, and multiple organ failure.

Prompt surgical treatment for severe extremity injuries benefits the whole patient by ameliorating the above systemic effects and promoting mobilization with attendant benefits to the respiratory and gastrointestinal systems. Fracture fixation should be delayed or modified if the patient is in unresuscitated shock, is coagulopathic, or is hypothermic. Recent data suggest that fracture fixation surgery may not be without extra risk for the patient with a severe acute head injury, but surgical judgment is required because of the potential for secondary brain injury due to hypotension or hypoxia.

It is important to view an extremity as an integrated whole that may involve multiple components. The injury from a fracture often depends more on the damage done to the soft tissues of the limb than on the bony injury. Thus understanding an extremity injury requires assessment of all soft tissues as well as the bony injury. The basic principles of treatment for extremity injuries are listed in Table 38-1 in general order of priority, but this may require variations in sequencing according to the patient's needs. Open fractures require urgent surgical treatment (Fig. 38-1).

In situations involving a choice between limb salvage and amputation, the two primary concerns are the systemic consequences of the alternative for the patient, and the likelihood of achieving a functional limb. One absolute indication for primary amputation is an avascular open fracture with warm ischemia time over 6 hours. Another is an ischemic open fracture with anatomic loss of tibial nerve. Relative indications include associated polytrauma, serious ipsilateral foot injury, and requirement for a prolonged reconstruction. Revascularization in the face of severe neuromuscular injury may result in a viable but dysfunctional limb.

OPEN FRACTURES

All open fractures require urgent surgical treatment to reduce the risk of infection. The preferred algorithm for open fracture care is provided in Fig. 38-1. Evaluation and treatment of life-threatening injuries takes precedence. Radiographs of the limb may be deferred until more urgent care is completed. Bleeding is controlled during the primary survey with pressure dressings. A careful examination of the entire injured limb is part of the secondary survey, during which limb realignment and application of a sterile dressing and a

TABLE 38-1 Assessment of Severely Injured Lower Extremity

1. Realign (straighten) limb
2. Careful examination for open wounds or threatened skin
3. Complete neurologic examination
4. Thorough vascular examination including:
   a. Limb perfusion
   b. Pulses
   c. Ankle-brachial index, if pulses diminished, or high-risk injury
5. Betadine dressings over all open wounds
6. Radiolucent splint
7. 90° Opposed radiographs of any fractured bone or joint disruption
8. Tetanus prophylaxis
9. First-generation cephalosporin +/− aminoglycoside if open fracture
   suspected

well-padded splint are completed. Intravenous antibiotics and tetanus prophylaxis are routine. Once the emergent injuries are dealt with, operative wound care is carried out. This should be done within 6 hours of injury if possible, because longer delays probably increase the risk of infection. The open fracture wound, extended as required for debridement, is left open initially. Delayed primary closure, generally after 3 or 4 days, reduces the risk of wound infection. Aside from open fractures, other emergent lower extremity injuries may be present (Table 38-2).

INJURY COMBINATIONS

Knowledge of typical combinations of lower extremity injuries aids diagnosis and may decrease the risk of missing important injuries. A list of common orthopedic injury combinations is listed in Table 38-3.

PHYSICAL SIGNS

Virtually all fractures will demonstrate at least one physical sign such as: deformity, swelling, tenderness, and/or instability. Displaced long-bone fractures result in shortening, malrotation, or angulation. Intra-articular injuries usually cause a hemarthrosis, unless the joint capsule is disrupted. Compartment syndromes must always be suspected with a swollen limb and if motor or sensory function is disturbed, and may develop several hours after injury (Fig. 38-2). Distal pulses *can* be present even after a significant arterial injury, and are typically seen after injury to the popliteal artery (Table 38-3). Any alteration of pedal pulses, before or after manipulation of a fracture or dislocation, mandates an investigation for a vascular injury (Fig. 38-3). The neurologic status of the extremity should be documented before any definitive treatment. Bleeding, even after amputation, can generally be managed with a pressure dressing, and use of a tourniquet should be discouraged.

RADIOGRAPHY OF EXTREMITY INJURIES

Chest and cervical spine radiographs are indicated early in the evaluation of the injured patient. Because pelvic injuries may be very difficult to identify by physical findings alone, a screening anteroposterior (AP) pelvic x-ray is required, as it may reveal clues to potentially exsanguinating hemorrhage (Table 38-4). X-rays of extremities are of lower priority. Patient resuscitation should not be delayed or interrupted to make x-rays of extremities. If adequate

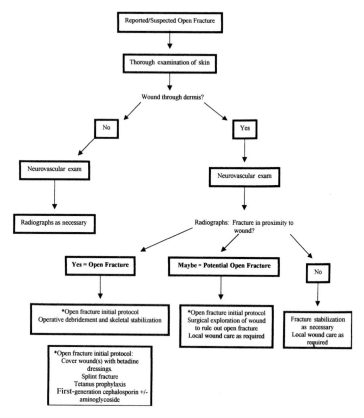

FIG. 38-1.   Algorithm for assessment of open fracture.

extremity radiographs can be obtained without delaying other essential tasks, however, they can usually help in planning the patient's overall care. Extremity x-rays should show both AP and lateral views of the entire bone in question, and be centered over the injured area. Pelvic fractures and certain complex articular fractures are best visualized with computed tomography (CT) scans. If a patient is hemodynamically stable and will be sent for other CT studies, it may be appropriate to obtain all of the extremity CTs at the same time.

TABLE 38-2 Lower Extremity Orthopedic Emergencies

- Pelvic ring fracture with exsanguinating hemorrhage
- Closed fracture or dislocation with vascular disruption
- Compartment syndrome
- Open fracture
- Traumatic hip dislocation
- Displaced femoral neck fracture in nonelderly patients
- Displaced talar neck fracture

TABLE 38-3 Injuries Commonly Associated with Lower Extremity Fractures
or Dislocations

Injury	Common association
"Open book" pelvis fracture	Severe bleeding, usually venous
	Bladder or urethral injury
"Vertical shear" pelvis fracture	Severe bleeding, usually venous
	Lumbosacral plexus injury
"Lateral compression" pelvis fracture	Head, chest, or abdominal injury
	Fasciocutaneous shear injury
Acetabular fracture	Head, chest, or abdominal injury
	Fasciocutaneous shear injury
Posterior hip dislocation/posterior wall acetabular fracture	Femoral head fracture
	Sciatic nerve injury
	Knee injury (typically isolated posterior cruciate ligament disruption)
Femoral shaft fracture	Femoral head fracture
	Femoral neck fracture
Multiligamentous knee injury/knee dislocation	Popliteal artery disruption
Medial tibial plateau fracture	Arterial injury
	Nerve injury
Proximal fibular fracture	Peroneal nerve injury
	Knee ligament injury
Tibial shaft fracture	Compartment syndrome
Calcaneal fracture	Thoracolumbar junction compression/burst fracture

MANAGEMENT OF COMMON FRACTURES AND DISLOCATIONS

Pelvic Ring Injuries

High-energy pelvic ring injuries carry a significant risk of morbidity and mortality. Injuries that deform the pelvic ring or render it unstable must involve at least two different foci of damage (bone, joint, or both components). The radiographic appearance of anterior pelvic injuries (pubic ramus or symphyseal injuries) is quite obvious. However, they are less significant than the posterior ring disruption that accompanies them. The character of the posterior injury determines the degree of pelvic instability. Anterior pelvic ring injury thus requires a careful search for posterior disruption. Subtle radiographic injuries may be found on an AP pelvic x-ray, and should be actively sought (Table 38-4).

Pelvic ring disruptions can be grouped according to the mechanism of injury. Lateral compression, AP compression, and vertical shear are the three basic types. While vertical shear displacement always creates instability, the extent of pelvic instability associated with lateral compression and AP compression injuries varies greatly. Pelvic ring injuries may have associated life-threatening hemorrhage, the source of which is usually low-pressure bleeding from pelvic veins. Only 10 percent of patients with significant bleeding have an embolizable artery as the source. Therefore, most pelvic fracture bleeding should first be addressed by promoting tamponade by reducing any pathologically increased pelvic volume. Miliary antishock trousers, pelvic binders, or pelvic external fixation all control hemorrhage via this mechanism. Means of initial stabilization are shown in Table 38-5.

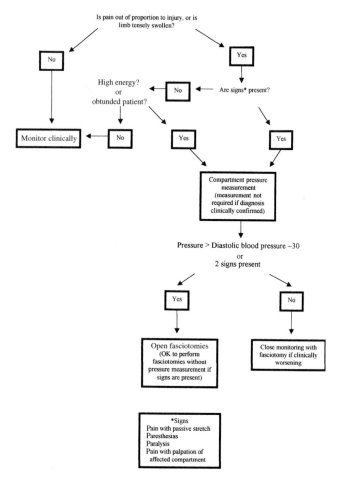

FIG. 38-2.   Algorithm for assessment and treatment of compartment syndrome.

Posterior pelvic stabilization surgery is indicated for displacement or instability. Anterior fixation alone appears to provide enough stability to stop hemorrhage. Vertical displacement can be corrected by applying skeletal traction to the proximally displaced limb. It is essential for all health care providers involved in treatment to develop a plan for management before any team member chooses a method that may preclude optimal care (e.g., a colostomy in the location of a surgical approach to the pelvis).

Acetabular Fractures

Fractures of the acetabulum are articular injuries with profound implications for long-term function of the hip joint. Successful open reduction and internal fixation of displaced acetabular fractures significantly improves the progno-

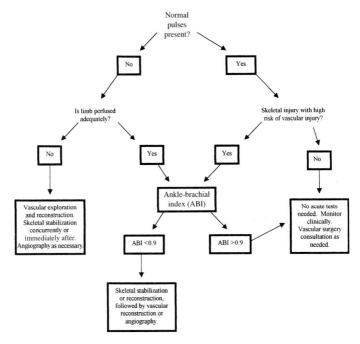

FIG. 38-3. Algorithm for assessment and treatment of vascular injury.

sis. Oblique x-rays and CT scans are used to classify the acetabular fracture. A precise anatomic reduction must be achieved and made stable, generally with screws and plates (Table 38-5). Acetabular fractures are rarely open. Delaying repair a few days permits adequate preparation and may reduce intraoperative bleeding. Patients with pelvic and acetabular fractures have a significant risk of thromboembolic disorders. Anticoagulation and/or inferior vena cava filters should be considered.

TABLE 38-4 AP Radiograph Pelvic Assessment

- Unless rotated to one side, the pelvis should be symmetric, right to left, with the symphysis directly in line with the middle of the sacrum
- Proximal displacement of either side of the pelvis relative to the other indicates fracture
- Fracture of bony structures (look carefully for fracture line across sacral foramina)
- Sacroiliac joint congruity (second sacroarcuate line should be at level of iliopectineal line and brim of true pelvis)
- Pubic symphysis widening indicates fracture
- Avulsion fractures (these suggest failure of ligaments that stabilize the pelvic ring)
    a. L5 transverse process
    b. Ischial spine
    c. Ischial tuberosity
- Hip dislocation
- Proximal femoral fracture

TABLE 38-5 Methods of Provisional Stabilization by Type of Injury

Injury	Stabilization technique
Pelvic ring fracture	Pelvic binder (or bedsheet wrapped tightly around pelvis)
	Anterior external fixator +/− proximal tibial pin traction
Acetabulum fracture	Knee immobilizer +/− Buck's traction (stable)
	Proximal tibial pin traction (unstable)
Hip dislocation	Knee immobilizer +/− Buck's traction (stable)
	Proximal tibial pin traction (unstable)
Femoral neck fracture	Buck's traction (elderly)
	Immediate fixation (nonelderly)
Intertrochanteric fracture	Buck's traction
Subtrochanteric/femoral shaft fracture	Proximal tibial pin traction
Distal femur fracture	Proximal tibial pin traction
	External fixator across knee
Patella/tibial spine fracture	Knee immobilizer
Tibial plateau fracture	Knee immobilizer (stable)
	Calcaneal pin traction or external fixator across knee (unstable)
Tibial shaft fracture	Long leg cast/splint
Tibial pilon fracture	Long leg splint (stable)
	External fixator (unstable)
Malleolar ankle fracture	Long leg splint or cast (dislocation)
	Short leg splint (no dislocation)
Calcaneus fracture	Padded Buck's traction boot
Hindfoot/midfoot fracture	Short leg splint
Forefoot/phalangeal fracture	Short leg splint/cast with toe plate extension

Dislocations of the Hip

Posterior dislocations of the hip result from direct blows to the front of the knee or upper tibia of a seated individual. Posterior wall acetabular fractures occur if the leg is more abducted, and pure dislocations result if it is adducted at the time of impact. The typical appearance of a patient with a posterior hip dislocation is with a hip that is flexed, adducted, and internally rotated. An associated sciatic nerve palsy must be suspected. An AP pelvic x-ray usually shows obvious signs of a hip dislocation. A CT scan is required after reduction of a dislocated hip to assess the integrity of the acetabulum, as well as to exclude the presence of intra-articular fragments. Femoral head fractures occasionally occur with hip dislocations (Table 38-3).

Dislocations of the hip demand immediate reduction, usually with intravenous analgesia, or with general anesthesia and muscle relaxation. A rapid reduction is urgent (less than 6 to 8 hours), as delay increases the risk of avascular necrosis of the femoral head. This complication results in destruction of the hip joint, with the future need for arthroplasty or arthrodesis. Both these options have a poor outcome for young, active people. The reduced joint must be checked for stability. Skeletal traction is required only for unstable hips (Table 38-5).

Femoral Neck Fractures

Intracapsular fractures involve the part of the upper femur below the femoral head. They have a high risk of nonunion and of avascular necrosis of the femoral head, especially when its blood supply is disrupted by displaced fractures. Avascular necrosis is less frequent if the femoral neck fracture is reduced and fixed as a surgical emergency (Table 38-2). Urgent anatomic reduction, decompressive capsulotomy, and secure fixation are required. Prompt internal fixation procedures can achieve high rates of fracture union, but still have a 20 percent incidence of avascular necrosis. In elderly osteoporotic patients, fixation failure and/or nonunion are more common, and render internal fixation less attractive. For these individuals, hip arthroplasty may be a better alternative. Undisplaced femoral neck fractures are generally at risk of displacing, and are thus best treated with internal fixation with several screws.

Intertrochanteric Fractures

Nearly half of hip fractures involve the wider intertrochanteric region of the proximal femur. With modern internal fixation devices properly applied, union is typically achieved within 3 or 4 months, with acceptable alignment and a low incidence of fixation failure. Initial stabilization is with skin traction (Table 38-5), and the risk of avascular necrosis is negligible, making surgical treatment nonemergent.

Subtrochanteric Fractures

Subtrochanteric fractures can be separated into those due to low-energy trauma, usually in osteoporotic elderly patients, and those due to high-energy trauma (e.g., motor vehicle crashes). Provisional stabilization of these injuries generally requires skeletal traction (Table 38-5). Healing is rapid and reliable, as with femoral shaft fractures, when the fracture can be fixed with an intramedullary nail.

The location of a subtrochanteric fracture is important to determine the proper means of fixation. If there is a large enough proximal femoral segment to insert an intramedullary nail, this type of fixation is preferred. Often a cephalomedullary (reconstruction-type) nail is used, with locking screws inserted proximally into the femoral head. If the fracture involves the nail entry site, a blade-plate or screw-plate device may be more appropriate. Significant bleeding may be associated with a subtrochanteric fracture, particularly in a young, muscular patient.

Fractures of the Femoral Shaft

Fractures of the femoral shaft are almost always caused by high-energy trauma. Open fractures of the femur are rare, but a closed soft tissue injury may involve significant muscle contusion and bleeding into the thigh. Occasionally, a compartment syndrome may occur. The systemic consequences of femoral fractures are significant, with shock, fat embolism, and adult respiratory distress syndrome well recognized. Emergent application of a temporary traction splint or skeletal traction improves comfort and reduces local and distant effects of these severe injuries (Table 38-5).

Prompt surgical fixation provides comfort and mobility for the patient, and reduces the risk of systemic complications in multiply injured patients. If possible, femoral fracture fixation should be done during the early surgical care of any trauma patient. The vast majority of femoral shaft fractures are treated with intramedullary nailing, which provides generally reliable fixation.

Recent awareness of intravasation of reaming debris (fat, marrow fragments, etc) has raised concerns that embolization to the lung might increase the risk of postoperative pulmonary complications, particularly in patients with multiple injuries or thoracic involvement. The prevalence of pulmonary problems, however, is no higher in nailed than in plated femur fractures. This raises questions about the clinical relevance of this debris. Nonetheless, it may still be wiser to use temporary external fixation for femur fractures in severely injured patients, delaying nailing until they have recovered sufficiently (usually at least 4 days after injury). After adequate wound debridement, most open femoral shaft fractures can be managed with intramedullary nailing, though the risk of infection increases with the severity of the wound. Delayed closure of the open fracture, after excision of all nonviable tissue, is safest.

Fractures of the Distal Femur

Distal femoral fractures are often articular fractures. Principles of management for articular fractures include anatomic reduction of the articular surface, with sufficiently stable fixation to permit early motion of the joint, but delayed weight bearing. Undisplaced fractures of the distal femur can be managed nonoperatively. Displaced fractures, particularly if the articular surface is involved, are best managed surgically. In some cases, intramedullary fixation can be used advantageously. Retrograde intramedullary nails inserted across the fracture site via the knee joint are a recent helpful advance. Open plate fixation, however, remains the most common method of fixation for displaced, intra-articular distal femoral fractures. Bridging external fixation, from the femur above the injury to the tibia below, adequately stabilizes the open fracture. This temporary approach, as an alternative to skeletal traction, simplifies patient care including transfer, while awaiting an appropriate time and place for definitive intra-articular fracture fixation.

Fractures of the Patella

Patellar fractures usually result from a direct blow to the flexed knee. With displacement, there is loss of continuity of the quadriceps mechanism, and therefore knee extension. The function of the quadriceps mechanism is assessed by asking the patient to lift his or her leg off the bed without allowing the knee to bend. While nonoperative treatment is successful for closed, undisplaced fractures in patients who can perform this maneuver, surgical treatment is necessary if quadriceps function is absent or if the articular surface is incongruous.

Dislocations and Ligamentous Injuries of the Knee

Dislocations may involve either the patellofemoral or the tibiofemoral joints. Patellar dislocations are common and typically occur in adolescent females. True tibiofemoral dislocations are much less common, and often require significant injury forces, though these may occur in the elderly with a simple slip and fall. These injuries are important to recognize because of their extensive ligamentous disruption and associated risk of arterial and neurologic injuries. The potential for limb loss because of popliteal artery injury must always be kept in mind when evaluating a patient with a tibiofemoral dislocation. Patellar dislocations are lateral. Reduction, if necessary, is performed by extending the knee, flexing the hip, and applying medially-directed pressure to the patella. Immobilization for 4 to 6 weeks follows. Knee dislocations usually produce obvious deformity, as well as a radiographically evident dislocation. Multiligamentous knee injuries are often considered to be "dislocation equivalents," and have neurovascular concerns similar to those of true dislocations. This may be due to a purely ligamentous injury or may involve both ligament disruption and a fracture as might occur from an avulsion injury. Gross knee instability in more than one direction is the key diagnostic finding. A knee dislocation should be reduced emergently and splinted, with careful periodic reexamination of perfusion and sensorimotor function.

Any pulse deficit or measurable reduction in ankle-brachial index, before or after manipulation, should be considered evidence of a vascular injury (Fig. 38-3). If pulse pressures are normal, and the patient's distal circulation can be monitored adequately, routine arteriography is probably not indicated in unstable knee injuries. Stabilization of the knee dislocation is highly advisable at the time of any vascular reconstruction. This can be accomplished simply and quickly with external fixation spanning the knee joint.

Fractures of the Proximal Tibia

Fractures of the tibial plateau are generally due to falls or direct blows, such as when an auto bumper strikes a pedestrian. Displaced fractures involving both condyles of the proximal tibia typically involve extensive soft tissue injury. Many of these fractures occur from less forceful injuries in osteoporotic patients. Medial tibial condyle fractures have a worse prognosis and are associated with injuries to neurovascular structures (Table 38-3).

Whereas routine x-rays are usually adequate for diagnosis, complete characterization of the injury may require a CT scan. Undisplaced proximal tibial fractures can usually be treated with early motion, and delayed weight bearing with a hinged knee brace. Provisional limb stabilization, especially in a multiply injured patient, is best achieved with a bridging external fixator across the knee (Table 38-5). Significant articular surface displacement or knee instability are indications for surgical treatment, generally with open reduction and fixation.

Fractures of the Shaft of the Tibia

Tibial shaft fractures range from low-energy indirect injuries to severe high-energy fractures with extensive closed or open soft tissue damage. Determining the severity of a tibial fracture radiographically is essential for establishing prognosis and planning treatment. Radiographic signs of severe injuries include displacement of more than the shaft diameter, a segmental fracture, or a transverse fracture line. The severity of the soft tissue wound, whether open or closed, is perhaps most important. The amount of muscle damage is much more significant than the size of any skin opening. A small skin wound may be the only external sign of a large cavity of crushed muscle and bone in a leg that has been caught between two automobile bumpers. Compartment syndromes develop in a variable percentage of tibial fractures (Table 38-3) and are more frequent in more severe injuries, including open fractures. Compartment syndromes must be sought immediately and repetitively during the first few days after injury (Fig. 38-2).

Treatment of tibial fractures varies with injury severity and with associated problems. Limb-threatening complications (open wounds, vascular injuries, and compartment syndrome) require prompt surgery (Table 38-5, Fig. 38-1).

In tibial shaft fractures of minor severity, casting is the method of choice. Intramedullary nailing is the fixation of choice for most tibial fractures that need surgical treatment. External fixation remains a valuable technique for selected tibial fractures. It can often be applied more simply than an intramedullary nail and can be used for very proximal and distal fractures of the tibia, particularly when ring fixators are chosen. Plate fixation of acute tibial shaft fractures is also generally reserved for fractures not amenable to intramedullary nailing.

Pilon Fractures

These injuries involve the distal tibial metaphysis and usually its horizontal weight-bearing surface, the articular plafond. The fibula may or may not be involved. Pilon fractures typically involve significant soft tissue damage, whether or not an open wound is present. Calcaneal pin traction, or a bridging external fixator from the midtibia to the foot, can provide stability prior to definitive fracture reduction and fixation (Table 38-5). Severe pilon fractures are very challenging injuries that are treated with either open or external fixation techniques.

Malleolar Ankle Fractures

Malleolar fractures are produced by indirect forces, generally caused by the body's twisting momentum when the foot is planted on the ground. Restoration of the proper relationship between the lateral malleolus and the distal tibia is the key to treating malleolar injuries. Medial ankle disruptions may involve the medial malleolus or the deltoid ligament. The posterior lip of the tibial plafond (posterior malleolus) is frequently fractured in these injuries. The basic principles of treatment remain open reduction of displaced injuries, with anatomic reduction and rigid fixation. If significant displacement or a dislocation is present, prompt closed reduction is urgent, while open reduction and internal fixation can be delayed unless the injury is open or satisfactory closed reduction is impossible. As with pilon fractures, significant swelling is an indication for delay of surgery to decrease complications of wound healing.

Fractures and Dislocations of the Foot

Injuries of the foot may result from a direct blow or crushing force. These injuries may be unrecognized or underestimated, especially in a multiply injured patient (Table 38-6). Compartment syndromes occasionally develop in the foot, and often go unrecognized due to the severe pain that accompanies many foot injuries. A foot compartment release should be performed for any severely swollen foot that has been caused by a crush injury or multiple fractures. Major injuries such as tarsometatarsal dislocations often have subtle x-ray findings (Table 38-6). Undisplaced and extra-articular fractures of the calcaneus can be managed nonoperatively, while displaced fractures are more often operated on, although treatment of this injury remains controversial. Displaced fractures of the talus require precise reduction and rigid fixation. This decreases the risks of avascular necrosis with collapse of the talar body. Isolated, minimally displaced, or undisplaced metatarsal fractures may be treated with immobilization in a stiff shoe, brace, or cast for comfort. Phalangeal fractures generally require little specific treatment. Loss of skin in

TABLE 38-6 Commonly Missed Severe Lower Extremity Injuries

- Sacroiliac joint injury
- Femoral neck fracture, potentially associated with ipsilateral femoral shaft fracture, or hip dislocation.
- Arterial injury, typically associated with ligamentous knee injury or knee dislocation
- Occult open fracture
- Unstable ligamentous injury of knee
- Lisfranc fracture/dislocation
- Compartment syndrome, especially in the foot
- Talar fracture (may need foot as well as ankle x-ray)

the foot is a serious problem and may require free tissue transfer or even amputation.

ADDITIONAL READING

Ciraulo DL, Cowell V, Jacobs L: Evaluation and treatment of the multiple-injured patient, in Browner BD, Jupiter JB, Levine AM, et al (eds): *Skeletal Trauma,* 2nd ed. Philadelphia, WB Saunders, 1998, pp 131-150.

Bosse MJ, Kellam JF: Orthopaedic management decisions in the multiple-trauma patient, in Browner BD, Jupiter JB, Levine AM, et al (eds): *Skeletal Trauma,* 2nd ed. Philadelphia, WB Saunders, 1998, pp 151-164.

Extremity Trauma. Advanced Trauma Life Support Course for Physicians, 6th ed. Chicago, American College of Surgeons, 1997, pp 243-262.

Bosse MJ, MacKenzie EJ, Riemer BL, et al: Adult respiratory distress syndrome, pneumonia, and mortality following thoracic injury and a femoral fracture treated either with intramedullary nailing with reaming or with a plate. A comparative study. *J Bone Joint Surg* 79A:799, 1997.

Butcher JL, MacKenzie EJ, Cushing B, et al: Long-term outcomes after lower extremity trauma. *J Trauma* 41:4, 1996.

39 | Peripheral Vascular Trauma

EPIDEMIOLOGY

In patients treated at urban trauma centers, 80 percent of peripheral vascular injuries are from penetrating wounds (50 to 53 percent gunshot wound; 25 to 28 percent stab wound), 15 percent are from blunt trauma, and 5 percent from other causes (2 to 3 percent iatrogenic). At rural trauma centers, blunt trauma accounts for 40 percent of vascular injuries.

Because of the low wounding power of civilian handguns and improvements in prehospital emergency medical services, there are now more patients treated with truncal vascular injuries (45 to 50 percent of all) than peripheral vascular injuries (37 to 48 percent) in some urban centers. Injuries to the brachial artery in the upper extremity account for 6 to 14 percent of all vascular injuries and 16 to 28 percent of all peripheral vascular injuries in urban centers. Injuries to the femoral artery in the lower extremity account for 7 to 15 percent of all vascular injuries and 19 to 32 percent of all peripheral vascular injuries.

PATHOPHYSIOLOGY

A laceration is the most frequent type of injury to both arteries and veins. It may be a simple puncture wound or may extend obliquely or axially for several centimeters. Transection results in a complete loss of vessel continuity. Injuries between these two extremes are classified as mild when less than 25 percent of the vessel wall is involved, moderate when 25 to 50 percent is involved, and severe when more than 50 percent is involved. Occasionally, the severed arterial ends of a transected vessel will retract and produce proximal and distal thrombosis. Exsanguination can follow either transection or partial transection, especially when associated with a large soft tissue wound. Bleeding can be contained within muscle and fascial compartments to create an acute pulsatile hematoma, which is frequently termed a false aneurysm. If there are contiguous wounds to both the artery and the vein, a direct communication between them can result in an arteriovenous fistula.

Thrombosis interrupts arterial flow and can cause regional ischemia. Pseudoaneurysms compress adjacent structures and may cause pain. In addition, they contain thrombus, which can fragment and embolize distally, producing regional ischemia. Intimal defects may acutely thrombose or be a source of peripheral emboli. Arteriovenous fistulae can cause high-output cardiac failure or lead to chronic arterial or chronic venous insufficiency.

Acute interruption of arterial flow results in regional ischemia in the organ or limb served by the artery. Ischemia occurs because oxygen delivery fails to meet metabolic need. Interruption of flow for relatively short periods of time can result in ischemic neural damage. Because peripheral nerves are so vulnerable to interrupted substrate delivery, neuropathic symptoms (e.g., paresthesias) or neuropathic signs (e.g., the loss of light touch sensation) are often the first to manifest in the patient with an arterial injury. Skeletal muscle, on the other hand, is relatively tolerant to decreased arterial flow. Complete interruption of all arterial inflow (including all arterial collaterals) will result in ischemic damage after 3 hours that can be extended, rather than reversed, by reperfusion.

This "reperfusion" injury is initiated by biochemical events that occur during ischemia. During ischemia, xanthine dehydrogenase is converted to xanthine oxidase. As a result of this conversion hypoxanthine accumulates. When oxygen is reintroduced during reperfusion, the accumulated hypoxanthine is converted to xanthine by xanthine oxidase with the generation of relatively large amounts of superoxide anion, a highly reactive oxygen free radical. Because skeletal muscle contains relatively little xanthine oxidase, the major source of the free radicals producing the reperfusion injury is thought to be the polymorphonuclear leukocyte. Superoxide anion injures the microvascular endothelial membrane by lipid peroxidation. The events associated with reperfusion after complete ischemia can extend the magnitude and severity of the original ischemic insult and lead to a reperfusion injury of the skeletal muscle and the peripheral nerve.

Incomplete interruption of arterial flow with preservation of collaterals will substantially extend the "ischemia" time. Because collateral vessels may provide sufficient nutrient flow to temporarily maintain basal aerobic metabolism and abrogate the conversion of xanthine dehydrogenase to xanthine oxidase, the risk of a reperfusion injury is lessened if they remain patent. If prolonged and severe, ischemia will lead to necrosis of the skeletal muscle, or rhabdomyolysis, which will release potassium and myoglobin into the circulation. Myoglobin, an oxygen-transporting protein similar in structure to hemoglobin, is harmless, but can dissociate into hematin, which is nephrotoxic in an acidic milieu. Myoglobinemia and myoglobinuria in this setting can lead to acute tubular necrosis and renal failure.

DIAGNOSIS

History

A history of pulsatile, bright red bleeding from the wound that ceases after a period of minutes suggests arterial injury, while the history of a steady flow of dark blood from the wound suggests a venous injury. Because peripheral pulses may be palpable in up to 33 percent of patients with arterial injuries, a history suggesting vascular injury may be the most important diagnostic indicator at the time of initial evaluation.

An algorithm for the diagnostic work-up for suspected vascular injury is shown in Fig. 39-1.

Physical Examination

If there is a large, firm, pulsatile hematoma with ill-defined margins surrounding the wound, arterial injury should be suspected. Venous bleeding may also create a tense hematoma, but it will be nonpulsatile. The presence of a thrill or a bruit over a hematoma suggests an associated arteriovenous fistula.

The absence of palpable peripheral pulses and the presence of pallor, poikilothermia, pain, paresthesia or anesthesia, and paralysis are findings indicative of severe ischemia. The most significant of these are the neurologic signs of paresthesia and paralysis, because as discussed earlier, peripheral nerves are very sensitive to anoxia.

Signs *indicative* of ischemia or ongoing hemorrhage, commonly referred to as the "hard" signs (Table 39-1), signify the need for immediate arterial exploration. Signs *suggestive* of vascular injury, but without definite evidence of ischemia or hemorrhage, are called the "soft" signs (Table 39-2). In patients with blunt trauma or multiple penetrating wounds in whom only soft signs are present, diagnostic imaging or noninvasive studies of flow and pressure can be helpful to either confirm or exclude arterial injury.

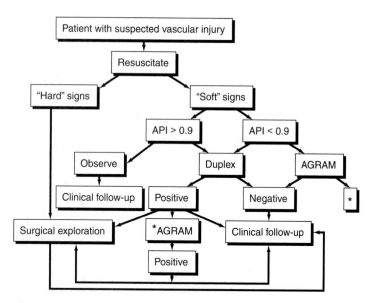

FIG. 39-1. Suggested algorithm for the diagnostic work-up of a patient with suspected vascular injury. "Positive" indicates that the lesion is symptomatic or, in the judgment of a surgeon, has significant likelihood of becoming symptomatic. (API, arterial pressure index; AGRAM, arteriogram; *, reenter algorithm at *AGRAM.)

Noninvasive Studies

Ultrasonic Flow Detection

The lack of enthusiasm for this technology by trauma surgeons has not been entirely inappropriate. First, the diagnostic criteria that apply to chronic occlusive disease cannot be directly extrapolated to acute arterial trauma. Second, wounds and discomfort may restrict application of pressure cuffs at multiple sites, thus limiting use of the flow detector in the measurement of segmental systolic pressure in an injured limb. Third, hemorrhage around vessels may impair transmission of Doppler signals and may limit appropriate interrogation

TABLE 39-1 "Hard" Signs: Physical Findings Indicating the Need for Operative Exploration

Pulsatile bleeding
Expanding hematoma
Palpable thrill
Audible bruit
Evidence of regional ischemia
    Pallor
    Paresthesia
    Paralysis
    Pain
    Pulselessness
    Poikilothermia

TABLE 39-2 "Soft" Signs: Physical Findings Suggestive of the Need for Further Evaluation

History of moderate hemorrhage
Injury (fracture, dislocation, or penetrating wound) in proximity to a
    major artery
Diminished but palpable pulse
Peripheral nerve deficit

of the vessel. Finally, not all trauma surgeons are completely familiar with the technology and have little experience in interpreting the audible signal.

Despite these apparent drawbacks, much can be learned from the hand-held continuous wave ultrasonic flow detector. First, the complete absence of Doppler signals objectively establishes the hard sign of pulselessness, which may be helpful for the inexperienced physician, nurse, or paramedic. Second, the determination of phasic Doppler signals by an experienced examiner provides much qualitative evidence regarding collateral flow. Triphasic signals indicate no significant obstruction, while a low-pitched monophasic signal strongly suggests an obstruction. Third, ultrasonic flow detection allows measurement of the systolic pressure, which can objectively establish the presence and severity of ischemia.

Johansen and colleagues have found the Doppler-determined arterial pressure index (API), determined by dividing the systolic pressure in the injured limb by the systolic pressure in an uninjured arm) to be highly reliable in excluding arterial injury after both blunt and penetrating trauma. They recommend that patients with an API of less than 0.9 undergo contrast angiography. Similar recommendations have been made by others, but with slightly different threshold criteria.

Examination of the analog waveform (obtained by connecting a directional Doppler flow detector to a strip chart recorder) from an injured extremity can provide additional objective information when compared to the uninjured limb. Proximal obstruction will reduce acceleration (decrease the slope) and reduce the peak velocity of forward flow.

Duplex Scanning

Duplex ultrasonography combines real-time B-mode (brightness modulation) ultrasound imaging with a steerable pulsed-Doppler flow detector. It provides the capacity to image a blood vessel and to sample the velocity spectra of the flowing elements in that vessel. When the reflected ultrasound image is processed for direction, amplitude, and frequency, and a Doppler shift frequency is calculated for each pixel in the image, a colorized image can be generated. The addition of color to duplex scanning has been termed "triplex" or color-flow Doppler.

In addition to screening for arterial trauma, duplex scanning has also been utilized to accurately diagnose specific injuries such as thrombosis, pseudo-aneurysm; intimal flap, and arteriovenous fistula.

Arteriography

Similar to noninvasive studies, arteriography may be indicated in patients with signs and symptoms suggestive of vascular injury, but without any evidence of obvious ischemia or ongoing hemorrhage. An exception is the patient with an ischemic extremity that has multiple sites of injury. In such a case, formal arteriography with its inherent delay should be supplanted by either emergency center arteriography or an arteriogram performed on the operating table just prior to exploration. After a scout film of the anticipated field is obtained, the artery to be studied is cannulated with an 18-gauge catheter (antegrade in the common femoral; prograde in the axillary or brachial) and 20 to 50 mL of contrast is injected. For visualization of more distal (popliteal or tibial) arteries, exposure should be delayed for several seconds after the contrast injection. The use of fluoroscopy, especially if equipped with subtraction capability, greatly simplifies the technique because it takes the guesswork out of coordinating the timing of the injection with the timing of the exposure. This is particularly useful for imaging of the distal vessels in which the appearance of contrast may be quite delayed.

A positive interpretation means that the arteriogram revealed one of the following abnormalities, which may or may not have clinical significance depending on the artery injured: occlusion, extravasation, pseudoaneurysm, arteriovenous fistula, intimal flap, intimal irregularity, spasm, or extraluminal compression. The clinical significance of any abnormal finding should be determined by the surgeon, who must *always* review the arteriograms with the angiographer, and based on available studies, proximity should no longer be considered as the *sole* indication for arteriography.

Arteriography is not without risks. Complications occur in 2 to 4 percent of patients. Most are minor, such as groin hematomas, and have no significant impact on care. Major complications such as iatrogenic embolic occlusion or iatrogenic pseudoaneurysm occur in up to 0.6 percent of patients. Further, there is an inherent delay in obtaining a formal arteriogram.

Digital Contrast Studies

Intra-arterial digital subtraction arteriography (IADSA) has a sensitivity and specificity similar to arteriography and has several advantages, including a shorter time to complete the examination, less exposure to radiation, reduced cost, reduced dye load, and less discomfort.

Venography

Life- or limb-threatening venous injuries are usually readily apparent or are associated with significant arterial injuries. As such, venography is seldom needed or indicated, and may be hazardous if it delays the treatment of more severe injuries.

Summary of the Diagnostic Approach

In the patient with hard signs, physical examination is highly reliable and no other diagnostic tests are needed. In the patient with soft signs, additional diagnostic studies *may* be needed, but each of these tests has limitations in terms of accuracy, morbidity, and resource utilization.

MANAGEMENT

Nonoperative

Observation

A substantial body of clinical and laboratory evidence now exists showing that some arterial injuries will remain asymptomatic and some will progressively heal. These reports have led to the selective use of nonoperative observation in the management of *angiographically* demonstrated arterial lesions, such as intimal flaps, intimal defects, pseudoaneurysm, and arteriovenous fistulae.

Current clinical and experimental evidence would suggest the following criteria for nonoperative management of asymptomatic patients with soft signs: (1) low-velocity injury, particularly a stab wound or iatrogenic puncture wound; (2) minimal (<5 mm) intimal defect; (3) small (<5 mm) pseudoaneurysm; (4) intact distal circulation; and (5) a compliant patient likely to understand the need for compulsive follow-up. Follow-up must include frequent physical examination and objective assessment of both the anatomy and the flow characteristics of the injured artery and the distal arterial bed. Carefully performed noninvasive studies coupled with duplex imaging are mandatory for adequate follow-up.

The use of adjuvant medical therapy, such as antiplatelet agents or anticoagulants, in patients managed nonoperatively has not been extensively studied. Although the use of such agents may seem intuitively advantageous, they are not without risk of bleeding. Thus their use should be individualized.

Ultrasound-Guided Therapy

Recent reports have documented the success of color flow duplex-guided compression of iatrogenic postcatheterization pseudoaneurysms of the femoral artery. The success rate of this modality has been 70 to 90 percent. Pseudoaneurysms of less than 3 cm in diameter are likely to close spontaneously within 4 weeks and require simple follow-up with ultrasound rather than therapy.

Postcatheterization femoral pseudoaneurysms can be treated using ultrasound-guided thrombin injection, as well. Large pseudoaneurysms (>3 cm in diameter) and those associated with arteriovenous fistulae have been effectively thrombosed in a matter of seconds with the injection of 0.5 to 1.0 mL of thrombin solution (1000 U/mL).

Endovascular Management

Therapeutic embolization and balloon or coil insertion under angiographic control, have been utilized to control hemorrhage and to treat arteriovenous fistulae and pseudoaneurysms. Intra-arterial pharmacotherapy has been used to treat severe vasospasm in small distal vessels.

Synthetic grafts sutured to balloon expandable stents (stent graft) can be introduced from a remote site where they are fluoroscopically directed to a site of injury. Endovascular grafting is likely to have its most frequent application in stable patients with delayed presentation who have a complex pseudoaneurysm or arteriovenous fistula.

Operative Management: General Principles

External bleeding must be controlled with digital pressure or compressive bandages. Temporary and intermittent use of a tourniquet should be a last resort to control exsanguinating hemorrhage. The importance of rapid resuscitation and treatment of shock cannot be overemphasized. Continuation of resuscitation may be necessary in the operating room, where urgent operations for associated life-threatening injuries can be appropriately timed.

Broad-spectrum antibiotics should be started as soon as possible after injury and continued for a minimum of 3 to 5 days depending on the degree of contamination and the amount of soft tissue injury. Patients with moderate contamination of open fractures and those with gunshot wounds should also receive tetanus prophylaxis. When there is advanced ischemia in an extremity and there is no evidence of intracranial injury or cavitary hemorrhage, consideration should be given to the administration of heparin in doses sufficient to produce systemic anticoagulation.

Preparation of the skin and draping of an entire *uninjured* extremity should be done to allow for the excision of a segment of superficial vein (cephalic in the upper extremity; greater or lesser saphenous in the lower) if needed for use as a vascular conduit. It is also helpful to prepare and drape the hand or foot of the injured extremity in order to evaluate pulses and color changes when an arterial repair is completed and perfusion re-established.

Immediate Amputation

There is a small group of patients who present with vascular disruption in combination with severe open, comminuted fractures and moderate loss of soft tissue. These "mangled limbs," usually produced by mechanisms of high-energy transfer or crush, are associated with a high morbidity and a poor prognosis in terms of function and often require late amputation (27 to 70 percent) despite initial limb salvage.

Objective scoring systems for use at the time of initial evaluation may assist in predicting ultimate amputation. Most systems combine an assessment of the individual components of the injury (soft tissue, bone, vascular, and nerve) with an evaluation of premorbid factors (age >40 years, associated illness) and an estimate of systemic and regional perturbation (presence of shock or prolonged limb ischemia).

Obtaining Vascular Control

The first operative priority is to obtain proximal and distal control of the injured vessel. This is best done, if possible, in uninjured tissue adjacent to the injury site using elective surgical incisions following the course of the injured vessel. If the patient is exsanguinating through a laceration or penetrating injury, control is often best obtained in this situation by direct means through the wound.

Occasionally, direct control of the vessel cannot be obtained quickly because of the distorted anatomy or because continuing hemorrhage obstructs the operator's vision. In this situation, bleeding can be controlled by inserting a balloon-tipped catheter into the open end of the vessel and inflating the balloon. Vessel obturation by balloon tamponade will provide a relatively dry field and allow careful dissection of the proximal and distal arteries.

Intraluminal Shunts

There are occasional instances when definitive treatment of an injured limb must be deferred because the life of a patient is endangered by systemic problems such as metabolic acidosis, hypothermia, or a coagulopathy. Similarly, orthopedic stabilization may preempt the vascular repair, potentially prolonging the time of warm ischemia past the "golden period" of 6 hours. In such circumstances, the insertion of a temporary shunt into the lumen of an injured artery or vein to maintain blood flow will ensure viability of the extremity until the patient or the fractures are stable. The intraluminal shunt can also be used while an amputated limb is being evaluated for replantation.

Techniques of Arterial and Venous Repair

Once proximal and distal control are obtained, the extent of the injury to both the artery and vein should be determined. Before definitive arterial repair, one must be assured that any thrombus that may have accumulated in either the proximal or distal artery during the period of ischemia is removed. As previously noted, thrombus can be removed using a balloon-tipped catheter, which is gently passed through until resistance is met. Extraction of the catheter is then begun *before* the balloon is inflated. Then, as the catheter is being *slowly* removed, the balloon is inflated just enough to cause the slightest resistance. Overinflation must be avoided because it may produce arterial injury. Immediately after thrombectomy, heparin should be instilled proximally and distally ("regional" heparinization with 15 to 30 mL of a solution of 50 to 100 U/mL).

It is recommended that the debridement of injured vessels and subsequent vascular repair be performed under loupe magnification ($2.5\times$) using coaxial lighting (headlamp). When arterial repair is performed, adjuncts such as small vascular clamps and forceps, as well as fine synthetic monofilament sutures (5-0 polypropylene for larger arteries such as the femoral or axillary, 6-0 or 7-0 for smaller arteries such as the popliteal or brachial arteries) on small atraumatic needles, are most valuable.

Lateral arteriorrhaphy is only recommended for repairing small puncture wounds or small iatrogenic lacerations that do not require debridement. These injuries can be closed by one or more interrupted sutures, placing each suture approximately 1 mm from the edge of the arterial laceration and 1 mm from the previous suture. To prevent constriction at the site of a lateral arteriorrhaphy, a patch of autogenous vein may be employed.

More extensive injury to the arterial wall that requires a segmental resection can occasionally be repaired using an end-to-end anastomosis. In the brachial and superficial femoral arteries, it is possible to perform an end-to-end anastomosis even after the loss of several centimeters of the original length of the artery. This will require significant mobilization of the proximal and distal artery, however, to avoid creating undue tension on the suture line. Major collaterals should not be interrupted to achieve sufficient length. If flexion of the joint is used during exposure of the vascular injury, the extremity should be returned to a straight position prior to the repair to ensure that there is adequate proximal and distal length to perform an end-to-end anastomosis.

Recently, interposition grafts have been used more frequently in both the military and civilian experience (Table 39-3). With contaminated wounds autologous greater saphenous vein from an uninjured lower extremity has been successfully used for many years with good long-term results, and remains the conduit of choice. The lesser saphenous and the cephalic are also acceptable. There are instances when autologous vein is not available or is of inadequate luminal size or quality. In such a situation, both Dacron® and poly-tetrafluoroethylene (PTFE) have been used successfully as synthetic conduits in replacing missing arterial and venous segments. Although the long-term patency rate appears to be less with synthetic conduits, previous concerns about infection have not been realized.

Completion arteriography should be performed in the operating room with the repair exposed. Arteriography allows one to evaluate the integrity of the repair, visualize arterial runoff, ensure that there are no additional vascular

TABLE 39-3 Method of Management of Acute Major Arterial Injuries in Vietnam and Recent Civilian Experience

Method	VNVR	Civilian
Autogenous interposition graft	462 (46.2%)	240 (39.3%)
End-to-end anastomosis	377 (37.7%)	115 (18.8%)
Lateral suture	87 (8.7%)	59 (9.7%)
Prosthetic interposition graft	4 (0.4%)	78 (12.8%)
Vein patch angioplasty	0 (0%)	23 (3.7%)
Questionable	55 (1.5%)	0 (0%)
Ligation	15 (1.5%)	96 (15.7%)
Total	1000 (100%)	611 (100%)

VNVR, Vietnam Vascular Registry.

injuries, and verify that no residual thrombus or embolus remains distal to the repair.

When faced with combined arterial and venous injury, the decision to repair the vein depends on the condition of the patient and the condition of the vein. If the patient is hemodynamically or metabolically unstable (acidotic, coagulopathic, hypothermic), controlling hemorrhage and preventing exsanguination is the priority and simple lateral venorrhaphy or ligation is the prudent choice. Venous ligation is always preferred in the upper extremity when the injury occurs distal to the axilla.

When the patient is metabolically stable, it is prudent to repair major veins when ligation would significantly impair venous drainage (i.e., popliteal, common femoral, or external iliac). The techniques are similar to those employed in the repair of arteries and include simple venorrhaphy, end-to-end anastomosis, vein patch grafting (where lateral venorrhaphy would compromise vein diameter) and autologous vein or PTFE interposition. Compilation grafts (creating a large venous conduit with a panel graft) and spiral vein grafts are reserved for common femoral and iliac injuries. Postoperatively, the injured extremity should be elevated and the venous repair monitored closely with either color Doppler or continuous-wave Doppler. If thrombosis of the repair is detected and there are no contraindications, the patient should be anticoagulated with heparin and converted to warfarin (coumadin). Anticoagulation should be maintained for a minimum of 3 months.

Management of the Wound

Copious irrigation of the wound with saline and antibiotic solution and debridement of all devitalized tissue and foreign material are essential to reduce the risk of postoperative infection.

Vascular repairs should be covered at the initial operation to prevent desiccation and infection. Large defects with an exposed vascular graft should be closed with vascularized tissue, preferably a transposed muscle flap or a free-tissue (muscular or myocutaneous) transfer. Local fasciocutaneous flaps have also been used. Rarely, the soft tissue defect will be so enormous that a local flap or free tissue transfer will be inadequate to completely cover the vascular repair. In such circumstances, the application of a porcine skin xenograft or cadaveric homograft to the wound has been successful. Extra-anatomic bypass of large defects is also a consideration, especially when there is extensive contamination or a graft infection has occurred.

Fasciotomy

A compartment syndrome is a common occurrence after trauma to an extremity. As described previously, reperfusion of the ischemic extremity plays a major role in the development of compartment syndrome. As such, the classic clinical findings may be absent prior to the vascular repair and may not appear until after the extremity has been reperfused. Once the diagnosis of a compartment syndrome is made, expeditious fasciotomy is necessary to relieve elevated compartmental pressure and prevent the sequela of neuromuscular disability.

The potential for development of a compartment syndrome after vascular trauma should be kept in mind. Although history and physical examination are helpful, the common clinical findings of paresthesia and paralysis are not sensitive and, when present, may indicate irreversible neuromuscular damage. Occasionally, because of an associated intracranial injury or drug ingestion, the physical examination is unreliable. In addition, the patient may have the need for prolonged anesthesia after a vascular repair to treat associated injuries, and repetitive physical examinations are impossible. After recovery from anesthesia, the clinical findings may become obvious, necessitating a second anesthetic for fasciotomy.

Items in the history that suggest the need for fasciotomy include a prolonged delay between injury and arterial repair and an episode of significant hypotension in the preoperative period. Hypotension reduces the "delta" pressure (difference between the mean arterial pressure and the compartmental pressure), and a reduced delta pressure has been associated with a depletion of high-energy phosphates and increased muscle damage. Operative findings suggesting the need for fasciotomy include massive preoperative swelling of the calf, associated crush injury, combined arterial and venous injuries, or the performance of a major venous ligation in the popliteal or femoral area.

The measurement of compartmental pressure is invaluable when doubt exists about the diagnosis or when physical examination is unreliable or cannot be performed. Normal intracompartmental pressure is less than 10 mm Hg. Although the threshold level of compartmental hypertension necessitating fasciotomy is controversial, it is generally agreed that a pressure of 30 mm Hg is abnormal and requires either fasciotomy or continuous monitoring. Fasciotomy should be performed *before* arterial exploration when an obvious compartment syndrome exists or when intracompartmental pressures are significantly elevated (>30 mm Hg) prior to reperfusion. In such instances, fasciotomies in the distal extremity can be performed rapidly and may be invaluable in preventing subsequent neurologic disability. The two-incision, four-compartment fasciotomy technique can be performed quickly and safely and is used by most trauma surgeons.

Role of Sympathectomy and Intra-arterial Vasodilators

On rare occasions when distal spasm threatens the viability of a limb, lumbar sympathectomy of the injured extremity should be considered, as laboratory data suggest that significant improvements in distal flow may be obtained in nonatherosclerotic vessels. An alternative approach is to infuse a mixture of 1000 mL normal saline containing 1000 units of heparin and 500 mg tolazoline into a major proximal artery at 30 mL/h.

Managing Combined Orthopedic and Vascular Injuries

Priorities in such situations should be established jointly by the vascular and orthopedic surgeons after a complete discussion of the nature of the combined injuries and duration of the planned repair of both the arterial and orthopedic injuries. If the fracture–dislocation is extremely unstable and will require extensive manipulation to achieve reduction and alignment, it is best to insert an intraluminal shunt and proceed with stabilization. During the orthopedic procedure, the vascular surgeon should continually monitor the integrity and patency of the shunt.

Managing Pediatric Vascular Injuries

Attempts at diagnosis should initially be made noninvasively, because arteriography has the potential of further injury. Arterial repair of major arteries should be undertaken to avoid growth retardation.

POSTOPERATIVE CARE

After systemic perfusion has been ensured, continual reassessment of the distal circulation in the injured extremity cannot be overemphasized. Frequently, peripheral pulses are not immediately palpable in either the injured or uninjured extremities. In such instances, the distal circulation can be evaluated by examining capillary refilling or comparing segmental Doppler pressures or transcutaneous PO_2 between the injured and uninjured limbs.

Elevation of the extremity will reduce the edema that accompanies resuscitation and reperfusion. Splinting of the extremities can be useful in preventing sudden movements that will stress vascular repairs.

Antibiotics should be given for at least 3 days. The presence of wound contamination or an open fracture mandates a longer duration of administration. The use of postoperative heparin should be avoided, particularly in patients with multiple injuries who might develop bleeding from other locations. The use of low molecular weight dextran, however, has been helpful in maintaining the patency of small arterial and venous repairs. Aspirin, which will decrease platelet adhesiveness, can also be given by suppository immediately after surgery when the patient can take nothing by mouth.

COMPLICATIONS

Disappearance of a pulse suggests the development of thrombus at the site of the arterial repair, whereas the rapid development of edema in the extremity may be associated with thrombosis at the site of the venous repair. A return to the operating room to perform a thrombectomy may once again secure a good result. If an arterial thrombosis occurs several days later and it is obvious that there is sufficient collateral blood flow to maintain viability of the extremity, revascularization may be performed at a later time.

Infection at the site of vascular repair is a dreaded complication that usually leads to ligation of the involved vessel. If ligation is required and it is obvious that the distal extremity will develop gangrene, an extra-anatomic bypass may be required. The graft, preferably autologous vein, can be placed subcutaneously or brought through a muscular tunnel.

Delayed complications of stenosis or late thrombosis can occur. In addition, some injuries deemed insignificant or frankly missed at the initial evalu-

TABLE 39-4 Factors Associated with Improved Limb Salvage After Vascular Trauma

Rapid prehospital transport
Penetrating injury with minimal soft tissue injury
Prompt diagnosis
Aggressive management
Earlier reperfusion using intraluminal shunts
Earlier stabilization of fractures
Venous repair
Liberal use of interposition grafts
Aggressive wound debridement
Immediate vascularized coverage
Liberal use of fasciotomy
Completion arteriography

ation may become symptomatic. Most common among the delayed injuries are a pseudoaneurysm or an arteriovenous fistula.

Although the experience with endovascular treatment is not large, it is growing and holds great promise for the management of these lesions. Finally, aneurysmal changes may occur in some autologous saphenous vein grafts used as arterial conduits, and intimal hyperplasia can develop at valve cusps or suture lines.

Chronic venous insufficiency has now been recognized in an increasing number of patients who have had four-compartment fasciotomy. The severity of symptoms is related to the elapsed time after fasciotomy and is probably due to a reduction in the efficiency of the calf muscle pump.

OUTCOME

The mortality rate following peripheral vascular trauma is low, with no fatalities reported in some series. The low mortality rate can be attributed to rapid and efficient prehospital care and transport, aggressive resuscitation, and expeditious diagnosis and treatment.

The amputation rate following peripheral vascular trauma continues to decrease. Early amputation, when it does occur, appears to be related to prolonged ischemia, but is clearly multifactorial. Late amputation is primarily done for disability or continued infection.

ADDITIONAL READING

Bondurant FJ, Cotler HB, Buckle R, et al: The medical and economic impact of severely injured lower extremities. *J Trauma* 28:1270, 1988.

Dennis JW, Fryberg ER, Veldenz HC, et al: Validation of nonoperative management of occult vascular injuries and accuracy of physical examination alone in penetrating extremity trauma: five to ten year follow-up. *J Trauma* 44:243, 1998.

Feliciano DV, Herskowitz K, O'Gorman RB, et al: Management of vascular injuries in the lower extremities. *J Trauma* 28:319, 1988.

Frykberg ER, Dennis JW, Bishop K, et al: The reliability of physical examination in the evaluation of penetrating extremity trauma for vascular injury: results at one year. *J Trauma* 31:502, 1991.

Johansen J, Lynch K, Paun M, et al: Non-invasive vascular tests reliably exclude occult arterial trauma in injured extremities. *J Trauma* 31:515, 1991.

In the last decade, there has been a tremendous revolution in repair and reconstruction after injuries to the musculoskeletal system. In spite of many technical advances, including intraoperative magnification, improved materials for suturing or bonding nerve ends, and perioperative monitoring, there has been very little improvement in the overall functional results after repair of peripheral nerves in recent years.

MICRONEURAL ANATOMY

The three basic elements of the peripheral nerves are the epineurium, perineurium, and endoneurium. The *external epineurium* contains collagenous tissues that surround the entire nerve. The *internal epineurium,* thickened in response to greater compressive forces where it crosses a joint, is an extension of the external epineurium, and surrounds the nerve fascicles to cushion them. The *perineurium,* an extension of the blood-brain barrier which lines the individual fascicles, is composed of closely packed cells united by tight junctions that control intercellular diffusion, maintain a positive intrafascicular pressure, and protect against infection. The *endoneurium* surrounds the individual axons and forms the structural component of the Schwann cell tube.

Fascicles are groups of axons within a perineurial sleeve, while anatomic *fascicular groups* are formed by condensations of internal epineurium. Interconnections between the fascicles form a *fascicular plexus.* While these interconnections are abundant in the proximal portions of peripheral nerves, they are fewer in number distally and provide for consistent neuroanatomy in the distal extremities. This, of course, aids the surgeon in aligning fascicles during repair. Because adjacent fascicles innervate sites in the extremities that are in close proximity, efforts to accurately align the nerves should result in more accurate reinnervation and better functional outcomes.

FUNCTION OF PERIPHERAL NERVES

Conduction of nerve impulses relies on the sodium-potassium (Na^+-K^+) pump on the inside of the cell membrane. The motor unit is made up of the neuron, its axons, and all the muscle fibers that it innervates (varying from 10 to 1000). The impulse is transmitted across the motor endplate by the neurotransmitter acetylcholine (ACh).

Fast antegrade transport is the movement of membrane-enclosed vesicles away from the neuron down the "railroad track" of microtubules (at a rate of 400 mm/d) while *slow antegrade transport* carries cytoskeletal elements at 0.5 mm/d. *Fast retrograde transport* returns scavenged components to the neuron.

The key organelles for sensation in the upper extremity are rapidly adapting Meissner corpuscles (which are suited for moving two-point discrimination) and pacinian corpuscles (which respond to constant touch or pressure), and the slower-adapting Merkel cells (which perceive static two-point discrimination).

NERVE DEGENERATION AND REGENERATION

Immediately after a nerve has been injured, a process of *wallerian degeneration* begins at the first node of Ranvier that is intact. Phagocytosis of the Schwann cell tube prevents obstruction of the regenerating axons. The proximal nerve end sends sprouts or axonal buds that form the regenerating nerve growth cone. This process is affected by a variety of growth factors and cytokines. Nerve growth factor can stimulate wallerian degeneration, increase neuronal activity, and enhance the rate of regeneration of sensory axons, but not motor axons. Calcium-activated neutral protease (calpain) disrupts the cytoskeletal elements of the motor endplates. Leupeptin inhibits the action of this protease and has been shown to enhance nerve regeneration by preventing the degradation of the receptors in skeletal muscle in laboratory animals.

Neurotrophism is the directed axon growth through a gradient of diffusible substances produced by the target (the distal end of the nerve). Motor axons send multiple buds per axon and show a preference for neural tissue, while aberrant sensory sprouts are eliminated during regeneration. The size of the distal fascicle appears to be the most important factor in determining the target of the regenerating growth cone.

DIAGNOSTIC STUDIES OF NERVE FUNCTION

Clinical Tests of Sensory Function in Peripheral Nerves

Threshold testing using Semmes-Weinstein monofilaments is the most sensitive test for nerve compression syndromes in which the number of functioning receptors is normal, but their level of activation is depressed. Both the moving two-point and static two-point tests require substantial cortical re-innervation and are best performed in patients who have a nearly complete sensory recovery after injury to a peripheral nerve.

Clinical Test of Motor Function in Peripheral Nerves

The British Medical Research Council (BMRC) devised a subjective staged level of motor recovery as follows: M0 = no muscle activity; M1 = contraction without movement; M2 = movement of extremity but not against gravity; M3 = movement against gravity; M4 = enough strength to move against gravity and additional resistance, but not normal strength; and M5 = normal strength.

Quantitative measurement of strength allows comparison of different techniques of neural repair. The force of an isolated muscle group is quantified using a load cell to determine the strength of the muscle group in the affected hand as a percentage of the uninjured extremity.

Laboratory Tests of Nerve Function

A 1 percent decrease in *nerve conduction velocity* (NCV) across a localized region (e.g., the carpal tunnel), or conversely, an increase in the delay or latency, indicates significant external compression producing partial nerve ischemia and is the most sensitive laboratory test to document a nerve compression syndrome. Injuries that disrupt all or a part of the nerve, or severe nerve compression syndromes, produce electromyographic (EMG) changes approximately 3 weeks after the injury.

Typically, if a stimulus is applied to a peripheral nerve such as the ulnar nerve, a signal can be recorded from a scalp electrode in the contralateral sensory cortex, known as a *somatosensory evoked potential* (SSEP). A disruption anywhere along the sensory pathway will result in a failure to detect a signal whether the injury is preganglionic or postganglionic. Preganglionic injuries, however, will demonstrate normal conduction velocities because the pathway from the neuron to sensory organelles in the skin is intact.

For magnetic resonance imaging (MRI) neurograms, the loss of T2-weighted signals indicates damage to the myelin sheath and the loss of water content in muscles, suggesting denervation.

CLASSIFICATION OF INJURIES TO NERVES

In the Sunderland classification, the following terminology and definitions are used.

Neuropraxia—a localized conduction block without axonal disruption. Tinel's sign is not present and complete recovery should occur.
Isolated axonotmesis—the axon is disrupted, but the Schwann cell tubes are intact. Wallerian degeneration occurs distal to the site of injury, and recovery is usually complete if the lesion is not too proximal for successful reinnervation.
Axonal injury with endoneurial scarring—the nerve is in continuity, but there is enough disruption of the axons that incorrect reinnervation occurs leading to a partial recovery, but one that is better than with excision and end-to-end repair.
Neuroma in continuity—the nerve sheath is intact, but the axons have been disrupted and there is scarring across the nerve. The treatment is excision and repair by end-to-end coaptation or interposition nerve grafting.
Neurotmesis—the nerve is completely divided and repair is required.
A combination of the above injuries may exist within a single nerve.

In the Seddon classification, the three categories are neuropraxia (same as above), axonotmesis (same as above), and neurotmesis (same as above plus neuroma in continuity).

SURGICAL APPROACHES TO INJURIES TO THE BRACHIAL PLEXUS AND ITS BRANCHES
Brachial Plexus

The brachial plexus is composed of the C5 through T1 nerve roots in the majority of cases. The most common type of injury is one involving a motor-cycle or bicycle crash in which forceful impact on the shoulder depresses the entire shoulder girdle and avulses a portion of the brachial plexus, usually injuring the upper trunk.

The sensory fibers of the brachial plexus are derived from the dorsal root ganglia lying outside the spinal cord, while the motor fibers are derived from the anterior horn cells of the spinal cord. Therefore it is quite common to have an injury with a preganglionic or central nervous system lesion—an injury proximal to the dorsal root ganglion, but outside the spinal cord—and a post-ganglionic or peripheral nerve injury of the motor nerve fibers. Preganglionic injuries can be associated with Horner's syndrome. Because preganglionic injuries do not regenerate, only the more distal postganglionic (peripheral nerve) injuries undergo repair.

Diagnosis

Diagnosis of an injury to the brachial plexus is suggested by the following: (1) elevation of the diaphragm on chest x-ray; (2) denervation of the cervical paraspinal muscles on EMG; (3) magnetic resonance neurogram demonstrating loss of signal of the proximal nerve trunks and the spinal roots; (4) cervical myelogram with myelomeningoceles; and (5) SSEPs showing disruption of sensory pathways.

Treatment

For postganglionic lesions, it is important to determine whether the lesion is complete or partial. The current recommendation is for exploration without delay when a complete lesion is documented using NCV and EMG testing to detect muscle denervation, usually 3 weeks after injury. Incomplete lesions can be explored and repaired if the entire upper or middle trunk of the brachial plexus has been injured.

One of the important goals of brachial plexus surgery is to restore elbow flexion in patients who have useful hand function. Exploration of the brachial plexus in patients with only partial neurologic deficit and functional hand and elbow flexion is not indicated. In such a case it is impossible to accurately isolate the injured portion without damaging functional portions of the brachial plexus. Lesions of the lower trunk are not amenable to repair because the distance of about 30 inches between the site of injury (the lower trunk in the cervical region) and the end organ (the intrinsic muscles in the hand) is too great for successful reinnervation. Nerves can regenerate for up to 18 months at a rate of 1 inch per month, for a total of 18 inches.

Median Nerve

The median nerve can be exposed with a medial incision in the arm, which then crosses the antecubital fossa transversely to extend longitudinally between the interval of the flexor carpi radialis (FCR) and the brachioradialis (BR). In the forearm, this allows exposure of the nerve using the internervous plane between the radial nerve and the median nerve-innervated FCR.

Ulnar Nerve

The medial intermuscular septum between the biceps and triceps is divided to expose the ulnar nerve. The incision is carried out posterior to the midaxial line to avoid injury to branches of the medial cutaneous nerve of the arm and the medial antebrachial nerves, which are both branches directly off the medial cord of the brachial plexus. The incision is continued posterior to the flexor carpi ulnaris (FCU), because the ulnar nerve travels beneath the FCU during its course in the forearm. In the palm, the approach to the carpal tunnel can be used to expose Guyon's canal, the ulnar nerve, and the superficial palmar arch.

Fifteen percent of patients have interconnections between the median and ulnar nerves (known as Martin-Gruber interconnections at the level of the forearm, and the more rare Riche-Cannieu interconnection in the palm). In both of these interconnections, the median nerve has received nerve fibers providing the innervation to the intrinsic muscles in the hand normally supplied by the ulnar nerve. The Martin-Gruber interconnection generally involves branches connecting between the anterior interosseous nerve and the ulnar nerve. These connections can explain why a patient who has a laceration of the ulnar nerve at the elbow still has the ability to use the intrinsic ulnar muscles in the hand.

Proximal injuries of the ulnar nerve have a very poor prognosis because the nerve can only regenerate 2.5 cm (1 inch) per month for a total of 12 to 18 months, for a total of 45 cm in an adult.

Radial Nerve

The radial nerve is best exposed by a posterior incision along the arm, with the patient placed in the prone position. Proximally, the incision exposes the nerve exiting from the posterior triangle, then splits the triceps to expose the nerve in the spiral groove before curving anteriorly to expose the radial nerve in the interval between the brachialis and brachioradialis muscle. At the level of the forearm, the posterior or Thompson's approach is recommended for exposure of the posterior interosseous nerve. This approach involves exposing the interval between the extensor digitorum minimi and the extensor carpi radialis brevis. This allows for exposure of the supinator muscle, which can be divided to expose the branches of the posterior interosseous nerve.

OPERATIVE REPAIR OF INJURIES TO PERIPHERAL NERVES

Primary Repair

Epineural repair involves simply suturing the external epineurium of the nerve. This technique works well for a sharp laceration with no loss of nerve substance and for partial nerve lacerations of the nerve when the proper alignment is already established. *Group fascicular repairs* work best when there has been a crushing component to the nerve injury or a delayed repair requiring the trimming of a portion of the nerve ends. *Fascicular repair* is not widely used because of the increased amount of suture material required at the site of repair and the difficulty of confirming the individual fascicle alignment. For most cases of isolated injury to a peripheral nerve, the use of fine nylon suture (8-0 nylon for a peripheral nerve; 10-0 for a digital nerve) is appropriate. The use of fibrin glue is most helpful when multiple cable grafts are required, as with repairs of the brachial plexus.

Secondary Repair: Overcoming Defects in Injured Peripheral Nerves

Shortening of bone is limited to use in the arm, and is most suitable for the repair of injuries to the radial nerve when there has been a delayed union or nonunion of an associated injury to the humerus. The technique is not used in the lower extremity because even one-half to one inch of shortening will result in a symptomatic alteration in adult gait. Transposition of the nerve for ulnar nerve injuries near the elbow is ideal for secondary repair when combined with elbow flexion. Joint positioning is one of the most successful means of obtaining increased length for nerve repair. The closer the nerve injury is to the joint, the more successful the joint positioning will be. Elongation or stretching of a peripheral nerve using these techniques can result in a 10 percent increase in available length, but an injured nerve can lose up to 8 percent of its length within 3 weeks of injury. The blood supply to the nerve, and not the strength of the suture, is the limiting factor in determining how much elongation a nerve can withstand. The blood flow to the nerve is inversely proportional to the applied tension. At 12 to 15 percent elongation of the nerve, blood flow decreases to approximately 30 percent of baseline and severe ischemia results. Injured nerves demonstrate a threefold increase in blood flow as part of the reparative process.

Nerve Grafts

Although there are reports of use of a variety of nerve grafts before the 20th century, the clinical use of nerve grafts was popularized by Bunnell for digital nerves in the upper extremity and by Duel for grafting of the facial nerve. The sural nerve is the gold standard for nerve autografts because of its favorable ratio of axons to epineurium, and because the loss of the nerve produces only a small area of sensory loss on the lateral side of the foot, which is generally well tolerated.

Because the supply of autograft nerve is limited, research has focused on the use of allograft nerves. Studies have confirmed that nerve grafts can survive if the patient is immunosuppressed, if tissue typing has been performed, and if the nerve allograft has been preserved to maintain cell viability. Once the nerve graft has become incorporated with an ingrowth of Schwann cells from the host nerve ends, immunosuppression no longer appears to be required on a permanent basis. Because the results for nerve autografts remain slightly superior, nerve allografts are limited primarily to clinical research investigations.

Group fascicular repairs are favored because the sural nerve graft is approximately the size of the fascicular group of most mixed motor and sensory nerves in the extremities. For both sensory and motor nerves, functional results after grafting decrease with increasing delays and increasing graft length. Optimum results are obtained with delays of less than 3 weeks from the time of injury, and with grafts that are 5 cm or less in length.

Artificial Conduits

Several investigators have evaluated the use of permanent or biodegradable artificial conduits with or without the impregnation of growth factors to "direct" nerve regeneration. Conventional autografts remain superior to these constructs.

RESULTS OF REPAIR

Eventual recovery of neural function after repair of a peripheral nerve depends in large measure on the overall status of the extremity. Significant associated injuries to the skin, muscle, tendons, and bony structures will jeopardize functional recovery by hampering reinnervation and increasing the formation of scar tissue, which adversely affects nerve healing. Interfascicular nerve repair is associated with approximately 70 to 100 percent return of sensation throughout an anesthetic area and 30 to 60 percent return of two-point discrimination. Epineural suturing has a reported 46 to 82 percent return of sensation, but only a 4 to 25 percent return of two-point discrimination.

NEUROMAS

Terminal Neuromas

By definition, every unrepaired laceration or avulsion of a nerve will produce a neuroma (disorganized axonal regeneration), which in areas with very little soft-tissue coverage can be so painful that the patient's hand or foot cannot be used.

Excision of a neuroma and repair can be very successful when both nerve ends can be identified and when the repair can be buried under ample soft tissue to provide the necessary mechanical padding. An alternative approach is to bury the neuroma, usually in muscle. The overall success rate for primary and revision attempts at burying or capping a neuroma with a piece of Silastic is 75 percent (but care must be taken because any Silastic debris can lead to a foreign body reaction). For neuromas in more inaccessible locations, proximal ligation of the nerve in combination with moving the neuroma to a more padded area may be useful.

Neuromas in Continuity

Dissection of the nerve proximal and distal to the site of repair separates the intact motor fibers from the disrupted sensory fibers, which is confirmed by electrical stimulation before resecting and grafting the neuroma.

Less symptomatic neuromas are those in which motor fibers are disrupted but sensory axons are in continuity, and these can be treated with tendon transfers in the upper extremity without exploring the neuroma.

SUMMARY

Achieving satisfactory functional recovery after injury to peripheral nerves in adults remains a significant challenge for reconstructive surgeons, and it is important to take every opportunity to optimize the patient's recovery after such an injury. It is critical to avoid delaying nerve repair in order to reduce the need for nerve grafts, and to allow the nerve the maximal time for regeneration of motor axons. The astute surgeon will help the patient with an acute and timely repair, proper rehabilitation to avoid losing joint mobility during nerve regeneration, and careful combinations of techniques to restore limb function (e.g., tendon transfers or transfers of innervated sensory pads). Basic science and clinical research into nerve regeneration and repair is a vital part of our growing effort to provide the most effective treatment for patients in the future.

ADDITIONAL READING

Badalamente MA, Hurst LC, Stracher A: Recovery after delayed nerve repair: influence of a pharmacologic adjunct in a primate model. *J Reconstr Microsurg* 8:391, 1992.

Bixby JL, Harris WA: Molecular mechanisms of axon growth and guidance. *Annu Rev Cell Biol* 7:117, 1991.

Brushart TM: Motor axons preferentially reinnervate motor pathways. *J Neurosci* 13:2730, 1993.

Dellon AL, Curtis RM, Edgerton MT: Evaluating recovery of sensation in the hand following nerve injury. *Johns Hopkins Med J* 130:235, 1972.

Lundborg G, Dahlin L, Danielsen N, et al: Trophism, tropism, and specificity in nerve regeneration. *J Reconstr Microsurg* 10:345, 1994.

IV | SPECIAL PROBLEMS

41 | Alcohol and Drugs

The personal and economic losses associated with trauma in part reflect our inadequate efforts to prevent injury. A major factor contributing to the continuing high incidence of both blunt and penetrating trauma is the association with substance abuse. This chapter examines the relationship of substance abuse with injury and altered pathophysiology.

MAGNITUDE OF THE ALCOHOL ABUSE PROBLEM

During 1995, 41,798 persons were killed as a result of traffic crashes. Alcohol intoxication with a blood alcohol concentration (BAC) above 100 mg/dL of either the driver or the pedestrian was present in 13,564 (32.5 percent) of these deaths. Alcohol contributed to 4000 additional fatal motor vehicle crashes (MVCs). Alcohol intoxication is more likely in a single-vehicle crash (42 percent) than in a multivehicle crash (21.9 percent), most of the involved drivers are males who are 20 to 45 years old, and these crashes occur most frequently on weekend evenings. Fatally injured pedestrians or cyclists are often intoxicated (25 percent). The societal tragedy is magnified when the severely maimed or killed victims are innocent bystanders with no alcohol in their blood.

Legal restriction of accessibility of alcohol has failed; sober victims are injured by their impaired neighbors. Prohibition of the sale of alcohol by the Eighteenth Amendment simply fostered bootlegging until it was repealed by the Twenty-First Amendment. Voluntary programs have had some impact, and from 1982 to 1995 the frequency of fatal MVCs involving alcohol decreased from 46.3 to 32.5 percent.

ADVERSE EFFECTS OF ALCOHOL: EXPERIMENTAL

Alcohol compromises the response to hemorrhagic shock, and the mortality from controlled shock is higher in dogs given alcohol. The impaired animals exhibit respiratory depression, and greater hypotension and myocardial irritability. Long-term alcohol exposure in man causes chronic cardiomyopathy with ventricular dysfunction and congestive failure. Alcohol-induced arrhythmias likely cause the increased mortality from hemorrhagic shock in man.

ADVERSE EFFECTS OF ALCOHOL: CLINICAL

Alcohol causes vasodilation and decreased peripheral vascular resistance, diuresis with increased salt and water excretion, and has a negative inotropic effect. The impaired victim is more likely to vomit and aspirate. The hypotension from vasodilation may lead to unnecessary surgery for control of perceived severe blood loss that is not present. Alcohol causes increased mortality after traumatic brain injury as well. Finally, long-standing alcohol abuse leads to Laennec's cirrhosis. Hemostasis after a hepatic injury in the cirrhotic patient is impaired by the hardened parenchyma which resists suture compression, the portal hypertension which promotes hemorrhage, and the coexistent coagulopathy. In addition, successful splenorrhaphy is rare in such patients.

EFFECT OF ALCOHOL ON OUTCOME

The increased extent of the hypotensive response to alcohol likely causes a higher death rate prior to arrival at the hospital. The combination of cocaine with alcohol may magnify this hypotensive response, especially during general anesthesia. Studies on large numbers of MVCs show a consistently higher mortality in comparable crashes matched for safety belt usage, vehicular weight, vehicular speed and deformation, and driver age when alcohol is involved.

WITHDRAWAL FROM ALCOHOL AND RELATED METABOLIC PROBLEMS

During or after binge drinking, the patient may develop convulsions referred to as rum or whiskey fits due to alcohol withdrawal (Table 44-1). While withdrawal is the most common cause of seizures in the alcoholic patient, the differential diagnosis includes craniocerebral trauma and alcohol-induced epileptic seizures. Withdrawal seizures have an abrupt onset at 7 to 48 hours after the last drink, and tend to be generalized tonic-clonic in nature with loss of consciousness. In contrast, focal seizures imply cerebral disease and recent craniocerebral trauma. Prevention of self-injury and aspiration pneumonitis are vital. The most common alcohol-related metabolic problem following operation for trauma is delirium tremens (DTs). The DTs usually appear 2 to 8 days after drinking ceases, may cause hypermetabolism, and the severity of the DTs correlates with morbidity (Table 44-1). Death during DTs may be from arrhythmia and cardiac arrest due to hypokalemia, as the serum potassium often falls below 3 mEq/dL and remains low despite aggressive intravenous replacement. Hyponatremia, hypophosphatemia, and hypomagnesemia may also occur during DTs.

A common nursing response to the hypermetabolic phase of DTs is four-limb restraint and increased sedation. This promotes aspiration pneumonitis, which occurs after the patient has entered the hypometabolic or postictal phase. Nutritional support in alcoholic patients should include glucose-containing solutions and vitamin B to prevent thiamine depletion and precipitation of Wernicke's encephalopathy. A toxicology screen helps identify other toxic agents.

THE REHABILITATION CHALLENGE

Rehabilitation must be offered to the injured patient with alcohol abuse to decrease the rate of recidivism. Such rehabilitation should be coordinated

---

TABLE 41-1 Symptoms of Withdrawal from Alcohol in the Injured Patient

Withdrawal syndrome
  Tremulousness
  Agitation
  Disordered perception
  Hallucinations
Withdrawal seizures or rum fits
  Sudden onset
  Tonic-clonic
  Multiple
Delirium tremens (2–8 days)
  Stage I: Hypermetabolism, confusion
  Stage II: Auditory hallucinations
  Stage III: Visual hallucinations
  Stage IV: Convulsions

closely with Alcoholics Anonymous and other regional alcohol rehabilitation programs.

DRUNK DRIVERS AND THE LAW

During 1994, 1,400,000 drivers were arrested for substance abuse. Historically, the societal approach to alcohol-related trauma has been haphazard, ineffective, and has failed to prevent the individual from causing subsequent alcohol-related injury. Societal attitudes are changing, and most citizens now claim they would avoid driving after imbibing. During the 1990s, over 500 drunk driving laws were enacted or strengthened, and all states have raised the drinking age to 21. For these reasons, there has been a progressive decline in deaths from alcohol-related MVCs. Recidivism, however, is still a serious problem. Over 20 percent of drivers involved in fatal crashes have a prior nonfatal MVC, and 13 percent were convicted for drunk driving. Surgeons must support groups devoted to removing the drunk driver from the road, mandatory incarceration of drunk drivers in an alcohol rehabilitation center, jail sentences for those who leave such centers prior to discharge, and use of taxis or other transportation by those too impaired to drive.

THE MAGNITUDE OF THE DRUG ABUSE PROBLEM

In recent years there has been an explosion of growth in the illicit drug trade and drug-related injury (DRI) (Table 44-2). Most acutely injured patients at Detroit Receiving Hospital use or have used cocaine, heroin, or both.

THE COCAINE RAGE

By 1988, the National Institute on Drug Abuse (NIDA) estimated that over 21 million Americans had tried cocaine, including 3 million Americans who had used the drug within the previous month. The Drug Abuse Warning Network (DAWN) of the U.S. Department of Health and Human Services appears to be underreporting this rising usage. Cocaine is usually inhaled, but it may be injected. Sharing of needles, syringes, and diluents must be prevented to stop the spread of the acquired immunodeficiency syndrome (AIDS). Cocaine can be purified into a more potent form and smoked (so-called "freebase"), or the

TABLE 41-2 Number of Americans Using Illicit Drugs

Drug	No. ever used (million)	No. used in past year (million)
Any illicit Drug	72.5	27.9
Marijuana	65.7	21.1
Cocaine	21.2	8.2
"Crack" cocaine	2.5	1.0
Hallucinogens	14.6	3.1
Psychotherapeutics*	23.5	11.4
Stimulants	14.1	5.0
Sedatives	7.0	3.1
Tranquilizers	9.5	4.4
Analgesics	10.3	5.3

*Includes nonmedical use of sedatives, tranquilizers, stimulants, or analgesics.
Source: From National Household Survey on Drug Abuse: population estimates: 1988. National Institute on Drug Abuse, Rockville, MD.

alkaloid can be dissolved, dried, and inhaled with a flammable vehicle. "Crack" cocaine is a neutral form like freebase that is made without solvent extraction. Cocaine absorption via inhalation is enhanced by a Valsalva maneuver, which may cause mediastinal emphysema with sudden midthoracic pain and shortness of breath. A "Hamman crunch" due to cardiac contraction adjacent to the mediastinal air is heard during systole. Treatment is expectant until symptoms abate. Crack cocaine is cheap, ubiquitous, easy to prepare, and yields rapid intense euphoria that can lead to addiction. As with other stimulants, the drug can cause impaired judgement, disinhibition, impulsiveness, compulsively repeated actions, paranoia, and extreme psychomotor agitation.

PHYSIOLOGIC EFFECTS OF COCAINE

The naturally occurring cocaine alkaloid from the shrub *Erythroxylon coca* has local anesthetic and sympathomimetic actions that affect multiple organs. Cocaine blocks presynaptic reuptake of the neurotransmitters norepinephrine and dopamine, thus augmenting the effects of circulating catecholamines. Unregulated vasoconstriction leads to multiple organ failure and occasional deaths.

MEDICOLEGAL IMPLICATIONS

A new hazard for the trauma surgeon and trauma centers is the widespread in-hospital use of narcotics, especially cocaine. When sudden unexpected death occurs on the trauma service, illicit narcotic exposure must be suspected, and blood samples drawn during unsuccessful CPR should be assayed for toxic agents. Proof of recent illicit drug exposure will augment the defense against later litigation.

HEROIN ABUSE

Heroin, a member of the opiate family, is derived from morphine, which is the principal product of the poppy *Papaver somniferum*. Heroin interacts with endogenous opiate receptors that function as neurotransmitters, neurohormones, and modulators of neural transmission throughout the central nervous system (CNS). Drug-related injuries from heroin include overdose, vascular aneurysms, and a myriad of infectious complications. The purity of heroin is often unknown, and deaths from overdoses occur with purer preparations that can cause respiratory depression. Like morphine, heroin induces peripheral vasodilation and a decrease in systemic vascular resistance. Ventilation must be supported and intravenous naloxone hydrochloride (0.4 mg, repeated every few minutes as necessary), an opiate receptor antagonist, is frequently beneficial. Long-term heroin use causes needle track scars from multiple injections, "skin pop" scars or ulcerations from prior subcutaneous injection, lymphedema and leg swelling due to lymphatic blockade from cellulitis, and scars of prior abscesses that were drained and allowed to heal by secondary intention. These signs portend that the resuscitative effort will be compromised by inaccessible peripheral veins and the need for large doses of anesthetic.

Heroin diluents include quinine, strychnine, lidocaine, various sugars, talcum powder, and starch. Bacterial contamination is common. Sequelae associated with injection include pulmonary embolization and respiratory failure, and CNS stimulation may cause tremors, agitation, and seizures. The diluent quinine may cause cardiac dysfunction with conduction delays, arrhythmias, or hypotension. Strychnine, a competitive antagonist of the central nervous system inhibitory neurotransmitter glycine, causes CNS stimulation with apprehension, nausea, muscle twitching, spasms, opisthotonos, seizures, rhabdomyolysis, and myoglobinuric acute renal failure.

Long-term use depletes the peripheral veins. Central venous injections cause pneumothorax, empyema, cellulitis, and cervical abscesses. *Staphylococcus,* enteric gram-negative bacteria, and oral flora resulting from reuse of needles and lack of sterile technique can be cultured. Aggressive treatment of cellulitis with antibiotics designed to cover methicillin-resistant *Staphylococcus aureus* and the gram-negative coliform bacilli should be maintained. Patients may develop an unusual or refractory pneumonia and endocarditis with inotropic compromise. Seeding of a hematoma in the abdominal wall, rectus sheath, liver, or spleen may convert a sterile lesion into an abscess.

Vascular injury from infected needles causes pseudoaneurysms or mycotic aneurysms of either arteries or veins, infected hematomas, and distal tissue ischemia when an artery is mistakenly injected with a solution containing particulate matter. Excision of a mycotic aneurysm may cause severe ischemia requiring an extra-anatomic arterial bypass if an unaffected tissue plane can be utilized. Venous pseudoaneurysms are associated with swelling, usually in the groin, that is refractory to elevation and antibiotic therapy. Venous aneurysms are best treated with excision and venous ligation. Bacterial embolization from the venous aneurysm often causes a refractory pneumonia.

DRUGS, TRAUMA, AND HIV

There is a high incidence of AIDS in drug addicts presenting with severe injury. The trading of sex for drugs, pandemic among female users, is another source of AIDS or hepatitis. Both prescription and nonprescription drugs such as paregoric or elixir terpin hydrate have a depressant effect that may compromise resuscitation. Trauma surgeons need at least a rudimentary knowledge of drug effects and overdoses.

Trauma due to the competitive and dangerous nature of distribution of illicit narcotics is rising. The profit motive has refined efficiency of distribution and has intensified the violence among competitors. Our medical responsibilities extend beyond care for injured patients into the realm of prevention. Physicians need to focus on prevention, and a policy of decriminalization of narcotics needs to be explored.

ADDITIONAL READING

Brookoff D, Campbell EA, Shaw LM: The underreporting of cocaine-related trauma: Drug abuse warning network reports vs. hospital toxicology tests. *Am J Public Health* 83:369, 1993.

Burgess M, Lindsey T: Alcohol involvement in fatal crashes—1995. Mathematical Analysis Division: National Center for Statistics and Analysis. Research and Development Division, National Highway Traffic Safety Administration, U.S. Department of Transportation, Washington, DC.

Kelen GR, Fritz S, Qaguish B, et al: Substantial increase in human immunodeficiency virus infection in critically ill emergency patients: 1986 and 1987 compared. *Ann Emerg Med* 18:378, 1989.

Wallace JR, Lucas CE, Ledgerwood AM: Social, economic, and surgical anatomy of a drug-related abscess. *Am Surg* 52:398, 1986.

Ward RE, Flynn TC, Miller PW, et al: Effects of ethanol ingestion on the severity and outcome of trauma. *Am J Surg* 144:153, 1982.

42 | Pediatric Trauma

RESUSCITATION AND STABILIZATION OF THE SEVERELY INJURED CHILD

Use the same sequence of primary survey, resuscitation, secondary survey, and definitive care as described for adults. Multiple system injury is the rule rather than the exception in pediatric trauma care; therefore, every organ system must be assumed injured until proven otherwise.

Airway Assessment

Adequate airway management begins with effective preoxygenation and then follows an ordered sequence as described in Figure 42-1.

Careful in-line cervical traction must be maintained. A reliable indicator of proper endotracheal tube size is the diameter of the child's fifth finger. The Broselow tape is a measurement device that indicates appropriate size of resuscitative equipment, proper drug doses, and drip concentrations.

Uncuffed endotracheal tubes that allow some air leakage are the most appropriate for use in children weighing less than 60 pounds. A critical part of the process of endotracheal intubation is concurrent pressure on the larynx to provide transient occlusion of the esophagus at the level of the cricopharyngeus.

Rarely, a child with acute airway obstruction requires a needle cricothyroidotomy performed with a 14- to 16-gauge catheter placed through the cricothyroid membrane. Surgical cricothyroidotomy is *not* used in the infant or small child because of the high association of secondary subglottic stenosis.

Infants and small children are primarily diaphragmatic breathers. Any compromise of diaphragmatic excursion significantly limits the child's ability to ventilate. A crying child may swallow large amounts of air, causing acute gastric distention and limitation of left diaphragmatic function. This is the reason for routine nasogastric decompression of every potentially severely injured child.

Circulation

A child with a significant hemorrhagic injury may initially present with normal blood pressure because of reflex tachycardia and peripheral vasoconstriction. Initial normal vital signs should not impart any sense of security regarding the child's circulating volume. Poor peripheral perfusion and decreased level of consciousness are classic stigmata of hypovolemia.

Vascular Access

Initial vascular access can usually be obtained by percutaneous intravenous catheters placed in the upper extremities. A single reliable venous line is far more important than multiple tenuous lines. If surgical cutdown is required, the site with which the operating physician is most familiar should be used. Most commonly this is the greater saphenous vein at the ankle. Subclavian venous catheterization should not be a primary consideration for initial venous access.

Intraosseous infusion through cannulation of the medullary cavity in the anteromedial aspect of the tibia in an uninjured extremity is a safe and efficacious method for emergency vascular access in the infant and small child. Using sterile technique, place the needle 2 to 3 cm distal to the tibial tuberosity on the anteromedial surface. The intraosseous approach can be used to

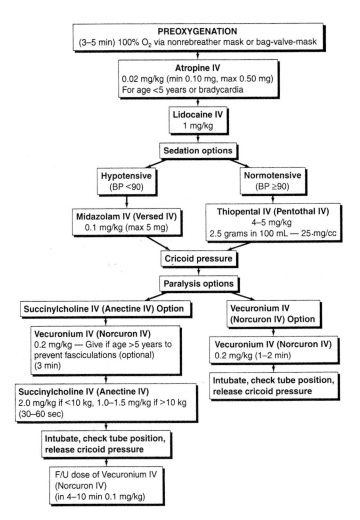

FIG. 42-1. Jacksonville Pediatric Injury Control System (JPICS). Rapid-sequence induction/intubation for pediatric airway management.

infuse saline, glucose, blood, bicarbonate, atropine, dopamine, epinephrine, diazepam, antibiotics, phenytoin, and succinylcholine (see Table 42-1 for drugs and dosages used in treating pediatric trauma). Fracture sites and areas of infection cannot be used. Avoid multiple attempts to place the needle in the medullary cavity because this results in leakage of fluid that may cause an iatrogenic compartment syndrome.

After adequate venous access is established, administer 20 mL/kg of normal saline to any hypotensive child. If there is no response to the first bolus, a second bolus is infused and immediate red cell transfusion should be considered. Massive exsanguination also mandates immediate transfusion of blood.

TABLE 42-1 Pediatric Drug Dosages

INTUBATION DRUGS	
Thiopental	4.0–6.0 mg/kg
Diazepam	0.5–1.0 mg/kg
Midazolam	0.1 mg/kg
Succinylcholine	1.0–3.5 mg/kg
Pancuronium	0.1–0.2 g/kg
Vecuronium	0.2 mg/kg
CARDIOVASCULAR DRUGS	
Atropine	0.02 mg/kg (min 0.10 mg, max 0.5 mg)
Calcium chloride (10%)	10–20 mg/kg
Calcium gluconate (10%)	15–60 mg/kg
Epinephrine	
Initial	1.0–10 mg/kg/min
Maintenance	0.1–2 mg/kg/min
Dopamine	2–5 μg/kg/min
Dobutamine	2.5–5 μg/kg/min
Sodium bicarbonate	1.0–4.0 mEq/kg
	Depends on pH and base deficit: Body weight (kg) $\times$ 0.3 $\times$ base deficit = total $NaHCO_3$

If in doubt, it is better to initiate transfusion than to exacerbate cerebral ischemia by inadequately treating hypovolemia.

Children who initially receive type O negative blood for resuscitation must continue to receive this until stabilized. Because the transfused blood may contain significant numbers of anti-A or anti-B antibody, it is not appropriate to change to type-specific blood after a massive transfusion of O negative blood.

Fresh frozen plasma is effective in replacing coagulation factors; however, it should never be used as a simple volume expander.

Hypothermia

Hypothermic stress is a significant problem in the infant and small child. Hypothermia stimulates catecholamine secretion and initiates shivering, resulting in significant metabolic acidosis. The hypothermic infant may be refractory to therapy for shock, may develop a bleeding diathesis, and may manifest a prolonged effect from anesthetic agents. For these reasons, all intravenous solutions including blood should be warmed. During surgical manipulations, extremities should be wrapped or covered with a warm-air heat exchange device. Fluids for irrigation of body cavities should be warmed and should not be allowed to soak the skin and back.

MANAGEMENT OF SPECIFIC INJURIES

Central Nervous System

Acute traumatic brain injury (TBI) initiates a multiphasic cascade of cyto-chemical events as a result of direct mechanical deformation of the brain and decreased cerebral perfusion. Children with a Glasgow Coma Scale (GCS) score of less than 9 need intracranial pressure (ICP) monitoring, usually with a combined drainage/monitoring device. Adequate ventilation to maintain oxygen saturation greater than 95 percent and CO_2 concentration of 35 to 40 torr prevents exacerbation of infarction in regions of poorly perfused brain that are present in the early phase of severe TBI. Hypocarbia less than 25 torr may produce vasoconstriction-induced ischemia in an injured brain. Cerebral perfusion pressure (CPP) should be at least 50 mm Hg in children less than 8 years, and 60 to 80 mm Hg in older children.

Electrolyte concentration must minimize free-water shift into the cerebral tissue. Normal saline is the primary solution used in resuscitation. Lactated Ringer's solution is an acceptable alternative; however, its lower sodium content (130 mEq/L) is not as effective in maintaining serum sodium concentrations within normal limits.

If CPP begins to decline, check the patient's volume status and hemoglobin concentration. If volume status and hemoglobin are within the desired range, start vasopressor support. Consider a repeat head computed tomography (CT) scan to rule out a new or evolving lesion.

In response to an ICP >20 to 25 torr, check any and all cerebrospinal fluid (CSF) drainage systems. Infuse mannitol 0.25 μg/kg every 4 to 6 hours. Monitor serum electrolytes and osmolarity and discontinue mannitol when osmolarity exceeds 310 mOsm.

If intracranial pressure remains abnormally elevated over 20 mm Hg for more than 5 minutes despite therapeutic maneuvers, start intravenous pentobarbital. Use a loading dose of 1 to 5 mg/kg administered over 20 to 30 minutes, with careful observation of blood pressure, followed by a maintenance dose of 1 to 4 mg/kg/h. In young children, use a central venous catheter to maintain central venous pressure (CVP) around 10 to 12 mm Hg. In older children, consider a Swan-Ganz catheter to confirm a CVP of 10 mm Hg or greater, or a pulmonary capillary wedge pressure of 10 to 15 mm Hg. As the dosage of pentobarbital is increased, myocardial depression and peripheral vascular vasodilation may require vasopressor support. Mild hypothermia induced by pentobarbital is acceptable. Fever and seizures dramatically increase neuronal oxygen requirements and contribute to secondary brain injury. Treat hyperthermia greater than 38°C with acetaminophen, 10 mg/kg every 4 to 6 hours, and an external cooling blanket.

If a seizure occurs, prophylaxis should be initiated and maintained with phenobarbital or phenytoin during the first 7 days after brain injury. Phenobarbital is given intravenously to children less than 1 year of age, with a 10 to 15 mg/kg loading dose and a maintenance dose of 5 mg/kg/d in two divided doses. Phenytoin is administered intravenously as an initial bolus of 10 to 20 mg/kg, followed by a maintenance dose of 5 mg/kg/d in two or three divided doses.

Thoracic Injuries

The bony and cartilaginous structures of the child's chest wall are extremely flexible; hence, deep compression of the chest may produce severe internal injury, without fracture of the bony thorax. The mediastinum of infants is very mobile, resulting in rapid ventilatory failure from tension pneumothorax. Thoracic injuries frequently require immediate correction of acute physiologic derangement before anything is known about the mechanism of injury or the child's prior physical condition. This is usually accomplished by tube decompression of a pneumothorax or hemothorax. Since aspiration of gastric contents frequently occurs in injured children, any clinical or radiologic evidence of this entity must be treated aggressively.

Abdominal Injuries

Because the abdominal wall and protective musculature of the young child are quite thin, a minor force may result in a serious compression or disrupting injury. Definitive evaluation of a child with blunt abdominal trauma begins with a history focused on the exact mechanism of injury. Physical examination of the abdomen should focus on evidence of external injury, tenderness, and distension. In the absence of intraperitoneal free air or frank peritonitis, diagnosis of hollow viscus disruption is often delayed. Thus, all children with equivocal physical findings should be observed for at least 24 hours. There are no laboratory tests that reliably diagnose solid or hollow visceral injury. With the evolution of nonoperative management of blunt abdominal trauma, diagnostic CT imaging has become a key component in the evaluation of injured children. Focused abdominal sonography for trauma (FAST) is an excellent screening tool for initial determination of the presence of fluid in the peritoneal cavity or pericardial sac. The absence of free fluid in a hemodynamically stable child may eliminate the need for an abdominal CT scan.

Hemodynamic instability mandates operative intervention. A child may be treated nonoperatively only if:

• The patient is monitored appropriately
• An experienced surgical team is prepared to intervene at any time
• Adequate support from anesthesia and transfusion services is immediately available

Children who require transfusion of more than half of their blood volume (40 mL/kg) within 24 hours of injury will almost always require operative intervention. Diagnostic peritoneal lavage (DPL) in the young child is potentially a major procedure and should be performed only when the results will affect therapeutic decisions.

Unique Pediatric Abdominal Injuries

Duodenal intramural hematoma results from the disruption of the vessels between the submucosa and muscularis. The child presents with gastric distension, bilious vomiting, a decreasing hematocrit, and an epigastric mass. A "coiled-spring sign" and cutoff on an upper gastrointestinal contrast study are diagnostic. The stomach should be decompressed, and the patient should be supported by total parenteral nutrition. Most duodenal hematomas will resolve within 10 days of injury; however, complete resolution of the obstruction may take up to 3 weeks. Follow-up includes measurement of nasogastric drainage and sonography to assess resolution of the hematoma.

A child with a lap belt hyperflexion injury, especially if it is associated with a Chance fracture of a lumbar vertebra, should be assumed to have a rupture of the small bowel until proven otherwise.

Rectal injuries are frequently very painful and require examination under anesthesia for complete assessment. Except for the occasional straddle injury, abuse causes the majority of isolated rectal injuries in children. Rectal mucosal or superficial anal injuries usually resolve with conservative treatment. Full-thickness injuries below the internal sphincter may be treated by primary repair.

The spleen of a hemodynamically stable child will often stop bleeding spontaneously; therefore, the vast majority of splenic injuries are managed nonoperatively.

An isolated hepatic injury, without disruption of the portal vein, hepatic veins, or suprarenal inferior vena cava, behaves clinically like a splenic injury and is usually managed nonoperatively.

Hyperamylasemia related to blunt pancreatic injury may not occur for at least 12 hours postinjury. Children with no evidence of major ductal disruption or clinical deterioration may require only expectant management.

Many series have demonstrated that all but gross disruption of the renal pedicle can be managed nonoperatively with full recovery of renal function. The absence of gross hematuria or less than 20 red cells per high-power field does not warrant any further diagnostic evaluation.

Vascular Injuries

The mechanism of vascular trauma in children is similar to that in adults. Unique pediatric injuries include arterial trauma associated with supracondylar long-bone fractures. Because the arterial intima is a cellular monolayer, transient deformity from external force may produce an intimal flap. Ischemia to adjacent nerves may result in pain, paresthesia, hyperesthesia, and even anesthesia within a few hours of injury. Arteriography has its own inherent risks in the small child, and it should only be performed by someone experienced in the technique, and only if repair of the injured vessel is indicated.

The most important differential diagnosis in pediatric vascular trauma is between thrombosis and spasm of the injured vessel (which usually disappears within 3 hours). Pulses absent longer than 3 hours suggest thrombosis or transection of the vessel. The diagnosis must be confirmed by arteriography or operative exploration, usually the latter in small children. Although a distal extremity may remain viable without pulsatile flow, potential growth retardation is an important factor in the decision to explore the site of major vascular injury in children.

Orthopedic Injuries

Associated skeletal injury puts additional stress on the entire healing process. Inadequate splinting of long-bone fractures provides a spherical dead space, which can rapidly fill with a fracture-related hematoma. Every limb must be carefully assessed for the presence of a distal pulse. Accurate documentation of intact sensation is critical.

SUMMARY

Care of the injured child is a complex process that requires understanding of the pathophysiology, unique characteristics, and special requirements of the pediatric population. It is an exercise in psychomotor skill, surgical judgment, and intellectual reasoning, but the results can be rewarding.

ADDITIONAL READING

Kissoon N, Dreyer J, Walia M: Pediatric trauma: Differences in pathophysiology, injury patterns and treatment compared with adult trauma. *Can Med Assoc J* 142:27, 1990.

Prough DS: Therapy of patients with head injuries: Key parameters for management. *J Trauma* 42:S10, 1997.

Rogers FB: Technical note: A quick and simple method of obtaining venous access in traumatic exsanguination. *J Trauma* 34:142, 1993.

Tepas JJ: Blunt abdominal trauma in children. *Curr Opin Pediatr* 5:317, 1993.

People over the age of 65 years are hospitalized for trauma at twice the rate of the general population, and account for one-quarter of all trauma-related deaths in the United States. The mortality rate in elder trauma victims has been estimated to be six times greater than in younger victims when controlling for degree of injury.

The combination of chronic diseases (comorbid conditions), senescence of cognitive and motor functions, and loss of physiologic reserve (physiology of aging) makes older patients uniquely susceptible to injury. This process begins earlier and is present to a much greater extent than has been generally appreciated. No single age comprehensively defines the stage of increased vulnerability for injury (Table 43-1).

PHYSIOLOGY OF AGING AND THE IMPACT OF COMORBIDITY

Aging is characterized by the progressive loss of organ function and decreased functional reserve in times of physical or metabolic stress. One-third of trauma patients older than 65 years have a comorbid condition or chronic disease. Comorbid conditions are associated with increased mortality varying with the type and number of conditions and with significantly longer lengths of stay in the hospital.

Cardiovascular System

Cardiovascular dysfunction is the most prevalent medical problem in the elderly and represents the greatest cause of death. Patients are often unaware of the degree of functional impairment until a time of acute stress. Functional cardiac decline results from changes intrinsic to the myocardium and from generalized effects of arteriosclerotic disease.

Prescription medications, including beta blockers, calcium channel blockers, diuretics, and afterload reducing agents may impair augmentation of myocardial function in response to injury, especially in the hypovolemic patient.

The very early use of invasive hemodynamic monitoring has been advocated to better identify patients at risk and direct their cardiovascular management. It is unclear at what age this approach should be done, but physiologic reassessment is critical as the limits of therapeutic and diagnostic tolerance are narrow, and overresuscitation may be as harmful as underresuscitation. A history of congestive heart failure, recent myocardial infarction, previous cardiac surgery or other circulatory disorder should prompt consideration of invasive monitoring as part of resuscitation.

Respiratory System

Decreased chest wall compliance and lung elasticity and chronic emphysematous changes contribute to the progressive loss of pulmonary reserve with aging. Impaired cough and laryngeal reflexes, diminished cough strength, swallowing disorders, and diminished lower esophageal sphincter tone all impair local airway protection and increase the risk of aspiration.

Therapy should be directed at supporting gas exchange, especially avoiding hypoxemia, optimizing chest wall mechanics by control of pain, and mini-

TABLE 43-1 Presumed Clinical Differences in the Evaluation and Management of Aging Patients

Age	55–64	65–74	>75
Physiologic reserve	+/−	−	− −
Organ function	+	+/−	− −/+
Preexisting diseases	+/−	+	+ +
Medication use	+/−	+	+ +
Competency of history	+	+/−	− −/+
Central nervous system alteration (imaging detection)	−/+	+	+ +
Diagnostic and therapeutic plans	S/A	A	A*
Outcome from severe injury	+	+/−	+/− −

S, standard; A, aggressive; *, with early re-evaluation.
Source: Schwab CW, Kauder DR: Trauma in the geriatric patient. *Arch Surg* 127:701, 1992.

mizing the risks of airway contamination. Evidence that early tracheostomy decreases nosocomial pneumonia and duration of ventilatory support has recently been disputed.

Pulmonary hygiene and appropriate analgesia are mutually supporting goals. Regional analgesia such as continual epidural and intercostal nerve blocks for injuries to the chest, torso, pelvis, and lower extremities may minimize the respiratory depressant effects of systemic analgesics.

Central Nervous System

The brain atrophies with age, with approximately 10 percent loss of weight between the ages of 30 and 70 years. Relatively minor injuries may lead to subdural or subarachnoid hemorrhage, and the extra space created by brain atrophy may allow a significant amount of blood to accumulate before causing any symptoms. Computed tomography (CT) scanning is essential for prompt diagnosis and is recommended for all patients over 55 years of age with injuries to the brain.

Functional changes with aging include deterioration in cognitive ability, memory, and processing of information. Deterioration of vision and hearing, loss of visual acuity, color perception, and depth perception, intolerance of bright light, and loss of vibration and position sense all occur and predispose to injury.

Injury to the brain is known to be a predictor of poor outcome in the elderly.

Renal System

Glomerular loss and sclerotic and degenerative changes with aging cause a reduction in glomerular filtration rate, with progressively declining creatinine clearance.

Measurement of serum creatinine may be misleading because as we age, we undergo a parallel decline in muscle mass. Creatinine clearance declines by up to 80 to 90 percent over the adult life span. Drugs that are excreted through the kidneys should be dosed according to measurements of renal function (creatinine clearance). Acute renal failure is associated with a 50 percent mortality rate, and is higher in the setting of progressive multiple-organ dysfunction.

Musculoskeletal System

Changes in strength and flexibility contribute to a progressive limitation of movement. Compensating changes, such as an alteration in gait in response to kyphosis, may replace the normal mechanisms used to maintain balance.

Loss of muscle mass and bone loss due to osteoporosis increase susceptibility to fracture, especially in the hip, pelvis, wrist, and ribs. Vertebral collapse is associated with progressive kyphosis.

Ability to Influence Outcome

The ability to influence patterns of injury before they occur or to promote optimal functional recovery is clearly important, but thus far is not well defined. Mixed results have been reported in trials of exercise regimens, behavior modification, and education. However, physical therapy programs have been shown to be effective in reducing falls. An inventory of individual impairments and environmental risk factors in the home may be useful to optimize safety and prevent injury.

Recovery from injury is limited by the patient's functional level and premorbid conditions prior to injury. A multidisciplinary response, including family support and social services; rehabilitative medicine; physical, occupational, and speech therapy; and nutritional guidance is essential to optimize the speed, and completion of recovery.

PATTERNS OF INJURY

While the elderly experience the same types of injuries as younger people, there are differences in mechanism and injury pattern with advancing age (Table 43-2).

Falls

Approximately 70 percent of all deaths due to falls occur in the geriatric population. Of those who are hospitalized after a fall at home, up to 50 percent are subsequently discharged to a nursing home. Only 50 percent of all elderly patients hospitalized after falling will be alive 1 year later.

Falls occur for reasons that are inherent to the aging process. Postural instability results from declining visual acuity, hearing loss, disorders of balance and coordination, and loss of memory. Falling in the elderly is often a manifestation of an acute or chronic occult illness characterized by syncope and

TABLE 43-2 Mechanism of Injury in Patients Over 45 Years of Age

Age	45–54	55–64	65–74	75–84
Number of patients	9276	6384	7328	7380
Incidence of injury by mechanism (%):				
Motor vehicle accident	36.2	35.2	33.4	25.5
Pedestrian struck by vehicle	4.9	5.9	5.7	5.3
Fall	25.3	39.3	49.8	63.0
Assault/abuse*	13.1	7.8	3.9	2.1
Burn†	1.1	1.9	1.0	0.8

*Includes gunshot and stabbing wounds.
†Data for two years only, 1995–1996.
Source: Pennsylvania Trauma Systems Foundation registry, 1992–1996.

"drop attacks." Postural hypotension may result from cerebrovascular disease, cardiac dysrhythmia, or autonomic dysfunction related to aging, medications, or in association with diseases such as diabetes mellitus or parkinsonism. Metabolic derangements such as hyperglycemia, hypoglycemia, and anemia are especially common. Falling may also be a nonspecific presentation of acute illness such as dehydration, urinary tract infection, or pneumonia.

Medications linked with falling include narcotics, sedatives, antidepressants, diuretics, and antiarrhythmics. Falling is associated with both recent changes in dose and the total number of medications prescribed.

Vehicular Trauma

Motor Vehicle Crashes

Motor vehicle crashes represent the leading mechanism of injury that brings an elderly person to a trauma center. It is the leading cause of trauma-related death between the ages of 65 and 74, and the second highest cause (after falls) in those over age 75.

The elderly are more likely to be involved in crashes in good weather, close to home, during daylight hours, and at intersections. Crashes in this latter category are frequently with another vehicle, are often due to traffic signals that were not seen, or are caused by poor judgment. Dementia and more subtle changes in memory and judgment impair the ability to recognize and navigate potentially hazardous situations. Deterioration in visual and auditory acuity slow recognition and reaction.

Pedestrians Struck by Vehicles

The population over 65 years of age has the highest population-based fatality rate for pedestrians at any age, accounting for more than 20 percent of fatalities in vehicular-pedestrian encounters. Nearly 50 percent of all pedestrian fatalities in those over 65 years of age occur within a crosswalk.

Declines in direct and peripheral vision, hearing, memory, and judgment make crossing a busy street hazardous. Diminished strength, reaction time, and coordination make it more difficult for the elderly to navigate these hazards safely.

Assault and Domestic Abuse

Violent assaults are becoming more common in the elderly (Table 43-2). Deterioration in vision, hearing, strength, coordination, cognition, and judgment contribute to the inability of the elderly to defend themselves.

As our population ages and requires more assistance with activities of daily living, elder abuse and neglect are on the rise. Detection requires a high degree of suspicion, particularly in those patients with signs of neglect, physical abuse, or a pattern of injury that is inconsistent with the mechanism described.

Burns

The over-65 population makes up approximately 20 percent of admissions to burn units. The over-75 population has the highest rate of death from domestic fires caused by cooking, heating, smoking, and electrical mishaps. Scalding is the most common form of burn injury in this population, typically from bath water.

Poor wound healing often complicates efforts to debride and graft skin onto burn wounds, while sepsis remains the predominant cause of late death.

OUTCOMES AND APPROACH TO CARE

The death rate in hospitalized geriatric trauma victims ranges from 15 to 30 percent, which is far greater than the 4 to 8 percent mortality rate seen in a younger population with comparable injuries. Elderly trauma patients are more likely to develop multiple-organ failure and sepsis leading to death than less-frequently injured younger patients. Further, trauma patients over 65 have an increased risk of subsequent new trauma; for example, age over 81 is associated with twice the likelihood of readmission for new injury after a previous admission.

Cost

Persons over age 65, estimated to be 12 percent of the U.S. population, are reported to consume 33 percent of health care expenditures and 25 percent of hospital costs for trauma. A larger proportion of injured elderly patients require intensive care for at least part of their hospitalization. The presence of any and all comorbid conditions is associated with greatly extended hospital length of stay. In general, standard third-party payments for trauma care are inadequate to cover the hospital costs of older trauma patients. The system of diagnosis-related group (DRG)-based coverage (Medicare) grossly underestimates costs, especially in the severely injured.

Withholding Care

The survivability of injury in the elderly is usually not clear at the initial presentation. The presence of an advance directive may be helpful in clarifying the patient's desires and expectations. As the head of the team, the trauma surgeon must keep all caregivers focused on realistic outcomes and the wise use of resources.

SUMMARY

- Chronological age does not predict physiologic age.
- Our understanding of the physiologic changes of aging has defined a much broader population at risk by highlighting the onset of some limitations at a younger age than was previously appreciated.
- Organ function and the decrease in physiologic reserve vary greatly between and within individuals. Individual organ systems are subject to decreases in physiologic reserve at differing rates, and each patient must be approached individually. The expected physiologic changes of aging and the presence of comorbid conditions are common and affect care and outcome.
- As age advances, patterns of injury, responses to injury, and related complications emerge that are different than those seen in younger victims of similar types of trauma. Elderly patients require a more aggressive approach, utilizing invasive monitoring when nonoperative management is appropriate.
- There is a correlation between increased age, decreasing injury severity, and poorer outcome. Early prediction of outcome in patients with moderate injuries, however, is imprecise.

- Advance directives are important in determining if continued aggressive care is warranted.

ADDITONAL READING

Gubler KD, Maier RV, Davis R, et al: Trauma recidivism in the elderly. *J Trauma* 41:952, 1996.

McMahon DJ, Schwab CW, Kauder DR: Comorbidity and the elderly trauma patient. *World J Surg* 20:1113, 1996.

National Safety Council: *Accident Facts* (1993 Edition). Itasca, IL, National Safety Council, 1993.

Projections of the Resident Population by Age, Sex, Race, and Hispanic Origin: 1999 to 2100. Washington, DC, U.S. Census Bureau, 2000.

Scalea TM, Simon HM, Duncan AO, et al: Geriatric blunt multiple trauma: Improved survival with early invasive monitoring. *J Trauma* 30:129, 1990.

Schwab CW, Shapiro MB, Kauder DR: Geriatric trauma: patterns, care, and outcomes, in Mattox KL, Feliciano DV, Moore EE (eds): *Trauma,* 4th ed. New York, McGraw-Hill, 2000, pp 1099–1113.

44 | Wounds, Bites, and Stings

WOUNDS

Basic Biology of Wound Healing

The physiologic phases of wound healing are:

1. Coagulation and inflammation;
2. Migratory phase;
3. Proliferative phase; and
4. Remodeling.

At 2 weeks, approximately 10 to 20 percent of the preinjury tensile strength has returned, at 4 to 6 weeks approximately 50 percent, and at 10 weeks approximately 80 percent. Increased collagen turnover continues for at least several years.

In open wounds there is a prolonged inflammatory, migratory, and proliferative phase, and in large defects epithelialization may not completely occur. Open wounds that heal by secondary intention do so by developing granulation tissue, with eventual epithelial migration and contraction. The granulation tissue seen in such wounds consists microscopically of collagen, fibroblasts, leukocytes (especially macrophages), and new blood vessels.

Figure 44-1 presents an algorithm for treating an acute wound. Diabetes, malnutrition, collagen vascular disease, chronic lung disease, and chronic corticosteroid therapy represent a few of the affiliated medical problems commonly encountered in injured patients.

Threats to Infection-Free Wound Healing

A number of fundamental variables set the stage for wound infections following trauma. Included among these are:

- Bacterial contamination from the patient's resident flora and the environment
- Damaged nonviable tissue, especially following high-velocity wounds
- Inadequate hemostasis leading to the development of a hematoma
- Presence of a foreign body, as this prevents adequate phagocytosis
- Wound ischemia caused by local or systemic factors
- Systemic factors such as shock, hypoxemia, and immunosuppression from the injury alone

Priorities in Wound Management

The first phase of wound management includes an assessment of the injured patient, directed toward identifying and rapidly treating life-threatening injuries. The most readily apparent wound is not always the most important. Wound management in this phase deals only with preventing major hemorrhage by the direct application of pressure.

Once life-threatening injuries are treated or are being treated, the second phase of wound management concerns how to deal with the given wound. The key questions in this phase are: (1) Should the wound be managed in the operating room? (2) Are these associated injuries related to the wound (fracture, tendon injury, vascular injury, visceral injury)? (3) Can the wound be closed primarily, or should it be managed by delayed primary closure or by healing through secondary intention? (4) Should preventive antibiotics be used? (5) Does the patient need tetanus or rabies immunization and/or prophylaxis?

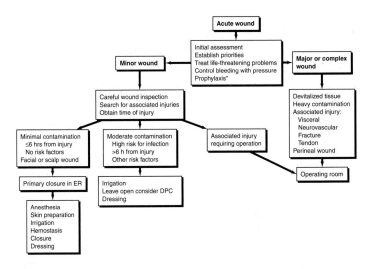

FIG. 44-1. Algorithm for the treatment of an acute wound. *Appropriate tetanus, rabies, and antibiotic prophylaxis. †Intermediate-risk wounds require more judgment. DPC, delayed primary closure.

The third phase of wound management relates to the type and technique of management and dressing (type of antiseptic, closure technique, choice of suture, and type of dressing to be applied).

The Search for Associated Injuries

Wounds should be locally explored for associated injuries. Scalp lacerations are gently probed, seeking a depressed skull fracture. Neck wounds are examined to see if they penetrate the platysma. Chest radiography is done for all thoracic wounds, and the wound is inspected for crepitance. Penetration of the anterior fascia and peritoneum in cases of abdominal stab wounds is determined by local wound exploration. Wounds of the extremities are examined to identify any associated fracture, tendon injury, and vascular or nerve injury.

Primary Closure Versus Open Management

Four options are available with respect to wound closure. First, the wound may be closed immediately with sutures, tapes, or staples to allow healing by primary intention. Second, the wound may be left open to heal on its own, by secondary intention. Third, the wound may be initially left open and then closed on the third to fourth day following injury (a procedure known as delayed primary closure or healing by tertiary intention). Fourth, a wound that cannot be closed because of tissue loss may be closed with a skin graft or tissue flap.

A number of variables affect the decision to close a wound primarily or to leave it open. A "golden period" of 6 to 8 hours follows wounding. During this period, primary closure should be considered. After 8 hours, bacterial colonization and proliferation, either by resident or external flora, impede infection-free primary closure. In general, wounds older than 6 to 8 hours should be managed by secondary intention or delayed primary closure. Exceptions to this rule are wounds of the face and scalp.

In summary, wounds more than 6 to 8 hours old, those associated with significant contamination (farm accident; human bite) or soft-tissue injury (crush; high-velocity gunshot wound; close-range shotgun wound), and those in patients with major associated systemic conditions pose a high risk of infection-related treatment failure. In general, these wounds should be managed with an open technique. Delayed primary closure is often an option with these wounds.

Skin Preparation

Several practical hair clippers are now commercially available and may be used in the emergency department and operating room. When hair does not have to be removed it should be left in place; when its removal is necessary, it should be removed in the least traumatic way possible.

Foreign bodies and debris on the skin surrounding the wound are removed, and the skin around the wound is cleansed and treated with one of a variety of skin antiseptics such as povidone-iodine solution or chlorhexidine gluconate solution. Both have immediate bactericidal effects, but chlorhexidine leaves a bactericidal skin residue that povidone-iodine solution does not. Both agents are toxic to normal tissue. The third most commonly used topical antiseptic preparation in the United States is a hexachlorophene solution. It is an effective skin antiseptic, but its immediate bactericidal action is not as apparent as that of the other two agents.

Local Anesthesia

The class of drugs for local anesthesia consists of polar weak bases that either have an amide or ester linkage. They appear to block nerve conduction by decreasing the permeability of the axon to sodium ions. Because they have the potential to affect all excitable membranes, their toxicity primarily involves the central nervous system (CNS) and the heart. Since it is the freebase forms of the anesthetics that penetrate the nerve membrane, a decreased tissue pH (as in acute inflammation) decreases their effectiveness.

The two most commonly used local anesthetic agents in the United States are lidocaine and bupivacaine. These agents are both amide-type local anesthetics, and both are available in combination with epinephrine (1:100,000 or 1:200,000). Lidocaine has a more rapid onset and shorter duration of action than bupivacaine, and is more commonly used. The most common technique used for their administration is local infiltration. The use of epinephrine prolongs the action of the local anesthetic drugs and allows them to be given in an increased total dose, since the resulting vasoconstriction delays the systemic absorption; however, there is evidence that epinephrine increases the risk of infection in contaminated wounds. Epinephrine is also contraindicated for use around the digits, the nose, ears, or penis, since it may produce vasospasm and severe ischemia or even necrosis.

Allergic reactions to bupivacaine and lidocaine are rare. The main risk with these drugs is dose-dependent CNS and cardiovascular toxicity. The maximum dose of lidocaine for infiltrative anesthesia is 4.5 mg/kg without epinephrine and 7 mg/kg with epinephrine added. Bupivacaine is not recommended for use in children. The maximum recommended dose in adults is 175 mg without epinephrine and 225 mg with epinephrine.

Various regional blocks are extremely valuable as an alternative to infiltrative local anesthesia, especially with respect to injuries and wounds of the extremities. Blocking the afferent sensory nerves from an affected region is the underlying principle of local block anesthesia.

Wound Preparation

A variety of substances have been used for wound irrigation. Two solutions, 0.9% saline and Polaxamer-188, are not significantly toxic to the host. Neither has significant antibacterial actions, but neither is associated with a significant impairment of wound healing.

Following irrigation, the wound should be debrided of all nonviable injured tissue. Debridement is rarely required for facial wounds, but is often needed with extensive soft-tissue injuries of the limbs or torso. With extensive or heavily contaminated wounds we schedule daily or alternate-day examinations in the operating room. This is particularly true for wounds in which pain, exposure, or both prevent adequate wound care and inspection on the ward. Muscle viability is assessed on the basis of bleeding, contractility, consistency, and color. Normal muscle contracts with a light pinch of the forceps, whereas stunned but viable muscle will frequently contract only with stimulation by an electrocautery device. Contractility is an unreliable sign in cases of acute ischemia, since muscle may be contractile for up to 8 hours after complete ischemia.

Hemostasis must be complete in order to avoid wound hematomas, which are excellent culture media for the bacteria associated with wound sepsis. If adequate hemostasis is not achievable in the emergency department, the wound should be managed in the operating room.

Use of Antibiotics for Acute Wounds

Most surgeons would recommend the use of preventive antibiotics in the following situations:

* In the presence of an open joint or open fracture
* When there is heavy contamination or major soft-tissue injury
* When there is a delay before debridement or treatment
* In patients with special problems, such as cardiac valvular disease or immunosuppression

Wound Repair

Wounds may be primarily closed with sutures, staples, or tapes. The use of nonabsorbable monofilament sutures for skin closure and absorbable monofilament sutures for closure of the deeper (fascial) tissue layers are recommended. The technique used should allow precise alignment of the skin edges, with the minimum amount of foreign material in the wound.

For a cosmetic closure of facial wounds, 6-0 monofilament suture with 1- to 2-mm bites in either a running or interrupted fashion is used. These sutures are removed in 3 to 5 days to minimize suture marking. Complicated wounds are pieced together where the pieces fit, and sutures are then placed between these key landmarks. This principle also applies to repair of the vermilion border of the lip and the skin over the eyebrows, where any misalignment is very noticeable.

Wound Dressings

Wound dressings can be broken down into several major groups, which include gauze, semipermeable film dressings, foam dressings, alginates, and hydrocolloids. A number of solutions (acetic acid, sodium hypochlorite, etc) have been added to the basic gauze dressing in an attempt to minimize bacterial growth, but unfortunately, almost all of them impair wound healing by damaging host tissues.

Hydrocolloid dressings are also attractively easy to manage for wounds that are closed primarily. Although their single-application cost is higher, both hydrocolloid and alginate dressings require much less-frequent changes than wet-to-dry dressings, which may make them cost-effective.

BITES AND STINGS

Mammalian Bites

Human Bites

The main clinical problem in human bites relates to soft-tissue infection. Human saliva contains up to 10^{11} bacteria/mL, and plaque on teeth has even greater numbers of bacteria. Therefore, bite-wound infection is common. Common infecting organisms include *Streptococcus viridans, Staphylococcus* spp, *Eikenella corrodens, Bacteroides* spp, and microaerophilic streptococci. The most common serious human bite-wound infections develop when there has been penetration of the joint capsule. This commonly happens when a clenched fist strikes the tooth of the person being assaulted ("fight bite"). These wounds commonly involve the metacarpophalangeal (MCP) joint or the proximal interphalangeal joint (PIP). They are usually benign-appearing wounds and will be missed unless the examiner is aware of the potential problem of joint penetration.

Antibiotic prophylaxis for human bites consists of ampicillin plus a beta-lactamase inhibitor (intravenous ampicillin/sulbactam or amoxicillin/clavulanic acid). Alternative agents include cefoxitin, erythromycin, penicillin, or ampicillin.

If the biting human is known or available for evaluation, it is recommended that serologic testing be done for HIV and hepatitis B and C. If the biting human is unavailable for testing, gamma globulin with hepatitis B vaccination should be considered. Tetanus immunization should be given if indicated.

Cat Bites

Commonly isolated organisms include *Pasteurella multocida* and *Staphylococcus* spp. Ampicillin plus a beta-lactamase inhibitor provides reasonable empiric coverage. Tetanus and rabies prophylaxis should be given if indicated.

Dog Bites

Large dogs can generate tremendous force with their muscles of mastication, producing devastating soft-tissue injuries. Soft-tissue infection following dog bites is not as common as after cat and human bites, but it does occur. After irrigation, facial dog-bite wounds are closed and other wounds are treated by delayed primary closure or allowed to heal by secondary intention. Common infecting organisms include *Pasteurella multocida, Streptococcus viridans, Bacteroides* spp, *Fusobacterium,* and *Capnocytophaga.* As in the case of human- and cat-bite wounds, ampicillin plus a beta-lactamase inhibitor provides reasonable empiric coverage for dog-bite wounds. Tetanus and rabies prophylaxis should be administered if indicated. (Table 44-1).

Rabies Prophylaxis

A number of different strains of highly neurotropic viruses cause clinical rabies infection. Susceptibility to rabies infection varies according to species, although most wild mammals can become infected with the virus. Foxes, coyotes, wolves, and jackals are most susceptible, while skunks, raccoons, bats, bobcats, mongooses, and monkeys are moderately susceptible. The epidemiology of human rabies reflects the animal geographic distribution, emphasizing the fact that rabies is primarily a disease of nonhuman mammals. Domestic animal vaccination programs in the United States have been responsible for a dramatic decline in rabies acquired from domestic dog and cat bites. Internationally, the majority of human rabies is still acquired from dog bites, where canine rabies is still endemic.

In humans, the established disease is almost always fatal. Clinical symptoms of human rabies include pain at the bite site, dysphagia, pharyngeal spasms, paralysis, hydrophobia, and seizures. An effective vaccine is available for preventing the onset of clinical rabies. The dismal prognosis of rabies encephalitis strongly emphasizes the importance of appropriate use of the vaccine and immunoglobulin preparation to prevent infection (Table 44-2).

The risk of acquiring rabies depends on the probability of rabies infection in the animal and the amount of inoculum delivered into the wound. The risk of rabies transmission between an animal and a human is greatest when the exposure is from a bite. All animal wounds should be irrigated and cleansed with soap or detergent. This has been shown to protect 90 percent of experimental animals from infection following inoculation of rabies virus into a wound.

Snake Bites

Venomous snakes indigenous to the continental United States fall into two major categories: crotalids, which include rattlesnakes, copperheads, and cot-

TABLE 44-1 Tetanus Prophylaxis

	Non–tetanus-prone wounds		Tetanus-prone wounds	
History of adsorbed tetanus toxoid (doses)	Td*	TIG	Td	TIG
Unknown or less than three doses	Yes	No	Yes	Yes
Three or more doses[†]	No[‡]	No	No[§]	No

*For children younger than 7 years old: diphtheria, tetanus, pertussis (DPT) vaccination (DT, if pertussis vaccine is contraindicated) is preferred to tetanus toxoid alone. For persons 7 years old or more, Td is preferred to tetanus toxoid alone.
[†]If only three doses of fluid toxoid have been given, a fourth dose of toxoid, preferably an adsorbed toxoid should be given.
[‡]Yes, if more than 10 years since last dose.
[§]Yes, if more than 5 years since last dose.
Td, tetanus and diphtheria toxoids adsorbed (for adult use); TIG, tetanus immune globulin (human).
Tetanus toxoid and TIG should be administered with different syringes at different sites.

TABLE 44-2 Schedule of Prophylaxis Recommended in the United States
After Possible Exposure to Rabies

Vaccination status	Regimen*
Not Previously Vaccinated	
Local wound cleansing	Immediate cleansing with soap and water
Rabies immune globulin	20 IU/kg of body weight (If anatomically feasible, up to half the dose should be infiltrated around the wound or wounds and the rest should be administered intramuscularly in the gluteal area. Never give more than the recommended dose. Do not use the syringe used for vaccine or inject into the same anatomic site.)
Vaccine	1.0 mL of HDCV or RVA intramuscularly in the deltoid area[†] on days 0, 3, 7, 14, and 28
Previously Vaccinated[‡]	
Local wound cleansing	Immediate cleansing with soap and water
Rabies immune globulin	Should not be given
Vaccine	1.0 mL of HDCV or RVA intramuscularly in the deltoid area[†] on days 0 and 3

HDVC, human diploid cell vaccine; RVA, rabies vaccine adsorbed.
*The regimens are applicable to all age groups, including children.
[†]The deltoid area is the preferred site of vaccination for adults and older children. For younger children, the outer aspect of the thigh may be used. Vaccine should never be administered in the gluteal area.
[‡]"Previously vaccinated" indicates previous vaccination with HDCV or RVA, or any other type of rabies vaccine, and a documented history of antibody response.
Source: Reproduced, with permission, from Fishbein D, Robinson L: Rabies. *N Engl J Med* 329:1636, 1993.

tonmouths; and elapids, of which coral snakes are the only indigenous species in the United States. Figure 44-2 shows an algorithm for treatment of snake bite.

Identification of the Snake

There are three important genera of Crotalidae in the United States: *Crotalus* and *Sistrurus* (rattlesnakes), and *Agkistrodon* (copperheads and water moccasins). These snakes are characterized by a broad triangular head, relatively thick body, elliptical pupils, and facial pits. All but one species of rattlesnakes have rattles, which distinguishes them from copperheads and water moccasins. The only other snakes of clinical importance in the continental United States are the coral snakes. Two species of these are indigenous to the United States: *Micrurus fulvius* fulvius (Eastern coral snake), and *Micrurus fulvinius* tenere (the Texas coral snake). These snakes are brightly colored, with red, yellow, white, and black rings. They are relatively small bodied, and have small, nontriangular heads without facial pits. The rings encircle the body and the mouth area is black. Their characteristic coloring pattern of a red band adjacent to a yellow one distinguishes coral snakes from other snakes that are brightly colored but nonvenomous. ("Red on yellow, kill a fellow, red on black, venom lack.") Coral snakes belong to the family Elapidae, or elapids, which includes cobras, kraits, mambas, and the poisonous snakes of Australia.

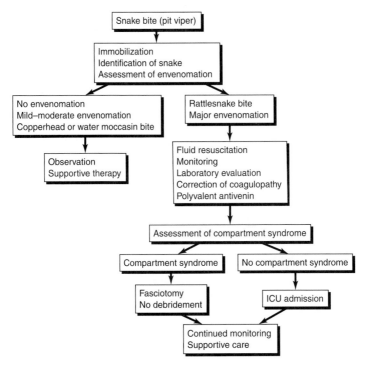

FIG. 44-2.   Algorithm for the treatment of a snake bite. Antivenin should only be used in a setting in which anaphylaxis can be treated.

Crotalid Envenomation

Determination of Envenomation   If there are no fang marks, there has not been envenomation. Even with the presence of fang marks, approximately 20 to 25 percent of patients will not have been envenomated. It is estimated that another 50 percent have minimal to mild envenomation, which would not be a threat to life or limb. Agkistrodon (moccasin and copperhead) bites tend to be less severe than rattlesnake bites, and rarely require antivenin or invasive treatment. With rattlesnake bites, it is usually easy to assess whether envenomation has occurred. A great deal of pain, edema, and frequently discoloration or bulla formation is associated with envenomation. Because these signs and symptoms have a rapid onset, it is probable that if by the time the patient arrives for treatment there is no edema or pain, a significant envenomation has not occurred, or the patient was bitten by a moccasin or copperhead.

First Aid   The most common potentially harmful treatments include incision and suction, electrical shock therapy, use of a tourniquet, and ice immersion. Instead of any of these, current recommendations include immobilization, neutral positioning, and a compression dressing on the bite site, followed by rapid transport of the patient to a hospital.

Definitive Care The principal debate concerns: (1) the use of antivenin therapy; (2) aggressive debridement and fasciotomy; and, more recently, (3) observation with supportive care alone. For severe bites antivenin use is favored, with fasciotomy only in cases of compartment syndrome, and the aggressive use of supportive care. Antivenin is not appropriate therapy for mild or even moderate envenomations, since in such cases the patient will almost certainly do well without any therapy.

Antivenin Therapy A polyvalent equine antivenin has previously been commercially available for the treatment of crotalid envenomations (Wyeth-Ayerst Laboratories, Philadelphia, PA). This product was manufactured by immunizing horses to crotalid venoms and then pooling the horse-serum globulin fraction containing the antibodies. It has been shown to be effective if given up to 4 hours after envenomation, although there is little evidence to support its use beyond 4 hours. However, it was recommended for use in life-threatening envenomations for up to 24 hours following a crotalid bite. Information on the new agent, polyvalent crotalid antivenin ovine FAB, is soon to be available in hospital pharmacies and poison control centers.

Crotalid antivenin is a foreign, impure horse-serum protein fraction and was associated with severe and even life-threatening anaphylactic reactions. The exact incidence of such reactions is unclear, ranging from 1 percent to as high as 30 percent. The antivenin also caused a dose-dependent, delayed-type serum sickness, which is much less severe than an anaphylactic response, although probably more common with massive infusions of antivenin.

In addition to being given as early as possible and in doses large enough to effect a difference, the antivenin was not to be administered in any setting in which anaphylaxis cannot be treated (i.e., in the field), and was initially infused very slowly, with the infusion stopped with signs of hypersensitivity. The dose of antivenin that was given was empiric and based on the physician's assessment of the amount of venom injected. The dose is the same in children as in adults, again being based on the amount of venom to be neutralized rather than on the weight of the patient. Many centers started with a minimum of 5 to 10 vials for severe bites and increased the amount as needed.

Fasciotomy Excellent results have been claimed in clinical series in which fasciotomy has been used. Unfortunately, no controlled trials of it have been conducted, and there are large series in which excellent results have been reported without operative intervention. At this time, fasciotomy should be reserved for the usual indication of compartment syndrome.

Supportive care should consist of fluid resuscitation, tetanus prophylaxis, appropriate monitoring, the administration of antibiotics, and the correction of any coagulopathy. The bacteriology of rattlesnake mouths has been studied. Commonly present organisms include *Pseudomonas* spp, Enterobacteraciae, *Staphylococcus* spp, and clostridia. Ticarcillin with clavulanic acid provides reasonable empiric coverage. Coagulopathy due to fibrinolysis is a common sequela of envenomation, and should be corrected with fresh-frozen plasma and cryoprecipitate.

Coral Snake Envenomation

Coral snake venom has primarily systemic effects consisting of respiratory depression and changes in CNS function. Supportive care, along with commercially available antivenin for sub-species of *Micrurus fulvius* (the Eastern and Texas coral snake), are the mainstays of treatment. This product probably has little cross-reactivity with the venom of *Micrurus euryxanthus* (the Sonoran coral snake). Patients with fang marks or fang scratches should be admitted for observation. Any signs or symptoms should be treated with from 3 to 5 vials of antivenin. If signs of respiratory distress develop, the patient should be intubated and ventilated mechanically.

BITES AND STINGS BY MARINE ANIMALS

Marine Invertebrates

Marine invertebrates of the phylum Cnidra include Schyphozoa (true jelly-fish), Hydrozoa (Portuguese man-of-war and hydras), and Anthozoa (corals and anemones). These animals all have specialized organelles known as nematocysts for poisoning and capturing prey. Most nematocysts cannot penetrate human skin and therefore cause only a painful superficial skin reaction; however, full-thickness penetration can lead to serious illness and even death. Common manifestations of jellyfish stings include local pain and eruption, edema, urticaria, anaphylaxis, and rarely, cardiorespiratory arrest. The principles in the management of such stings are to (1) minimize the number of nematocysts being discharged and (2) minimize the harmful effects of discharged nematocysts. Any adherent tentacles should be carefully removed. Unexploded nematocysts should be deactivated with either a baking soda slurry, papain (meat tenderizer), or a vinegar soak. Hypotension is treated with fluids and inotropic agents if necessary, while pain should be controlled with systemic narcotics. Calcium gluconate may improve the muscle spasms sometimes seen in cases of stings by marine invertebrates.

Venomous Fish

Envenomation by a stingray usually occurs when this fish is stepped on by a swimmer. The wounds are a combination of laceration and puncture, and much of the venom may be removed by simple mechanical irrigation.

INSECT BITES

Allergic reactions are the most common serious problem following insect bites. Because of their widespread distribution and proximity to humans, bees and wasps kill more people per year through fatal anaphylactic reactions to their venoms than do all other venomous animals combined.

Bites by Imported Fire Ants

Solenopsis richteri (the black fire ant) was the first species to be imported, and it has a limited range along the Mississippi-Alabama border. *Solenopsis invicta* (the red fire ant) has had tremendous success in colonization and now has a range extending over most of the southeastern United States. *Solenopsis invicta* tends to give multiple bites, which are initially vesicular, followed by the development of sterile pustule. Fire ant bite allergy is relatively common, and anaphylaxis is probably the most common major problem. Treatment consists of immediately scrubbing the wounds with soap and water, since much of the venom may be removed by mechanical action.

Spider Bites

The brown recluse spider (*Loxosceles reclusa*) has three pairs of eyes and a violin-shaped mark on its carapace. Usually, there is minimal pain following a brown recluse bite, which often makes exact identification of the bite location difficult. In serious bites, a hemorrhagic blister progresses to a dark black necrotic area that may extend over several centimeters. Systemic symptoms may be present, but these are usually mild. Treatment is usually supportive. Early treatment with dapsone may prevent ulceration or hasten healing.

The female black widow spider (*Cactrodecrus macrotans*) has a black body with a red hour-glass mark on the underside of her abdomen. Symptoms of envenomation, begin within an hour of the bite, and include pain, muscle rigidity, altered mental status, and seizures. Treatment is supportive, although there is an equine antivenin available for use in severe cases. Dantrolene has been used as have calcium and methacarbamol. The death rate from severe bites has been reported to be as high as 5 percent.

Bee and Wasp Stings

The most serious problem in cases of bee and wasp stings relates to the development of an immediate hypersensitivity reaction. Bees sting with double-barbed lancets, which tend to anchor the bee to the victim's skin. When the bee dislodges itself, it usually leaves its stinging apparatus behind, thus killing the bee. The exuded venom sac of the bee should be scraped with a knife, instead of squeezing the skin to get the poison sac out. Application of an ice pack to the local area tends to alleviate the associated pain. Some have advocated the local application of papain following removal of the venom sac. Patients who have a known sensitivity to bee or wasp stings should carry an emergency kit for the injection of epinephrine and should wear a medical identification bracelet.

ADDITIONAL READING

A Symposium. Wound infection and occlusion—separating fact from fiction. *Am J Surg* 167:1A, 1994.

Fishbein D, Robinson L: Rabies. *N Engl J Med* 329:1632, 1993.

Russell FE, Carlson RW, Wainschel J, et al: Snake venom poisoning in the United States: Experiences with 550 cases. *JAMA* 233:341, 1975.

Stewart RM, Page CP, Schwesinger WH, et al: Antivenin and fasciotomy/debridement in the treatment of the severe rattlesnake bite. *Am J Surg* 158:543, 1989.

Thomas S: *Wound Management and Dressing.* London, Pharmaceutical Press, 1990.

45 | Burns and Radiation Injuries

BURNS

Over 1.2 million people are burned in the United States every year. Most of these burns are minor and treated in the outpatient setting; however, approximately 60,000 burns are moderate to severe and require hospitalization. The American Burn Association has established guidelines to determine which patients may be treated in a general hospital setting and which should be transferred to a specialized burn unit. Patients meeting the following criteria should be treated at a designated burn center:

- Second- and third-degree burns of greater than 10 percent total body surface area (TBSA) in patients <10 or >50 years of age
- Second- and third-degree burns over 20 percent of TBSA in patients ages 10 to 50
- Full-thickness burns over 5 percent of TBSA in any age group
- Any burn involving the face, hands, feet, eyes, ears, or perineum that may result in cosmetic or functional disability
- High-voltage electrical injury including lightning injury
- Inhalation injury or associated trauma
- Chemical burns
- Burns in patients with significant comorbid conditions (e.g., diabetes mellitus, chronic obstructive pulmonary disease [COPD])

Pathophysiology

Burns are classified by cause into five different categories, into three zones of injury, and by five different depths of injury (Table 45-1). Most of these induce cellular damage primarily by the transfer of energy that induces coagulative necrosis. Direct injury to cellular membranes is the cause of injury in chemical and electrical burns. Clinical characteristics of the different burn levels are described in Table 45-2.

Initial Care and Resuscitation

The immediate treatment of a burn patient should proceed as with any trauma victim. Airway is the first priority after removing the patient from the inciting cause. If the patient is not breathing or has labored respirations, immediate orotracheal intubation is performed with in-line stabilization of the neck. Patients who are not intubated should be given oxygen by mask. All burned patients are placed on oxygen saturation monitors, but normal readings should be interpreted with caution. The presence of carbon monoxide (CO) in the blood, which has an affinity 280 times that of oxygen for hemoglobin, can falsely elevate oxygen saturation. The treatment for CO inhalation is 100 percent O_2 by endotracheal tube or face mask. This will decrease the half-life of CO from 4 hours (when breathing room air) to 45 minutes. Measurement of carboxyhemoglobin levels will give an estimate of the amount of CO in the blood. It must be emphasized that as generalized edema develops in the course of resuscitation, compromise of the airway may increase and mandate early intubation.

Intravenous access is the next priority. Venous access is best attained through peripheral catheters in unburned skin, though veins in burned skin can be used. The initial rate of intravenous fluids can be estimated by multiplying the estimated TBSA burned by the weight in kilograms and dividing by

TABLE 45-1 Definition of Burn Types, Zones, and Depth of Injury

Burn categories	Zones of injury	Burn depth
Flame	Zone of Coagulation	First degree (epidermal)
Scald	Zone of Stasis	Superficial second degree
Contact	Zone of Hyperemia	(superficial dermal)
Chemicals		Deep second degree (deep dermal)
Electricity		Third degree (full thickness)
		Fourth degree (deep organ
		involvement)

8. Thus the rate of infusion for a 80-kg man with 40 percent TBSA burned would be 80 kg × 40% TBSA/8 = 400 mL/h.

Most burn units around the country use something similar to either the Parkland or Brooke formula for initial resuscitation estimates. For burned children, formulas are modified to account for changes in surface area:mass ratios (Table 45-3). These formulas are guidelines to direct physicians in the amount of fluid necessary to maintain adequate perfusion. All of these formulas calculate the amount of volume given in the first 24 hours, one-half of which should be given in the first 8 hours. Responses are monitored by monitoring the volume of urine output, which should be at 1.0 mL/kg/h. Appropriate changes in infusion should be made hourly.

Patients should initially be placed on clean sheets with cotton gauze placed on the wounds. Cold water and ice do not reduce the level of injury. Initial treatment in addition to keeping the wounds clean should be left to the physicians

TABLE 45-2 Clinical Characteristics of Burn Levels

Burn depth	Clinical characteristics
First degree (epidermal)	Erythematous
	Blanch
	Painful to touch
	Will heal with minimal effort, treatment directed at symptomatic relief with NSAIDs, soothing salves
Superficial second degree (Partial-thickness)	Erythematous
	Wet and often blistered
	Painful to touch
	Will heal in 7–14 days by re-epithelialization
	Require coverage with topical antimicrobials or artificial skin covering
Deep second degree (Partial-thickness)	Pale and mottled
	Do not blanch
	May have a pseudoeschar that is soft
	Remain painful to pinprick
	Will heal in 14–28 days with severe scarring
Third degree	Hard leathery eschar that is white or cherry red in color
(Full-thickness)	
	Painless
	Will require excision and grafting for healing
Fourth degree	Thermal injury to underlying organs in addition to the skin

TABLE 45-3 Resuscitation Formulas

Formula	Crystalloid volume	Colloid volume	Free water
Parkland	4 mL/kg/% TBSA burn	None	None
Brooke	1.5 mL/kg/% TBSA burn	0.5 uL/kg/% TBSA burn	2.0 Liters
Galveston (Pediatric)	5000 mL/m² burned + 1500 mL/m² total	None	None

responsible for definitive care of the burns. Nasogastric tubes and bladder catheters are placed on admission to decompress the stomach, treat any early ileus, and to monitor the progress of resuscitation through urine output.

Determination of burn size is assessed by the "rule of nines" (Fig. 45-1). Another method of estimating smaller burns is by using the area of the patient's palm, which is approximately 1 percent TBSA; the palm is transposed visually on the wound to determine its size. This method is helpful when evaluating splash burns and other burns of uneven distribution. Children have a relatively larger portion of the body surface area on the head and neck, and the Berkow formula is used to determine burn size in pediatric patients (Table 45-4).

When deep second- and third-degree burn wounds encompass the circumference of an extremity, peripheral circulation to the limb can be compromised. Development of generalized edema beneath a nonyielding eschar impedes venous outflow and will eventually affect arterial inflow to the distal beds. Extremities at risk are identified on either clinical examination or by measurement of tissue pressures greater than 40 mm Hg. These extremities

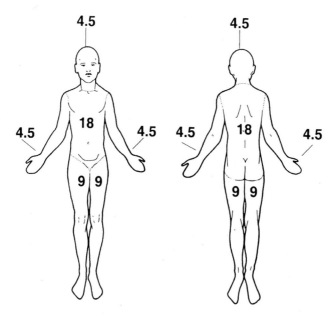

FIG. 45-1.   Determining burn size by the "rule of nines."

TABLE 45-4 Berkow Chart for Estimation of Burn Size in Children

Area	Up to 1 y	1–4 y	5–9 y	10–14 y	15 y
Head	19	17	13	11	9
Neck	2	2	2	2	2
Anterior trunk	13	13	13	13	13
Posterior trunk	13	13	13	13	13
Buttock	2.5	2.5	2.5	2.5	2.5
Genitalia	1	1	1	1	1
Upper arm	4	4	4	4	4
Lower arm	3	3	3	3	3
Hand	2.5	2.5	2.5	2.5	2.5
Thigh	5.5	6.5	8	8.5	9
Leg	5	5	5.5	6	6.5
Foot	3.5	3.5	3.5	3.5	3.5

require escharotomy, which is performed by incising the lateral and medial aspects of the eschar. The constricting eschar must be incised completely to relieve the impediment to blood flow. The incisions are carried down onto the thenar and hypothenar eminences, and along the lateral sides of the digits to completely open the hand if it is involved. If vascular compromise has been prolonged, reperfusion after an escharotomy may cause reactive hyperemia and further edema formation in muscle compartments. A standard fasciotomy in the involved extremity may then be needed.

A constricting truncal eschar can cause a similar phenomenon, except the effect is to decrease ventilation by limiting chest excursion. Decreased ventilation of a burn patient should prompt inspection of the chest with appropriate escharotomies to relieve the constriction and allow inspiration of adequate tidal volumes.

Chemical Burns

In the case of chemical burn, the wound is copiously irrigated with several liters of water or saline to neutralize the offending agent. Care must be taken to direct the drainage of the irrigating solution away from unburned areas to limit the area of skin exposed to noxious chemicals. Attempts at neutralization of acidic or basic solutions will only result in heat production and extend the injury. Acids cause coagulative necrosis and are therefore confined. This is in contrast to basic solutions, which will cause liquefactive necrosis and extend further into the tissues until the offending agent is removed.

Hydrofluoric acid is a toxic substance. When exposed to biological tissues, the fluoride ion precipitates all available calcium, making hypocalcemia the immediately life-threatening complication. In addition to copious irrigation, the exposed skin should be treated with 2.5 percent calcium gluconate gel to provide pain relief and limit the spread of the fluoride ion. All these patients should be monitored closely for prolongation of the QT interval with continuous electrocardiographic monitoring. Changes in the QT interval should be treated with 20 mL of 10 percent calcium gluconate per liter of lactated Ringer's solution used in resuscitation.

Electrical Burns

Electrical burns are unique in that the location of the injury is mostly internal. Electrical current proceeds down the path of least resistance, which is via nerves, blood vessels, and muscle, thus sparing the skin. With any significant electrical injury, vigorous intravenous resuscitation should be given with attention to myoglobinuria from muscle damage. Urine output should be maintained at greater than 1 mL/kg/h, with intravenous mannitol and bicarbonate given to increase renal tubular flow, alkalinize the urine and decrease precipitation of hemochromogens in the renal tubules. Patients should also be monitored for cardiac arrhythmias. Serial examinations of the extremities are necessary to detect any vascular compromise, and fasciotomies are often necessary.

The Burn Wound

The choice of dressing should be individualized based on the characteristics of the treated wound. Wounds from first-degree burns are minor with minimal loss of barrier function. These wounds require no dressing and are treated with topical salves to decrease pain and keep the skin moist. Wounds from second-degree burns can be treated with an antibiotic ointment such as silver sulfadiazine covered with several layers of cotton gauze under elastic wraps. The dressing should be changed daily. Alternatively, the wounds can be treated with a temporary biologic or synthetic covering (e.g., Biobrane®).

Deep second- and third-degree burns will not heal in a timely fashion without autografting. In fact, the dead tissue only serves as a nidus for inflammation and infection that may ultimately be fatal. Most burn surgeons now follow a practice of early excision and grafting for full-thickness wounds. This technique has made conservative treatment of full-thickness wounds a practice to be used only in the elderly and when anesthesia and surgery are contraindicated.

After a burn wound has been excised, the wound must be covered. This covering is ideally the patient's own skin. Wounds involving 20 to 30 percent of the TBSA can usually be closed at one operation with autograft split-thickness skin. In these operations, the skin grafts are either not meshed, or are meshed with a small ratio (2:1 or less) to improve the cosmetic result. In major burns, the amount of available autograft skin may be limited such that the wound cannot be completely closed. One method of treatment is to use widely expanded autografts (4:1 or greater) covered with cadaver allograft to completely close the wounds for which autograft is available. The 4:1 skin heals underneath the cadaver skin in approximately 21 days, and the cadaver skin will fall off. The portions of the wound that cannot be covered with even widely meshed autograft are covered with allograft skin in preparation for autografting when donor sites are healed. Ideally, areas with less cosmetic importance are covered with the widely meshed skin to close most of the wound prior to using nonmeshed grafts at later operations for the cosmetically important areas, such as the hands and face.

Occasionally, skin grafts will not adhere. Loss of skin grafts is due to one or more of the following reasons: (1) fluid collection under the graft, (2) shearing forces that disrupt the adhered graft, (3) presence of infection, or (4) an inadequate excision of the wound bed with remaining necrotic tissue.

Antimicrobials

Topical antibiotics can be divided into two classes, salves and soaks (Table 45-5). Salves are generally applied directly to the wound with cotton dressings placed over them, and soaks are poured into cotton dressings on the

TABLE 45-5 Common Salves and Soaks Used to Treat Burn Wounds

Salves	Advantages	Disadvantages
Silver sulfadiazine (Silvadene 1%)	Broad spectrum Relatively painless on application	Transient leukopenia Does not penetrate eschar May tattoo dermis with black flecks
Mafenide acetate (Sulfamylon 11%)	Broad spectrum Penetration of eschar	Painful on application to partial thickness burns May cause an allergic rash Carbonic anhydrase activity
Polymyxin B/ neomycin/bacitracin	Wide spectrum Painless on application Colorless allowing direct inspection of the wound	Antimicrobial coverage less than alternatives
Mupirocin (Bactroban)	Broad spectrum (especially species)	Expensive
Nystatin	Broad antifungal coverage	May inactivate other (Sulfamylon) antimicrobials

Soaks	Advantages	Disadvantages
Silver nitrate (0.5%)	Complete antimicrobial coverage Painless	Black staining when exposed to light Electrolyte leaching Methemoglobinemia
Mafenide acetate (Sulfamylon 5%)	Same as salve	Same as salve
Sodium hypochlorite (Dakins' 0.05%)	Broad-spectrum coverage	Inactivated with protein contact Cytotoxic
Acetic acid	Broad-spectrum coverage (especially *Pseudomonas*)	Cytotoxic

wound. Each of these classes of antimicrobials has its advantages and disadvantages. Salves may be applied once or twice a day, but may lose their effectiveness between dressing changes. Soaks will remain effective because antibiotic solution can be added without removing the dressing; however, the underlying skin can become macerated.

Inhalation Injury

One factor that contributes to mortality in burns is the presence of inhalation injury. Smoke injury adds another inflammatory focus to the burn, and impedes the normal gas exchange vital to critically injured patients. In most inhalation injuries, damage is caused primarily by inhaled toxins. Heat is generally dispersed in the upper airways, whereas the cooled particles of smoke and toxins are carried distally into the bronchi and alveoli. Thus the injury is principally chemical in nature.

A patient with smoke inhalation often presents with a history of exposure to smoke in an enclosed space, hoarseness, wheezing, and carbonaceous sputum. It may also be associated with facial burns and singed nasal vibrissae. Because each of these findings has poor sensitivity and specificity, the diagnosis is often established by the use of bronchoscopy or [133]xenon ventilation scanning.

Management of inhalation injury is directed at maintaining open airways and maximizing gas exchange while the lung heals. A coughing patient with a patent airway can clear secretions very effectively, and efforts should be made to treat patients without mechanical ventilation if possible. If respiratory failure is imminent, intubation should be instituted, with chest physiotherapy and suctioning performed frequently. Mechanical ventilation should be used to provide gas exchange with as little barotrauma as possible.

Inhalation treatments have been effective in improving the clearance of tracheobronchial secretions and decreasing bronchospasm. In addition to routine respiratory treatments, heparin administered directly into the lungs in a nebulized form (5000 units in 3 mL normal saline every 4 hours) decreases formation of fibrin casts.

RADIATION INJURIES

Radiation consists of both particles (α, β, and neutrons) and photons (γ- and x-rays) which have differing energies and tissue penetrance. The potential for biologic injury with each depends on the amount of energy transmitted by the particle or photon when it interacts with the target, which is referred to as *linear energy transfer* (Table 45-6).

Exposure to radiation can be classified into three types:

- Small contained events affecting one or more persons;
- An industrial incident affecting large numbers of people with varying degrees of severity (e.g., a nuclear power plant meltdown); and
- Detonation of a nuclear device.

Radiation Incidents

A significant radiation incident is one in which an individual receives an injury that meets at least one of the following criteria:

- A whole-body radiation dose of at least 25 rem (0.25 Sv);
- A skin dose of at least 600 rem (6 Sv);
- An absorbed dose of at least 75 rem (7.5 Sv) to tissues other than the skin; or
- Internal contamination of at least one-half the maximum permissible body burden (MPBB) as defined by the International Commission on Radiological Protection (ICRP). This number is different for each radionuclide and can be found in the ICRP manual.

Radiation incidents must be reported to the Radiation Emergency Assistance Center/Training Site (REAC/TS) in Oak Ridge, Tennessee. The telephone number for REAC/TS is (615) 482-2441.

TABLE 45-6 Types of Radiation, Relative Energies, Penetrance, and Relative Hazard

	Relative energy (MeV)	Penetrance into tissue (cm)	Relative hazard
α (Two protons and two neutrons)	1–5	.0007–0044	Low
β (One electron)	0.2–1.0	.017–34	Moderate
γ (One photon)	0.1–10	20–150	High

Pathophysiology

Radiation damage to cells is caused by the transfer of kinetic energy from particles or photons to other molecules, causing ionization of mostly oxygen, and the formation of free radicals (such as the hydroxyl radical). These highly toxic compounds then react with normal biologic molecules to cause cellular damage, mostly to the phospholipid membranes and DNA. Different cell types have different sensitivities to radiation based on characteristics of the individual cell (Table 45-7).

Treatment

Once resuscitation has begun and the initial trauma assessment is complete, decontamination of any open wounds should be begun. These wounds are assumed to be contaminated with radioactive material, and should be gently irrigated with copious quantities of water or saline. The irrigant should be disposed of properly. Irrigation is continued until the area reaches a steady state or absence of radiation is detected by a Geiger counter. Attention should then be turned to the intact skin, where decontamination proceeds with gentle scrubbing with a soft brush under a steady stream of water for 3 to 4 minutes. Following this, an application of hexachlorophene solution for a 2-minute scrub is recommended. After two more rounds of the above procedure are done, diluted hypochlorite bleach (3 percent) (1 part commercial bleach to 10 parts water) can be used to remove more radioactive particles.

During stabilization of the patient, important information to gather includes the type of radiation, whether the source was sealed, the duration of the exposure, and the distance from the source. These data are necessary to calculate the dose. A complete blood count should be performed as soon as possible, with particular attention to the total lymphocyte count (TLC), as this is the most accurate indication of degree of radiation injury (Table 45-8).

Localized Radiation Injury

Radiation injuries are either localized or whole-body, depending on the circumstances of the exposure. The term *localized radiation injury* refers to an

TABLE 45-7 Radiosensitivity of Human Cell Types

Radiosensitivity	Cell Types
Very high	Lymphocytes Hematopoietic cells Intestinal epithelium Spermatogonia, ovarian follicular cells
High	Urinary bladder epithelium Esophageal epithelium
Intermediate	Endothelium Fibroblasts Pulmonary epithelium Renal epithelium Hepatocytes
Low	Hematopoietic stem cells Myocytes Chondrocytes Neural cells

TABLE 45-8 Significance of Absolute Lymphocyte Count on Prognosis

Lymphocyte count	Significance and prognosis
>2000/mm^3	Normal; no injury suspected; prognosis good
1200–2000 mm^3	Mild exposure; significant but probably not lethal
500–1200 mm^3	Moderate exposure; prognosis guarded
100–500 mm^3	Severe exposure; prognosis poor
<100 mm^3	Lethal

injury involving a relatively small portion of the body. Erythema of the skin is often the first sign, and the sooner it appears, the higher the dose of exposure. Depilation is also helpful in determining the extent of localized injury and may occur as soon as 7 days after exposure. Moist desquamation equivalent to a second-degree burn develops over a period of 3 weeks, and occurs with doses of 12 to 20 Gy. The latency period is shorter with higher doses. Full-thickness ulceration and necrosis are caused by doses in excess of 25 Gy, and onset varies from weeks to months after exposure.

Management of Localized Injuries

After decontamination, mild erythema should be treated conservatively with light dressings if needed. Any dry desquamation can be treated with lotions to moisturize the skin, while moist desquamation should be treated as a second-degree burn wound. Wounds with high radiation exposure may ultimately convert to full-thickness necrosis from obliterative endarteritis and require skin grafting, flap coverage, or amputation.

Whole-Body Exposure

As with localized injury, the extent of manifestation of whole-body exposure depends on the dose of radiation received. The effects are primarily on the hematopoietic, gastrointestinal, cardiovascular, and central nervous systems. With relatively lower doses (<15 Gy), bleeding, infection, and electrolyte loss can occur from damage to the intestinal mucosa and blood cell components. Higher doses (>15 Gy) will cause cardiovascular collapse and circulatory failure.

The dose absorbed will determine which one or all of the three courses described below transpires:

1. Hematopoietic symptoms—exposure to 1 to 4 Gy causes pancytopenia with an onset of 48 hours and a nadir at 30 days. Opportunistic infections and spontaneous bleeding can also occur.
2. Gastrointestinal symptoms—exposure to 8 to 12 Gy will cause gastrointestinal symptoms in addition to pancytopenia. Severe nausea, vomiting, cramping, and watery diarrhea occur within hours of the exposure. This resolves, then in 4 to 7 days, the epithelium of the bowel sloughs, which causes bloody diarrhea and loss of the intestinal barrier mechanisms. Sepsis and massive fluid losses ensue.
3. Neurovascular symptoms—exposure to >15 Gy causes immediate total collapse of vascular tone superimposed on the above symptoms.

Management of Whole-Body Injuries

The management of whole-body irradiation is aimed primarily at symptoms of cellular loss until these systems can regenerate themselves. Except for removal of internal radiation, no treatment can speed up the process. Resuscitation needs may also be high to maintain euvolemia and urine output because of volume losses.

Patients with less than 1 Gy of exposure can be treated as outpatients if there are no other injuries. For those with more than 1 Gy exposure, they should be admitted and kept until the symptoms have subsided. Gastrointestinal bleeding, diarrhea, infections, anemia, and diffuse bleeding from pancytopenia may occur with varying degrees of severity. If the exposure is more than 2 Gy, a bone marrow transplant as a salvage maneuver should be considered. If this is considered, the blood analysis and cell typing should be completed promptly because severe radiation exposure may so rapidly deplete the peripheral lymphocytes that none remain to serve as a basis for identification.

ADDITIONAL READING

Brigham PA, McLoughlin E: Burn incidence and medical care in the United States: estimates, trends, and data sources. *J Burn Care Rehab* 17:95, 1996.

Browne D, Weiss JF, MacVitte TJ, Madhavan VP (eds): Consensus summary. p. 10. In *Treatment of Radiation Injuries.* New York, Plenum, 1990.

Nenot JC: Medical and surgical management for localized radiation injuries. *Int J Radiation Biol* 57:784, 1990.

Warden GD: Fluid resuscitation and early management. pp. 53-60. In Herndon DN (ed): *Total Burn Care.* Philadelphia, WB Saunders, 1996.

Wolf SE, Rose JK, Desai MH, et al: Mortality determinants in massive pediatric burns: an analysis of 103 children with greater than 80% TBSA burns (70% full-thickness). *Ann Surg* 225-554, 1997.

SYSTEMIC HYPOTHERMIA

Primary Accidental Hypothermia

Primary hypothermia is defined as a core temperature below 35°C caused by excessive exposure to snow, wind, water, or altitude. It is considered primary because thermoregulatory mechanisms remain intact, and the patient becomes cold due to environmental stress. Patients typically have a number of physiologic abnormalities, including acidosis, electrolyte disturbances, dehydration, hypoxia, respiratory failure, intense vasoconstriction, and cardiac dysfunction. These complications may not be apparent until rewarming is initiated, and may become progressively worse as body temperature increases. Control of these abnormalities may be more important determinants of outcome than the specific method of rewarming used. If the physiologic problems are corrected and cardiopulmonary function is maintained, mortality is relatively low, and primarily depends upon associated comorbidity.

Body temperature may continue to decrease (afterdrop) even after removal from the cold. Since the risk of fibrillation rises rapidly as the core temperature drops to 30°C, rewarming should be more aggressive as the core temperature approaches this level. The afterdrop was previously believed to be due to peripheral vasodilatation, with washout of cold, acidotic blood sequestered in the periphery, but there is little evidence to support this mechanism. Only a small amount of blood remains in the vasoconstricted periphery of a hypothermic patient. Several studies have measured peripheral blood flow, and noted no change in flow through skin or muscle during the afterdrop, and this phenomenon has been observed in fibrillating patients without any circulation.

Heat always flows from an area of higher temperature to one of lower temperature. Therefore, heat naturally flows from the core to the periphery, causing the central temperature to decrease. Intensive core rewarming to offset the dissipation of central heat, and aggressive external rewarming to reduce the abnormally elevated core to periphery temperature gradient are the best methods for eliminating or decreasing the duration of the afterdrop.

In determining whether or not to resuscitate a patient without cardiac activity, it is reasonable to attempt to determine if cooling preceded or caused cardiac arrest, or if hypothermia occurred afterwards. However, there are several reports of hypothermic patients who have been successfully resuscitated after several hours of cardiopulmonary resuscitation (CPR). Therefore resuscitation should generally be continued until the absence of cardiac activity is documented after raising the body temperature to a level that does not preclude defibrillation (30°C).

Secondary Accidental Hypothermia

Secondary hypothermia occurs when the patient has abnormal heat production and heat-conserving mechanisms, and becomes hypothermic while being subjected to only relatively mild cold stress. The mortality rate is far higher than that of primary hypothermia due to its association with severe underlying diseases (e.g., trauma, stroke, hypoglycemia, hypothyroidism). This very high mortality is especially true for the trauma patient. One study demonstrated a mortality of 40 percent when the core temperature was less than 34°, 69 percent when the temperature dropped to less than 33°, and 100 percent with hypothermia of 32°C or less. Shock appears to be the primary risk factor in injured patients. Heat production is due to oxidation, and is therefore proportional to oxygen consumption. Aggressive resuscitation is the key management priority for prevention and treatment of secondary hypothermia in the injured patient.

Hypothermia and Outcome

Due to the strong correlation between hypothermia and injury severity, it is difficult to use retrospective data to determine if mortality is due to the hypothermia, or to the severity of the underlying injuries. A recent randomized trial used an extracorporeal arteriovenous warmer to rapidly reverse hypothermia in cold, critically injured patients to determine if rapid rewarming improved outcome. During resuscitation, 43 percent of patients randomized to standard (slower) rewarming methods died, compared to 7 percent randomized to rapid rewarming ($p < 0.01$). Rapid rewarming also reduced crystalloid and blood requirements. This suggests that hypothermia has a particularly detrimental effect during resuscitation, and survival can be improved by aggressive rewarming. A suggested treatment algorithm is shown in Fig. 46-1.

Hypothermia and Coagulation

Coagulation assays are performed by heating both the blood and the reagents to 37°C before conducting the assay, regardless of the patient's core temperature. When assays are performed at the patient's body temperature the results are significantly prolonged in comparison to the 37°C test result. This appears to be due to a reduction in the reaction rates of the enzymes involved in the clotting process. Platelet dysfunction may also occur. Systemic hypothermia to 32°C nearly triples the bleeding time (Ivy method).

Protective Effects of Hypothermia

There has been recent interest in the use of hypothermia for neuroprotection after traumatic brain injury. However, two recent randomized prospective trials showed no improvement in neurologic outcome, and an increase in infections and length of hospital stay. Given the detrimental effects of systemic hypothermia on critically injured patients, hypothermia should be prevented or aggressively treated in all patients. Strategies for utilizing the potential benefits of hypothermia have not yet been identified.

Rewarming Methods

Specific heat is the amount of heat required to raise the temperature of 1 kilogram of a substance by 1 degree centigrade. The specific heat of the human body is 0.83 kcal/kg/°C. Thus a 70-kg patient must acquire 58.1 kcal (70 kg × 0.83 kcal/kg/°C) to increase body temperature by 1 degree.

Airway Rewarming

At 41°C, fully saturated air can hold 0.05 mL H_2O/L. At 32°C, air can hold only 0.03 mL H_2O/L. When a patient with a body temperature of 32°C inspires a liter of saturated air at 41°C, 0.02 mL of H_2O condenses within the airway. With a minute ventilation of 10 L/min (600 L air/h), 12 mL H_2O/h

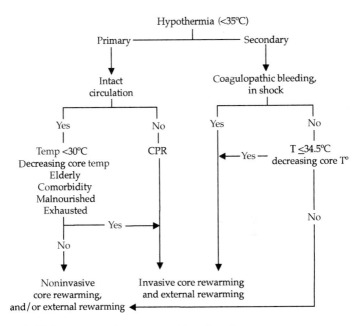

FIG. 46-1. Algorithm for treatment of hypothermia.

condenses within the airway. Condensation liberates 0.58 kcal/mL of conden-sate (latent heat of vaporization). Thus the amount of heat provided by airway rewarming under these conditions is 6.96 kcal/h (12 mL H_2O/h × 0.58 kcal/mL H_2O), which is only sufficient to raise the body temperature by 0.12°C/h (6.96 kcal/58.1 kcal/°C).

Convective Rewarming

Air blankets emit 24,000 L/h of warm (43°C) air. Since the density of air is 0.0012 kg/L, roughly 28.8 kg of air is emitted. The specific heat of air is 0.24 kcal/kg/°C. Given the high flow rate, the temperature of the air decreases by only 1 to 2 degrees as it passes over the body. Thus this method provides only 6.9 to 13.8 kcal/h (28.8 kg air/h × 0.24 kcal/kg/°C).

However, when two masses are in contact, heat always flows from the warmer object to the colder one, regardless of the differences in their heat content. If the air surrounding the skin is warmer than the skin, the patient cannot lose heat except by sweating. Since most heat is lost through the skin, these devices are effective at limiting heat loss by creating a warm environ-ment around the patient, but little heat is actively transferred to a patient by the use of warm air.

Body Cavity Lavage

Since the specific heat of water is 1 kcal/kg/°C, when a liter of 42°C water exits the body at 37°C, 5 kcal of heat is left in the body, which increases body temperature by 0.08°C. As the patient warms, the temperature of the exiting water increases, resulting in less heat transfer unless longer dwell times are used. Continuous irrigation is advisable, using thoracic cavity lavage via two ipsilateral chest tubes.

Warm Intravenous Fluids

The amount of heat transferred is equal to the temperature difference between the fluid and the patient. A liter of 42°C fluid infused into a 32°C patient provides 10 kcal of heat, which will increase body temperature by 0.17°C/L (10 kcal/58.1 kcal/°C). Due to the high specific heat of water, warm intravenous fluid can have a significant effect on cold patients with high fluid resuscitation requirements.

Extracorporeal Rewarming

Cardiopulmonary bypass relies on the principle of continuous warm intravenous fluid infusion, but circumvents the patient's fluid requirement limitations by recirculating the patient's blood. The specific heat of blood is 0.9 kcal/L/°C. If 32°C blood is warmed to 41°C and reinfused, 8.1 kcal/L of heat is transferred. At a flow rate of 2.5 L/min, the initial heat transfer rate will equal 1250 kcal/h. Using a similar calculation method, an extracorporeal arteriovenous fistula with a flow rate between 200 and 350 mL/min will provide an initial heat transfer rate of between 97 and 170 kcal/h.

Spontaneous Rewarming

Normal oxygen consumption produces 1 kcal/kg/h. A 70-kg patient will generate sufficient heat to rewarm at a rate of 1.2°C/h. With shivering, heat production can increase threefold. The patient's own heat production is the most important source of heat gain.

FROSTBITE AND NONFREEZING COLD INJURIES

Frostbite is defined as local freezing of tissues, resulting in ice crystal formation within the extracellular space. This causes osmotic transport of water out of the cell and cellular dehydration, and if prolonged leads to mechanical tissue injury due to enlarging ice crystals. Pain and numbness are the typical symptoms, and pain usually becomes severe during thawing. The frozen body part appears waxy or white. During thawing, severe hyperemia, edema, and blistering occur. Edema, as well as red cell and platelet dumping, cause profound circulatory stasis, which may lead to ischemia, with progression to gangrene. Autonomic dysfunction due to nerve damage is also a common sequela. The absence of edema during rewarming, or cyanosis that does not blanch with pressure are poor prognostic signs. The depth and extent of damage to frostbitten tissue is often not apparent for days or even weeks after injury.

Decreasing the time the tissues are frozen by rapid rewarming significantly decreases the extent of damage and reduces the progression of injury. Standard treatment consists of immersion in a warm water bath (40 to 42°C) until rewarming is complete and flushing is observed down to the tips of the fingers or toes and sensation returns. Early debridement should be avoided, even in the face of obvious necrosis, unless infection occurs. Postponement for as long as 2 to 3 months, and allowing spontaneous amputation of tissues, maximizes tissue preservation. Significant healing usually takes place, and the amount of resection required is considerably less than initially anticipated. Early surgical treatment is limited to treatment of compartment syndrome, which sometimes occurs after thawing.

Local treatment while awaiting demarcation consists of elevating the body part to minimize edema, gentle daily nonabrasive cleaning, preferably in a whirlpool bath, air drying of tissues, placing cotton between the digits to minimize maceration, using a tent to prevent abrasion, and avoiding pressure spots. Prophylactic antibiotics are not indicated. Blisters should be left intact, as they provide sterile coverage of underlying tissues. After resolution of edema, digits should be exercised during the whirlpool bath, and physical therapy begun.

Trench foot, or nonfreezing cold injury, is due to repeated long-term exposure to cold water at near-freezing temperatures. There is no ice crystal formation, and the pathophysiology appears to be due to intense arterial vasospasm. Peripheral myelin sheaths are particularly sensitive to cold and ischemia, and undergo degeneration and chronic neuropathic changes. The feet initially feel cold and painful, and appear waxen, but not frozen. After rewarming, a hyperemic phase ensues, with intense burning and blister formation. Local warmth and pain may last for weeks. Chronic pain and cold sensitization, Raynaud's phenomenon, numbness, and motor nerve abnormalities are the most common sequelae. Treatment consists of rapid rewarming, elevation, pain control, and range-of-motion exercises to minimize disability.

HEAT OVERLOAD SYNDROMES

There are two main categories of heat-related illness: heat exhaustion and heat stroke. Heat exhaustion is characterized by profuse sweating and progressive hypovolemia, with tachycardia, tachypnea, dizziness, and profound fatigue. Treatment consists of removing the patient from the heat, oral or intravenous hydration, removal of clothing, and increasing evaporative and convective heat losses by fanning with mist, by dry fanning after moistening the body with water or alcohol, or by placing the patient in an artificially cooled environment or in a cool bath. It should be noted that with high ambient temperatures ($\geq$37.8°C, 100°F) fanning will actually increase heat stress. Fanning can also be rendered ineffective by high humidity. If the ambient temperature exceeds 90°F, fanning does not result in cooling if the humidity exceeds 35 percent.

Heat stroke is a much more serious illness characterized by complete thermoregulatory dysfunction, with hyperpyrexia and absence of sweating. Mortality is between 17 and 80 percent in most reports. The two key signs that distinguish heat stroke from heat exhaustion are the absence of sweating and the presence of neurologic findings ranging from stupor to coma and convulsions, which are present in all patients. The duration of hyperpyrexia, rather than its magnitude, appears to be the more critical determinant of outcome. Therefore, early, rapid cooling is essential, and usually results in complete neurologic recovery, while delays in treatment usually result in permanent sequelae.

The adverse effects of heat on the heart are common, with many patients demonstrating ischemia or conduction defects. However, multiple organ failure with acute respiratory distress syndrome, hepatic failure, disseminated intravascular coagulation, rhabdomyolysis, and renal failure are the most frequent causes of death after cooling. High circulating levels of endogenous pyrogens with proinflammatory effects, such as tumor necrosis factor, interleukin-1, and gamma interferon have been detected in victims of heat stroke, and have been proposed as mediators of the multisystem organ failure which often occurs, and which has striking similarities to the systemic inflammatory response syndrome (SIRS).

Treatment consists of intravenous therapy with fluids at 18°C, whole-body cooling, control of neurologic symptoms such as seizures, treatment of acid-base and electrolyte abnormalities, and treatment of multisystem involvement. Due to the effects of hyperpyrexia on cardiac function, fluid replacement may need guidance with central pressure monitoring. At the point of collapse patients may be peripherally dilated, but during cooling vasoconstriction may occur, making accurate determination of volume status difficult.

Surface cooling is adequate in most cases, and internal cooling and peritoneal or pleural lavage is generally not necessary except in cases thought to be due to malignant hyperthermia or neuroleptic malignant syndrome, in which there is an ongoing abnormal rate of heat production. Fanning after moistening the body surface with water or alcohol, or cold water immersion are the most commonly used treatments. Excessive cold should be avoided, as this may prompt vasoconstriction and reduce the rate of cooling, and potent vasoconstricting drugs to treat hypotension should probably also be avoided.

ADDITIONAL READING

Clifton GL, Miller ER, Choi SC, et al: Lack of effect of induction of hypothermia after acute brain injury. *N Engl J Med* 344:556, 2001.

Gentilello LM, Jurkovich GL, Stark MS, et al: Hypothermia in the trauma patient. Is it protective or harmful? *Ann Surg* 226:439, 1997.

Jurkovich GJ, Greiser VVB, Lutennan A, et al: Hypothermia in trauma victims: An ominous predictor of survival. *J Trauma* 27:1019, 1987.

Mills WJ Jr, O'Malley J, Kappes B: Cold and freezing: A historical chronology of laboratory investigation and clinical experience. *Alaska Med* 35:89, 1993.

Reed RL II, Johnston TD, Hudson JD, et al: The disparity between hypothermic coagulopathy and clotting studies. *J Trauma* 33:465, 1992.

Shiozaki T, Hayakata T, Taneda M, et al: A multicenter prospective randomized controlled trial of the efficacy of mild hypothermia for severely head injured patients with low intracranial pressure. *J Neurosurg* 94:50, 2001.

47 | Rehabilitation

INTRODUCTION

Although major strides have been made in the acute care of the injured, the availability of rehabilitative services and their integration into systems of trauma care have been slow. Each year more than 2.5 million people hospitalized for injury survive to hospital discharge. Trauma care systems must strive to reduce impairment, not just mortality, and must return individuals to the highest functional level possible (Table 47-1).

Brain and spinal cord injury have a tremendous impact on function, and necessitate the greatest application of rehabilitation resources. Orthopedic injuries, notably those of the spine, lower extremities, and hand, also require special services, and can lead to significant disability.

The Rehabilitation Team

An interdisciplinary team orchestrating different therapies in a coordinated fashion is required for optimal rehabilitation (Table 47-2). Physician supervision and interaction between the physician and therapists is crucial. Involvement of the trauma physician in recognizing the need for rehabilitation and fostering the process through communication with the other team members is paramount. The team must identify the needs of each individual patient and assign the needed services. The team must address mobility, activities of daily living, communication, cognition, psychological well-being, and sexual function. A qualified physician (often a physiatrist) should lead the interdisciplinary team, but any member of the team may take the lead in their area of expertise. The trauma surgeon should be an active participant in this team.

SPECIFIC ORGAN SYSTEM INJURY

Brain Injury

In the United States, more than 100,000 individuals per year suffer disability due to brain injury. Although a small percentage of brain injury survivors are vegetative, the majority regain some measure of independence, and many return to work after appropriate rehabilitation.

Assessment of the needs of brain-injured patients is an ongoing process. Initial prediction of neurologic outcome is unreliable. Early assessment of needs may be possible in patients with mild injury (Glasgow Coma Scale score [GCS] >12), but initial appraisal of those with moderate (GCS 9 to 12) and severe (GCS <9) injury can be misleading. In comatose patients, serial evaluation of their response to brain-directed therapy must be part of planning for rehabilitation. Prolonged posttraumatic coma is associated with poor survival, and as duration of coma increases, chances of functional recovery decrease.

Initial rehabilitative efforts for the moderate to severely brain-injured patient focus on physical needs. Abnormal muscle tone due to posturing or spasticity may occur. Early efforts must also address prevention of decubitus ulcers. Frequent changes in position and the use of special beds may be of benefit, but must be tailored to acute brain-directed therapy, avoiding increases in intracranial pressure due to position. Careful attention to cervical orthosis care is necessary to prevent occipital decubitus ulcers. Passive range of motion and splinting of major extremity joints may prevent contractures.

TABLE 47-1 Definitions

Impairment
Any loss of or abnormality of psychological, physiologic, or anatomic structure or function.
Disability
Any restriction or lack resulting from an impairment of ability to perform any activity in the manner or within the range considered normal for a human being.
Handicap
A disadvantage for a given individual resulting from an impairment or disability.

In less-severely injured patients, and those with severe injury who recover, evaluation for cognitive deficits must take place. Shock and multiple extracranial injuries have been demonstrated to reduce cognitive outcome, and efforts to prevent secondary brain injury must have priority. Following this, early initiation of cognitive rehabilitation in severely injured patients leads to improved outcome. An integrated brain injury recovery program should be started once life-threatening physiologic disturbances have been corrected and critical brain injury management has been completed. Behavioral abnormalities are common among patients recovering from severe brain injury. During acute care, agents such as haloperidol or chlorpromazine may be required to control agitation or aggressive behavior.

Minor head injury cannot be ignored. Some patients with minor head injury develop postconcussive syndrome and its attendant significant disability. Persistent subjective neurologic complaints such as headache, vertigo, nausea, emotional lability, or other nonspecific symptoms should alert the clinician to this disorder. Evaluation by a neurologic specialist and appropriate therapy should be initiated.

Spinal Cord Injury

There are approximately 8000 to 10,000 new cases of spinal cord injury in the United States yearly, and about 200,000 paraplegics and tetraplegics. Acute care is focused on stabilization of bony and ligamentous injury, and prevention of extension of neurologic injury. Rehabilitative efforts should be begun as soon as physiologic stability is secured. Mobility is of primary concern for patients

TABLE 47-2 Members of the Rehabilitation Team

Physiatrist
Orthopedist
Physical therapist
Occupational therapist
Speech therapist
Rehabilitation nurse
Psychologist
Neuropsychologist
Psychiatrist
Recreational therapist
Prosthetist/orthotist
Vocational counselor
Nursing staff
Social worker
Respiratory therapist
Trauma surgeon

with paralysis. Passive range of motion and splinting for joints below the level of paralysis should be started as soon as possible. Active range of motion of upper extremities should be begun, particularly in low tetraplegics and paraplegics. Patients' families should be involved in this effort as much as possible. As in head-injured patients, contractures and decubiti are a significant risk, and steps to prevent them are necessary. In the supine patient, the occiput, scapulae, vertebrae, elbows, sacrum, coccyx, and heels are pressure points at risk. Lifelong decubitus ulcer prophylaxis is necessary for these patients.

As soon as bony stability is established, active mobilization of the patient should be initiated. Early in acute hospitalization, a regimen of daily stool softeners and suppositories should be instituted to develop bowel training and control. Bladder training should begin when the patient is stable and urine output is low enough to allow intermittent catheterization less than 6 times a day. Whenever possible, the patient should be trained to do self-catheterization until reflex voiding patterns develop.

Planning with inpatient social services, insurance company rehabilitation nurses, and community support services must be started early, to prepare the patient for reintegration into society.

Orthopedic Injuries

Although the early fixation of lower-extremity fractures is frequently undertaken to reduce respiratory and infectious complications, it affords the opportunity to institute early rehabilitative care. Teaching transfer and gait training may be the only requirements for patients with isolated injury, but those with multiple fractures may require extensive physical rehabilitation. Early use of continuous passive motion devices to maintain joint mobility may be of benefit, particularly in patients with multisystem injury.

Multisystem Injury

Multisystem trauma victims pose challenges to the rehabilitation system, just as they do to the acute care system. Prioritization of needs and sequential introduction of treatments should be used to optimize outcome. As many as 70 percent of survivors of severe trauma can return to their prior work status. Severity of injury is a poor predictor of return to work, but specific injuries such as brain, spinal cord, and major extremity fractures may be predictive. Return to social function is likely after multisystem trauma; this emphasizes the need for organized acute rehabilitation services.

The need for vocational rehabilitation must be emphasized for this population. A significant number must change their employment, particularly those with cognitive deficits. Vocational rehabilitation is critical to either adapting for return to previous work, or identifying and developing another work skill. Psychological support is also important for these patients.

PEDIATRIC TRAUMA

Systems for pediatric trauma care have developed more recently than those for adults, and rehabilitation systems for children have also been slow to develop. Availability and integration of acute rehabilitation services for children is critical to their postinjury function. Without rehabilitative services, injured children with impairments may not recover or adapt, resulting in accentuated disability or handicap. Fifty-five percent of children are found to have functional limitations 1 year after severe injury, and those with good outcome after brain injury frequently have major functional deficits. Social and psychological factors must play a major role in planning pediatric rehabilitation. The child's family should be intimately involved in all phases of the rehabilitation of their child. Psychosocial support should be available for the family. Transfer to inpatient or outpatient specialized pediatric rehabilitation rather than a general rehabilitation facility is especially important for children with severe injury.

AMPUTEE REHABILITATION

Injuries are responsible for 75 percent of upper-extremity amputations and 20 percent of lower-extremity amputations in the United States. In many cases, the need for amputation after trauma is clear. While salvage of a damaged limb is desirable, it should not be attempted if it appears likely that the limb will not be functional or if attempted salvage may threaten the patient's survival. Unsuccessful limb salvage attempts can prolong hospitalization, rehabilitation, and return to function, particularly for severe lower-extremity injury. Below-knee amputation has a better functional result than above-knee amputation, but a tibial length of 6 cm or more must be preserved for prosthetic fitting. Knee disarticulation leads to good function but poor cosmesis. In the upper extremity, wrist and elbow disarticulations have poor cosmesis and function. In children less than 12 years of age, bony overgrowth at the amputation point can be a major problem. These stumps become painful and often require surgical revision. It is often better to amputate through a joint in children.

Postinjury function and pain control can be improved by sharp transection of nerves, beveling of bone ends, placement of skin incisions to avoid adhesions to bone, and careful muscle layer closure. Effective postinjury dressings also contribute to good recovery. Soft elastic dressings provide even pressure to help shrink the stump. Rigid dressings of stumps can provide for early application of a prosthesis for mobilization and may reduce the incidence of phantom sensation. Unfortunately, they reduce the possibility of wound inspection.

Immediate postoperative goals include maintenance of range of motion, control of swelling, pain management, and strengthening of uninvolved extremities. As the wounds heal, strengthening of the residual limbs is helpful. In traumatic lower-extremity amputation, transfer training and ambulation with crutches or walker should be started early. Training in activities of daily living should also begin quickly for the upper-limb amputee.

Perioperative pain that fails to resolve is often due to neuroma, adhesions, or inadequate muscle padding over bone ends. Phantom sensation occurs in 70 to 80 percent of amputees, but generally fades away. However, phantom limb pain occurs in less than 20 percent of cases, and occurs more commonly when the limb was painful prior to amputation. Modalities such as transcutaneous electrical nerve stimulation (TENS), massage, biofeedback, and acupuncture may be helpful, but this pain is very difficult to treat. Analgesics, antidepressants, anticonvulsants, and beta blockers may also be of some benefit, as may nerve blocks or steroid injections.

HAND INJURIES

Hand injuries are quite common, and the keys to treatment are edema and pain control, maintenance of range of motion, splinting, scar suppression, and muscle reeducation. Significant hand edema can occur with or without direct hand trauma. The keys to controlling this edema are range-of-motion exercises, massage, elevation, splinting, and elastic wraps. Two types of splinting are useful after hand injury. Static splints are used to maintain position, prevent contracture, and reduce swelling. Dynamic splints allow motion over a controlled range. Precise fitting of these orthotics is crucial. Range-of-motion machines may be helpful in the rehabilitation process. Strengthening, coordination, and muscle reeducation are important to the functional rehabilitation of hand injury.

Pain is a common problem after hand injury, and can be disabling. Desensitization is often successful in managing this pain. Fluidotherapy, hot packs, ultrasound, paraffin, and TENS may also be helpful for hand pain, but heat should not be used in patients with infection, impaired sedation, or impaired cognition. As with phantom pain after amputation, drugs for pain control may be helpful. Nerve block may be necessary for severe pain.

NERVE INJURY

Peripheral nerve and plexus injuries occur more frequently than commonly recognized in multitrauma patients. As many as 20 percent of patients in motor vehicle crashes sustain peripheral nerve injury. The majority of vehicle crash-related injuries occur in the upper extremity in drivers. Median nerve injury at the wrist and ulnar nerve injury at the elbow are also common.

Complete brachial plexus injuries are usually secondary to auto crashes, and cause complete upper-extremity paralysis and sensory loss below the shoulder. The lower brachial plexus is most commonly injured, and results in a claw-hand deformity, with loss of ulnar sensation. Brachial cord injuries are common in penetrating trauma. Bony injuries around the shoulder may be associated with axillary nerve injury, and the musculocutaneous nerve or radial nerve are injured in humerus fractures. Median nerve injury may be associated with shoulder dislocation, wrist fracture, and penetrating trauma. Ulnar nerve injuries are seen in wrist and elbow fractures and penetrating trauma.

Lumbosacral plexus injuries are usually seen in pelvic fractures and are rarely complete. The sciatic nerve may be injured by pelvic or femur fractures or hip dislocation, as well as by penetrating trauma. The common peroneal nerve is frequently injured in fibular head fractures, and the tibial nerve is occasionally injured in tibia or ankle fractures.

The clinical examination is crucial in diagnosing peripheral nerve injury. Magnetic resonance imaging (MRI) may be helpful in diagnosing plexus injuries when they are suspected. Electrodiagnosis is crucial to diagnosis of both peripheral nerve and plexus injuries. These studies, however, may not be diagnostic until 3 weeks after injury.

Surgery may be useful to relieve compression and for nerve repair or grafting. Bracing is used to maintain range of motion and limb function, particularly with medial, ulnar, and peroneal nerve injury. It is crucial that the patient be informed that nerve injuries require many months to resolve, and that deficits may be permanent.

COMORBIDITY AND AGE

There have been few studies regarding the impact of preexisting conditions or age on functional outcome in trauma, and their results are contradictory. The reported rate of return to function of injured elderly ranges from 8 to 70 percent. Injury-related factors that impact most on outcome in older patients are central nervous system injury, shock, and sepsis.

Preexisting conditions such as drug or ethanol dependency, or psychiatric or chronic medical disorders may necessitate modification of the rehabilitation plan. The neuropsychiatric and dependency problems must be addressed as part of rehabilitation, and care must be taken to reduce the physical expectations of those with limits imposed by neurologic, cardiac, pulmonary, vascular, or other disease. Age alone is not a contraindication to rehabilitation efforts, but those over 75 years of age have a higher risk of poor outcome, particularly with brain injury.

ECONOMICS OF REHABILITATION

Recent advances in rehabilitation services have allowed disabled individuals to lead more productive lives, but with a significant cost. Rehabilitation services are expensive. The total cost of care for spinal cord injury in the United States was more than $6.2 billion in 1989, and the 1988 costs for traumatic brain injury exceeded $25 billion.

Rehabilitation services are often difficult or impossible to arrange for patients with limited financial resources and/or poor social support. Medicare and Medicaid generally do not pay for traumatic brain injury programs. In some states, funds for auto crash victims may not be available until legal cases have been settled, leading to delays in services. Other patients may exhaust their resources during acute care hospitalization.

For these reasons, it is crucial to begin planning for rehabilitation early in the patient's course. Social services should be consulted early in order to investigate insurance and other resources available to the patient, as well as support systems and patient and family preferences. Monitoring of the patient's progress by payors and potential rehabilitation facilities is routinely conducted in order to assess the patient's suitability for rehabilitation. Patients with severe brain injury who remain in deep coma for prolonged periods may not be candidates for rehabilitative services.

Different patients require different resources. The choice of inpatient or outpatient programs and acute or subacute programs should be based on patient needs. On average, acute rehabilitation centers provide 5 hours per day of therapy. Patients must be motivated and able to tolerate this level of activity to benefit from these programs. Subacute programs generally provide about half as much coordinated therapy, with less intensity, and may be more appropriate for patients with reduced stamina or medical problems for use as a stepping-stone to acute rehabilitation. For patients with limited potential, nursing homes may be appropriate. Day therapy or home services may be appropriate for patients recovering well from traumatic brain injury, or after a short acute rehabilitation inpatient stay. For home services to work to the patient's benefit, however, family support and supervision must be available, particularly for the brain-injured patient.

ADDITIONAL READING

Anke AGW, Stanglelle JK, Finset A, et al: Long-term prevalence of impairments and disabilities after multiple trauma. *J Trauma* 42:54, 1997.
Butcher JL, MacKenzie EJ, Cushing B, et al: Long term outcomes after lower extremity trauma. *J Trauma* 41:4, 1996.

National Research Council: *Accidental Death and Disability: The Neglected Disease of Modern Society.* Washington, DC, U.S. Government Printing Office, 1966.

Rhodes M, Aronson J, Moerkirk G, et al: Quality of life after the trauma center. *J Trauma* 28:931, 1988.

Rice DP, MacKenzie EJ, et al: *Cost of Injury in the United States: A Report to Congress.* San Francisco, University of California, 1989.

VanAalst JA, Morris JA, Yates HK, et al: Severely injured geriatric patients return to independent living: A study of factors influencing function and independence. *J Trauma* 31:1096, 1991.

A reasonable question to be raised by the reader of a book devoted to trauma is why it should contain a separate section on the management of battle casualties. The reasons for this are many, and one of the most important is controversy over the differences and similarities in the management of civilian and battle casualties. The controversy is probably specious. On the one hand, there are clear similarities between civilian wound management and battle wound management. On the other hand is the fact that differences in the management of battle casualties are simply reflections of the unique features of war surgery. It is for this reason that civilian surgeons must have preparation before attempting to care for battle casualties.

The purposes of this chapter are multiple. We will point out the similarities and differences in the management of civilian and battle casualties, as well as some of the problems identified in providing optimal battle-casualty management, and tell how civilians can best prepare for and participate in this process when called upon. In addition, we will briefly review the threat of terrorism.

SIMILARITIES IN TRAUMA MANAGEMENT

Severe wounds, no matter what their etiology, have a similar pathophysiology and are subject to the same principles of wound repair. A civilian shotgun blast and burn injury involve kinetic energy and destruction similar to those encountered in military wounds. All wounds will initiate certain components of the inflammatory cascade. The most severe wounds are capable of causing an imbalance in this cascade that contributes to the pathophysiology of multiple organ failure.

The resuscitation of patients with civilian and war wounds is remarkably similar. Many of the current resuscitative techniques used in civilian trauma centers were learned during wartime surgery. It is useful to follow the most recent history of fluid resuscitation. During World War I, fluid resuscitation was accomplished mainly with normal saline, gelatin solution, and blood. The amount of fluid given was based on the estimated blood loss. Cannon recognized that the degree of shock in the severely injured patient always seemed worse than would be explained by the measured or estimated amount of blood loss. Experimental studies done after the war did not provide a resolution to this question, which Cannon termed *exemia*. During World War II, resuscitation continued to be accomplished mainly with normal saline, plasma, protein solution, and whole blood. Fluids were restricted and did not compensate for losses into the intracellular space or for the interstitial edema surrounding a wound. As a consequence, many patients arriving at battalion aid stations in severe shock ultimately developed renal failure, and up to 80 percent subsequently died as a consequence of this. The same principles held during the Korean Conflict, but between the Korean and the Vietnam conflicts, studies by Shires and others showed that during shock there was a significant intracellular sequestration of fluids that required an exaggerated initial resuscitation and appropriate amounts of blood. According to Lucas, this resulted in three distinct phases of resuscitation. As a consequence of this better understanding of fluid resuscitation, the Vietnam Conflict saw patients survive who would not previously have done so, and renal failure was not as common as previously experienced. In contrast, a new phenomenon occurred: the so-called "Da Nang lung." This represented a form of adult respiratory distress seen in severely injured patients. The pulmonary failure responsible for this distress, and what later was to become recognized as sequential organ failure, were consequences of more critically injured patients surviving beyond surgery, and to some extent probably also represented overzealous fluid administration. It was not initially recognized that in these critically injured patients, the management of fluid hydrostatic pressure in the pulmonary circulation was important in helping to prevent capillary leakage in the lung. From this, it can be appreciated that concepts developed in peacetime and put in practice during wartime led to the evolution of modern fluid resuscitation.

In general, the surgical techniques used in critically injured patients, whether civilian or military, are essentially the same. A neurosurgeon's craniotomy does not differ whether it is performed in a modern trauma center or in a field hospital.

The approach to managing penetrating neck injuries is somewhat different in a military than in a civilian trauma center. The availability of arteriograms is limited, and wounds of proximity will therefore be explored, even more so for high-energy fragment wounds and high-velocity wounds than those generally seen in civilian medicine, because they may damage surrounding tissues even if they do not directly hit them. Because of this, most neck injuries will be explored and debrided. Although precise data are unavailable, the rate of thoracotomy for war wounds is probably higher than in a civilian setting. The operative approach and control of hemorrhage are no different.

Celiotomy, including the approach to the retroperitoneum and pelvis and the general principles for control of bleeding, is precisely the same in the military and civilian setting. It is in orthopedic injuries that some major differences in management exist between peacetime and wartime situations. External fixators are more commonly used in war, and almost all wounds are closed secondarily or skin grafted at a later date. In general, peripheral vascular injuries, whether in wartime or peacetime, are managed in a similar manner.

Intensive care and organ support are provided using the same principles and equipment whether one is in a level 1 trauma center or a combat support hospital. The major differences relate to how long one can keep a patient close to the combat zone, and the rapidity with which a severely injured patient's condition permits evacuation of the patient. This creates special problems that will be addressed in the section on differences in military and civilian trauma management.

Optimally, rehabilitation is instituted as soon as possible after severe injury, even in a theater of war. Obviously this is limited in a war zone because of the austerity of resources.

DIFFERENCES IN TRAUMA MANAGEMENT

A significant difference in the management of civilian and war injuries is in the amount of prehospital time. Even in rural areas of the United States, prehospital time does not usually exceed 30 minutes. In urban areas, on-scene and transport times are often less than 15 minutes. In contrast, to remove a battle casualty from a fire zone usually requires more than an hour under even the best of circumstances—a delay that is more serious in the case of high-velocity rifle wounds and multiple fragmentation wounds. It can thus be appreciated that wounds to the torso, head, and neck can have much higher mortality rates in the prehospital combat setting.

Differences also exist in resuscitation in a wartime situation. Because of the number of casualties that may arrive simultaneously at a treatment center, surgeons may not be able to participate directly in resuscitation since they are busy with lifesaving surgery. Resuscitation may be delegated to nonsurgeon physicians, corpsmen, and nurses who have been trained in resuscitation. Clearly, it is prudent to train such individuals prior to arrival in the theater of war.

The kinds of wounds seen in a military situation have obvious differences from those seen in civilian settings. In addition to differences in the velocity of wounding projectiles, high-energy fragment wounds are fairly common, and during Operation Desert Storm they accounted for 42 percent of the wounds of 204 soldiers, as compared to only 10 percent caused by gunshots.

Prehospital resuscitation in a combat zone obviously differs from that in a civilian setting. In the Persian Gulf War, soldiers wounded in action gave high praise to the combat medics, and the Combat Lifesaver Program was thought to be very valuable. Unfortunately, although the U.S. Army has invested heavily in studies of hypertonic saline, this was not investigated in the combat setting of the Persian Gulf War. The use of saline for resuscitation remains controversial, particularly in desert warfare. However, it should be noted that during Operation Just Cause, many parachutists had hypotensive episodes during the induction of anesthesia, probably as a consequence of not having taken any fluids for 8 to 12 hours prior to their surgery. Pneumatic antishock garments (PASGs) are bulky and not currently available in situations involving heavy combat. Hemoglobin solutions may be optimal in the prehospital setting in combat, but their use will have to await the results of clinical trials in a civilian setting. At present, resuscitation in a combat prehospital setting is primarily accomplished with Ringer's lactate and the control of bleeding where possible. Once the patient arrives in a casualty-collecting point, MASH, or combat support hospital, resuscitation is done much as in a civilian setting. The exception may lie in the personnel who perform the resuscitation.

Although surgical approaches to the control of bleeding are similar for civilian and war injuries, major differences exist in the way in which various wounds are handled. Soldiers often wear protective headgear, and the management of penetrating injuries to the head almost always includes obligatory surgical exploration. Abdominal injuries are also treated with techniques different from the standard ones developed for civilian practice. A colon injury would never be closed primarily; colostomy is mandatory. No attempts are made to save the spleen. Vascular injuries must be approached differently in a combat setting because arteriograms and other diagnostic modalities are usually unavailable. Thus proximity injuries would be explored, and although synthetic grafts have been used in civilian practice, autologous tissue would be used in a war zone. A major difference in the operative management of trauma in a war zone as opposed to the civilian setting has to do with injuries involving soft tissue. In a war zone, soft-tissue injuries must be debrided relatively extensively in order to remove clothing and debris associated with the battlefield. Antibiotics are routinely used, and the patient is always hospitalized for a period of observation and wound care.

It can be appreciated from the foregoing that a major difference between military and civilian wound care is the lack of continuity of care surrounding military surgery. A primary goal in treating battlefield casualties is to evacuate them as soon as possible. Accordingly, the surgeon cannot follow the patient's postoperative care. Wound management must be standardized by protocol in order to minimize complications and mortality. As the patient is evacuated to higher levels of care, there must be an explicit understanding of how wounds have been managed at prior levels. If a surgeon in a forward combat support hospital has performed a primary closure of the colon in a patient who develops a fever on the fourth or fifth postinjury day at an evacuation hospital, it might not be appreciated that the patient had surgery, thus setting the stage for an adverse outcome. Protocols are also necessary for wound debridement, irrigation, and antibiotic treatment. In a theater of war it is often impossible to maintain the complete antibiotic armementarium that a surgeon may have access to in civilian practice. Although it is not difficult to appreciate these relatively minor differences in operative care, it seems that they must be learned by the surgeons first entering combat at the start of every new conflict.

UNIQUE FEATURES OF MILITARY SURGERY

One of the unique features of surgery in war is the number of patients that can arrive simultaneously at a treatment center. Following a firefight or forward action, the casualty rate may be as high as 30 percent. Depending on the number of combat units involved, it can be appreciated that this may temporarily overwhelm the nearest medical facilities. Triage becomes critical. Optimally, the casualties should be distributed to multiple medical units, but this may be impossible because of geography, the battlefield situation, and resources for evacuation. Triage at the medical center becomes equally critical, since patients whose lives are most at risk may often wait hours for lifesaving surgery. It makes no sense to spend an inordinate amount of time trying to salvage one individual when 10 others could be saved with shorter procedures or more simple lifesaving surgery.

Another feature unique to combat surgery is the mobility of forward medical units. This was particularly appreciated in Operation Desert Storm, in which armor and mobile cavalry units moved more than 100 miles a day. Having medical resources keep up with these units poses incredible logistic problems. A MASH or combat support hospital takes time to move. Moreover, in modern conflict the enemy must be assumed to have surface-to-air missiles, which makes the evacuation of casualties by helicopter impossible. Because of the need for mobility, plans are already being made to have fast-forward surgical teams accompany the lead troops and provide lifesaving surgery in a war zone.

Surgery under combat conditions is often austere. It is impossible to provide all of the modern diagnostic equipment and supplies found in a civilian trauma center. The surgeon may not have a wide choice of antibiotics or suture materials. It may be impossible to provide air conditioning in the operating room or for patients in recovery and intensive care units. Nevertheless, despite these austere conditions, it is possible to deliver surgical care of a quality essentially equal to that in any modern civilian hospital.

Evacuation of casualties may be the most unique feature of combat surgery. It is often difficult for the surgeon to understand why a critically injured patient must be transferred postoperatively to a higher-level care center. The purpose of far-forward surgical units is simply to provide lifesaving surgery. After this has been accomplished, it is in the best interest of the wounded soldier to be evacuated to a higher-level care facility away from the battlefield. Often, it is difficult to precisely determine the best time for the evacuation.

The military tactical situation, nature of the patient's wounds, anticipation of new casualties, and overextension of resources are all part of the equation in deciding an evacuation time. In general, patients in a forward area should be held there for no longer than 24 to 36 hours postoperatively, and approximately 40 percent of bed capacity should be kept open for anticipated new casualties.

Another feature of surgery during wartime is the environment. Wars are frequently fought in environmentally hostile areas. The problem can be compounded by persistent rain, snow, mud, or tropical heat. Desert warfare creates unusual problems that may influence resuscitation, as well as additional needs for fluid in the postinjury period. The cleanliness and tidiness of a large university hospital are not achievable in a tent or combat support hospital.

Some wounds are obviously unique to surgery during war. Fragments and high-velocity missiles cause most such wounds. The locations of wounds are quite different than those seen in civilian trauma care. Blast injuries from airbursts or in confined spaces will produce pulmonary injuries. Underwater explosions cause their own type of injury to hollow intra-abdominal viscera. Mixtures of fuel and air produce a combination of blast and burn injuries and hypoxia. Thermal burns are inevitable in a setting in which fuels and high explosives are universally employed. Most conflicts cause a 10 to 11 percent burn rate among all casualties. Penetrating injuries may result not only from high-velocity missiles, but also from peculiarly shaped fléchettes or cluster-bomb fragments specifically designed to cause maximum tissue damage. Inhalation injuries may be secondary to the combustion of ammunition, various plastics, or rocket fuel. Aerosols of metal fragments are used to cloud electromagnetic transmissions, and if inhaled cause pulmonary damage. The increasing use of directed-energy beams such as laser beams, charged-particle beams, and high-powered microwaves is certain to lead to new and unique injuries in conflicts of the future. Finally, there are the problems of nuclear, biologic, and chemical warfare. These three potential causes of injury emphasize the need for reserve surgeons to have appropriate training and preparation prior to combat duty.

TERRORISM

Military surgery and civilian trauma surgery now face a common problem: terrorism. The bombing of the Marine barracks and the two terrorist bombings of U.S. military facilities in Saudi Arabia show the vulnerability of our troops to terrorist activities. How realistic is the threat of terrorist activity in the United States? Between 1980 and 1990 there were 12,216 bombing incidents in the United States. The majority of these were pipe bombs. In 1990 alone there were 1582 bomb incidents (53 percent were pipe bombs). There were 222 injuries in 1990 and 27 deaths. The trend over this 10-year period was for bomb incidents to increase each year. More recently, powerful explosive devices have been constructed with seemingly mundane materials and exploded in public buildings. This is illustrated by the massive destruction following the detonation of a 1800-kg ammonium nitrite (fertilizer) and diesel fuel bomb in Oklahoma City in 1995, which killed 167 individuals and destroyed the 9-story Alfred P. Murrah Federal Building. That explosion, plus the one in the World Trade Center in 1993, make large bombs not only a threat but also a reality. Finally, the terrorist attacks of September 11, 2001 on the Pentagon and the World Trade Center demonstrated how far we have to go before we are ready to deal with a large number of trauma patients in a very short time period in the civilian sector.

Since terrorist organizations operate outside of the law, they are not restricted in their choice of weapons or targets. Conventional weapons and explosives are the most commonly used. However, weapons systems that utilize radioactive, chemical, and biological components can and have been used. A vivid example occurred when the Aum Shinrikyo cult in Japan used sarin nerve gas in the subway system of Tokyo (see below). It is now evident that both military and civilian surgeons must be prepared to deal with conventional weapons as well as nuclear, biological, and chemical weapons. Military units are not immune to terrorist activities such as those that occurred in Beirut, Lebanon and a military housing facility in Saudi Arabia.

The threat of terrorism from biological weapons is already a reality. One incident occurred in September 1984, when 750 people became sick after eating in restaurants in The Dalles, Oregon. A member of the cult founded by the Bahgwan Shree Rajneesh had spread *Salmonella* bacteria on salad bars in four local restaurants in an attempt to disrupt the electoral process in eastern Oregon. There are other examples of biological weapons being confiscated in other parts of the United States. The intent was to use these agents in terrorist activities.

One of the most serious examples of the threat posed by chemical terrorism occurred in Japan. In June of 1994, the Aum Shinrikyo cult either accidentally or intentionally released sarin gas in the community of Matsumoto, leading to several deaths and 200 casualties. This was followed in March of 1995 by a widespread attack on the Tokyo subway system. Sarin gas was placed in five subway cars on three separate lines. The attack was planned for the early morning rush hour and coordinated to occur beneath the Japanese National Government Office buildings. Twelve people were killed and there were 5500 casualties related to this single attack. The cult had also purchased a Russian helicopter with the intent using it for aerial spraying of nerve gas. The chemical and biological weapons available are summarized in Tables 48-1 and 48-2.

Injuries caused by explosives can be divided into primary, secondary, tertiary, and miscellaneous blast injury. Often casualties will sustain a mixed type of injury, although secondary blast injury usually predominates. Most terrorist bombings generate low mortality rates, although there are several notable exceptions. Frykberg and Tepas provided an excellent overview of the injuries sustained by a group of 3357 casualties from 220 explosions. Of the 2934 immediate survivors, 881 (30 percent) were hospitalized and only 40 deaths (1.4 percent) were noted in this group. Soft-tissue (55.4 percent), head (31.4 percent), and bony extremity (10.9 percent) injury predominated. The majority of operations were performed for soft-tissue (67.0 percent) and skeletal (17.5 percent) injuries. Despite the preponderance of injury to and operation for soft-tissue and skeletal injury, no mortality was observed in patients with injury confined to these areas. Mortality was highest in those casualties with abdominal (19.0 percent) and chest injury (15.1 percent). Because of the high percentage of casualties with minor injuries, one of the major challenges for medical personnel will be the rapid identification of the small number of patients who are severely injured.

The risk of terrorism has increased worldwide and the United States is not immune from these acts, committed by both internal and external perpetrators. Most disaster plans anticipate a large number of casualties from natural

TABLE 48-1 Chemical Agents

Class	Examples	Mechanism	Symptoms	Treatment
Nerve agents	Tabun (GA) Sarin (GR)	Inhibition of acetylcholinesterase	Weakness Salivation	Atropine 2-PAM
	Soman (GD) VX		Miosis Paralysis Hypoxia Eye inflammation	
Vessicants Decontamination (blister agents)	Mustard (HD) Nitrogen mustards (HN1, HN2, HN3)	Alkalation	Upper respiratory tract irritation Skin blisters	
Choking agents	Phosgene Diphosgene	Variable	Tearing Coughing Dyspnea Pulmonary edema	Supportive
Cyanide (blood) agents	Hydrogen cyanide (AC) Cyanogen halides (i.e., cyanogen chloride, CK)	Form stable complexes with metalloporphyrins	Hypoxia	Nitrites
Incapacitating agents	Quinuclidinyl benzilate Cannabinols Barbiturates	Variable	Central nervous system alterations	Physostigmine

2-PAM, 2-pyridine aldoxime methochloride

TABLE 48-2 Biological Agents

Agent	Class	Transmission	Symptoms	Treatment
Anthrax (*Bacillus anthracis*)	Bacteria	Inhalation of bacillus or spores	Dyspnea Cyanosis Pulmonary edema Respiratory failure	Vaccination Antibiotics
Bubonic plague (*Yersinia pestis*)	Bacteria	Fleas	Fever Delirium Cutaneous lesions	Vaccination Antibiotics
Salmonella spp.	Bacteria	Ingestion	Gastrointestinal symptoms Fever	Antibiotics
Botulinum toxin (*Clostridium botulinum*)	Bacterial neurotoxin	Inhalation Contact (skin or wound)	Paralysis	Supportive
Gas gangrene (*Clostridium perfringens*)	Bacteria	Wound infection	Necrotizing soft-tissue infection	Antibiotics Surgical debridement
Ebola	Virus (Filoviridae)	Body fluids	Fever Hemorrhage Convulsions	Supportive No specific treatment

disasters such as earthquakes, transportation accidents, and even large industrial explosions and fires. We believe it is prudent to now include disaster medical care planning for blast as well as nuclear, biological, and chemical (NBC) attacks.

Secondary and tertiary blast injuries should not require changes in our current disaster plans, other than preparing for the possibility of being overwhelmed with the sheer numbers of patients involved in the blast. However, surgeons and other health care providers do not commonly see primary blast injuries. The unique damage to air-containing organs and the risk of air embolism need to be incorporated into our educational programs for physicians, nurses, and prehospital personnel.

Casualties from NBC terrorism will challenge our disaster medical plans and health professionals to the extreme. Not only will the large number of casualties be potentially overwhelming, there is the added risk of contamination from the patients and the environment. Protective devices are available to minimize contamination of health care providers. Mission-oriented protective posture (MOPP) gear is available for military use and, in theory, civilian use. MOPP is indispensable for protection against chemical vapors and also provides protection for biological aerosols. It is even somewhat protective against nuclear fallout. Surgical masks and cloth collectors can filter particles smaller than one-tenth of a micron, thus reliably providing fairly effective protection against a biological terrorist attack.

For surgeons, nurses, or paramedics working in the actual disaster area, some type of protective clothing will be necessary. Unfortunately, studies by the military have shown that claustrophobia, difficulties with breathing apparatus, overheating, dehydration, failure to recognize danger, and anxiety commonly occur in this type of setting. In studies of simulated chemical and biological warfare environments, between 4 and 10 percent of participants terminated the exercise because of psychological symptoms (predominantly claustrophobia, anxiety, or panic). These studies have profound implications for the civilian sector, where minimal (if any) training is conducted in the delivery of emergency health care utilizing protective clothing. Inability of care providers to tolerate prolonged periods within protective clothing will only result in secondary casualties among the health care workers secondary to patient contamination.

The other component of NBC terrorism that has to be incorporated into disaster medical care is detection of the various agents. Gas chromatography and other types of chemical detectors are fairly sensitive and specific for chemical agents. Detectors for biological agents are available, and the recent development of polymerase chain reaction (PCR) technology has increased sensitivity. The downside is that the process takes a long time to perform and the apparatus is quite elaborate. Enzyme-linked immunosorbent assay (ELISA) and mass spectrometry are more practical, the equipment needed is relatively small, and it can be produced at low cost. Measurement of radioactivity is easy and cheap.

Although the first priority at the disaster scene or in a triage area would be detection, the second priority is decontamination and maintaining the safety of those individuals doing the decontamination. Very few disaster plans include a comprehensive decontamination component. This decontamination would require large quantities of water, the ability to apply it to the casualty, and a means of disposing of contaminated waste water and clothing. If the health care workers doing the triage are not wearing MOPP gear, it will be unsafe for them to render lifesaving resuscitation until the patient has been decontaminated.

After triage detection and decontamination have taken place, the patient would be admitted to an acute care facility, and treatment appropriate for the cause of injury would commence. It is imperative that treatment protocols for blast, nuclear, biological, and chemical injuries be incorporated into the disaster medical plan. Physicians and nurses who have never treated such casualties must have a reference easily available, not only to assist in diagnosis, but to aid in the choice of appropriate treatment.

ADDITIONAL READING

Bellamy RF: The causes of death in conventional land warfare: Implications for combat casualty care research. *Mil Med* 149:55, 1984.

Frykberg ER, Tepas JJ: Terrorist bombing: Lessons learned from Belfast to Beirut. *Ann Surg* 208:359, 1988.

Fullerton CS, Ursano RJ: Health care delivery in the high-stress environment of chemical and biological warfare. *Mil Med* 159:524, 1994.

Karmy-Jones R, Kissinger D, Golocovsky M, et al: Bomb-related injuries. *Mil Med* 159:536, 1994.

Mallonee S, Shariat S, Stennies G, et al: Physical injuries and fatalities resulting from the Oklahoma City Bombing. *JAMA* 276:383, 1996.

V MANAGEMENT OF COMPLICATIONS AFTER TRAUMA

49 | Principles of Critical Care

The term *critical care* pertains to care given as part of the crisis or turning point of a disease or injury. While initial operative management of traumatic injury has historically been regarded as the live-or-die turning point, this literal definition reflects the contemporary importance of postoperative management of the trauma patient. Critical care may be defined loosely as the process of high-frequency physiologic monitoring coupled with short-response-time pharmacologic, ventilatory, and procedural interventions. This activity is designed to reestablish normal homeostasis and minimize complications of primary, secondary, and iatrogenic injury. Surgical critical care is inherently different from medical intensive care in that surgical patients, and particularly trauma patients, require intensive care as the result of an acute surgical intervention or injury, and not as part of the (often inexorable) progression or exacerbation of chronic disease. This fundamental difference affects a multitude of patient management practices and decisions.

The inherent integration between surgical critical care and the management of severe traumatic injury is reflected by the organization and contents of this manual in that numerous elements of critical care are discussed in the context of the management of specific injuries. This chapter will focus on elements of critical care essential to the management of the acutely injured patient and briefly review some of the more recent developments in the management of specific organ-system dysfunction.

DISEASE SEVERITY SCORING IN THE INTENSIVE CARE UNIT

A number of scoring systems for critically ill patients have been developed. Of these, the APACHE scoring system, introduced in 1981, is one of the most widely used scoring systems, using indices of chronic illness as well as acute physiologic measures. APACHE II (1985) was an attempt to trim the number of variables, focusing on those with higher predictive powers. The APACHE II system, with scores ranging from 0 (least ill) to 71 (most ill), was subsequently evaluated using hospital deaths in over 5000 patients in 13 centers. APACHE II was less effective in predicting mortality in surgical patients, in moderate risk patients, and for specific subgroups such as patients with sepsis and major trauma.

APACHE III (1991) was created to further refine the ability of this scoring system to assess ICU patients. The wide distribution and validation of this version, however, has been limited because of the proprietary nature of the product, with the statistical analysis and weights not in the public domain.

Other critical illness severity scoring systems include: the Therapeutic Intervention Scoring System (TISS), which assigns point values to therapeutic interventions rather than physiologic abnormalities like APACHE; the Simplified Acute Physiology Score (SAPS II), based on a logistical model that includes 17 total ICU variables; and the mortality probability model (MPM II), also based on a logistical model, but providing a prediction of mortality at various times following ICU admission.

In addition to general models for the prediction of ICU mortality, several investigators have proposed scaled scores of specific organ dysfunction in order to grade and compare the severity. Sauia and coworkers (1994) updated their previously proposed postinjury multiple-organ failure score (Denver

MOF Score). Another organ dysfunction score reflecting lung dysfunction was developed by Murray, and is used widely in clinical research studies as a means for quantifying the severity of acute lung injury and acute respiratory distress syndrome (ARDS).

PHYSIOLOGIC MONITORING IN THE INTENSIVE CARE UNIT

Monitoring, for purposes of the early detection of organ system deterioration, is an essential component of critical care. Most ICU-specific monitoring involves invasive hemodynamic monitoring, ventilatory monitoring, intracranial dynamic monitoring, and surveillance for ICU infections.

Hemodynamic Monitoring

Hemodynamic monitoring is directed at assessing the results of resuscitation and maintaining adequate tissue and organ perfusion. It is generally recognized that we continue to lack reliable, direct measures of tissue perfusion, and must rely on more global physiologic measurements that may or may not accurately reflect events at the tissue level. Most routine hemodynamic monitoring in the ICU is performed using indwelling vascular catheters: arterial lines, central venous pressure lines, and pulmonary artery lines.

While central venous pressure (CVP) lines are useful in assessing intravascular volume in the majority of trauma patients, the utility of CVP pressures decreases in the setting of left heart disease or failure, and severe acute lung injury. Modified pulmonary artery catheters now allow both continuous cardiac output monitoring, and assessment of right heart ejection fraction and the secondary calculation of right ventricle end-diastolic filling volume, which provides a more accurate measure of potential preload-recruitable increases in cardiac index, as well as assessment of right heart failure.

The arterial base deficit (BD) is a value calculated using the Henderson-Hasselbalch relationship between pH, $Paco_2$, and serum bicarbonate that represents the stoichiometric equivalent of base that has to be added to the pH to return the patient to a normal pH of 7.40. Arterial BD is routinely calculated by blood gas analyzers and provides perhaps the best accessible metabolic indicator of shock states in the setting of major hemorrhage. It has been shown to be superior, as an indicator of hemorrhagic shock, to other parameters such as blood pressure, pulse, and urine output. In the setting of major hemorrhage, normalizing BD should be a primary goal of resuscitation in the operating room or ICU. BD is a nonspecific indicator of metabolic acidosis, however, and levels may be elevated with ethanol, cocaine, and methamphetamine ingestion, as well as seizures.

Transesophageal echocardiography (TEE) has been used for a number of years as an intraoperative monitor for high-risk cardiovascular patients. Its use as a potential monitoring device in the ICU has been limited by expense and lack of available expertise and well-defined indications, but it has been used successfully in some centers in lieu of the pulmonary artery catheter for the acute assessment of cardiac function.

Monitoring of Mechanical Ventilation

The principal focus of a great deal of critical care is the management and monitoring of mechanical ventilation. Ventilatory monitoring involves five areas: (1) gas exchange (the level of arterial oxygenation and the ability of the lungs to oxygenate the blood); (2) ventilation (the ability of the lungs to exchange CO_2), (3) lung mechanics (the elastic and resistive properties of the lungs); (4) inspiratory/expiratory pressures (the degree of positive pressure applied to the lungs during mechanical ventilation); and (5) the ventilatory capacity of the patient. Ventilatory and hemodynamic monitoring are inextricably linked due to the ability of transmitted mean intrathoracic pressures to impair cardiac output and the effect of cardiac output on deadspace ratios, shunt fraction, and arterial oxygenation.

Arterial oxygen tension (PaO_2) and continuous oximetric saturation provide the most readily available assessment of oxygenation, but do not provide information relative to the oxygen concentration being administered. Other measures of gas exchange include the alveolar arterial oxygen gradient, the (calculated) intrapulmonary shunt fraction, and the ratio between the PaO_2 and FIO_2. Arterial CO_2 tension remains the most accurate means of assessing ventilation. Continuous on-line determination of the end-expiratory PCO_2 is also being used increasingly as an indirect reflection of $PaCO_2$. The accuracy of end-tidal PCO_2 over time depends on a constant alveolar-arterial CO_2 gradient. This gradient is known to vary considerably with cardiac output, deadspace ratios, airway resistance, and metabolic rate. As a result, longer-term ETCO$_2$ monitoring in patients with more severe cardiac or pulmonary insufficiency is not recommended.

The mechanical properties of the airways and lungs are static and dynamic compliance. Compliance, the change in volume produced by a given change in pressure, is typically calculated from measured intratracheal (or ventilator circuit) pressures, and includes both lung and chest wall compliance. Compliance may be calculated based on peak inspiratory pressures (PIP) and incorporate any tube, airway, or bronchial resistance (dynamic compliance), or on the basis of inspiratory hold pressures (static compliance). Compliance is nonlinear and is increased at very low and very high lung volumes. The normal compliance of the lung and the chest wall (static) is approximately 100 mL/cm H_2O. Compliance is an important indicator of other disease states and is often a reflection of intra-alveolar injury.

GENERAL MANAGEMENT OF MECHANICAL VENTILATION

Acute respiratory failure constitutes the most common indication for admission to many surgical critical care units, and is a common sequela of major injury. Principal indications for endotracheal intubation and mechanical ventilation include the following:

1. Airway control and maintenance
2. Need for mechanically augmented ventilation
3. Need to improve oxygenation via increased FIO_2 or positive end-expiratory pressure (PEEP)
4. Need to tightly control PaO_2 and $PaCO_2$ for traumatic brain injuries
5. Prophylactic intubation for shock, neurologic injuries, inhalation injuries, etc

Ventilatory Modes

The principal physiologic effect produced by mechanical ventilation is related to positive versus negative airway pressures, as is the case during spontaneous ventilation. Positive pressure has a number of salutary effects on gas exchange produced mainly by the recruitment of marginal alveolar air spaces, increasing functional residual capacity, improving ventilation-perfusion matching, and decreasing intrapulmonary shunt. Adverse effects of positive pressure relate to its ability to produce barotrauma and ventilator-induced lung injury through the use of either excessive inflation volumes or inflation pressures, and the potential for impairment of cardiac output produced by increases in mean intrathoracic pressure. In general, some degree of both salutary and adverse effects of mechanical ventilation are common to all modes of mechanical ventilation since they all utilize, to varying degrees, positive insufflation pressures. The most common ventilatory modes and techniques and their descriptions are shown in Table 49-1.

TABLE 49-1 Common Modes of Mechanical Ventilation

Ventilatory mode or technique	Description
Assist control (AC)	Volume-controlled mode with preset V_t and minimum rate. Cycles may be triggered by patient with delivery of full TV. Not appropriate as a weaning mode.
Intermittent mandatory ventilation (IMV)	Similar to AC, with minimum preset rate. Additional machine cycles are not triggered by patient, but spontaneous breathing, subject to set EEP, is allowed between machine cyles. May be used as a weaning mode. Synchronous mode (SIMV) used to avoid breath "stacking."
Pressure support ventilation (PSV)	Pressure-limited, pressure-triggered by patient, without preset rate of TV. Allows machine-augmented spontaneous ventilation. Used commonly as a weaning mode. May be used with SIMV. Rate is entirely patient-derived.
Time-cycled pressure control (PCV)	Pressured controlled/limited, time-cycled with minimal preset rate. Used commonly with inverse ratio (inspiratory time > expiratory time) ventilation. Used frequently in the setting of acute lung injury. Not appropriate for weaning.
Airway pressure release ventilation (APRV)	Pressure-controlled/limited, time-cycled. Allows spontaneous breathing, but releases ambient airway pressure, lowering lung volume and limiting barotrauma.
Inverse ratio ventilation (IRV)	Technique whereby normal inspiratory: expiratory (I:E) ratios of between 1:2 and 1:1.2 are reversed, prolonging the inspiratory phase. Depending on respiratory rate, this may result in the establishment of intrinsic (auto) PEEP, caused by air trapped in constricted (ARDS-injured) airways. This controlled air trapping may improve oxygenation by increasing FRC and decreasing intrapulmonary shunt.
Permissive hypercapnea	Technique whereby low tidal volumes ± lower ventilatory rates are used in order to limit volutrauma and ventilatory-induced lung injury. $PaCO_2$ may increase to >60–70 mm Hg with pH limited to $\geq$7.2.

ARDS, acute respiratory distress syndrome; EEP, end-expiratory pressure; FRC, functional residual capacity; PEEP, positive end-expiratory pressure; TV, tidal volume; V_t, total ventilation.

Ventilator-Induced Lung Injury

It has become increasingly recognized that the process of positive pressure insufflation of the lungs may, in the setting of ARDS and decreased compliance, produce a secondary injury. This so-called ventilator-induced lung injury may further contribute and prolong the inflammatory injury to the lung by overdistention of injured airspaces. Overt barotrauma with spontaneous pneumothorax is the most obvious result of this process, but many now believe that the inflammatory injury may also be amplified by high tidal volume volutrauma to the lung, based on a series of recent comparative studies of high versus low tidal volume.

Limiting airway pressures and/or tidal volume, while straightforward from a ventilator standpoint, often produces secondary hypercapnea and corresponding acidosis. The practice of allowing this to occur in the setting of acute lung injury and low tidal volume ventilation is called permissive hypercapnea. The acidosis produced may be countered a variety of ways, assuming that there is incomplete renal compensation.

Weaning from Mechanical Ventilation

One of the primary and unique functions of a critical care team, and one that often occupies considerable time and effort, is the management of weaning from mechanical ventilation. Ventilator weaning is the transition process by which the patient, as opposed to the mechanical ventilator, assumes the function of the ventilatory pump—moving air into and out of the lungs. The process is typically gradual, and may or may not incorporate a directed program of respiratory muscle strength and endurance conditioning. Weaning should not be equated with extubation, although there is frequently a strong temporal association in the course of critical illness. Ventilator weaning may be complex and require the careful analysis of a variety of conditions and factors pertaining to the function of other organ systems.

The group of patients that require prolonged, directed efforts at weaning from mechanical ventilation are those with longer-term or permanent decreases in ventilatory work or ventilatory capacity. This group might include patients with high spinal cord injury, those with post-ARDS pulmonary fibrosis, and elderly patients recovering from prolonged respiratory failure or malnutrition. In many cases, this patient population is distinguished by their need for some sort of respiratory muscle strength conditioning to compensate for chronically increased ventilatory work or decreased capacity.

Under normal circumstances, it is thought that the ratio of resting ventilatory reserve compared to normal ventilatory work is approximately 10:1, creating a large margin of safety in most patients. Ventilatory failure, a failure of the ventilatory pump, occurs when this safety margin is overcome and ventilatory capacity is exceeded by the work requirements. In analyzing the treatable causes of ventilatory failure as part of the weaning process, it is useful to separate the various causes into those acting to increase ventilatory work and those acting to reduce ventilatory capacity (Table 49-2). Efforts at ventilatory weaning should be directed at reversing or decreasing injury and iatrogenically related increases in work of breathing, and instituting measures that will improve the patient's ventilatory capacity.

TABLE 49-2 Factors Pertaining to Ventilatory Capacity and Work of Breathing

Decreased ventilatory capacity	Cause	Treatment
Malnutrition	Chronic respiratory muscle weakness caused by protein-calorie insufficiency and catabolism	Establish anabolic state. Ensure adequate nutrition. Recovery may be prolonged. [anabolic steroids]
Metabolic derangements: PO_4, Mg^{++}, Ca^{++}, etc	Typically associated with hyperalimentation and inadequate replacement	Replenishment. Adjustment of hyper/enteral alimentation. Evaluate other causes
Cardiac insufficiency	Underlying disease, myocardial infarction, blunt myocardial injury	Establish diagnosis and appropriate monitoring to evaluate function and volume status. Treat under-lying cause of myocardial insufficiency. May require inotropic agents
Spinal cord injury	Primary injury	Abdominal binding to improve function and tussive capacity. Upright posture. Establish program for respiratory muscle conditioning
Chest wall injury, thoracotomy incision/pain	Dysfunctional respiratory patterns caused by pain, splinting or mechanical instability of the chest wall	Directed analgesia: epidural opiates ± bypivacaine or other methods. [surgical stabilization of chest wall in selected cases]
Abdominal injury/laparotomy	Dyssynchronous respiratory pattern associated with laparotomy ± opiate agents	Pain control. Ambulation (if possible). Early respira-tory muscle exercise (e.g., incentive spirometry)
Critical illness polyneuropathy	May be associated with prolonged use of paralytic agents and steroids. Nonspecific	Confirm diagnosis and exclude other causes. Limit/discontinue use of paralytic agents + steroids. Establish program for respiratory muscle conditioning. Expectant.
Decreased muscle strength/atrophy	Nonspecific. Disuse atrophy associated with prolonged mechanical ventilation, prolonged critical illness, prolonged catabolic state	Exclude other causes. Treat other reversible causes of decreased ventilatory capacity or increase WOB. Early establishment of program for respiratory muscle conditioning.
Functional limitation: fear/anxiety, lack of motivation, lack of understanding	Lack of understanding process and goals. Poor tolerance of decreased tidal volumes/rate	Reassurance, encouragement, "coaching," careful use of anxiolytics. Use of different weaning ventilatory modes

TABLE 49-2 *continued*

	Cause	Treatment
Increased ventilatory work		
Decreased pulmonary and chest wall compliance	Surfactant depletion/sepsis/ARDS, chronic/acute pulmonary fibrosis, endobronchial hemorrhage, massive fluid resuscitation and chest wall edema, high FRC ventilation/overdistention	Restrict high pressure/volume ventilation. Assess PEEP/TV compliance grid. Active or passive diuresis NG decompression. Restriction of enteral alimentation temporarily. Diagnose and treat. IACS, fluid/salt restriction, diuresis as needed
Decreased abdominal compliance	Ileus/abdominal distention, intra-abdominal compartment syndrome (IACS), ascites	
Increased airway resistance	Endotracheal tube size/obstruction/narrowing. Bronchospasm, bronchial mucus plugging	Consider up-sizing ETT. Wean with pressure support sufficient to overcome tube resistance. Bronchodilators as needed. Suctioning and mucolytic agents as needed. [bronchoscopy] Restrict high pressure/volume ventilation. Treat myocardial dysfunction as above. [tracheostomy]
Increased minute volume requirements: increases in physiologic/anatomic deadspace.	Acute lung injury, barotrauma, emphysema, decreased cardiac output, excessive breathing circuit deadspace	
Increased minute volume requirements: CO_2 production, metabolic acidosis	Infection, SIRS, high carbohydrate substrates, excessive hyper or enteralimentation	Diagnose infection. Pyrolytics. Alter nutritional substrate to higher lipid content. Adjust hyper/enteral alimentation.

ARDS, acute respiratory distress syndrome; ETT, endotracheal tube; FRC, functional residual capacity; NG, nasogastric; PEEP, positive end-expiratory pressure; SIRS, systemic inflammatory response syndrome; TV, tidal volume; WOB, work of breathing.

The Weaning Process

A weaning method consists of the application of a specific ventilatory mode with the goal of reduction and eventual removal of mechanical ventilatory support. A weaning ventilatory mode is typically one that allows stepwise decrements in the amount of machine support of the work of breathing (e.g., intermittent mandatory ventilation [IMV], pressure support ventilation [PSV], or a combination). The mode of ventilation used for the weaning process is probably less critical than the method used.

The critical distinction between weaning methods is those that incorporate a conditioning regimen for respiratory musculature and those that do not. Ventilatory reconditioning programs should involve the common elements of periods of vigorous muscle work, separated by periods of complete ventilatory muscle rest. Ventilatory rest may be accomplished by the use of several modes, but is most easily accomplished through the use of assist control with a rate set just slightly lower than the patient's demand rate. This approach of periodic ventilatory reconditioning exercises separated by rest periods has been associated with faster ventilator weaning in controlled trials.

Decisions regarding the specific method, mode, and initial settings may be individualized and incorporated into a formal weaning protocol for difficult patients. The use of such protocols for ventilator weaning has been associated with reduced ventilator days and reduced ICU costs. A general approach to ventilator weaning involving reconditioning is shown as a protocol in Fig. 49-1.

Weaning Versus Extubation

A clear distinction should be made between weaning from mechanical ventilation (stepwise reduction in machine-related ventilatory work) and actual removal of the endotracheal tube (extubation). In most circumstances, the weaning process should begin as soon as actual or anticipated organ system instability has resolved. High FIO_2 requirements or low compliance should not necessarily constitute a contraindication to begin the weaning process, particularly for patients with longer-term decreases in ventilatory capacity or increases in ventilatory work.

Factors entering into the decision to discontinue endotracheal intubation, in addition to increasing ventilatory capacity and decreased demands, include tussive capacity, the extent of mucous secretions, and anticipated organ-system stability (Table 49-3).

Analgesia and Conscious Sedation

During the last decade, there has been a fundamental change in the perception of the role of pain and anxiety in the outcome of critically ill patients. These patients have historically been perceived as being at risk primarily from the adverse effects associated with treatment. More recently, the contribution of pain and anxiety to morbidity and possibly even mortality is better appreciated, particularly in the ICU. The development of improved analgesic and sedative agents, and the expanding use of regional anesthetic techniques have led to greater efforts to develop uniform approaches to the management of conscious sedation and postinjury pain. Consensus recommendations to guide analgesic and sedative therapy in the ICU are available. It is now recognized that analgesia and sedation are important components of quality critical care.

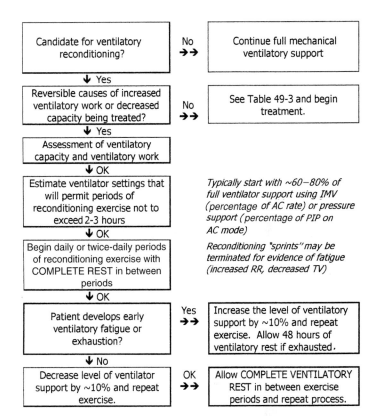

FIG. 49-1. Generalized example of ventilator weaning protocol. AC, assist control; PIP, positive inspiratory pressure; IMV, intermittent mandatory ventilation; RR, respiratory rate; TV, tidal volume.

Opioid agents (e.g., morphine, fentanyl) are mainstays in the treatment of pain in the ICU. Recently, an executive panel has published recommendations regarding preferred parenteral opioid agents in the treatment of pain in adult ICU patients. This analysis, based on an exhaustive review of the literature, supports the use of parenteral morphine, fentanyl, and hydromorphone as agents of choice for the treatment of pain in the ICU.

In addition to pain, it is often necessary to treat anxiety arising from prolonged or uncomfortable ICU care. The benzodiazepines (midazolam, lorazepam, and diazepam) have been the cornerstone of anxiolytic, amnestic, and sedative therapy for adult ICU patients, but the introduction of propofol has expanded the number of agents available for this indication. Recent recommendations suggest the use of propofol or midazolam for routine short-term ICU sedation, and lorazepam for long-term sedation.

COMPLICATIONS OF CRITICAL CARE

A discussion of the wide variety of critical illness complications is beyond the scope of this brief overview. Two of the most common ICU complications are

TABLE 49-3 Suggested Criteria for Extubation

Extubation criteria (all must be met)	Associated physiological parameters or physical findings
Ability to maintain and protect airway	• Adequate laryngeal function • Intact gag and swallowing reflexes • Adequate leak around deflated endotracheal tube balloon • No evidence for cord/laryngeal edema • Exclusion of possible cord/laryngeal function/edema by laryngoscopy as needed • Mental status commensurate w/airway protection
Ability to maintain adequate oxygenation	• FiO_2 ≤.4 and adequate O_2 saturation (>97%) • No requirement for PEEP • Adequate independent ventilation
Ability to maintain adequate ventilation	• Minute ventilation <10–12 L/min • Respiratory rate <30–35 • Maximum inspiratory flow >−30, PEEP ventilatory capacity >12–15 mL/kg • Toleration of minimal ventilator support of T-piece without clinical evidence of ventilatory fatigue
Ability to clear secretions	• Adequate tussive capacity (subjective) • No significant impairment of mucocilliary function • Secretions not excessive • Postextubation tracheal suctioning not difficult and suctioning requirements not excessive
No expected deterioration in organ system function (reintubation not anticipated)	• No developing major infection, sepsis, etc • Adequate cardiac reserve • No anticipated deterioration in neurological, pulmonary, or cardiac function • No short-term need for reoperation

ventilator-associated pneumonia (VAP) and central venous catheter (CVC) infection.

VAP occurs frequently in patients with prolonged mechanical ventilation, and is associated with a variety of factors and injuries, including

• Prolonged endotracheal intubation
• Nasogastric tubes
• The prolonged use of chemical paralytic agents
• Traumatic brain injury with immobility, upright position, and limited pulmonary functioning
• Use of H_2 blockers or proton pump inhibitors for the prevention of stress gastritis

There is evidence that pneumonia may exacerbate multiple organ failure and ARDS, and sepsis from pneumonic sources as a secondary factor might also be expected to substantially worsen outcome. A number of approaches to preventing VAP have been used over the years, including reestablishing normal gastric acidity, selective contamination of the GI tract, prophylactic use of antibiotics, and the use of modified endotracheal tubes designed to allow subglottic suctioning of fluid thought to contribute to VAP. Despite the apparent efficacy of some of these methods in reducing the incidence of VAP, effects on overall mortality have been more difficult to demonstrate.

In the United States, it is estimated that between 35,000 and 50,000 patients are affected annually by CVC bacteremia, representing roughly 2 to 9 percent of all catheters. Some of the variability in incidence is related to a lack of a consistent definition of catheter-related sepsis or catheter-related infection. A CVC infection may be diagnosed on the basis of the presence of clinical sepsis, the presence of an indwelling CVC, and identical organisms isolated from peripheral cultures and catheter tips. Factors that have been associated with or causal to CVC infections include:

- Suboptimal aseptic line placement and site preparation
- Multiuse lines and multilumen catheters
- Polypropylene or PVC versus Silastic catheters
- Hyperalimentation lines
- Use of occlusive dressings
- Antibiotic-impregnated cuffs or catheters
- Duration of placement

Migratory skin colonization, hub colonization, contaminated insertion, and bacteremic seeding are all mechanisms whereby organisms gain access to indwelling catheters. Depending on patient population, ICU practices, severity of illness, and protocols for placement and maintenance of CVCs, variable rates of infection and different sites of colonization have been reported. This inherent heterogeneity has acted to perpetuate the substantial confusion that exists in many critical care units with respect to developing optimal management protocols for CVCs.

The question of prophylactic rotation of CVC sites with or without changes over a guidewire has yet to be definitively resolved. The conventional routine of frequent (every 3 days) rotation of sites has given way to a more selective approach involving CVC change over a guidewire, with site rotation based on catheter tip culture results. Protocols governing the management of CVC infections are helpful in standardizing and optimizing management, but must be tailored to each individual ICU.

It is important to note that each individual intensive care unit will have varying combinations of line insertion protocols, dressing change protocols, catheter manipulation usage rates, patient demographics, and severity of illness, all of which interact to create unique CVC infection epidemiology in each unit. The most rational approach to prevention of CVC infections should typically begin with careful analysis of the standards and practices within a given unit, catheter colonization rate data (if available), and the clinical incidence of suspected and documented CVC-related sepsis.

ADDITIONAL READING

Esteban A, Frutos F, Tobin MJ, et al: A comparison of four methods of weaning patients from mechanical ventilation. Spanish Lung Failure Collaborative Group. *N Engl J Med* 332:345, 1995.
Groeger JS, Strosberg MA, Halpern NA, et al: Descriptive analyses of critical care units in the United States. *Crit Care Med* 20:846, 1992.
Hinson JR, Marini JJ: Principles of mechanical ventilator use in respiratory failure. *Ann Rev Med* 43:341, 1992.
Lemeshow S, Klar J, Tares D, et al: Mortality prediction models for patients in the intensive care unit for 48 or 72 hours: A prospective, multicenter study. *Crit Care Med* 22:1351, 1994.
Parker JC, Hernandez LA, Peevy KJ: Mechanisms of ventilator-induced lung injury. *Crit Care Med* 21:131, 1993.
Shapiro B, Warren J, Egol A, et al: Practice parameters for intravenous analgesia and sedation for adult patients in the intensive care unit: an executive summary. *Crit Care Med* 23:1596, 1995.

50 | Bleeding and Coagulation Problems

Important to the concept of rapid control of surgical bleeding is an understanding of the physiology of bleeding and coagulation complications. The complex interactions between formed blood elements, plasma constituents (Table 50–1), and the blood vessel wall act to prevent undue hemorrhage and preserve vascular integrity while maintaining the fluid nature of blood. Derangements of hemostasis during the acute resuscitation of the severely injured trauma patient may contribute significantly to death. Prompt attention to and correction of these factors is necessary if such patients are to be salvaged. Moreover, disorders of natural anticoagulant systems that occur hours or even days after the initial traumatic insult are important to consider. These processes may lead to venous thromboembolic complications and serve as a major cause of late morbidity and even mortality in the trauma patient.

PHYSIOLOGY OF HEMOSTASIS

Blood Vessel Contraction

Transection of small vessels is followed by intense spasm and resultant vasoconstriction. Both catecholamines and thromboxane A_2 (TXA_2) act to produce vasoconstriction and platelet aggregation. This results in a decrease in the total number of platelets needed for plug formation, ultimately leading to decreased bleeding.

Primary Hemostasis

Formation of the platelet plug is referred to as primary hemostasis. Exposure of the subendothelium initiates primary hemostasis, with platelet adhesion, aggregation, and plug formation occurring in the first few minutes after injury. Subsequent consolidation and stabilization occur as the coagulation cascade leads to fibrin formation and stabilization.

Secondary Hemostasis

The conversion of fibrinogen to fibrin, culminating in the formation of an insoluble fibrin clot, constitutes secondary hemostasis. The mechanisms involved in secondary hemostasis are complex and best described as a waterfall effect or the coagulation cascade (Fig. 50-1). The extrinsic pathway and the intrinsic pathway are critical in forming thrombin, fibrin monomers, and ultimately a stable fibrin clot. A number of checks and balances are normally present, which serve to control the process of coagulation and prevent massive thrombosis. These include blood flow, circulating protease inhibitors, and some proteolytic enzymes which have antithrombotic properties.

Fibrinolysis

Tissue plasminogen activator (tPA), released from endothelial cells adjacent to a thrombus, converts plasminogen to plasmin, the most potent fibrinolytic protein in the body (Fig. 50-2). Venous stasis, exercise, and thrombin may also lead to the release of tPA. Pharmacologic agents such as urokinase (UK) and streptokinase (SK) also convert plasminogen to plasmin, which actively degrades both fibrinogen and fibrin at the sites of deposition. The result is the

TABLE 50-1 Human Clotting Factors

Name	Synonym	Pathway	Levels	Half-life
Factor I	Fibrinogen	Common	250 mg/dL	120 h
Factor II	Prothrombin	Common	100 μg/mL	72 h
Factor V	Proaccelerin	Common	10 μg/mL	36 h
Factor VII	Proconvertin	Extrinsic	1 μg/ml	5 h
Factor VIII	Antihemophillic factor	Intrinsic	7 μg/mL	10 h
Factor IX	Christmas factor	Intrinsic	4 μg/mL	24 h
Factor X	Stuart-Prower factor	Common	5 μg/mL	40 h
Factor XI	Plasma thromboplastin antecedent	Intrinsic	4 μg/mL	65 h
Factor XII	Hageman factor	Intrinsic	30 μg/mL	60 h
Factor XIII	Fibrin-stabilizing factor	Common	10 μg/mL	150 h
Platelets		Primary hemostasis	225,000/mm³	8–11 days

formation of fibrin degradation products, the smallest of which is termed the D dimer. A number of nonplasmin fibrinolytic mechanisms are also present. Protein C and cofactor protein S act to inactivate factors V and VIII, thus inhibiting clotting. Both are produced in the liver. Antithrombin III binds to thrombin in such a way that it prevents factors V and VIII, as well as platelets, from being activated. Again, as a result, clotting is inhibited.

TESTS OF COAGULATION

The complex system of primary hemostasis, secondary hemostasis, and fibrinolysis cannot be completely assessed with any single test. Some of the criti-

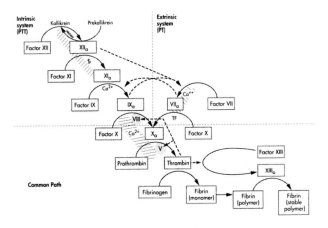

FIG. 50-1. Secondary hemostasis. (Reproduced, with permission, from Thompson AR, Harker LA (eds): Manual of Hemostasis and Thrombosis, 3rd ed. Philadelphia, FA Davis, 1983, p. 25.)

TABLE 50-2 Common Tests of Coagulation

Test	Normals	Comments
Platelet count	150–400 K/mm³	Quantitative test
Bleeding time	4–7 min	Qualitative test of platelet function
Prothrombin time	11–14 sec	Extrinsic and common pathways
Partial thromboplastin time	22–30 sec	Intrinsic and common pathways
Fibrinogen level	170–410 mg/dL	Quantitative test
Fibrin degradation products	<18 µg/mL	Nonspecifically detects fibrin degradation
D dimer	<0.5 µg/mL	More specific than fibrin degradation products for pathologic thrombolysis

cal tests available for modern coagulation assessment are summarized in Table 50-2. Understanding the fundamental purpose of these tests is important to the understanding of coagulation in general.

The most frequently used test of primary hemostasis is the bleeding time, which measures the time to formation of the platelet plug. Tests of secondary hemostasis include the prothrombin time (PT) and the partial thromboplastin time (PTT). The PT measures the function of the extrinsic and common pathways of the coagulation cascade and is most sensitive to low levels of factors VII (one of the vitamin K-dependent factors, along with factors II, IX, and X). The PTT evaluates the intrinsic and common pathways of the coagulation cascade. It can detect deficiencies of all coagulation factors except factors VII and XIII.

There are a number of tests that measure the presence of fibrinogen degradation products (FDP). These include the measurement of FDP, as well as the more specific testing for the presence of D dimer, which is usually indicative of lysis of stable, crosslinked fibrin, and does not react with derivatives originating from fibrinogen or uncrosslinked fibrin. As a result, the D dimer assay may be a more reliable marker of pathologic thrombolysis.

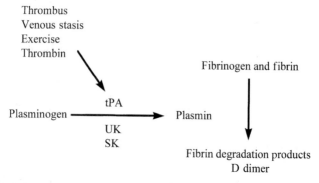

FIG. 50-2. Fibrinolysis. tPA, tissue plasminogen activator; SK, streptokinase; UK, urokinase.

COMORBID COAGULATION DEFECTS

Studies have demonstrated that preexisting disease in the trauma victim may predict outcome independent of age and injury. The presence of a coagulation defect in trauma patients also significantly increases hospital length of stay, especially in older patients. Regardless of the cause of the comorbid coagulation defect, each can have far-reaching implications in the overall outcome of the injured patient. Some of the comorbid conditions potentially leading to coagulation defects are summarized in Table 50-3. These include hepatic insufficiency, renal insufficiency, hemophilia, coumadin therapy, aspirin use, and alcohol intoxication.

HYPOCOAGULABILITY AFTER MAJOR TRAUMA

Ongoing bleeding, despite control of all surgical hemorrhage, is common in the severely injured trauma patient. Such coagulopathic bleeding has been recognized as a major cause of early death after major trauma. Most believe that a number of specific injuries may lead to a rapid development of a coagulopathic state in the trauma patient. Brain injury, severe pulmonary contusion, and severe hepatic injury have been implicated as specific injury complexes, which result in the release of thromboplastin leading to intravascular activation of the extrinsic cascade, activation of thrombin, and formation of fibrin clots. With the subsequent vigorous fibrinolysis, D-dimer levels are elevated, coagulation factors and fibrinogen are depleted, and disseminated intravascular coagulation develops.

Of even greater concern is the potential development of the so-called "bloody vicious cycle." This cycle of coagulopathy after exsanguination occurs through a number of mechanisms and can lead to progressive hypothermia and acidosis. This then leads to additional bleeding and a progressive spiral may develop, ultimately resulting in the demise of the patient.

Recognition of this cascade leading to physiologic exhaustion led to the development of a "damage control" approach in the massively exsanguinating patient. Damage control calls for abbreviation of laparotomy and other operative procedures after initial control of hemorrhage and contamination has been secured. Aggressive attempts to control the physiology targeted at improvement of coagulation function are then undertaken in the intensive care unit. The algorithm in Fig. 50-3 can be utilized for most injured patients. Specific blood products can be given to correct identified abnormalities and effect hemostasis, and in virtually all cases massive transfusion of blood products is required. In this situation, both clinical and laboratory coagulopathy is usually noted. Massive transfusion protocols may be necessary to meet the needs of the exsanguinating patient.

A third type of hypocoagulable state can exist in the injured patient. Disseminated intravascular coagulation (DIC) typically results from the combination of shock and a clotting stimulus. It occurs as a result of the release of thromboplastic substances secondary to this stimulus, which initiates the coagulation cascade and reflexively activates systemic fibrinolysis. If the clotting stimulus escalates, intravascular coagulation factor consumption increases and a critical depletion of factors can occur. Moreover, as fibrinolysis occurs and fibrinogen is degraded by thrombin and plasmin, split fibrin degradation products accumulate. As a result, hemostatic failure occurs and the consumptive coagulopathy of DIC becomes clinically evident. Treatment centers on resuscitation of the patient and prompt removal of the inciting stim-

TABLE 50-3 Common Comorbid Coagulation Disorders

Disorder	Lab Findings	Treatment	Comments
Hepatic insufficiency	Increased prothrombin time	Fresh frozen plasma/vitamin K	Associated with increased mortality
	Decreased platelets	Platelet transfusion	Secondary to hypersplenism
Renal insufficiency	Increased bleeding time	Desmopressin/dialysis	Desmopressin effect transient
Hemophilia	Increased partial thromboplastin time	Factor replacement	Fresh frozen plasma replacement inefficient
Warfarin (coumadin) therapy	Increased prothrombin time	Fresh frozen plasma/vitamin K	Vitamin K therapy makes reanticoagulation with coumadin difficult
Aspirin use	Increased bleeding time	Platelet transfusion	Irreversibly "poisons" platelets
Acute alcohol intoxication	Increased bleeding time	Hydration	Transient effect

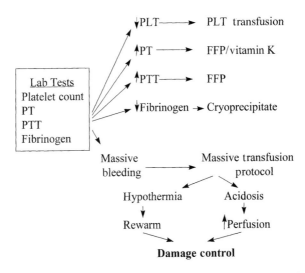

FIG. 50-3. Algorithm for bleeding trauma patient. FFP, fresh frozen plasma, PLT, platelet; PT, prothrombin time; PTT, partial thromboplastin time.

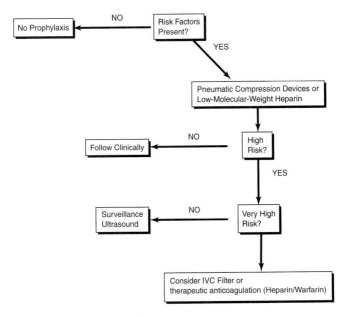

FIG. 50-4. Algorithm for venous thromboembolism prophylaxis. IVC, inferior vena cava. (Source: Division of Trauma and Surgical Critical Care, Hospital of the University of Pennsylvania, Philadelphia.)

ulus. If these measures are ineffective, a heparin bolus may be warranted, followed by platelet and FFP administration. There may also be a role for ε-aminocaproic acid (EACA). EACA may abolish or reduce the tendency toward fibrinolysis and allow for some hemostasis to occur.

HYPERCOAGULABILITY AFTER TRAUMA

Although coagulopathic bleeding represents a dramatic manifestation of the acute pathophysiologic changes after major trauma, the insidious onset of a hypercoagulable state is equally important in the postinjury period. As a result, venous thrombosis, pulmonary embolism (PE), and even death can occur. Recent reviews of trauma populations suggest an incidence of lower extremity thrombosis of greater than 50 percent when no prophylaxis is employed, with nearly one-third of these thromboses extending to the popliteal vein or above. The incidence of pulmonary embolism, despite prophylactic measures, may approach 5 percent in association with some injury complexes. The pathophysiology of venous thrombosis is based on the triad of stasis, endothelial damage, and hypercoagulability. The injured patient often demonstrates all three of these elements, and as a result, is at exceptional risk for venous throm-

TABLE 50-4 Risk Factors for DVT and PE

At Risk
Age >40 years
Injury Severity Score >9
Blood transfusion(s)
Surgical procedure ≥2 h
Lower-extremity fracture(s)
Pelvic fracture
Spinal cord injury
Immobilization
Pregnancy
Estrogen therapy
History of DVT/PE
Malignancy
Hypercoagulable state (e.g., ATT III deficiency)
Extensive soft-tissue trauma
Congestive heart failure
At High Risk
Age >50 years
Injury Severity Score ≥16
Femoral central venous catheter
Abbreviated injury Score ≥3 (any one body region)
Glasgow Coma Scale score ≤8
Spinal cord injury
Pelvic fracture
Femur/tibia fracture
Venous injury
At Very High Risk
Spinal cord injury with paralysis
Abbreviated injury Score-Head/Neck ≥3 + long-bone fracture (upper/lower)
Severe pelvic fracture (posterior element) + long-bone fracture
Multiple (≥3) long-bone fractures

Source: Division of Trauma and Surgical Critical Care, Hospital of the University of Pennsylvania, Philadelphia, PA.

bosis. While both stasis and endothelial damage play a clear role in the pathophysiology of venous thrombosis, the hypercoagulable state is complex and incompletely understood. Low levels of antithrombin III, protein C, and protein S have all been implicated in the process. Moreover, increased platelet adhesiveness and alteration of the coagulation cascade may well be important.

The diagnosis of both deep venous thrombosis (DVT) and pulmonary embolism can be difficult and is based on a preponderance of both clinical and diagnostic evidence. Most important for both is the need for prophylaxis, prompt recognition, and treatment. Prophylaxis algorithms for deep venous thrombosis are being developed and implemented in many institutions. One such algorithm is described in Fig. 50-4. High-risk patients are followed with serial duplex ultrasonography. Very high-risk patients undergo placement of a prophylactic vena cava filter. Table 50-3 lists the risk factors for DVT and PE. Using an approach such as this, a fatal pulmonary embolism in the high-risk and very high-risk groups can be greatly reduced. Despite this success, additional research in the field of hypercoagulable states and their sequelae after a major trauma is needed.

ADDITIONAL READING

Blaisdell FW: Bleeding, in Wilmore DW, Cheung LY, Harken AH, et al (eds): *Scientific American Surgery*. New York, Scientific American Inc., 1998, p 1.

Knudson MM: Coagulation disorders, in Ivatury RR, Cayten CG (eds): *The Textbook of Penetrating Trauma*. Baltimore, Williams & Wilkins, 1996, p 1016.

Rhodes M, Cipolle MD: Deep venous thrombosis and pulmonary embolism, in Maull KI, et al (eds): *Complications in Trauma and Critical Care*. Philadelphia, WB Saunders, 1996, p 81.

Rotondo MF, Zonies DH: The damage control sequence and underlying logic. *Surg Clin North Am* 77:761, 1997.

Wakefield TW: Hemostasis, in Greenfield LJ, et al (eds): *Surgery, Scientific Principles and Practice*. Philadelphia, JG Lippincott, 1993, p 102.

51 | Cardiovascular Failure

Cardiac failure is defined as cardiac output that is inadequate relative to the input of the heart and the metabolic needs of the body. Blood flow may be inadequate for several reasons, including global decreases in cardiac output, decreases in regional microvascular perfusion despite adequate global cardiac output, and increases in metabolic demand without an appropriate compensatory increase in perfusion.

DETERMINANTS OF CARDIAC OUTPUT

In the absence of significant regurgitant flow, cardiac output is equal to average ventricular stroke volume (SV) multiplied by heart rate. When managing patients with a pulmonary artery catheter (or other means of determining cardiac output), clinicians should routinely calculate the SV, thereby isolating the effects of therapeutic manipulations on ventricular performance independent of heart rate. SV, which is equal to the end-diastolic volume minus the end-systolic volume, is a function of three variables: preload, afterload, and contractility. The normal SV in adults is approximately 50 to 100 mL.

Preload

Increasing preload increases the force of contraction. In the intact ventricle, the force of contraction is determined by end-diastolic volume (EDV) and not end-diastolic pressure (EDP), although the latter is often used as a proxy for the former in clinical practice. Although it cannot be conveniently measured directly in patients, left ventricular EDP (LVEDP) is well approximated by left atrial pressure or pulmonary artery wedge pressure (PAWP), parameters that can be assessed in the clinical setting using a pulmonary artery (Swan-Ganz) catheter floated through the right heart at the bedside. In clinical practice, the most important determinant of preload is intravascular volume. Hypovolemia can be caused by any of the following factors (alone or in combination): external or internal losses of whole blood (i.e., hemorrhagic shock); contraction of the (cell-free) intravascular space due to external fluid losses (e.g., diarrhea or inappropriate polyuria); and contraction of the intravascular fluid compartment due to internal sequestration as edema fluid.

Venous return, and hence preload, is also a function of vasomotor tone of the major venous capacitance vessels. Venous return (i.e., preload) is adversely affected by increased intrathoracic pressures. This is the primary mechanism leading to shock and hypotension in patients with tension pneumothorax. Intrathoracic pressure is also increased to a variable extent by intermittent positive-pressure ventilation (IPPV) and the application of positive end-expiratory pressure (PEEP).

Afterload

Ventricular afterload describes the forces that retard ventricular ejection of blood and is best expressed in terms of ventricular wall stress at the end of systole. It is approximated by systemic vascular resistance (SVR).

SVR (in dyne $\cdot$ sec $\cdot$ cm^{-5}) is calculated using the hemodynamic equivalent of Ohm's law:

$$SVR = 80 \, (MAP - CVP)/CO$$

where MAP is mean arterial pressure (in mm Hg), CVP is central venous pressure (in mm Hg), and CO is cardiac output (in L/min). The normal value for SVR is 770 to 1500 dyne $\cdot$ sec $\cdot$ cm^{-5}.

Contractility

Contractility describes the performance of the cardiac muscle independent of preload and afterload. Using a pressure-volume diagram and end-systolic volume at several afterload states, the inotropic state or contractility of the myocardium can be determined. For any given stroke volume, increasing afterload increases the external work performed by the heart during a cardiac cycle. Reducing afterload is an important clinical tool to improve the balance between myocardial oxygen demand and delivery (provided that the arterial blood pressure is not reduced so much as to impair diastolic perfusion of the coronary arteries).

Heart Rate

Heart rate is a determinant of cardiac output. Ordinarily, increasing heart rate increases output by simply increasing the number of ejections per unit time. When heart rate is very high, the diastolic interval is shortened enough to interfere with ventricular filling, and cardiac output is compromised. In the clinical setting, rapid ventricular rates often occur in patients with preexisting ischemic heart disease; tachyarrhythmias can also adversely affect cardiac output by upsetting the balance between myocardial oxygen delivery (Do_2) and oxygen utilization (Vo_2), leading to impaired contractility from ischemia.

Myocardial Dysfunction

Inadequate cardiac output in surgical and trauma patients is most often due to systemic hypovolemia (i.e., inadequate preload). However, inadequate global perfusion also can be caused by a deterioration in the intrinsic performance of the heart regardless of loading conditions. Most often, acute reduction of myocardial performance occurs as a complication of acute myocardial infarction.

In treating myocardial dysfunction, whether in trauma patients or in other individuals with critical illness, consideration should be given to all of the four factors affecting cardiac output (i.e., heart rate, preload, afterload, and contractility). The effect of volume infusion on pressure measurements should be assessed; for example, a volume expander can be infused until the CVP increases by some target value (e.g., 3 cm H_2O). Manipulation of afterload, contractility, or heart rate generally requires pharmacologic intervention (Table 51-1).

Pharmacologic Agents Useful in the Management of Myocardial Dysfunction

Dopamine

Dopamine is an endogenous catecholamine that is capable of stimulating cardiac β_1 receptors, peripheral α-adrenoreceptors, and dopaminergic receptors in the splanchnic, renal, and other vascular beds. The effects of dopamine are dose dependent. At low doses (2 to 3 μg/kg/min), dopamine

TABLE 51-1 Inotropic Agents and Vasodilators Used in the Treatment of Cardiac Failure

Drug	Function	Add mg to 250 mL	μg/mL	μg/kg/min
Epinephrine	α_1, β_1, β_2 agonist	2	8	1–20
Norepinephrine	α, β_1 agonist	4	16	8–64
Phenylephrine	α_1 agonist	60	240	40–180
Dopamine	Dopamine, α_1, β_1 agonist	400	1600	2–20
Dobutamine	α_1, β_1 agonist	250	1000	2–20
Amrinone	Phosphodiesterase	800	3200	5–10
Milrinone	inhibitor	40	160	0.375–0.75
Nitroglycerine	NO donor	50	200	0.1–8
Nitroprusside	NO donor	100	400	0.1–7
Vasopressin	V1, V2, V3, oxytocin	100 U	0.4 U/mL	0.04 U/min

NO, nitric oxide.

increases renal blood flow (RBF), glomerular filtration rate (GFR), and urine output in normal human volunteers. At higher infusion rates (5 to 20 μg/kg/min), dopamine increases heart rate, cardiac output, and systemic arterial blood pressure. The value of low-dose dopamine as a renal protective agent is a topic of enormous controversy. Low-dose dopamine has been shown to improve urine flow in critically ill patients.

Dobutamine

Dobutamine is a synthetic catecholamine that binds to α_1-, β_1-, and β_2-adrenergic receptors. Dobutamine is structurally related to isoproterenol. In vivo, dobutamine exerts a powerful inotropic effect, but unlike isoproterenol, it is only a weak chronotrope. Because increasing heart rate increases myocardial oxygen demand, marked tachycardia is undesirable in the management of low cardiac output states, particularly in patients with coronary occlusive disease. Compared with most other sympathomimetic amines in clinical use, dobutamine has relatively minimal effects on peripheral vasomotor tone, perhaps because of opposing α_1 (vasoconstricting) and β_2 (vasodilating) effects. The increase in cardiac output, induced by dobutamine, clearly is partly due to decreased vascular impedance (i.e., afterload reduction due to peripheral vasodilation) leading to improved ventricular-vascular coupling (Fig. 51-1). Though dobutamine is clearly valuable in the management of many critically ill patients, it should not be employed thoughtlessly. In one recent study, using intravenous volume loading to increase preload was preferable to infusion of dobutamine as the primary intervention to improve visceral Do_2 in trauma patients.

Epinephrine

Epinephrine is an endogenous catecholamine with both α- and β-adrenergic activity. Epinephrine is occasionally used to treat low-output states after cardiopulmonary bypass or myocardial infarction, but its superiority over other agents (e.g., dobutamine) for these indications is not well documented. Certainly, epinephrine is far more potent than many other agents; whereas dobutamine is commonly infused at 5 to 20 μg/kg/min, epinephrine significantly increases heart rate at doses as low as 10 ng/kg/min. In patients with ventricular dysfunction secondary to sepsis refractory to treatment with dobu-

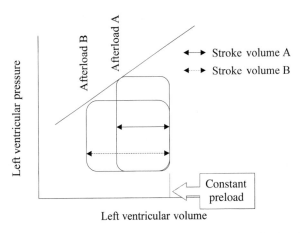

FIG. 51-1. The effect of changes in afterload at constant preload and constant inotropic state on stroke volume. Decreasing afterload (from A to B) increases stroke volume.

tamine and dopamine, infusion of epinephrine has been shown to improve mean arterial pressure (MAP), cardiac output, and right ventricular ejection fraction. Infusion of epinephrine can provoke the development of metabolic derangements, including hypokalemia, hyperglycemia, and ketoacidosis.

Norepinephrine

Norepinephrine is another endogenous catecholamine with α- and β-adrenergic activity. Clinicians have been reluctant to use norepinephrine for the treatment of shock because of concern about adverse effects on visceral (particularly renal) blood flow, because it is a potent vasoconstrictor. Nevertheless, there is increasing evidence that judicious use of norepinephrine may be valuable in certain shock states, especially those characterized by hypotension and right ventricular pressure overload. In the setting of right ventricular failure, norepinephrine, carefully titrated, may improve right ventricular perfusion and function without adversely affecting peripheral perfusion. In sepsis and septic shock, norepinephrine may be preferable to dopamine for providing cardiovascular support.

Amrinone and Milrinone

Amrinone and milrinone are synthetic bipyridines with potent inotropic and vasodilating actions. These agents inhibit the enzyme phosphodiesterase III, and thereby increase intracellular concentrations of cyclic adenosine monophosphate (cyclic AMP). The positive inotropic effects of these agents, however, may be due to secondary changes in intracellular ionized calcium metabolism rather than alterations in intracellular cyclic AMP. The positive hemodynamic actions of these drugs are due both to positive inotropic effects and peripheral vasodilation leading to decreased ventricular afterload. Unlike dopamine, dobutamine, and other catecholamines, the pharmacologic effects of intravenous amrinone and milrinone persist for a prolonged period after the drugs are discontinued. In contrast to dobutamine and other catecholamines, minute-to-minute titration of the dose of amrinone or milrinone does not make pharmacologic sense. Moreover, milrinone and amrinone tend to be "self-weaning" agents, since circulating levels decrease gradually over a period of several hours.

Bipyridine inotropes have been shown to improve cardiac performance in a wide variety of clinical situations, including low cardiac output following cardiopulmonary bypass, severe congestive heart failure, cardiogenic shock after myocardial infarction, hypoperfusion after trauma, and in other forms of critical illness in adult patients. In some settings, additive improvements in cardiac performance may be achieved by combining a bipyridine phosphodiesterase III inhibitor with a catecholamine (e.g., dobutamine).

Vasopressin

Arginine vasopressin (AVP), the antidiuretic hormone in humans, is a potent vasoconstrictor. AVP may be a very useful vasopressor in the management of septic shock refractory to the effects of other, more commonly employed agents.

Nitrovasodilators

Afterload reduction is widely used in the management of ventricular dysfunction. The most commonly used intravenous, titratable vasodilators are sodium nitroprusside (SNP) and nitroglycerine (NTG). By releasing nitric oxide, both of these compounds mimic the actions of this potent endogenous endothelial-derived vasorelaxing factor. NTG is generally thought to have a greater effect on capacitance than resistance vessels; i.e., NTG is said to be venoselective, whereas SNP is thought to be a more "balanced" vasodilator. Both NTG and SNP tend to increase intrapulmonary venous admixture and thereby worsen arterial P_{O_2}; accordingly, in some instances, switching to an alternative vasodilator (e.g., labetalol) may improve systemic oxygenation. In managing patients with ventricular dysfunction, inotropic agents are often best used in combination with a carefully titrated nitrovasodilator.

Diastolic Dysfunction

Clinicians commonly focus on the systolic performance of the left ventricle. Clearly, however, in order to function as a pump, the left ventricle must fill during diastole. For the most part, filling of the left ventricle during diastole is driven by the passive pressure in the pulmonary veins and the active contraction of the left atrium. A component of ventricular filling, however, also occurs as a result of the elastic recoil of the muscular chamber producing diastolic "suction." Diastolic dysfunction can occur as a result of increased resistance to passive filling and/or diminished elastic recoil. Causes of diastolic dysfunction include excessively high heart rate, valvular heart disease (mitral stenosis), and diminished diastolic compliance. Extraventricular factors, notably pericardial tamponade due to effusion or hemorrhage, can also impair diastolic performance. Diastolic dysfunction is best diagnosed by echocardiography. Treatment consists of afterload reduction, restoration of normal sinus rhythm if possible, and maintenance of a normal atrial rate.

Pulmonary Artery Catheter

The flow-directed pulmonary arterial (Swan-Ganz) catheter can provide clinicians with a wealth of hemodynamic data. With a standard thermodilution Swan-Ganz catheter, the following parameters are easily measured or calculated: right atrial (central venous) pressure; systolic, diastolic, and mean pulmonary arterial pressure; PAWP; cardiac output; mixed venous oxygen saturation; systemic Do_2; systemic Vo_2; and systemic oxygen extraction. Using more sophisticated catheters, it is possible also to estimate right ventricular ejection fraction and measure cardiac output and/or mixed venous oxygen saturation on a continuous basis. Selective utilization of pulmonary artery catheterization improves outcome for patients with trauma, sepsis, or other forms of critical illness.

OPTIMAL ENDPOINTS FOR RESUSCITATION

Porter and Ivatury recently reviewed the available data regarding endpoints in the acute resuscitation of victims of trauma. The conclusions are probably applicable to critically ill and high-risk patients in general. Most clinicians would agree that heart rate, systemic arterial blood pressure, skin temperature, and urine flow (i.e., the primary endpoints of resuscitation used by clinicians prior to the era of invasive hemodynamic monitoring) provide relatively little information about the adequacy of oxygen delivery to tissues. Instead of titrating patients to a hemodynamic endpoint such as cardiac output, another approach is to use a biochemical endpoint, such as arterial base deficit or blood lactate concentration. These endpoints recognize that tissue hypoperfusion leads to increased anaerobic metabolism. Accordingly, increases in arterial base deficit and/or blood lactate concentration are evidence of an increase in the rate of anaerobic metabolism. Numerous studies have documented that high blood lactate levels portend an unfavorable outcome in patients with shock, but it has not been proven that survival is improved when therapy is titrated using blood lactate concentration as an endpoint.

Base deficit is more quickly and easily measured than lactate concentration, and has been shown to have prognostic value in patients with shock. Although intuitively reasonable, it remains to be proven that titrating therapy to a base deficit endpoint improves survival.

Perhaps the most rational way to titrate resuscitation is to use a measure of the adequacy of regional tissue perfusion. There are a number of highly complex approaches to achieve this goal, such as using near infrared spectroscopy or tissue capnometry. Given the present state of knowledge, the availability of monitoring technologies, and the constraints on costs faced by all clinicians, the most economical and effective way of determining the adequacy of resuscitation probably is to combine routine hemodynamic monitoring (i.e., measurements of intra-arterial and central venous pressure and urine flow) with serial measurements of arterial base deficit and tissue Pco_2.

ADDITIONAL READING

Davis JW, Kaups KL, Parks SN: Base deficit is superior to pH in evaluating clearance of acidosis after traumatic shock. *J Trauma* 44:114, 1998.

Landry DW, Levin HR, Gallant EM, et al: Vasopressin deficiency contributes to the vasodilation of septic shock. *Circulation* 95:1122, 1997.

Le Tulzo Y, Seguin P, Gacouin A, et al: Effects of epinephrine on right ventricular function in patients with severe septic shock and right ventricular failure: a preliminary descriptive study. *Intensive Care Med* 23:664, 1997.

Miller RR, Meredith JW, Chang MC: Randomized, prospective comparison of increased preload versus inotropes in the resuscitation of trauma patients: effects on cardiopulmonary function and visceral perfusion. *J Trauma* 44:107, 1998.

Porter JN, Ivatury RR: In search of the optimal end points for resuscitation in trauma patients: a review. *J Trauma* 44:908, 1998.

52 | Respiratory Insufficiency

Postinjury respiratory insufficiency can result from a variety of insults, including direct chest trauma, abdominal trauma complicated by abdominal compartment syndrome, and sepsis. These diverse topics are discussed in the textbook. This chapter will focus on postinjury acute respiratory distress syndrome (ARDS).

EPIDEMIOLOGY AND RISK FACTORS

The epidemiologic study of ARDS has been hampered by the lack of a uniform definition as well as the heterogeneity of causes. The recognition of ARDS as a distinct clinical entity resulted from the description by Ashbaugh and Petty in 1967. Until then, ARDS was variously referred to by other names, such as shock lung, Da Nang lung, and traumatic wet lung. Subsequent descriptions have outlined five principal criteria: hypoxemia refractory to oxygen administration; diffuse, bilateral infiltrates on chest radiograph; low static lung compliance; absence of congestive heart failure; and presence of an appropriate at-risk diagnosis. Despite overall agreement regarding these general criteria for the diagnosis of ARDS, considerable variability remains in their specific application. In 1994, a consensus conference of American and European investigators agreed that ARDS should be viewed as the most severe end of the spectrum of acute lung injury. They also recommended diagnostic criteria for acute lung injury and ARDS (Table 52-1).

The 1972 report of the National Heart and Lung Institute Task Force of Respiratory Diseases reported that there were approximately 150,000 cases of ARDS per year (60 to 71 cases per 100,000 person-years). Several subsequent reports suggested that the actual incidence of ARDS was much lower, ranging from 1.5 to 3 cases per 100,000 person-years. Based on a more recent Scandinavian study and screening results from the National Institutes of Health ARDS Network using the 1994 American-European Consensus Conference on ARDS definition of ARDS, the original estimate of 70 cases per 100,000 person-years may be most accurate.

Multiple clinical risk factors have been identified and can be broadly categorized into direct and indirect groups (Table 52-2). Direct factors are those primarily associated with local pulmonary parenchymal injury and include pulmonary contusion, aspiration, and pulmonary infection. Indirect factors are those thought to be associated with systemic inflammation and resultant lung injury. These include sepsis syndrome, multiple transfusions, and multiple long bone fractures. Although hypovolemic shock occurs frequently in trauma patients, it has not been demonstrated to be an independent risk factor for ARDS. Unless shock is associated with significant tissue injury or other known risk factors, it has not been shown to result in ARDS. Studies have consistently found an increased incidence of ARDS when more than one risk factor is present.

PATHOLOGY AND PATHOGENESIS

The pathologic features of ARDS are related to injury to the alveolocapillary interface, which has been termed diffuse alveolar damage. The histologic appearance of this damage can be divided into three overlapping phases: (1) the exudative phase with edema and hemorrhage; (2) the proliferative phase with organization and repair; and (3) the fibrotic phase with end-stage fibrosis.

TABLE 52-1 American-European Consensus Conference Definitions of Acute Lung Injury and Acute Respiratory Distress Syndrome (ARDS)

Acute Lung Injury Criteria
  Timing: Acute onset
  Oxygenation: $Pao_2/Fio_2 \leq 300$ mm Hg (regardless of positive end-expiratory pressure)
  Chest radiograph: Bilateral infiltrates on anteroposterior chest radiograph
  Pulmonary artery occlusion pressure: ≤ 18 mm Hg or no clinical evidence of left atrial hypertension

ARDS Criteria
  Same as acute lung injury except:
  Oxygenation: $Pao_2/Fio_2 \leq 200$ mm Hg (regardless of positive end-expiratory pressure)

Obtaining a better understanding of the mechanisms responsible for acute lung injury continues to be an important challenge. This complex process involves disturbances of inflammation, clotting, vascular control, and other physiological systems. Better understanding of these cellular and molecular events allows for the development of novel therapeutic approaches. Mechanisms of lung injury include both cellular and humoral components. Neutrophils, macrophages, and endothelial cells participate in the inflammatory response in the lungs, resulting in release or activation of multiple mediators of ARDS. Pathophysiologic features of ARDS are summarized in Table 52-3.

PATHOPHYSIOLOGY

Increased capillary permeability and pulmonary edema are hallmarks of ARDS. The balance between pulmonary capillary fluid flux and lung lymph flow governs pulmonary edema formation and is characterized by the Starling equation. While ARDS is the most common cause of pulmonary edema from increased permeability, a hydrostatic component may also be present in these patients. This may result from aggressive volume resuscitation in patients with shock in combination with pulmonary venous hypertension related to release of inflammatory mediators.

ARDS frequently presents as hypoxemia that is refractory to increasing supplemental oxygen administration. Hypoxemia results from ventilation-perfusion mismatching and right-to-left intrapulmonary shunting of blood flow.

TABLE 52-2 Clinical Risk Factors for ARDS

Risk Factor	Frequency of ARDS (%)
Direct	
Aspiration	12–36
Pneumonia	12–31
Pulmonary contusion	5–22
Toxic inhalation	2–17
Indirect	
Sepsis syndrome	11–80
Multiple transfusions	5–36
Multiple fractures	2–21
Pancreatitis	7–18
DIC	23

DIC, disseminated intravascular coagulation.

TABLE 52-3 Pathophysiologic Changes of Modern Acute Respiratory Distress Syndrome (Low-Pressure Pulmonary Edema)

Radiographic change	Clinical finding	Physiologic change	Pathologic change
Phase 1 (Onset of parenchymal changes)*			
Patchy alveolar infiltrates beginning in dependent lung	Dyspnea, tachypnea, cyanosis, tachycardia, coarse rales	Pulmonary hypertension, normal wedge pressure, increased lung permeability, increased lung water, increasing shunt, progressive decrease in compliance, moderate-to-severe hypoxemia	Neutrophil infiltration, vascular congestion, fibrin stands, platelet clumps, alveolar septal edema, intra-alveolar protein, white cells, type 1 epithelial damage
No perivascular cuffs (unless a component of high-pressure edema is present) Normal heart size			
Phase 2 (Acute respiratory failure with progression, 2–10 days)			
Diffuse alveolar infiltrates	Tachypnea, tachycardia, hyperdynamic state, sepsis, syndrome, signs of consolidation, diffuse rhonchi	Phase 1 changes persist, progression of symptoms, increasing shunt fraction, further decrease in compliance, increased minute ventilation, impaired oxygen extraction of hemoglobin	Increased interstitial and alveolar inflammatory exudate with neutrophil and mononuclear cells, type II cell proliferation, beginning fibroblast proliferation, thromboembolic occlusion
Air bronchograms Decreased lung volume No bronchovascular cuffs Normal heart			

TABLE 52-3 *continued*

Phase 3 (Pulmonary fibrosis–pneumonia with progression, >10 days)†

Persistent diffuse infiltrates	Symptoms as above, recurrent sepsis, evidence of multiple-system organ failure	Phase 2 changes persist, recurrent pneumonia, progressive lung restriction, impaired tissue oxygenation, impaired oxygen extraction, multiple-system organ failure	Type II cell hyperplasia, interstitial thickening, infiltration of lymphocytes, macrophages, fibroblasts, loculated pneumonia and/or interstitial fibrosis, medial thickening and remodeling of arterioles
Superimposed new pneumonic infiltrates		
Recurrent pneumothorax		
Normal heart size		
Enlargement with cor pulmonale		

*Process readily reversible at this stage, if initiating factor controlled.
†Multiple-system organ failure common; mortality rate >80% at this stage, as resolution is more difficult.
Reproduced, with permission, from Demling RH: Adult respiratory distress syndrome: Current concepts. *New Horiz* 1:388, 1993.

Shunting results from perfusion of nonventilated alveoli, and the total amount of pulmonary blood flow that perfuses nonventilated areas is termed the *shunt fraction*. Normally, the shunt fraction is less than 5 percent, but in ARDS it may exceed 25 percent. Because blood flowing through a shunt is not exposed to alveoli participating in gas exchange, supplemental oxygen is ineffective in increasing arterial oxygen concentration. Other techniques designed to restore ventilation to nonventilated lung regions, such as positive end-expiratory pressure (PEEP) or continuous positive airway pressure (CPAP), are thus necessary to improve oxygenation. In ARDS, shunting is the result of continued perfusion of atelectatic or fluid-filled alveoli. Hypoxic pulmonary vasoconstriction is a protective mechanism that limits perfusion to poorly ventilated alveoli and minimizes shunting. In ARDS, hypoxic pulmonary constriction is impaired, resulting in greater intra-pulmonary shunting. Multiple factors may contribute to loss of hypoxic pulmonary vasoconstriction in acute lung injury, including local prostaglandin or nitric oxide production.

In early ARDS, most patients are tachypneic from hypoxemia and are secondarily hypocapneic. With disease progression, hypercapnia may become a prominent feature because of physiologic deadspace and CO_2 production. Increased deadspace ventilation is invariably present. Deadspace is defined as pulmonary parenchyma that is ventilated but not perfused. The normal deadspace:tidal volume ratio is 30 percent, but in ARDS it can approach 90 percent. Moreover, high minute ventilation requirements may be related to persistent hypermetabolism and ongoing systemic inflammation with increased CO_2 production.

Lung compliance is defined as the change in lung volume per change in transpulmonary pressure. Normal lung compliance in a mechanically ventilated patient ranges from 60 to 80 mL/cm H_2O. With ARDS, it is not unusual to see greatly diminished lung compliance on the order of 10 to 30 mL/cm H_2O. Initially, reduced compliance is the result of interstitial and alveolar edema with alveolar flooding. Surfactant dysfunction and terminal bronchiolar spasm contribute to loss of ventilated alveoli. In later ARDS, interstitial fibrosis and parenchymal loss further reduce pulmonary compliance.

ARDS is characterized by diffuse pulmonary infiltrates on plain chest radiograph, which were previously thought to be homogeneously distributed throughout the lung. Computed tomography of the chest, however, subsequently demonstrated the parenchymal changes to be inhomogeneous with the dependent lung regions most affected.

An alternative method to describe the mechanical properties of the lung is to determine the static pressure-volume curve during inflation and deflation (Fig. 52-1). In early ARDS, the lower inflection point represents the airway pressure at which considerable alveolar recruitment occurs. The upper inflection point is where near-maximal inflation occurs such that further increases in airway pressure result in alveolar overdistension and little change in volume. The "open lung approach" to mechanical ventilation in ARDS advocates setting PEEP at or just above the lower inflection point to avoid repetitive alveolar recruitment and collapse with each breath. In the later stages of ARDS, the inflection points frequently disappear due to fibrosis.

PRESENTATION

The diagnosis of ARDS is based on the criteria used to define the syndrome. Clinical findings are summarized in Table 52-3. Initially, dyspnea and

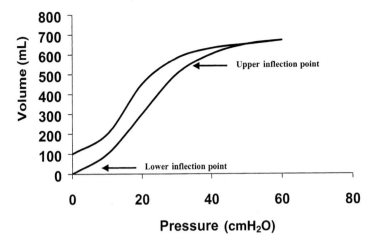

FIG. 52-1.   Idealized static pressure-volume curve demonstrating upper and lower inflection points. The lower inflection point denotes the pressure where alveolar recruitment occurs. The upper inflection point is the pressure where alveolar overdistension occurs.

tachypnea are evident with a remarkably normal chest examination (radiographically and clinically). Arterial oxygen saturation is preserved and hypocapnia from hyperventilation is frequently noted. Physiologic and pathologic evidence of lung injury quickly follows (12 to 24 hours later). The chest x-ray shows bilateral patchy alveolar infiltrates with hypoxemia evident on arterial blood gas determination. Heart size is normal with a lack of perivascular cuffing unless the patient has concomitant cardiac disease or received vigorous volume resuscitation. If ARDS persists and progresses, acute respiratory failure necessitates mechanical ventilation with increasing inspired oxygen concentrations. There is an increase in physiologic deadspace and rising minute ventilation. Patients at this point may develop sepsis syndrome with a hyperdynamic hemodynamic pattern. The radiographic picture worsens with more diffuse infiltrates, consolidation, and air bronchograms. Without resolution, progressive pulmonary failure and fibrosis result. Pneumonia, often recurrent, is frequent. Hypercapnia may worsen and become more difficult to control. Multiple organ failure commonly develops and is the most common cause of death.

MANAGEMENT

Because there is no proven specific treatment for ARDS, therapy primarily involves supportive measures to maintain life while the lung injury resolves. Such measures include identifying and treating predisposing conditions, mechanical ventilatory support with oxygen, nutritional support, nonpulmonary organ support, and hemodynamic monitoring as necessary. Attention to detail is necessary to avoid nosocomial infection and iatrogenic complications.

Fluid Management and Hemodynamic Support

The appropriate use of fluids in managing patients with ARDS has been controversial for more than two decades. Some investigators believe that hydrostatic intravascular forces contribute significantly to pulmonary edema in ARDS, and favor early diuresis and fluid restriction to minimize interstitial and alveolar edema. With this approach, pulmonary capillary wedge pressure is maintained at 5 to 8 mm Hg. If necessary, cardiac output and blood pressure are supported with vasopressors. Several nonrandomized studies suggest that this approach may improve outcome. A careful randomized, controlled clinical trial of this approach is warranted.

There is no clear evidence that the use of colloids for resuscitation in ARDS improves outcome. It has been well documented that patients with acute lung injury leak albumin and other high-molecular-weight proteins into the alveolar space. Thus, colloids administered early in ARDS are likely to leak into the pulmonary interstitium and are unlikely to be beneficial in reducing tissue edema. Theoretically, this increase in interstitial tissue albumin could delay the resolution of pulmonary edema. The use of colloids later in ARDS (when the capillary permeability has been restored) has not been well studied. The use of pulmonary artery catheters in patients with ARDS remains controversial. These catheters are expensive, have significant potential morbidity, and have not been reliably proven to improve outcome. Central hemodynamic monitoring may be helpful, however, in the diagnosis and fluid management of ARDS. Multiple studies have documented the inability to reliably predict the volume status of patients with pulmonary edema. Moreover, the pulmonary artery catheter allows the assessment of therapeutic intervention (such as PEEP) on oxygen delivery and the rational use of vasopressors.

Mechanical Ventilation

Respiratory support is a cornerstone of the supportive management of patients with or at risk for ARDS. It has become increasingly clear, however, that mechanical ventilation can perpetuate or worsen lung injury, as well as result in more readily recognized forms of barotrauma (mediastinal emphysema, pneumothorax, etc). Traditional ventilation strategies used in the ICU have evolved directly from anesthetic and surgical applications. Relatively large tidal volumes (10 to 15 mL/kg) were used to achieve normal gas exchange while avoiding microatelectasis and patient discomfort. With little modification and the addition of PEEP, this approach was applied as the standard for most critically ill patients. In the setting of ARDS, the conventional goals of mechanical ventilation have been to achieve adequate oxygenation using the least PEEP possible and a nontoxic FIO_2. This strategy was intended to minimize or avoid hyperoxic lung injury and the adverse effects of PEEP. A growing number of intensivists are shifting their primary priority from optimizing tissue oxygen delivery to ensuring adequate lung protection (Table 52-4).

In patients with ARDS, the aerated lung volume able to participate in gas exchange is markedly reduced to one-third of the original volume. Thus, in nonfibrotic stages of ARDS, the lungs may be thought of as small rather than stiff. The use of conventional tidal volumes in this setting may result in alveolar overdistension with further impairment of gas exchange, frequent barotrauma, and ventilator-induced lung injury. One approach is to reduce tidal volume in order to limit peak and plateau airway pressures while maintaining adequate alveolar ventilation. The safe upper limit of airway pressure is not

TABLE 52-4 Ventilatory Strategies in ARDS

	Conventional	Lung Protective
Goals	Normal ABGs Nontoxic F_{IO_2} (≤.50) Adequate O_2 delivery	Acceptable ABGs Prevent alveolar damage Facilitate healing Nontoxic F_{IO_2} (≤.50)
Ventilator mode	Volume-cycled	Pressure-limited
Settings		
Tidal volume	10–15 mL/kg	5–7 mL/kg
PEEP	5–20 cm H_2O as needed	Sufficient to prevent tidal recruitment/derecruitment, and achieve acceptable PaO_2/F_{IO_2} ratio
I:E ratio	1:2–1:4	1:4–4:1
Plateau airway pressure	As required by PEEP and tidal volume	<35 cm H_2O

I:E ratio, inspiratory: expiratory ratio; PEEP, positive end-expiratory pressure.

known. Maintaining a transalveolar pressure gradient lower than 35 to 40 cm H_2O has been suggested for two reasons. First, pressures in excess of this have been shown to cause lung injury in animal models. Additionally, the normal lung is at total capacity with a transalveolar pressure gradient of 35 to 40 cm H_2O. The plateau airway pressure is a rough approximation of the peak alveolar pressure and represents a convenient target for lung-protective ventilatory strategies. A recent prospective, randomized trial by the NIH ARDS Network has validated this approach and demonstrated a 22 percent reduction in mortality in ARDS patients ventilated with lower tidal volumes (6 mL/kg compared to 12 mL/kg of body weight).

PEEP is one of several methods of increasing mean airway pressure and improving oxygenation and has become a key element of all ventilator management strategies for ARDS. PEEP improves oxygenation by enhancing lung volume, increasing functional residual capacity (FRC), and recruiting collapsed alveoli. Moreover, extravascular lung water is redistributed from the alveolar to the interstitial space. The net effect is an increase in total alveolar surface available for gas exchange and a decrease in the shunt fraction. Lung compliance may also be improved. It should be emphasized that PEEP is solely a supportive measure with no direct therapeutic effects. Prophylactic PEEP has not been shown to prevent the development of ARDS in at-risk patients or to alter the outcome in established ARDS. The use of PEEP in patients with ARDS has two primary goals: adequate tissue oxygen delivery and the reduction of F_{IO_2} to nontoxic levels. However, increasing PEEP above a certain level may have significant adverse effects, including impaired venous return, falsely elevated PCWP, decreased cardiac output, alveolar overdistension, increased intracranial pressure and deadspace, decreased oxygenation, and barotrauma.

With recent ventilatory strategies emphasizing pressure-limiting techniques, using the lowest level of effective PEEP seems logical. This approach has been associated with less barotrauma and cardiac compromise. The use of minimal PEEP, however, does not address the potential damage from repeated alveolar opening and collapse with each breath. This forms the basis for the "open lung" ventilation strategy, in which static pressure-volume curves are used to select a PEEP level above the lower infection point to prevent alveolar end-expiratory collapse. Confirmatory clinical trials of the open lung approach are in progress.

With improvement in the patient's lung injury, PEEP should be withdrawn as quickly as can safely be accomplished to avoid the complications of PEEP. However, premature attempts at PEEP reduction will only delay resolution of lung injury and prolong the need for ventilatory support. PEEP weaning should be performed in an orderly fashion; PEEP is reduced slowly in 2.5- to 5-cm H_2O increments with serial monitoring of arterial oxygen saturation using ABGs or oximetry. A significant decrease in Pao_2 should prompt a quick return to previous levels of PEEP. Once alveolar collapse and loss of FRC occur, higher levels of PEEP for more prolonged periods may be needed. Generally, PEEP should not be reduced by more than 3 to 5 cm H_2O in a 12-hour period.

Traditional ventilation of ARDS patients has stressed the avoidance of hypercapnia and respiratory acidosis. This goal can be difficult to meet with the increased physiologic deadspace and hypermetabolism frequently associated with ARDS. Moreover, pressure-limited ventilatory strategies may lead to decreased minute ventilation and hypercapnia. Controlled hypoventilation with increased $Paco_2$ is referred to as *permissive hypercapnia*. Gradual increases in $Paco_2$ are usually well tolerated, provided renal compensation is adequate and severe acidosis (pH <7.1) does not occur. Several reports document that permissive hypercapnia in the setting of ARDS is remarkably well tolerated. Ideally, this strategy should be implemented slowly over several hours to allow compensatory mechanisms to act. The role of sodium bicarbonate infusion is unclear. In most institutions, sodium bicarbonate would not be administered unless the pH was lower than 7.2. With increased experience, however, many centers reserve bicarbonate infusion for pH less than 7.0. Sedation is mandatory with permissive hypercapnia in mechanically ventilated patients in order to control respiratory drive and prevent discomfort. Even with heavy sedation, however, respiratory drive may be insufficiently suppressed, resulting in patient-ventilator dyssynchrony. Neuromuscular blockade may be necessary in these patients. Contraindications to permissive hypercapnia include increased intracranial pressure or other cerebral disorders in which intracranial hypertension may be detrimental. Uncorrected hypovolemia and significant cardiac disease are relative contraindications due to the negative inotropic effects of permissive hypercapnia.

Clinical experience with other nonconventional modes of ventilatory support (such as prone ventilation, high-frequency ventilation, partial liquid ventilation, extracorporeal life support, or tracheal gas insufflation) is too limited and their use cannot be routinely recommended.

PHARMACOLOGIC THERAPY

No specific medications have been shown to be efficacious in the treatment of ARDS. The ability of corticosteroids to attenuate the inflammatory response would seem to make them ideal treatment for ARDS, but large prospective clinical trials showed no survival benefit with high-dose steroids in early ARDS. Several anecdotal reports, however, support the use of steroids in late ARDS. The ARDS Network is currently enrolling patients in a multicenter, prospective, randomized, double-blind, clinical trial of steroids in late ARDS.

With the success of surfactant replacement in neonatal respiratory distress syndrome, exogenous surfactant replacement has been suggested for treatment of ARDS. Clinical trials to date have been disappointing but interest in this therapy remains strong.

Studies of other drugs such as ibuprofen, inhaled nitric oxide, prostacyclin, prostaglandin E_1, and lisophylline have been uniformly disappointing. Further investigation and clinical trials are underway.

OUTCOME

Mortality associated with ARDS has historically ranged from 40 to 60 percent. The majority of deaths are related to sepsis and multiple organ failure. Respiratory failure is a cause of death in only 15 percent of patients. Over the past 4 to 5 years, several reports have suggested that mortality in ARDS has improved. Varying definitions and heterogenous patient populations make assessment of outcome changes difficult. In an attempt to address some of these problems, Milberg and colleagues analyzed temporal trends in ARDS fatality rates from 1983 to 1993 at the same institution. They used the same ARDS definition over the entire 10-year period. Overall mortality rates declined starting in 1987 and reached a low of 36 percent in 1993. The decline in mortality was strongest in sepsis-related ARDS.

ADDITIONAL READING

Ware LB, Matthay MA: The acute respiratory distress syndrome. *N Engl J Med* 342:1334, 2000.

The Acute Respiratory Distress Syndrome Network: Ventilation with lower tidal volumes as compared with traditional tidal volumes for acute lung injury and the acute respiratory distress syndrome. *N Engl J Med* 342:1301, 2000.

Bernard GR, Artigas A, Brigham KL, et al: The American-European Consensus Conference on ARDS. Definitions, mechanisms, relevant outcomes, and clinical trial coordination. *Am J Respir Crit Care Med* 149:818, 1994.

Amato MB, Barbas CS, Medeiros DM, et al: Effect of a protective-ventilation strategy on mortality in the acute respiratory distress syndrome. *N Engl J Med* 338:347, 1998.

Meduri GU, Headley AS, Golden E, et al: Effect of prolonged methylprednisolone therapy in unresolving acute respiratory distress syndrome: a randomized controlled trial [see comments]. *JAMA* 280:159, 1998.

Milberg JA, Davis DR, Steinberg KP, et al: Improved survival of patients with acute respiratory distress syndrome (ARDS): 1983–1993. *JAMA* 273:306, 1995.

53 | Acute Renal Failure

Acute deterioration of renal function often complicates care of trauma patients, increasing morbidity and mortality through effects on nearly all other organ systems. The most common etiologies of renal dysfunction are renal hypoperfusion and toxin-mediated (radiocontrast, antimicrobials) renal parenchymal injury. This intrinsic renal failure—most often manifesting as acute tubular necrosis—has a gradual onset, requires time to resolve, and has major therapeutic and prognostic implications.

DEFINITIONS

Acute renal failure (ARF) is abrupt (hours or days) deterioration of renal function with a decrease in glomerular filtration rate (GFR), or renal tubular injury compromising the kidneys' ability to maintain fluid or electrolyte homeostasis. Most commonly, investigators define ARF as an increase in serum creatinine (P_{Cr}) of 0.5 mg/dL or greater from baseline, and a 50 percent reduction in calculated creatinine clearance (C_{Cr}). Acute azotemia is any increase in serum blood urea nitrogen (BUN) or creatinine of greater than 50 percent over baseline in 24 hours.

Acute renal failure may or may not include a decrease in urine output. Acute oliguria is typically defined as urine output (UOP) less than 400 mL in any 24-hour period. Nonoliguric and high-output renal failure refer to accumulation of nitrogenous waste products or failure to maintain water or electrolyte homeostasis in the face of a 24-hour UOP of 400 to 1000 mL and greater than 1000 mL, respectively. Anuria is any urine volume lower than 50 mL/d.

RISK FACTORS

Primary risk factors for development of ARF include renal hypoperfusion, exposure to nephrotoxins, and preexisting renal insufficiency.

NORMAL RENAL PHYSIOLOGY

The major aspects of renal function are renal blood flow, glomerular filtration, and tubular excretion and reabsorption. Normally, renal blood flow (RBF) is 20 to 25 percent of cardiac output and is directed primarily to the renal cortex to optimize glomerular filtration with proportionate perfusion of the renal medulla. Both total RBF and distribution of blood flow within the kidney are maintained relatively constant over a wide range of arterial blood pressure (autoregulation), and are governed by neural, hormonal, and local paracrine influences. Mechanisms regulating RBF and GFR include tubuloglomerular feedback (TGF), the renin-angiotensin system, vascular myogenic responses, sympathetic innervation, and circulating catecholamines.

The primary role of the renal tubules is concentration of the urine via reabsorption of sodium and water. In addition, glucose, potassium, chloride, and phosphate are actively reabsorbed in the tubules. Urea undergoes passive reabsorption in the tubules, depending on tubular flow rates. Creatinine, on the other hand, depends chiefly on GFR for elimination, allowing its use to estimate GFR. Hydrogen and ammonium ions are secreted in the proximal and distal tubules, depending on serum and urine pH.

Within the medulla, tubules and vasa recta are arranged in parallel bundles allowing maximum concentrating ability by a countercurrent exchange system.

The medullary thick ascending limb (MTAL) is responsible for the generation of an osmotic gradient by active reabsorption of sodium, a process that generates a large oxygen demand. If oxygen demand is increased from basal conditions, the cells of the medulla, particularly the cells of thick ascending limbs, are at risk for severe hypoxia. This combination of low regional oxygen delivery and high cellular oxygen consumption creates a tenuous oxygen supply-demand relationship, placing renal tubules at risk for ischemic injury and contributing to the pathophysiology of acute renal failure.

PATHOPHYSIOLOGY OF ACUTE AZOTEMIA AND ACUTE TUBULAR NECROSIS

Etiologies of acute azotemia are typically categorized according to anatomic location (prerenal, postrenal, or intrinsic) (Table 53-1). Prerenal azotemia is the most common cause of declining urine output and accumulation of nitrogen wastes. GFR declines when effective circulating volume, mean arterial pressure, and renal blood flow decrease below levels at which renal autoregulation can maintain flow to the glomerulus. In response to hypovolemia, aldosterone and antidiuretic hormone (ADH) are secreted to conserve sodium and water, respectively. As a result, the kidney produces a small volume of concentrated urine with low sodium content. Due to low urine flow rates, BUN is reabsorbed in the tubules, resulting in azotemia. Prompt recognition and rapid treatment usually rapidly reverses prerenal azotemia. While renal tubular cell integrity is maintained in reversible prerenal azotemia, severe and prolonged azotemia can result in tubular cell dysfunction or cell death resulting in acute tubular necrosis.

In the critically ill inpatient, the most common source of postrenal azotemia is blockage of a neglected Foley catheter. Intrinsic renal azotemia in trauma patient is most commonly due to renal tubular damage, particularly to the cells of the ascending limb of the loop of Henle located in the outer renal medulla. These cells are particularly vulnerable to hypoxia and nephrotoxins, and damage to these cells is central to the pathophysiology of acute tubular necrosis (ATN).

Aminoglycosides are the single most common cause in drug toxicity-induced ATN. An estimated 10 to 25 percent of patients treated with aminoglycosides develop some degree of renal insufficiency. Aminoglycosides such as gentamicin are directly toxic to renal proximal tubular cells.

Risk factors for development of aminoglycoside nephrotoxicity include prolonged exposure to aminoglycosides (high serum trough levels), volume depletion, sepsis, and advanced patient age. Synergistic toxicity may also occur with other drugs, such as amphotericin B, nonsteroidal anti-inflammatory drugs, cyclosporine, radiographic contrast, and antimicrobials such as the cephalosporins and vancomycin. Because nephrotoxicity is more closely related to trough concentrations, and antimicrobial efficacy varies with peak concentrations of the drugs, once-a-day dosing of aminoglycosides may be less nephrotoxic with equal efficacy in patients with normal renal function.

Polyene antimicrobials such as amphotericin are particularly nephrotoxic. Amphotericin B damages tubular cell and lysosomal membranes, and causes profound renal vasoconstriction. Amphotericin toxicity depends on total dose: Less than 600 mg rarely produces significant alterations in renal function, whereas cumulative doses exceeding 3 g cause significant renal toxicity in over 80 percent of patients. Maintaining adequate hydration with intravenous

TABLE 53-1 Common Etiologies of Acute Oliguria

Prerenal	Hypovolemia
	Hemorrhage
	Gastrointestinal fluid loss (nasogastric suction, high-output fistula, diarrhea, etc)
	Renal loss (excessive diuretic use, diabetes insipidus, diabetes mellitus)
	Surgery
	Burns
	Decreased effective vascular volume
	Sepsis
	Hepatic failure
	Anaphylactic shock
	Neurogenic shock
	Vasodilators
	Impaired cardiac function
	Myocardial infarction
	Pulmonary embolus
	Cardiac tamponade
	Congestive heart failure
	Mechanical ventilation
Dysfunction due to renal parenchymal injury	Glomerulonephritis
	Poststreptococcal glomerulonephritis
	Systemic lupus erythematosus and other connective tissue disorders
	Scleroderma
	Malignant hypertension
	Eclampsia/preeclampsia
	Others
	Vasculitis
	Interstitial nephritis
	Drugs (e.g., methicillin)
	Infection
	Neoplasm (e.g., lymphoma, leukemia, or sarcoidosis)
	Acute tubular necrosis
	Ischemia (prerenal events)
	Antibiotics (amphotericin, aminoglycoside)
	Radiocontrast agents
	Pigment load (e.g., myoglobin as in rhabdomyolysis)
	Heavy metals (mercury)
	Solvents (carbon tetrachloride, ethylene glycol)
Postrenal/ obstructive	Ureteral obstruction
	Stone
	Infection (pyelonephritis)
	Traumatic disruption
	Urethral obstruction
	Obstruction of Foley catheter
	Mucus
	Blood clots

saline over the course of treatment is the most effective means of reducing this dose-dependent toxicity. Lipid-encapsulated preparations of amphotericin have reduced toxicity, but at a markedly increased cost. Lists of dialyzable and nondialyzable drugs are found in Table 53-2.

Radiocontrast-induced acute renal failure is common in hospitalized patients. Risk factors contributing to radiocontrast-induced ARF include pre-

TABLE 53-2 Dialyzable and Nondialyzable Drugs

Negligible clearance by IHD		
Antibiotics	Cardiovascular agents	Miscellaneous
Amphotericin B	Amiodarone	Benzodiazepines
Azidothymidine	Digoxin	Cimetidine
Cefotetan	Diltiazem	Cyclosporine A
Ciprofloxacin	Disopyramide	Famotidine
Clindamycin	Esmolol	Morphine
Cloxacillin	Labetalol	Omeprazole
Doxycycline	Metoprolol	Phenytoin
Erythromycin	Propafenone	Prednisone
Itraconazole		Propoxyphene
Ketoconazole		
Nafcillin		
Vancomycin		

Significant clearance by IHD	
Antibiotics	Miscellaneous
Acyclovir	Allopurinol
Aminoglycoside	Atenolol
Ampicillin	Captopril
Aztreonam	Cyclophosphamide
Trimethoprim–sulfamethoxazole	N-acetylprocainamide
Flucytosine	Ranitidine
Ganciclovir	Sotalol
Imipenem	
Isoniazid	
Metronidazole	
Most cephalosporins	
Piperacillin	

IHD, intermittent hemodialysis.

existing renal insufficiency, diabetes mellitus, and depletion of extracellular volume. Radiocontrast agents produce local (medullary) ischemia related to endothelin release and depressed nitric oxide–mediated vasodilatation.

Contrast-induced renal failure can be ameliorated by pre- and postimaging saline and volume loading or avoiding contrast studies altogether. Loop diuretics and mannitol have been proposed but not proven as useful prophylaxis. Indeed, mannitol appears to increase the risk for contrast nephropathy in diabetic patients with preexisting renal disease. Fortunately, the clinical course of contrast nephropathy is usually self-limited. Oliguria is rare, and serum creatinine usually peaks within 72 hours after administration. The majority of patients return to baseline renal function by 7 to 10 days. However, up to 30 percent of patients, especially those with the known risks described above, sustain permanent functional loss. In any case, adequate saline fluid loading before infusion of radiocontrast remains the mainstay of prophylaxis against damage from these agents.

Common etiologies of oliguria are outlined in Table 53-1. Laboratory criteria for azotemia and oliguria are set forth in Table 53-3.

Many injuries can set the stage for pigment-induced renal injuries. Rhabdomyolysis is the release of free myoglobin from skeletal muscle after muscle necrosis. Besides major crush injuries and prolonged limb ischemia, seizures, drugs (heroin, cocaine, amphetamines), toxins (isopropyl alcohol,

TABLE 53-3 Laboratory Indices of Intrinsic Renal Dysfunction and Prerenal
Azotemia/Oliguria*

	Prerenal azotemia	Renal dysfunction
Plasma Cr:BUN	>20	<10
Urine osmolality	>500 mOsm/L or >100 over plasma	<350 mOsm/L or < plasma
Urine specific gravity	>1.020	>1.010
Urine sodium	<20 mEq/L	>30 mEq/L
Fractional excretion of sodium	<1%	>2%
U_{Cr}/P_{Cr}	>40	<20

*Laboratory values unreliably distinguish between intrarenal and obstructive
pathology.

BUN, blood urea nitrogen; P_{Cr}, serum creatinine; U_{Cr}, urinary creatinine.

ethylene glycol), streptococcal infections, and myositis can cause rhabdomyolysis.

Once filtered, pigment accumulates in proximal tubule cells by endocytosis. If urine pH is below 7.0, myoglobin is converted to ferrihemate, which is directly toxic to renal cells. Diagnosis is secured by the finding of heme pigment in the urine in the absence of red blood cells, and an elevated serum creatinine phosphokinase in patients with clinical findings consistent with rhabdomyolysis or hemoglobinuria. The diagnosis can be suspected with the appearance of dark (cola-colored) urine containing dark brown granular casts.

Treatment is by aggressive volume resuscitation, careful hemodynamic monitoring, and diuresis of at least 100 mL/h. While mannitol is often employed to maintain diuresis, little evidence supports this practice. Because both pigment precipitation and conversion to ferrihemate depend on aciduria, sodium bicarbonate (typically around 3 ampules in each liter of 5 percent dextrose in water [D5W]) is added to intravenous fluids to maintain an alkaline urine pH.

Other causes of intrinsic renal dysfunction include nonsteroidal antiinflammatory drugs, the abdominal compartment syndrome, and sepsis.

Few organ systems escape the effects of ARF. If ARF produces increased free water and sodium load, volume complications can occur, including congestive heart failure, pulmonary edema, and hypertension. Arrhythmias occur in 10 to 30 percent of patients and can be exacerbated during intermittent hemodialysis. Pericarditis may occur in severe uremia. Gastrointestinal complications of uremia include anorexia, nausea, emesis, and ileus. Gastrointestinal bleeding can occur in up to 30 percent of patients with acute renal failure, particularly as BUN levels exceed 80 mg/dL and platelet dysfunction ensues. Neurologic changes occurring in patients with uremia include confusion, asterixis, somnolence, and seizures. Neurologic manifestations are sometimes exacerbated by electrolyte shifts during intermittent hemodialysis. Conversely, such symptoms can be improved following dialysis therapy.

Uremia also produces hematologic abnormalities. Increased hemolysis in uremia leads to anemia compounded by decreased erythropoiesis as renal secretion of erythropoietin falls. While some advocate administration of recombinant erythropoietin, transfusion of packed red blood cells is clearly the better choice for correction of anemia in the trauma patient. Platelet dysfunction produces a risk of clinically significant bleeding as BUN rises above 60 to 80 mg/dL. Because this dysfunction is not corrected by platelet infusion, desmopressin or dialysis may be required to treat significant hemorrhage from the gastrointestinal tract or intracranial bleeds.

DIAGNOSIS AND MANAGEMENT

Prevention

The most important therapeutic modality in the management of ARF is prevention: maintenance of intravascular volume, avoidance of hypotensive episodes, minimization of toxic exposures, aggressive treatment of infection, and early intervention.

A general algorithm for diagnosis and management of acute renal dysfunction is shown in Fig. 53-1. In general, the objectives of ARF management include early identification of renal dysfunction, elimination of obstruction as a source of compromise, identification and treatment of prerenal failure, laboratory confirmation of renal parenchymal damage, optimization of intravascular volume and oxygen delivery, trial of loop diuretics, elimination of nephrotoxins, correction of associated metabolic abnormalities, institution of renal replacement therapies if indicated, provision of adequate nutrition, and adjustment of drug dosages to account for decreased clearance.

Renal Replacement

Despite decades of use, no consensus indications for the initiation or dosing (frequency and duration) of renal replacement therapy have been widely accepted, and aspects of its use are controversial. Early dialysis may avoid uremic complications, simplify fluid management, and facilitate nutrition delivery. On the other hand, hemodialysis is not a benign procedure. Patients routinely experience hypotension requiring increased pressor support, cardiac arrhythmias, hypoxemia, complications, and infections at dialysis catheter sites. Despite these arguments, dialysis has some clear indications.

Renal replacement therapy is indicated for any one of several life-threatening metabolic derangements: fluid overload, severe uremia, critical electrolyte abnormalities, metabolic acidosis that cannot be compensated by hyperventilation, and some toxins. Dialysis for clinical volume overload should be approached with care; in the trauma population, hypovolemia is more common and far more dangerous than fluid overload. As BUN approaches 100 mg/dL, patients exhibit mental status changes and coagulopathy secondary to platelet dysfunction. Some clinicians advocate earlier initiation of dialysis (e.g., when BUN reaches 60 mg/dL) in order to avoid complications of azotemia. The most common electrolyte abnormality treated with dialysis is hyperkalemia. Values greater than 7 mEq/dL are thought to be critical, but any value above normal accompanied by electrocardiographic changes is an emergency. Metabolic acidosis is best addressed by remedying the underlying cause of the acidosis. In general, timing and frequency of hemodialysis are best decided within a daily clinical context rather than simply by strict laboratory criteria.

Three forms of renal replacement therapy are commonly used in hospitals today: peritoneal dialysis, intermittent hemodialysis, and continuous renal replacement. Peritoneal dialysis (PD) is a poor choice to treat ARF in trauma patients. Established efficacy has made intermittent hemodialysis (IHD) the

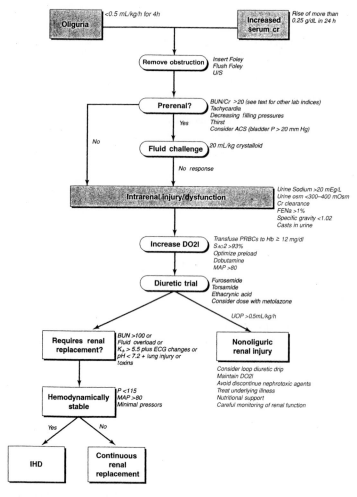

FIG. 53-1. General algorithm for diagnosis and treatment of oliguria and azotemia. ACS, abdominal compartment syndrome; BUN, blood urea nitrogen; DO2I, oxygen delivery; ECG, electrocardiogram; FENa, fractional excretion of sodium; IHD, intermittent hemodialysis; K_+, potassium; MAP, mean arterial pressure; P, pulse; PRBCs, packed red blood cells; UOP, urine output; U/S, ultrasound.

standard therapy for ARF. Besides ready availability in most hospitals, IHD rapidly removes fluid, solutes, and toxins; however, these advantages are tempered by dangers. Due to rapid volume solute shifts, intermittent dialysis in the critically ill patient in the intensive care unit is associated with episodes of hypotension, hypoxemia, hemolysis, and cardiac arrhythmias. Rapid solute shifts have also been associated with worsening of cerebral edema. Moreover, IHD is associated with increased oxygen consumption and decreased oxygen delivery, leading to intestinal mucosal acidosis that persists after the procedure is complete. Finally, hemodialysis activates the systemic inflammatory reaction by priming neutrophils, activating the complement system, causing generation of reactive oxygen species, and increasing release of leukotrienes and proinflammatory cytokines.

Continuous Renal Replacement Techniques

Even with biocompatible membranes, many patients are too unstable to tolerate IHD. To provide renal replacement to these patients, various continuous, low-flow replacement therapies have been devised. These methods differ in the method used as the driving force for blood flow through the device and of the mechanism of solute removal. Arteriovenous (AV) circuits use mean arterial pressure (MAP) as the driving force. Venovenous (VV) circuits use an external pump as the driving force and generally permit better control and higher flow rates. Arteriovenous systems (e.g., continuous arteriovenous hemofiltration [CAVH]) are the simplest and least expensive systems, but require more risky arterial access and depend on a MAP of at least 80 mm Hg for effective flow. VV systems utilizing external pumps add complexity and cost, but are generally more efficient. Both systems require anticoagulation of the external system via citrate or heparin.

Continuous renal replacement techniques (CRRT) use highly permeable, biocompatible, synthetic membranes that allow gradual, continuous removal of fluids and solutes. They are more effective than IHD in clearing nitrogenous wastes and providing nutrition without risk of volume overload. They also have a lower incidence of cardiac arrhythmias and decreased exacerbation of cerebral edema in patients with closed head injuries.

Nutrition

A common mistake in treating patients with renal dysfunction is withholding protein calories for fear of driving serum nitrogen levels upward. Nutritional support should take precedence over withholding renal replacement therapy.

Drug-Kidney Interactions

Because most drugs and their metabolites are at least partly metabolized and excreted by the kidney, pharmacokinetics of most drugs can be drastically altered in ARF. The following mechanisms are important in altering available drug levels during acute renal failure: *decreased filtration, decreased tubular secretion, decreased tubular reabsorption, and altered volume of distribution.* Drug therapy should be designed specifically for each patient in ARF. Dosing tables or the hospital pharmacist should be consulted for a dosing regimen. Many drugs are best avoided altogether in the setting of ARF. Aminoglycosides and amphotericin B may precipitate or aggravate renal dysfunction. Other drugs have active metabolites that accumulate to toxic levels in renal failure. For example, normeperidine, the renally excreted active metabolite of meperidine, can rapidly accumulate in ARF and cause neurotoxicity, including seizures. Morphine is the preferred analgesic in ARF, but it should also be used with caution; decreased protein binding in ARF increases the bioavailability of a given dose of morphine. As with meperidine, metabolites of diazepam can accumulate and cause prolonged sedation in patients with ARF. Other drugs carry large electrolyte loads, potentially exacerbating electrolyte disorders in ARF. Examples include carbenicillin and ticarcillin (sodium loads), potassium penicillin (potassium load), and many antacids (magnesium load). Hemodialysis also affects drug dosing. Postdialysis dosing is recommended for drugs that are cleared during dialysis.

OUTCOMES

Most patients with renal dysfunction can be managed without dialysis if treated early. If allowed to progress, ARF contributes significantly to morbidity and mortality. Older age and a higher number of dysfunctional organ systems have the strongest association with mortality in ARF. Higher mortality is also seen in ARF secondary to ATN than from other etiologies. Finally, patients with oliguric ARF have an eightfold increased risk of requiring dialysis and a correspondingly worse prognosis than nonoliguric patients. Patients who survive initiation of dialysis have less than a 25 percent chance of requiring chronic dialysis, demonstrating the ability of the kidney to recover from severe injury with time. Most survivors regain nearly normal renal function within 30 days.

ADDITIONAL READING

Brown C, Ogg C, Cameron J: High dose furosemide in acute renal failure: A controlled trial. *Clin Nephrol* 15:90, 1981.

Denton M, Chertow G, Brady H: "Renal-dose" dopamine for the treatment of acute renal failure: scientific rationale, experimental studies, and clinical trials. *Kidney Int* 49:4, 1996.

Thadhani R, Pascua M, Bonventre J: Acute renal failure. *N Engl J Med* 334:1448, 1996.

54 | Nutritional Support

Nutritional therapy is an integral part of the management of severely injured patients. Nutritional risk does not result from preexisting defects in protein stores but rather from the hypermetabolic response to injury and subsequent sepsis induced by the inflammatory and hormonal responses.

The modern era of nutrition support can be traced to the successful central venous infusion of hypertonic solutions of dextrose and protein hydrolysates, but recently there has been renewed interest in the enteral route in severely injured trauma patients.

THE ENDOCRINE RESPONSE TO STRESS AND INJURY

There are differences between hypercatabolism of injury, stress, or sepsis, and starvation. In starvation, amino acids provide the substrate for gluconeogenesis, but fatty acids, ketone bodies (KB), and glycerol become the primary substrate within 7 to 10 days as insulin levels drop. The respiratory quotient ([RQ], a ratio of CO_2 production to O_2 consumed) is approximately 0.6 to 0.7 during starvation, indicative of fat utilization.

In hypermetabolism, the RQ ranges from 0.80 to 0.85. Catecholamines induce hepatic glycogenolysis and gluconeogenesis and inhibit insulin release; elevated cortisol stimulates glycogenolysis, muscle proteolysis, and gluconeogenesis and induces a peripheral insulin resistance; and insulin anabolic effects for protein synthesis, lipogenesis, and glycogenesis are inhibited. Muscle provides the primary substrate for glucose.

The Nutrient Prescription: Issues Common to Enteral and Parenteral Feeding

Estimating Nutritional Needs

The most common calculation used to determine basal energy expenditure (BEE) is the Harris-Benedict formula, defined as follows:

For males: BEE = 66 + (13.8 × W) + (5 × H) − (6.8 × A)
For females: 665 + (9.6 × W) + (1.8 × H) − (4.7 × A)

where W is the weight in kilograms, H is the height in centimeters, and A the age in years. These values were increased by stress (ranging from 1.25 to 2) and activity factors, but indirect calorimetry has shown that these factors overestimate nutrient needs, which increase only 10 to 20 percent above the BEE.

Caloric density for nutrients is as follows: 1 g protein provides 4 kcal, 1 g of hydrated glucose in total parenteral nutrition (TPN) provides 3.4 kcal versus 4.0 kcal in enteral formulas, and 1 g of fat (as an enteral form) provides 9.1 kcal, but 1 g of intravenous fat emulsions (IVFE) contains 10 kcal/g because of emulsifiers. Standard TPN solutions are described in Table 54-1. If 30 kcal/kg is provided, 90 percent of patients will reach their energy requirement with overfeeding in only 15 to 20 percent. Our approach is to provide 30 kcal/kg/d after severe trauma and decrease to 25 kcal/kg as hypermetabolism decreases.

Glucose Requirements

Glucose should provide 50 to 60 percent of calories. The maximal rate of glucose oxidation is 5 mg/kg/min or 7.2 g/kg/d. In a 70-kg man, this is approxi-

TABLE 54-1 Examples of TPN Formulas Used in Trauma Patients

Type	Carbohydrate	Protein	Fat
Standard #1	D20W	AA 5%	Lipids 2%
Standard #2	D15W	AA 5%	Lipids 3%
Concentrated	D30W	AA 6%	Lipids 4%
ARF—no dialysis	D30W	AA 2%	Lipids 2%
ARF—dialysis	D30W	AA 4%	Lipids 2%

AA, amino acids; ARF, acute renal failure.

mately 500 g of glucose, which is met by 2 L of a 25 percent dextrose solution. Blood sugars should be maintained below 220 mg percent.

Fat Requirements

Fat should be given at a dose of 1 g/kg/d to provide 20 to 30 percent of calories if triglyceride levels are below 300 mg/dL. The maximum adult dose of IV lipid is 2.5 g/kg/d. Greater amounts may be used in hyperglycemic patients, but hyperlipidemia, cholestasis, increased risk of infection, and perhaps immunosuppression may occur.

Protein Requirements

The recommended dose of amino acids or protein for stressed or septic patients without renal dysfunction is 1.5 to 2 g/kg/d. If blood urea nitrogen (BUN) levels climb above 60 mg/dL, protein should be reduced to 1.3 to 1.5 g/kg/d. As stress resolves, protein is reduced to 1 to 1.5 g protein/kg/d. Burn patients typically receive 2 to 2.5 g/kg/d.

Formula Recommendations

For nonseptic, nonstressed patients provide a calorie:nitrogen (Cal:N) ratio of 130:1 to 160:1 with 1.5 g of protein/kg/d. For stressed or septic patients without renal failure, provide a Cal:N ratio of 80:1 to 120:1 with 1.5 to 2 g of protein/kg/d. For burn patients provide a low Cal:N ratio with 35 to 40 total kcal/kg/d and 2 to 2.5 g of protein/kg/d.

For severely injured patients, immune-enhancing diets (IEDs) with a Cal:N of 50:1 to 60:1 (due to supplemental glutamine [GLN] and/or arginine [ARG] and/or branched-chain amino acids [BCAA]) should provide 2.0 to 2.2 g/kg of protein (0.32 to 0.35 g of N/kg/d). BUN often rises to 50 mg/dL but rarely higher if renal function is normal.

For patients with renal failure, provide about 0.6 to 0.8 g of protein/kg/d predialysis with a Cal:N of 300:1 to 375:1. Specialized, essential amino acid solutions provide little if any additional benefit. A high Cal:N ratio may control K^+, Mg^{++}, and PO_4^{-2}, but they should be removed initially and added as necessary. With dialysis, increase protein to 1 to 1.2 g/kg/d and reduce the Cal:N ratio to ~200.

For pulmonary failure in trauma patients, overfeeding and resultant lipogenesis rarely pose clinically significant problems due to CO_2 production, and high fat pulmonary-specific formulas are not recommended.

With hepatic failure and multiple-organ dysfunction syndrome (MODS), avoid excessive protein restriction. Intravenous solutions are better tolerated (e.g., 1 to 1.5 g/kg/day) than the enteral protein. Although high-BCAA formulas for hepatic failure are available, severe failure with MODS usually does not respond.

Enteral Feeding

There appears to be immunologic benefit when nutrients are delivered enterally. Randomized studies show reduced rates of intra-abdominal abscess and pneumonia with enteral feeding compared to TPN or no feeding. The algorithm for nutrition support posttrauma is shown in Fig. 54-1.

Access During Celiotomy for Trauma

The abdominal trauma index (ATI) (Table 54-2) can be rapidly tabulated at the operating table and enteral access obtained in patients with an ATI of 25 or greater. Certain intra-abdominal injuries (colon, pancreas, liver, or duodenum) are at increased risk of developing septic complications. Patients requiring celiotomy with insignificant intra-abdominal injuries who will benefit from enteral access are also shown in Fig. 54-1. Principles of safe postpyloric access are listed in Table 54-3.

Closed-Head Injury Patients

There is no clear evidence that early administration of enteral or parenteral feeding reduces sepsis or improves outcome after severe head injury. Wait until GI tract function returns and gastroparesis resolves (generally within 3 to 4 days) and start intragastric enteral nutrition. Add a prokinetic agent on days 4 and 5, if necessary, and start TPN if gastroparesis persists.

Burn Patients

Start intragastric feeding within 12 hours to reduce the incidence of gastroparesis. Clinical data suggests a blunting of the hypermetabolic response.

Diet Choice By the Enteral Route

In critically ill patients at high risk of developing sepsis (ATI ≥25, Injury Severity Score [ISS] >20; Fig. 54-1), some clinical data support use of IEDs containing omega-3 fatty acids, nucleotides, BCAA, ARG, and/or GLN. Otherwise, in severely injured patients a Cal:N of approximately 80:1 to 120:1 should be used. As stress resolves, increase the Cal:N to 130:1 to 160:1 and reduce protein to 1 to 1.5 g protein/kg.

Diet progression is determined by the type of formula used. Table 54-4 provides an advancement protocol for chemically defined elemental formula diets. Start more complex diets full strength at 15 mL/h for the first 6 to 8 hours in patients with previous hemodynamic instability only after resuscitation and splanchnic perfusion is adequate. Advancement to 25 mL/h after 6 to 8 hours and at increments of 25 mL/h/day depending on tolerance. *Examine the abdomen daily!*

Patients with an ATI ≥ 40 and bowel injuries have increased bloating, cramps, and general intolerance when advanced quickly and may require slower advancement.

Prokinetic Agents

Impaired gastric emptying may limit intragastric feeding. If persistent beyond 3 to 4 days, a prokinetic agent such as metoclopramide or erythromycin may enhance emptying.

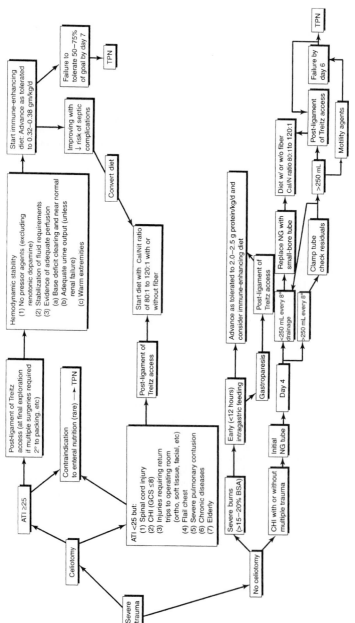

FIG. 54-1. Protocol for nutrition support at the Presley Trauma Center. ATI, Abdominal Trauma Index; BSA, body surface area; CHI, closed head injury; GCS, Glasgow Coma Scale; ISS, Injury Severity Score; NG, nasogastric; TPN, total parenteral nutrition.

TABLE 54-2 Calculated Sepsis Risk Using the Abdominal Trauma Index (ATI)

Organ injured	Risk factor	Scoring	Organ injured	Risk factor scoring	Scoring
High Risk			*Low Risk*		
Pancreas	(5)	1. Tangential 2. Through-and-through (duct intact) 3. Major debridement or distal duct injury 4. Proximal duct injury 5. Pancreaticoduodenectomy	Kidney	(2)	1. Nonbleeding 2. Minor debridement or suturing 3. Major debridement 4. Pedicle or major calyceal 5. Nephrectomy
Large intestine	(5)	1. Serosal 2. Single wall 3. ≤25% Wall 4. >25% Wall 5. Colon wall and blood supply	Ureter	(2)	1. Contusion 2. Laceration 3. Minor debridement 4. Segmental resection 5. Reconstruction
Major vascular	(5)	1. ≤25% Wall 2. >25% Wall 3. Complete transection 4. Interposition grafting or bypass 5. Ligation	Bladder	(1)	1. Single wall 2. Through-and-through 3. Debridement 4. Wedge resection 5. Reconstruction
Moderately High Risk					
Duodenum	(4)	1. Single wall 2. ≤25% Wall 3. >25% Wall 4. Duodenal wall and blood supply 5. Pancreaticoduodenectomy	Extrahepatic Biliary	(1)	1. Contusion 2. Cholecystectomy 3. ≤25% Wall 4. >25% Wall 5. Biliary enteric reconstruction

TABLE 54-2 *continued*

Liver	(4)	1. Nonbleeding peripheral 2. Bleeding, central, or minor debridement 3. Major debridement or hepatic artery ligation 4. Lobectomy 5. Lobectomy with caval repair or extensive bilobar debridement	Bone	(1)	1. Periosteum 2. Cortex 3. Through-and-through 4. Intra-articular 5. Major bone loss
Moderate Risk Stomach	(3)	1. Single wall 2. Through-and-through 3. Minor debridement 4. Wedge resection 5. >35% Resection	Small bowel	(1)	1. Single wall 2. Through-and-through 3. ≤25% Wall 4. >25% Wall 5. Wall and blood supply or >5 injuries
Spleen	(3)	1. Nonbleeding 2. Cautery or hemostatic agent 3. Minor debridement or suturing 4. Partial resection 5. Splenectomy	Minor vascular	(1)	1. Nonbleeding small hematoma 2. Nonbleeding large hematoma 3. Suturing 4. Ligation of isolated vessels 5. Ligation of named vessels

Sources: Adapted from Moore DE, Dunn EL, Moore JB, et al: Penetrating Abdominal Trauma Index. *J Trauma* 21:439, 1981; and Borlase BC, Moore EE, Moore FA: The Abdominal Trauma Index—A critical reassessment and validation. *J Trauma* 30:1340, 1990.

TABLE 54-3 Principles of Safe Enteral Feeding Access

Choose the tube appropriate for expected needs:
- Needle catheter: 3–4 weeks
- Large-bore tube: Chronic needs
- Transgastric jejunostomy: If contraindication to direct small bowel access or for simultaneous gastric drain. Read the instructions provided!

Obtain safe postpyloric access:
- Position jejunostomy to avoid afferent loop tension if distension occurs.
- Create lax Witzel tunnel.
- Suture 6–10 cm of jejunum to the anterior abdominal wall.
- Position at the lateral aspect of the rectus sheath away from the midline.

Complications of Enteral Feeding

Mild abdominal distension is not uncommon but does not necessitate discontinuation of feedings. If patients complain of severe discomfort or cramping, slow the rate if pain is not incisional. Daily abdominal examinations are mandatory.

The incidence of diarrhea is 5 to 25 percent in tube-fed patients, depending on the definition of diarrhea. Antibiotic-induced enterocolitis, magnesium medications, or sorbitol account for 75 percent of cases. Prokinetic drugs may cause diarrhea. If multiple antibiotics were given, *Clostridium difficile* should be suspected and proctosigmoidoscopy should be performed, particularly if patients are guaiac positive. *C. difficile* was found in over 50 percent of patients with diarrhea receiving multiple antibiotics and enteral nutrition.

Change the formula to isotonic formula with fiber if diarrhea occurs and reduce the rate by 50 percent. Stop prokinetic agents and all enteral medications. Perform sigmoidoscopy and test for *C. difficile*. If positive, start appropriate therapy.

Mechanical Complications

Occlusion of feeding tubes is not uncommon. Size 14 or 16 F tubes can be replaced, but clogged 5 and 7 F needle catheter jejunostomies (NCJ) may require removal. Occlusion of an NCJ within 24 to 48 hours is usually caused by a kink at the fascia. Withdraw the NCJ 5 or 6 cm while flushing, cut off the NCJ beyond the kink, and reconnect. Give no medications via an NCJ since elixirs coagulate feedings and occlude the tube.

Parenteral Feeding

The percutaneous subclavian vein approach is the best procedure. Alternative methods include the internal jugular vein and the femoral vein, but these carry

TABLE 54-4 Protocol for Advancement of Chemically-Defined Diet

Strength	Rate	Duration
1/4	50 mL/h	8h
1/4	75 mL/h	8h
1/4	100 mL/h	8h
1/2	100 mL/h	8h
3/4	100 mL/h	8h
Full	100 mL/h	8h
Full	125 mL/h*	

*If required.

an increased risk of catheter sepsis and deep venous thrombosis (with femoral lines). When starting central TPN, decide whether to: (1) use the current central line for TPN (e.g., triple-lumen catheter, Swan-Ganz catheter), (2) change the present catheter to a new catheter with the modified Seldinger technique and a flexible guidewire, or (3) place an entirely new central line. Swan-Ganz (SG) catheters may be used temporarily in hemodynamically unstable patients. Once stable, change the SG to a triple-lumen catheter using the modified Seldinger technique. Use silicone or polyurethane elastomers, which are less thrombogenic than polyethylene. Change the central catheter with a sterile guidewire and culture the tip after obtaining central and peripheral blood cultures if suspected catheter sepsis occurs with chills and shaking, hyperthermia, tachypnea, tachycardia, and leukocytosis with left shift. If a pathologic organism grows with > 15 colony-forming units, change the catheter site.

TPN Formulas

Preprinted order forms minimize confusion, especially when there are multiple prescribers. Table 54-1 lists several common TPN formulas.

IVFEs provide essential fatty acids. Essential fatty acid deficiency (EFAD) is prevented by giving 2 to 4 percent of calories as essential fatty acids (i.e., linoleic acid and linolenic acid). The maximum dose in adults is 2.5 g/kg/d, but should be limited to 1 g/kg/d as a continuous infusion or as part of a total nutrient admixture (TNA) given over 24 hours. Provide a lower dose (0.5 to 1 g/kg/d as a continuous infusion) with acute respiratory distress syndrome (ARDS) due to oxygenation problems with rapid infusions (3 mg/kg/min). Withhold lipids with hypertriglyceridemia (e.g., >500 mg/dL). Biochemical evidence of EFAD develops within 2 weeks on a fat-free TPN regimen and symptoms can occur within 1 week.

Electrolyte components of TPN (Table 54-5) may vary considerably in these patients depending on serum concentrations, concomitant drug therapy, acid-base status, preinjury nutritional status, and extrarenal losses of fluid and electrolytes.

Provide daily vitamins in the TPN solution as suggested by the American Medical Association Nutrition Advisory Group (AMANAG) (Table 54-6). Parenteral multivitamin products (e.g., MVI-12, Astra Merck) meet recommendations for 12 of the vitamins, but vitamin K is not included and must be added to the TPN individually (5 to 10 mg/wk or 0.5 to 1 mg/d).

Provide the trace elements zinc, chromium, copper, manganese, and selenium. Copper and manganese should be withheld in patients with cholestasis. Patients with substantial ostomy losses are prone to zinc deficiency and given at least 5 mg/d of zinc. Parenteral molybdenum and iodine are also available.

TABLE 54-5 Electrolytes in TPN

Electrolyte	Usual requirement per day	Standard TPN concentration/L
Sodium	100–150 mEq	40–60 mEq/L
Potassium	80–100 mEq (more if anabolic)	20 mEq/L as phosphate 20 mEq/L as acetate
Magnesium	8–30 mEq	8 mEq/L as sulfate
Calcium	10–15 mEq	5 mEq/L as gluconate
Phosphorus	20–40 mmol	15 mmol/L as K^+ salt or Na^+ salt

TABLE 54-6 Parenteral Vitamins Recommended by AMANAG Guidelines*

Vitamin	Dose
Vitamin A	3300 IU
Vitamin D_2	200 IU
Vitamin E	10 mg
Thiamin	3 mg
Riboflavin	3.6 mg
Pyridoxine	4 mg
Niacin	40 mg
Pantothenate	15 mg
Biotin	60 µg
Folate	400 µg
Cobalamin	5 µg
Ascorbic acid	100 mg

*Vitamin K must be given as a single entity in adults.

Most patients can be started on TPN and advanced to a desired goal over 2 to 3 days. A reasonable initiation rate is 25 to 50 mL/h with advancement by 25 to 40 mL/h/day to the desired goal.

Provide regular insulin with glucose ≥200 mg/dL due to stress and/or diabetes or with moderate to severe glucosuria (≥500 mg/dL). Add regular human insulin to the TPN solution, usually beginning with at least 15 U/L. Add an insulin drip and limit the TPN rate with extreme glucose intolerance.

Monitoring Therapy

TPN fluid provides 50 to 95 percent of the patient's intake at the goal rate. Concentrate the formula and reduce sodium in overloaded patients. Monitor electrolytes daily until stable. Add additional IV fluids for euvolemic patients requiring larger volumes due to unusual losses (e.g., fistula).

ADDITIONAL READING

Borlase BC, Moore EE, Moore FA: The Abdominal Trauma Index—A critical reassessment and validation. *J Trauma* 30:1340, 1990.

Frankel WL, Evans NJ, Rombeau JL: Scientific rationale and clinical application of parenteral nutrition in critically ill patients, in Rombeau JL, Caldwell MD (eds): *Clinical Nutrition,* Vol 2. *Parenteral Nutrition,* 2nd ed. Philadelphia, WB Saunders, 1993, p 597.

Hwang T-L, Hwang S-L, Chen M-F: The use of indirect calorimetry in critically ill patients—Relationship with measured energy expenditure to Injury Severity Score, Septic Severity Score, and APACHE II score. *J Trauma* 34:247, 1993.

Kudsk KA, Croce MA, Fabian TC, et al: Enteral vs. parenteral feeding: Effects on septic morbidity following blunt and penetrating abdominal trauma. *Ann Surg* 215:503, 1992.

55 | The Immune Response

The complex entity of inflammation and infection with ensuing organ dysfunction and failure continues to be the leading problem after injury and surgery. When systemic inflammation progresses to multiple and remote organ failure, the mortality rate increases, ranging from 30 to 80 percent despite state-of-the-art intensive care medicine. Major injury is thus a profound threat to survival, and nearly 50 percent of patients who survive the initial injury phase go on to suffer from subsequent inflammatory or infectious complications. The causes for these complications of multisystem injuries are extensive tissue necrosis, prolonged hemorrhagic shock, and significant alteration of circulating cytokines, prostaglandins, and coagulation factors.

Severe injury results in major dysfunction of host defense mechanisms, a consequence of a systemic, diffuse, nondiscriminant, and excessive inflammatory response, together with a failure of cell-mediated immune function. While parts of the immune system are stimulated, others are depressed in a complex series of events that is yet not completely understood (Fig. 55-1). On one hand, the nonspecific immune system is activated, as white blood cells and macrophages mobilize to the site of injury with activation of complement and opsonins. Following tissue injury acute-phase proteins are produced as a part of the immune response with interleukin-6 (IL-6) production and release of other proinflammatory cytokines. On the other hand, circulating immunosuppressive factors including suppressor T cells appear because of tissue necrosis and shock, and this may impede the activity of white blood cells as well as lung and liver macrophages. All of these factors may contribute to increased susceptibility to infection.

The immune system can cope with a modest injury, but when the injury is severe and overwhelming, with extensive tissue necrosis, the immune system is activated systemically and may become self-destructive. A response that should be localized to the area of the wound and is critical for healing and survival may become generalized and produce remote organ damage. It has been reported by a number of groups that remote organ failure usually affects the lungs first, followed by the liver, the gut, and the kidneys, while circulatory failure occurs in the later stages. Survival of septic patients is generally dependent upon identification of the septic focus. If a treatable cause for sepsis is not found, mortality often follows with frequency in direct proportion to the number of organs that fail. During recent years a number of clinical and experimental studies have reported significant gender differences regarding incidence and survival of septic complications in trauma patients. It appears that immune function after hemorrhagic shock and/or severe trauma is influenced by detrimental effects of male sex steroids, while female sex steroids appear to beneficially influence posttraumatic immune functions.

PRIMING

Neutrophil priming is initiated by exposure to antigens (e.g., lipopolysaccharide [LPS]) or proinflammatory cytokines (e.g., tumor necrosis factor-α [TNF-α]) as well as granulocyte macrophage colony-stimulating factor (GM-CSF), and results in an upregulation of reduced nicotinamide adenine dinucleotide phosphate (NADPH) oxidase activation. The priming process plays a crucial role in neutrophil-mediated tissue damage, and it has been shown that superoxide anion generation is markedly enhanced in primed neutrophils.

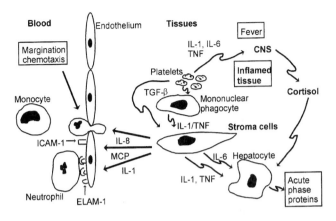

FIG. 55-1. Intercellular signal transduction of circulating and tissue-fixed immunocompetent cells with proinflammatory intercellular mediators during the development of the systemic inflammatory response. CNS, central nervous system; ELAM-1, endothelial leukocyte adhesion molecule; ICAM-1, intercellular adhesion molecule; IL-1, interleukin-1; IL-6, interleukin-6; MCP, monocyte chemotactic protein; TNF, tumor necrosis factor.

Although this process was thought to be irreversible, there are data that indicate that neutrophil priming is reversible.

IMMUNOLOGIC DERANGEMENTS FOLLOWING INJURY

Prostaglandin E₂ and Interleukin-2

There is a wide array of immunologic derangements after injury, shock, trauma, burns, and extensive surgical procedures. They are induced mainly by macrophage activation, a significant inhibition of the bone marrow, and changes in the specific (Table 55-1) and nonspecific (Table 55-2) immune system. Following major injury, lymphopenia (CD3$^+$ lymphocytes) and simultaneous monocytosis (CD14$^+$ cells) have been reported. Flow-cytometric analysis of lymphocyte subpopulations demonstrates a massive decline of CD4$^+$ T-helper cells, while interleukin-2 (IL-2) receptor expression on the surface of lymphocytes is also reduced. The CD8$^+$ cytotoxic and suppressor-active T cells that play a central role in posttraumatic immunosuppression are found to be unchanged or elevated, which leads to a conversion of the CD4:CD8 ratio to a value below 1. These alterations of circulating lymphocyte subpopulations have been reported to continue as long as 21 days after trauma. Shock, trauma, and burns have been shown to produce a severe inhibition of mitogenic stimulation of lymphocyte proliferation which appears to be related to the release of excessive prostaglandin E₂. A number of clinical studies have reported that the depression of lymphoblastogenesis after severe trauma may exacerbate the development of infectious complications. Moreover, depression of IL-2 biosynthesis has been observed instantaneously after injury and has been shown to persist for a longer period of time. The detrimental effects of depressed IL-2 synthesis are important since this effects T-cell replication, clonal T-cell expansion, and B-cell antibody pro-

TABLE 55-1 Specific Immune Functions That Are Altered Following Hemorrhage and Tissue Trauma

Myelodepression
Lymphopenia
$\dfrac{CD4}{CD8}$ ratio <1
T- and B-cell proliferation $\downarrow$
Release of lymphokines (IL-2, IL-3, γ-IFN) $\downarrow$
Lymphocyte IL-4 and IL-10 release $\uparrow$
IL-2 receptor expression
NK cell activity $\downarrow$
Alteration of Mϕ/T-cell interaction
HLA-DR antigen expression $\downarrow$
DTH skin test reactivity $\downarrow$
Inhibition of B-lymphocyte differentiation
Plasma cells: IgM synthesis and secretion $\downarrow$
Shift from IgM $\rightarrow$ IgG synthesis

DTH, delayed-type hypersensitivity; IgM, IgG, immunoglobulin M and G; NK, natural killer.

duction. Suppression of IL-3 and interferon gamma (IFN-γ) synthesis from lymphocytes has also been described after major trauma. In addition to the inhibition of IL-2 receptor expression, there is a striking decrease in HLA-DR antigen (human leukocyte antigen-DR, a class II major histocompatibility complex antigen) expression on macrophages after injury. HLA-DR expression appears to be more severely depressed in patients who developed or died of sepsis, when compared with patients who had an uneventful recovery from trauma. Addition of IFN-γ to peripheral mononuclear leukocyte cultures obtained from these patients induced an increase in HLA-DR antigen expression.

TABLE 55-2 Nonspecific Immune Functions That Are Altered Following Hemorrhage and Tissue Injury

Monocytosis
Plasma levels of TNF-α and IL-6 $\uparrow$
Mϕ TNF-α and IL-6 secretion accelerated
Mϕ L-1 secretion $\downarrow$
Mϕ PGE$_2$ synthesis $\uparrow$
PGE$_2$ plasma levels $\uparrow$
PMN
Chemotaxis $\downarrow$
Phagocytic capacity $\downarrow$
β_2-Integrin expression $\downarrow$
LTB$_4$ synthesis $\downarrow$
Release of O$_2$ radicals $\downarrow$ $\uparrow$
Release of elastase $\uparrow$
Acute-phase protein synthesis $\uparrow$
C3a plasma levels $\uparrow$
Cathepsin, lactoferrin, myeloperoxidase levels $\uparrow$
Neopterin plasma levels $\uparrow$
Depletion of fibronectin, opsonins, and AT III plasma levels $\uparrow$

AT III, antithrombin III; C3a, complement 3a; IL, interleukin; LTB, leukotriene B; PGE$_2$, prostaglandin E$_2$; PMN, polymorphonuclear neutrophils; TNF, tumor necrosis factor.

Delayed-Type Hypersensitivity Response

The delayed-type hypersensitivity (DTH) response to ubiquitous antigens provides a global assessment of the host defense response. Patients with infectious complications who show an intact DTH skin response usually respond appropriately to their infection, do not develop multiple-organ failure (MOF) and survive, whereas anergic patients fail to control their infections. After 20 years of experience with the DTH response it was concluded that anergy in this test has a strong association to sepsis-related mortality in intensive care or trauma patients; nonetheless, statistical significance was not seen in elective surgical patients due to a reduction in overall patient mortality.

B-Lymphocyte System

In patients with major surgery, a massive depression of B-cell differentiation and immunoglobulin M (IgM) synthesis has been observed when peripheral mononuclear cells were cultured and stimulated with pokeweed mitogen. The degree of suppression correlated well with the amount of macrophage suppression in the peripheral blood mononuclear cell (PBMC) cultures, while IgG and IgA synthesis were not affected by trauma. Additional studies in purified B-cell cultures confirmed these observations and showed a persistent IgM/IgG shift.

Activated Macrophages

There is evidence that altered behavior of activated macrophages plays a key role in the abnormal inflammatory and cell-mediated immune response after severe injury. Shock, trauma, burns, and hemorrhagic shock as well as endotoxemia and bacteremia induce profound monocyte and macrophage activation with increased synthesis and secretion of inflammatory mediators, which may contribute to remote organ as well as multiple-organ failure. Clinical studies have reported that increased release of proinflammatory cytokines (e.g., IL-6, TNF-α) by macrophage cultures from patients after major surgery is associated with septic complications as well as impaired outcome.

Cytokine Changes

The response to trauma is initiated within the immune system at the moment of injury, and all patterns of trauma (sepsis, hemorrhage, ischemia, reperfusion, soft tissue trauma, and burns) may activate macrophages and induce the release of proinflammatory cytokines. The production and release of all cytokines is altered by physiologic stress, and it is well recognized that changes in the synthesis and release of cytokines play an important role in mediating functional changes of the immune as well as the circulatory system. Nonetheless, clinical studies of the relationship between circulating proinflammatory cytokine levels and development or onset of septic complications have thus far failed to provide compelling data. The therapeutic targeting of elevated TNF-α levels in patients with severe sepsis did not provide any clinical benefit. Nonetheless, in patients with inflammatory bowel disease, significant benefit has been observed following administration of long-acting TNF-α antibodies.

Despite the inconsistent findings regarding the effects of severe trauma on circulating levels of pro- and anti-inflammatory cytokines as well as the lack of correlation between serum concentrations of these mediators and the development of infectious complications, it appears that increased generation of IL-1, IL-6, and possibly TNF-α contribute to the acute phase response and a hypermetabolic phase that accompanies trauma. The exact role of these mediators in the pathogenesis of multiple-organ failure, however, remains unclear. There is nonetheless evidence indicating that severe immunosuppression involving T- and B-cell function may result from the effects of stress-related alterations in cytokine release. With regard to this, it has been suggested that trauma causes a disintegration of the monocyte-T-cell interaction, which is associated with profound changes in macrophage forward regulatory capacities and substantial depression of T-cell function.

In addition to the above mentioned alterations of cytokine release, a profound deficit of IL-1 and IL-8 production which may last for several days has been observed after severe trauma. This deficit may contribute to the immunodeficiency of traumatized as well as septic patients, because these cytokines in low concentrations are involved in the upregulation of all essential humoral and cellular immune functions. Inadequate IL-1 synthesis appears to be a substantial component of defective IL-2 synthesis following trauma. Moreover, a significant shift of the cytokine response toward the T-helper lymphocyte (T_H2) direction following major trauma—as indicated by excessive upregulation of IL-4—has been observed, and it appears to originate from the CD8$^+$ rather than the CD4$^+$ phenotype.

Polymorphonuclear Neutrophil Antibodies

Abnormal function of polymorphonuclear neutrophils (PMNs) after severe trauma has been interpreted by some as a sign of unresponsiveness, while others have observed PMN hyperactivation. These contradictory findings most likely are time-dependent, since early postinjury (<6 hours) and delayed (>48 hours) PNM functioning are different. A significant correlation between the degree of PMN dysfunction and morbidity has been observed. PMN dysfunction after trauma includes decreased phagocyte activity, reduction of intracellular bacterial killing, a decrease of glucose oxidation and oxygen consumption, a reduction of hydrogen peroxide production, as well as loss of lysosomal enzymes.

Repair and healing or perpetuation of acute inflammation is characterized by a complex network of interacting cellular and humoral defense mechanisms. Among the numerous inflammatory mediators, the proteolytic lysosomal enzyme PMN elastase is highly destructive when released extracellularly and contributes to organ dysfunction after injury. A number of investigators have observed a correlation between increased circulating levels of elastase and the development of organ failure.

GOALS OF IMMUNOTHERAPY

The principal clinical goal of modem immunotherapy after major trauma must be to prevent the conversion of the systemic inflammation seen in an immunocompromised host into bacterial sepsis. Several strategic approaches to prevent the development of late multiple-organ dysfunction appear feasible (Table 55-3). Nonetheless, until now, all clinical trials in septic patients with or without gram-negative bacterial infections employing therapy such as anti-LPS monoclonal antibodies, anti-TNF antibodies, soluble TNF receptors, IL-1 receptor antagonists, or other agents have not shown a significant clinical benefit. The major reason all these sepsis trials failed is that they treated "sep-

TABLE 55-3 Crucial Issues in the Decision Process for Preventive
Immunotherapy in Trauma Patients

Patient selection (injury severity)
Timing
Choice of cellular targets
Downregulation but not complete shutdown of inflammatory response
Strengthening of specific immune response
Cost

sis" and not specific diseases. Moreover, patients differ in their immune
response and antigen exposure genetically, by gender, and in numerous other
ways that we do not yet understand (Table 55-4).

Ideally, the immunotherapy chosen should prevent the posttraumatic systemic inflammatory response from becoming an irreversible autodestructive
inflammation with or without infection. Such an intervention must be
employed as early as possible following trauma and it should protect multiple
cellular targets (e.g., lymphocytes, macrophages, granulocytes, and endothelial cells). It should protect the host from cell hyperactivation as well as
exhaustion. It is most likely that only a combination of several drugs will be
effective in controlling the posttraumatic dyshomeostasis. Crucial issues in
the complex field of preventive immunomodulation for the control of systemic inflammation include patient selection, timing of adminstration, the difficulty in avoiding a complete shutdown of inflammatory responses, and the
cost of therapy. It is clear that the increased susceptibility to infection after
injury correlates with injury severity and thus with the degree of uncontrolled
inflammation. A combined therapeutic strategy should include (1) a global
short-term (≤ 72 hours) downregulation of inflammatory macrophages and
PMN activity, (2) the prevention of excessive macrophage stimulation via
neutralization of circulating endo- and exotoxins with high doses of polyvalent immunoglobulins and soluble complement receptors, and (3) upregulation of cell-mediated specific immune activity to overcome posttraumatic
paralysis by administration of IFN-γ and granulocyte colony-stimulating factor (G-CSF).

Despite the progress that has been made in our understanding of the mechanisms of host defense dysfunction in trauma, shock, and sepsis, employing
immunotherapeutic interventions effectively in surgical patients in the near
future will depend on (1) our ability to measure the activation state of host
defenses accurately, (2) a clear comprehension of the interactions among the
various components of the immune system during health and disease, and
(3) a much more rapid and precise identification of pathogens and microbial
toxins.

TABLE 55-4 Reasons for the Failure of Sepsis Trials

- Treatment of different complex diseases in the same way
- Overlap and redundancy of mediators
- No single factor or mediator is consistently lethal
- Inconsistent timing of treatment
- Modulation of inflammation as an essential biologic function
- Uncertainty about whether immune deficiency or immune excess was treated
- Diversity of genetic background
- Diversity of "immunological experience"

ADDITIONAL READING

Baue AE, Durham R, Faist E: Systemic inflammatory response syndrome (SIRS), multiple organ dysfunction syndrome (MODS), multiple organ failure (MOF): are we winning the battle? *Shock* 10:383, 1998.

Baue AE: Multiple organ failure—the discrepancy between our scientific knowledge and understanding and the management of our patients. *Langenbeck's Arch Surg* 385:441, 2000.

Faist E, Wichmann M, Kim C: Irnmunosuppression and immunomodulation in surgical patients. *Curr Opin Crit Care* 3:293, 1997.

Wichmann MW, Inthorn D, Andress HJ, et al: Incidence and mortality of severe sepsis in surgical intensive care patients: the influence of patient gender on disease process and outcome. *Intensive Care Med* 26:167, 2000.

56 | Postinjury Multiple-Organ Failure

Multiple-organ failure (MOF) emerged as a new syndrome 25 years ago as a result of our ability to keep patients alive with advanced technology. Despite intensive investigation, it remains the leading cause of late postinjury deaths in the intensive care unit today.

DEFINITIONS

Systemic Inflammation Response Syndrome (SIRS):

To make this diagnosis, at least two of the following need to be present:

- Temperature above 38°C or below 36°C
- Heart rate >90 beats/min
- Respiratory rate >20 breaths/min or a $PaCO_2$ <32 mm Hg
- White blood cell count (WBC) >12,000 cells/mm^3 or <4000 cells/mm^3, or >10 percent immature (bands) forms

Sepsis:

SIRS in the presence of an identifiable source of infection.

Acute Respiratory Distress Syndrome (ARDS):

- Acute onset
- PaO_2/FIO_2 <200 (regardless of positive end-expiratory pressure [PEEP] level)
- Bilateral infiltrates seen on frontal chest radiograph
- Pulmonary capillary wedge pressure (PCWP) ≤18 mm Hg or no clinical evidence of left atrial hypertension

Multiple-Organ Failure:

The Denver MOF score includes four organ systems (pulmonary, renal, cardiac, and hepatic) and each system's function is graded on a scale of zero to three (0 normal, 1 mild, 2 moderate, and 3 severe) to reflect a continuum of physiologic derangement. Individual organ failure is defined as a dysfunction grade of two or more, while MOF is defined as the sum of simultaneous individual organ dysfunction grades, after 48 hours of admission, of four or more. (Table 56-1).

Current Epidemiology

Over a 4-year period, 457 patients were prospectively followed, and 70 (15 percent) developed MOF. A high Injury Severity Scale score (ISS), increasing number of units of red blood cell (RBC) transfusion, elevated base deficit, and elevated lactate levels were associated with MOF. MOF patients suffered significantly more major infections (87 percent versus 23 percent), minor infections) 41 percent versus 23 percent), and nonseptic complications (53 percent versus 12 percent) than patients without MOF (Table 56-2). Additionally, MOF patients required more mechanical ventilator days (18.6 ± 1.5 versus 3.1 ± 0.3), longer ICU stays (25.6 ± 2.2 versus 8.7 ± 0.5 days), and had a higher mortality rate (25 of 70 patients [36 percent] versus 13 of 387 patients [3 percent]). The mortality per number of failing organs was: one organ, 11 percent (7/16); two organs, 24 percent (7/30); three organs, 60 percent (6/10); and four

TABLE 56-1 Multiple-Organ Failure Score

	Grade 0	Grade 1 dysfunction	Grade 2 dysfunction	Grade 3 dysfunction
Pulmonary*	Normal	ARDS score >5	ARDS score >9	ARDS score >13
Renal	Normal	Creatinine >1.8 mg/dL	Creatinine >2.5 mg/dL	Creatinine >5 mg/dL
Hepatic†	Normal	Bilirubin >2 mg/dL	Bilirubin >4 mg/dL	Bilirubin >8 mg/dL
Cardiac‡	Normal	Minimal inotropes	Moderate inotropes	High inotropes

*ARDS score = A + B + C + D + E, pulmonary capillary wedge pressure (PCWP) ≤18 cm H_2O, or clinical setting where high PCWP is not anticipated.

A. Pulmonary findings by plain chest radiography
0 = Normal
1 = Diffuse, mild interstitial marking/opacities
2 = Diffuse, marked interstitial/mild airspace opacities
3 = Diffuse, moderate airspace consolidation
4 = Diffuse, severe airspace consolidation

B. Hypoxemia (Pao_2/Fio_2)
0 = Normal
1 = 175–250
2 = 125–174
3 = 80–124
4 = <80

C. Minute ventilation (L/min)
0 = <11
1 = <11–13
2 = <14–16
3 = <17–20
4 = >20

D. Positive end-expiratory pressure (cm H_2O)
0 = <6
1 = 6–9
2 = 30–39
3 = 14–17
4 = >17

E. Static compliance (mL/cm H_2O)
0 = >50
1 = 40–50
2 = 30–39
3 = 20–29
4 = <20

†Biliary obstruction and resolving hematoma excluded.

‡Cardiac index <3.0 L/min/m^2 requiring inotropic support. Minimal dose, dopamine or dobutamine <5 μg/kg/min; moderate dose, dopamine or dobutamine 5–15 μg/kg/min; high dose, greater than moderate doses of above agents.

TABLE 56-2 Septic Complications for Patients With and Without MOF

Complications	No. Infections/No. Patients (% Patients)		P Value
	MOF (n = 70)	No MOF (n = 387)	
Major infections	91/61 (87%)	103/88 (23%)	0.001
Pneumonia	60/55 (79%)	84/80 (21%)	<0.001
Empyema/lung abscess	2/2 (3%)	4/4 (1%)	0.230
Abdominal abscess	13/13 (20%)	4/4 (1%)	<0.001
Wound	11/11 (16%)	4/4 (1%)	<0.001
Other	5/5 (7%)	7/7 (2%)	0.024
Minor infections	50/29 (41%)	61/45 (23%)	0.001
Urine	13/12 (17%)	21/20 (5%)	0.001
Catheter	18/11 (16%)	11/11 (3%)	<0.001
Wound	9/9 (13%)	10/10 (3%)	0.007
Sinus	6/6 (9%)	5/5 (1%)	0.003
Other	4/4 (6%)	14/14 (4%)	0.499

organs, 62 percent (8/13). An analysis of the temporal distribution of the onset of the MOF revealed that in 27 patients (39 percent), MOF occurred early (i.e., was present on day 3), while in the remaining 43 patients (61 percent), MOF presented late (after 3 days). The risk factors for "early MOF" and "late MOF" identified by multiple logistic regression analysis were different (Table 56-3).

To determine the potential causal relationship between major infectious complications and early versus late MOF, the temporal relationship between the onset of infection and serial MOF scoring was examined. Major infections were classified in four categories: (1) "not related" because it was community acquired or occurred in the hospital 4 or more days before the onset of MOF; (2) a potential "trigger" if the MOF score on the day of diagnosis was less than 4 (i.e., no MOF) and rose 3 points or more within 72 hours; (3) "worsening MOF" if MOF was present on the day of diagnosis (i.e., MOF score ≥4) and rose 3 points or more within 72 hours; or (4) potential "symptom" if the major infection occurred after MOF was present and was associated with a rise in the MOF score of less than 3. The potential impact of major infections on the clinical course of early MOF compared with late MOF is shown in Table 56-4.

Unifying Hypothesis: Postinjury MOF Occurs as a Result of a Dysfunctional Inflammatory Response

Following major trauma, patients are resuscitated into an early state of systemic hyperinflammation (i.e., SIRS) (Fig. 56-1). The initial intensity of SIRS is dependent on the amount of tissue injury, the degree of shock, and the presence of host factors (such as age and comorbid disease). Mild to moderate SIRS is presumed to be beneficial and resolves as the host recovers. However, if the initial insult is massive (the "one-hit" model), the resulting severe SIRS

TABLE 56-3 Risk Factors for MOF

Early MOF (≤ day 3)	Late MOF (> day 3)
ISS ≥25	Age >55 years
Early PRBCs >6 units	Early PRBCs >6 units
ED systolic BP <90 mm Hg	Early base deficit >8 mEq/L
Lactate ≥2.5 nmol/L at 13–24 hours after admission	Lactate ≥2.5 nmol/L at 13–24 hours after admission

ISS, Injury Severity Score; PRBC, packed red blood cells; ED, energy department.

TABLE 56-4 Classification of Major Infection in Early and Late MOF

Early MOF (n = 27)	32 Major infections/23 patients (85%)			
	Not Related	Trigger	Worsen	Symptom
Pneumonia	2 (6%)	1 (3%)	3 (9%)	14 (44%)
Abdominal abscess			2 (6%)	2 (6%)
Wound infection		1 (3%)		4 (6%)
Other infections				3 (9%)
Total	2 (6%)	2 (6%)*	5 (16%)	23 (72%)

Late MOF (n = 43)	59 Major infections/38 patients (88%)			
	Not Related	Trigger	Worsen	Symptom
Pneumonia	15 (25%)	11 (19%)	1 (2%)	13 (22%)
Empyema/abscess	1 (2%)			1 (2%)
Abdominal abscess	2 (3%)	3 (5%)	1 (2%)	3 (5%)
Wound infection		2 (2%)	1 (2%)	3 (7%)
Other	1 (2%)			1 (3%)
Total	19 (32%)	16 (27%)*	3 (5%)	21 (36%)

*$P = 0.025$ number of major infections serving as "triggers" for early MOF compared to late MOF.

can precipitate early MOF. Alternatively, early MOF can occur when vulnerable patients are exposed to early secondary inflammatory insults (the "two-hit" model). At the same time, negative feedback systems (i.e., counter antiinflammatory response syndrome [CARS]) act to limit certain components of SIRS so that it does not become an autodestructive process. This results in delayed immunosuppression. Again, mild to moderate delayed immunosuppression is presumed to be beneficial, but when it is severe, it is associated with major infectious complications (principally pneumonia) and late MOF.

Evolving Concepts in the Pathogenesis of Postinjury MOF

Numerous mechanisms have been proposed and extensively studied. A comprehensive discussion is beyond the scope of this chapter. The following are mechanisms consistent with the above hypothesis:

1. Flow-dependent and -independent impaired oxygen consumption. The efficacy of maximizing DO_2 in traumatic shock is time-dependent, similar to that observed in septic shock. Early volume loading can dramatically increase DO_2 and VO_2. However, a significant subset of

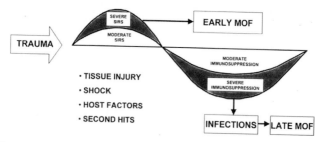

FIG. 56-1.   Unifying hypothesis for the cause of multiple-organ failure. SIRS, systemic inflammatory response syndrome; MOF, multiple-organ failure.

patients who are in the later stages of shock fail to increase VO_2. A persistent elevated lactate level despite above-normal DO_2 may be indicative of impaired mitochondrial function and is highly predictive of MOF and death.

2. Reperfusion injury:
   a. Xanthine oxidase-dependent reactive oxygen metabolites: With reperfusion, oxygen becomes available to catalyze the xanthine oxidase-mediated oxidation of hypoxanthine to uric acid. There is a concomitant burst of superoxide production which is converted into more toxic reactive oxygen metabolites.
   b. Neutrophil chemotaxis. Ischemia/reperfusion activates cytosolic phospholipase-A_2 which then generates platelet-activating factor and other eicosanoid derivatives that act as chemoattractants. Resident macrophages and mast cells have also been implicated in recruiting polymorphonuclear neutrophils.
   c. Neutrophil adherence to the endothelium is a necessary step in polymorphonuclear neutrophil (PMN)-mediated injury and is mediated by β_2-integrins on the PMN and members of the immunoglobulin superfamily (intercellular adhesion molecule-1; ICAM-1) on the endothelium. In basic laboratory models, blocking integrin-ICAM-1 interactions by specific antibodies can prevent PMN-mediated endothelial cell injury and improve organ function.

3. The "two-hit" hypothesis: PMN priming is defined as the amplification of a cellular physiologic response to a second stimulus. The priming response in the PMN is now recognized to include the upregulation of the CD11/CD18 adhesion molecule and enhanced release of reactive oxygen metabolites, proteases, elastases, and cytokines on activation. Many biological mediators relevant to postinjury MOF have been demonstrated in vitro to prime PMN responses, including interleukins (IL-1, IL-6, and IL-8), tumor necrosis factor, platelet-activating factor (PAF), leukotriene B_4 (LTB$_4$), lipopolysaccharide (LPS), and complement-derived C5a. The physiologic purpose of priming is to enhance bacterial killing at sites of infection; however, after severe trauma, the inflammatory response bombards PMNs with a multitude of priming and activating stimuli which can then lead to cytotoxic responses, resulting in tissue injury.

4. Fat embolism syndrome (FES) is characterized by the triad of mental confusion, acute lung injury, and petechiae. The role of FES in provoking ARDS and MOF remains unclear. The potential deleterious role of early fracture fixation in patients with associated head and chest injuries is an area of current investigation.

5. The gut hypothesis: In early MOF, shock can cause persistent gut hypoperfusion and sloughing of villus tips. Either or both of these events may allow bacteria and their by-products access to the mucosal-associated lymphoid tissue, which may become activated and release local and systemic proinflammatory mediators to amplify SIRS. The gut may serve as a reservoir for pathogens in late MOF-associated infections. It is not clear at this time, however, if late gut-associated infections are the cause of ongoing MOF.

6. Role of blood transfusions: Blood transfusions have been clearly identified to be a risk factor for MOF. Laboratory studies suggest that blood

TABLE 56-5 Steps To Minimize MOF in High-Risk Patients

Initial emergency department evaluation and management
Appropriate triage: Operating room, angiography suite, or intensive care unit
Early shock resuscitation (first 24 hours)
Maximize oxygen delivery
Early recognition of abdominal compartment syndrome, missed injuries, or ongoing bleeding
Early nutritional support (within 48 hours)
Enteral route preferred
Immune-enhancing enteral diet
Prevent secondary nosocomial infections
Appropriate prophylactic antibiotics and avoidance of prolonged use of therapeutic antibiotics
Minimize gastrointestinal tract colonization
Early fracture fixation
Early mobilization
Aggressive respiratory care to prevent pneumonia
Remove indwelling devices as soon as possible
Early diagnosis and treatment of late infections
If MOF occurs:
Control source of inflammation
Support failing organs
Provide nutritional support
Prevent further iatrogenic injury

transfusions may activate the primed PMN. If this holds true clinically, alternative transfusion strategies should be sought, including the further development of blood substitutes.

7. Role of initial trauma in promoting infection. Severely injured patients develop late immunosuppression and an increased risk for nosocomial infections. Intra-abdominal infections have become a less frequent inciting event for MOF while ventilator-associated pneumonia occurs frequently in MOF patients and has roughly a 30 percent attributable mortality.

8. Role of infection in promoting MOF. Basic laboratory studies have supported the clinical observation that infection with systemic sepsis can cause ARDS and MOF.

See Table 56-5 for a list of means to prevent or minimize MOF in high-risk patients.

ADDITIONAL READINGS

Bone BC, Balk RAA, Cerra FB, et al: American College of Chest Physicians/Society of Critical Care Medicine Consensus Conference: definitions for sepsis and organ failure and guidelines for the use of innovative therapies in sepsis. *Crit Care Med* 20:864, 1992.

Fabian TC, Hoots AV, Stanford DS, et al: Fat embolism syndrome: prospective evaluation in 92 fracture patients. *Crit Care Med* 18:42, 1990.

Kudsk KA, Minard G, Croce MA, et al: A randomized trial of isonitrogenous enteral diets after severe trauma: an immune-enhancing diet reduces septic complications. *Ann Surg* 224:531, 1996.

Moore FA, Sauaia A, Moore EE, et al: Postinjury multiple organ failure: a bi-modal phenomenon. *J Trauma* 40:501, 1996.

Sauaia AJ, Moore FA, Moore EE: Multiple organ failure can be predicted as early as 12 hours postinjury. *J Trauma* 45:291, 1998.

INDEX

Page numbers followed by the letters *f* and *t* indicate figures and tables, respectively.

Musculoskeletal assessment
  secondary survey, 58
Mycobacterium tuberculosis, 18
Myocardial contusion, 200
Myocardial infarction, cardiogenic
    shock and, 79-80

N
Nasal fractures, 144-145
National Academy of
    Sciences/National Research
    Council, 20
National Association of Emergency
    Medical Technicians
    (NAEMT)
  prehospital trauma life support
    course (PHTLS), 30
National Association of EMS
    Physicians (NAEMSP)
  conditions indicating that resus-
    citation should not be
    attempted, 28
National Emergency Medical
    Services education and
    practice blueprint
  emergency medical technician—
    basic, 22
  emergency medical technician—
    intermediate, 22
  emergency medical technician—
    paramedic, 22-23
  first responder, 22
  overview, 22
National Heart and Lung Institute
    Task Force on Respiratory
    Diseases, 465
National Institute on Drug Abuse
    (NIDA), 379
National Registry of Emergency
    Medical Technicians
    (NREMT), 22
Neck trauma
  penetrating
    anatomy, 148-149, 149*f*
    evaluation, 149-151, 151*t*
    management, 151-152, 152*f*
    operative approach, 153
    overview, 148, 153
  secondary survey
    cautions, 56
    diagnostic pearls, 56

overview, 55-56
Neisseria meningitidis, 18
Nerve conduction velocity (NCV),
    369
Nerve grafts, 372-373
Nerve injury
  peripheral nerves. *See* Peripheral
    nerve injury
  rehabilitation, 425
  secondary survey
    cautions, 59
    diagnostic pearls, 59
    overview, 59
Neurogenic shock
  spinal cord injury, 77
Neuromas
  in continuity, 370, 374
  terminal, 373-374
Neuromuscular blocking agents,
    68-69, 111, 112*t*
Neuropraxia, 370
Neurotmesis, 370
Neurotrophism, 369
New Injury Severity Score (NISS),
    5
Newton's laws of motion and
    energy, 31, 34, 36
NIDA (National Institute on Drug
    Abuse), 379
Nitrous oxide (contraindicated),
    111
Nitrovasodilators
  myocardial dysfunction, 463
Nondepolarizing relaxants, 111,
    112*t*
Non-ventilator-associated pneumo-
    nia (N-VAP), 120
Norepinephrine
  myocardial dysfunction, 462
Normal saline *versus* lactated
    Ringer's
  prehospital care, 25
Nosocomial infections
  Candida sepsis, 123-124
  Clostridium difficile enterocoli-
    tis, 124
  intravascular device infection,
    122-123, 123*t*
  overview, 120
  pneumonia, 120-122, 121*t*
  urinary tract infection, 122, 123*t*
Notification time, 19-20